CLINICAL MANUAL
OF OBSTETRICS

NOTICE

Medicine is an ever-changing science. As new research and clinical experience broaden our knowledge, changes in treatment and drug therapy are required. The editors and the publisher of this work have checked with sources believed to be reliable in their efforts to provide information that is complete and generally in accord with the standards accepted at the time of publication. However, in view of the possibility of human error or changes in medical sciences, neither the editors nor the publisher nor any other party who has been involved in the preparation or publication of this work warrants that the information contained herein is in every respect accurate or complete, and they are not responsible for any errors or omissions or for the results obtained from use of such information. Readers are encouraged to confirm the information contained herein with other sources. For example and in particular, readers are advised to check the product information sheet included in the package of each drug they plan to administer to be certain that the information contained in this book is accurate and that changes have not been made in the recommended dose or in the contraindications for administration. This recommendation is of particular importance in connection with new or infrequently used drugs.

CLINICAL MANUAL OF OBSTETRICS

SECOND EDITION

Editors

David C. Shaver, MD
Department of Obstetrics and Gynecology
University of Tennessee College of Medicine
Memphis, Tennessee

Sharon T. Phelan, MD
Department of Obstetrics and Gynecology
University of Alabama
Birmingham, Alabama

Charles R. B. Beckmann, MD, MHPE
Department of Obstetrics and Gynecology
University of Wisconsin,
Milwaukee Clinical Campus
Milwaukee, Wisconsin

Frank W. Ling, MD
Department of Obstetrics and Gynecology
University of Tennessee College of Medicine
Memphis, Tennessee

McGRAW-HILL, INC.
Health Professions Division
New York   St. Louis   San Francisco   Auckland   Bogotá   Caracas
Lisbon   London   Madrid   Mexico   Milan   Montreal   New Delhi
Paris   San Juan   Singapore   Sydney   Tokyo   Toronto

CLINICAL MANUAL OF OBSTETRICS

12345678910 DOCDOC 9876543

ISBN 0-07-105401-4

This book was set in Optima by Kachina Typesetting, Inc.
The editors were Gail Gavert and Mariapaz Ramos Englis;
the production supervisor was Clare B. Stanley;
the cover was designed by Marsha Cohen/Parallelogram.
The text was designed and the project was supervised by M 'N O
   Production Services, Inc.
R. R. Donnelley & Sons Company was printer and binder.

Library of Congress Cataloging-in-Publication Data

Clinical manual of obstetrics / editors, David C. Shaver . . .]et al.].
   —2d ed.
      p.   cm.
   Includes index.
   ISBN 0-07-105401-4
   1. Obstetrics—Handbooks, manuals, etc. I. Shaver, David C.
[DNLM: 1. Obstetrics—handbooks. 2. Pregnancy Complications—
handbooks.   WQ 39 C641]
RG531.C5   1993
618.2—dc20
DNLM/DLC
for Library of Congress   92-49503
                                                                   CIP

We dedicate this book to our children

Aaron, Daniel, Joseph, and Timothy

Andrew and Katherine

David and Katherine

Mandy and Trevor

Contents

Contributors   **xiii**

Foreword   **xvii**
Joe Leigh Simpson

PART I: NORMAL OBSTETRICS   **1**

1. History Taking and the Physical Examination   3
   Charles R. B. Beckmann
   Frank W. Ling
   Barbara M. Barzansky
   Barbara F. Sharf
   Daniel L. Clarke-Pearson

2. Care of the Patient   14
   Roger P. Smith

3. Basic Prenatal Care and Childbirth Education   23
   Sharon T. Phelan

4. Normal Labor and Delivery   38
   Susan Rice
   Sharon T. Phelan

5. Birthing Rooms: Alternative Styles of Labor
   and Delivery   56
   Patrick J. Sweeney

6. Care of the Newborn   63
   Charles Fitch

7. The Puerperium   76
    Sharon T. Phelan

8. Lactation and Lactation Suppression   82
    Truus Delfos-Broner
    Nancee Neel
    Sharon T. Phelan

PART II: OBSTETRIC INTERVENTION   **93**

9. Obstetric Analgesia and Anesthesia   95
    Michael N. Skaredoff

10. Operative Obstetrics   116
    David C. Shaver

11. Abnormal Labor   130
    Aldo D. Khoury
    Sharon T. Phelan

12. Abnormal Fetal Lie, Including the Breech   141
    Stanley Gall

PART III: FETAL ASSESSMENT AND MANAGEMENT   **151**

13. Drugs and Toxic Substances   153
    Sandra Ann Carson

14. Reproductive Genetics and Prenatal Diagnosis   168
    Lee P. Shulman

15. Management of Congenital Anomalies   195
    Joseph A. Spinnato

16. Antenatal Fetal Assessment   220
    Susan Baker

17. Intrapartum Fetal Assessment   236
    J. Martin Tucker

18. Altered Fetal Growth   244
    Ralph K. Tamura
    Rudy E. Sabbagha

19. Isoimmunization 252
David C. Shaver

20. Perinatal Infections 264
Jessica L. Thomason

PART IV: OBSTETRIC COMPLICATIONS **279**

21. Premature Labor and Delivery 281
David C. Shaver

22. Premature Rupture of the Membranes 293
Brian Mercer

23. Multifetal Pregnancy 303
John Dacus

24. Prolonged Pregnancy 313
John R. Barton

25. Peripartum Infections 322
Jessica L. Thomason

26. Antepartum Bleeding in Advanced Pregnancy 329
Jeffrey C. King

27. Postpartum Hemorrhage 340
Peter A. Grannum

**PART V: MEDICAL AND SURGICAL COMPLICATIONS
IN PREGNANCY** **353**

28. Cardiovascular and Thromboembolic Diseases 355
Jeffrey C. King

29. Hypertensive Disease and Preeclampsia/Eclampsia 368
Jeffrey C. King

30. Renal Disease 384
Ana Tomasi

31. Pulmonary Disease 394
Michael T. Parsons

32. Gastrointestinal Diseases 405
   Michael T. Parsons
   Shirley K. Sawai

33. Hepatobiliary Diseases 421
   Michael T. Parsons
   Marcello Pietrantoni

34. Diabetes Mellitus 430
   William N. Spellacy

35. Endocrine Disease 441
   Jeffrey C. King

36. Hematologic Disease 457
   Nina Boe

37. Immunologic Disease 498
   Milo B. Sampson
   Joaquin Santolaya

38. Neurologic Diseases 509
   Aldo D. Khoury
   Baha M. Sibai

39. Dermatologic Disease 524
   Iris K. Aronson
   Barbara N. Halaska

40. Cancer 535
   Gary H. Lipscomb

41. Psychological and Psychiatric Diseases in Pregnancy 545
   Henry Lahmeyer

42. Dental and Oral Diseases 558
   Trusten P. Lee

43. Obstetric Emergencies 563
   Sharon T. Phelan
   David C. Shaver

Appendix A 579

Immunization during Pregnancy

Appendix B 591

Ultrasound Values in Pregnancy

Index 603

Contributors

Iris K. Aronson, MD [39]
Associate Professor
Department of Dermatology
University of Illinois
College of Medicine
Chicago, Illinois

Susan Baker, MD [16]
Instructor/Fellow
Division of Maternal/Fetal Medicine
Department of Obstetrics and
  Gynecology
University of Alabama at Birmingham
Birmingham, Alabama

John R. Barton, MD [24]
Director of Antenatal Diagnostic
Department of Obstetrics and
  Gynecology
Central Baptist Hospital
Lexington, Kentucky

Barbara M. Barzansky, PhD [1]
Assistant Director
Division of Undergraduate Medical
  Education
The American Medical Association
Chicago, Illinois

Charles R. B. Beckmann, MD, MHPE [1]
Professor
Division of Gynecology
Department of Obstetrics and
  Gynecology
University of Wisconsin–Madison
Sinai Samaritan Medical Center
West Campus
Milwaukee, Wisconsin

Nina Boe, MD [36]
Instructor/Fellow
Division of Maternal/Fetal Medicine
Department of Obstetrics and
  Gynecology
University of Tennessee
College of Medicine
Memphis, Tennessee

Sandra Ann Carson, MD [13]
Associate Professor, Chief In Vitro
  Fertilization and Embryo Transfer
Division of Reproductive
  Endocrinology and Fertility
Department of Obstetrics and
  Gynecology
University of Tennessee
College of Medicine
Memphis, Tennessee

Daniel L. Clarke-Pearson, MD [1]
Professor and Head
Division of Gynecologic Oncology
Department of Obstetrics and
  Gynecology
Duke Medical Center
Duke S. Hospital
Durham, North Carolina

John Dacus, MD [23]
Associate Professor
Division of Maternal/Fetal Medicine
Department of Obstetrics and
  Gynecology
University of Tennessee
College of Medicine
Memphis, Tennessee

Truus Delfos-Broner, CNM [8]
Clinical Coordinator
Certified Nurse Midwifery Program
Department of Obstetrics and
  Gynecology
University of Alabama of Birmingham
Birmingham, Alabama

Charles Fitch MD [6]
Associate Professor
Department of Pediatrics
University of Tennessee
College of Medicine
Memphis, Tennessee

Stanley Gall, MD [12]
Professor and Chairman
Department of Obstetrics and
  Gynecology
University of Louisville
School of Medicine
Louisville, Kentucky

Peter A. Grannum, MD [27]
Late Associate Professor
Department of Obstetrics and
  Gynecology
Yale University Medical School
New Haven, Connecticut

Barbara N. Halaska, MD [39]
Assistant Professor
Department of Dermatology
Loma Linda Medical Center
Loma Linda, California

Aldo D. Khoury, MD [11, 38]
Assistant Professor
Department of Obstetrics and
  Gynecology
Seaton Hall University
South Orange, New Jersey

Jeffrey C. King, MD [26, 28, 29, 35]
Associate Professor
Assistant Chairman
Department of Obstetrics and
  Gynecology
Georgetown University
School of Medicine
Washington, DC

Henry Lahmeyer, MD [41]
Professor
Department of Psychiatry
Northwestern University Medical
  School
Chicago, Illinois

Trusten P. Lee, DDS [42]
Director
Lakeland Dental Center
Rush Medical Center
Merrillvile, Indiana

Frank W. Ling, MD [1]
Associate Professor and Director
Division of Gynecology
Department of Obstetrics and
  Gynecology
University of Tennessee
College of Medicine
Memphis, Tennessee

Gary H. Lipscomb, MD [40]
Assistant Professor
Department of Obstetrics and
  Gynecology
University of Tennessee
College of Medicine
Memphis, Tennessee

Brian Mercer, MD [22]
Assistant Professor
Department of Obstetrics and
  Gynecology
University of Tennessee
College of Medicine
Memphis, Tennessee

Nancee Neel, CNM [8]
Department of Obstetrics and
  Gynecology
University of Alabama at Birmingham
Birmingham, Alabama

Michael T. Parsons, MD [31, 32, 33]
Assistant Professor
Department of Obstetrics and
  Gynecology
University of South Florida
Tampa, Florida

Sharon T. Phelan, MD [3, 4, 7, 8, 11, 43]
Associate Professor
Department of Obstetrics and
  Gynecology
Division of Maternal/Fetal Medicine
University of Alabama at Birmingham
Birmingham, Alabama

Marcello Pietrantoni, MD [33]
Clinical Assistant Professor
Department of Obstetrics and
  Gynecology
University of Arizona
Tucson, Arizona

Susan Rice, CNM [4]
Department of Obstetrics and
  Gynecology
University of Alabama at Birmingham
Birmingham, Alabama

Rudy E. Sabbagha, MD [18]
Professor and Director
Ultrasound Department
Northwestern University Medical
  School
Chicago, Illinois

Milo B. Sampson, MD [37]
Obstetrics and Gynecology
In Private Practice
Chicago, Illinois

Joaquin Santolaya, MD, PhD [37]
Assistant Professor
Department of Obstetrics and
  Gynecology
University of Illinois
Chicago, Illinois

Shirley K. Sawai, MD [32]
Associate Director
Phoenix Perinatal Association
Good Samaritan Hospital
Phoenix, Arizona

Barbara F. Sharf, MD [1]
Associate Professor
Department of Medical Education
University of Illinois
Chicago, Illinois

David C. Shaver, MD [10, 19, 21, 43]
Associate Professor
Division of Maternal/Fetal Medicine
Department of Obstetrics and
  Gynecology
University of Tennessee
College of Medicine
Memphis, Tennessee

Lee P. Shulman, MD [14]
Assistant Professor
Division of Gynecology
Department of Obstetrics and
  Gynecology
University of Tennessee
College of Medicine
Memphis, Tennessee

Baha M. Sibai, MD [38]
Professor and Chief
Division of Maternal/Fetal Medicine
Department of Obstetrics and
  Gynecology
University of Tennessee
College of Medicine
Memphis, Tennessee

Michael N. Skaredoff, MD [9]
Director
Department of Anesthesia
Vencor Hospital
Northlake, Illinois

Roger P. Smith, MD [2]
Associate Professor and Chief
Department of Obstetrics and
  Gynecology
Medical College of Georgia
Augusta, Georgia

William N. Spellacy, MD [34]
Professor and Chairman
Department of Obstetrics and
  Gynecology
University of South Florida
Tampa, Florida

Joseph A. Spinnato, MD [15]
Associate Professor and Director
Division of Maternal/Fetal Medicine
Department of Obstetrics and
  Gynecology
University of Louisville
Louisville, Kentucky

Patrick J. Sweeney, MD, MPH, PhD [5]
Professor of Obstetrics and Gynecology
Brown University
Director of Ambulatory Care
Women's and Infant's Hospital
Providence, Rhode Island

Ralph K. Tamura, MD [18]
Associate Professor
Department of Obstetrics and
   Gynecology
Northwestern University
Medical School
Chicago, Illinois

Jessica L. Thomason, MD [20, 25]
Professor and Chief
Division of Infectious Diseases
Department of Obstetrics and
   Gynecology
University of Wisconsin–Milwaukee
Sinai Samaritan Medical Center
Milwaukee, Wisconsin

Ana Tomasi, MD [30]
Assistant Professor
Department of Obstetrics and
   Gynecology
University of Tennessee, Chattanooga
Chattanooga, Tennessee

J. Martin Tucker, MD [17]
Maternal Fetal Medicine
Obstetrics and Gynecology
In Private Practice
Jackson, Mississippi

Foreword

Obstetrics in the 1990s is an exciting discipline, one that never fails to pique the interest of medical student, trainee, and even experienced physician. The excitement of the birth process and the exhilaration of being involved in such a defining event leaves an impact upon all in the health care field. Clearly this experience was pivotal in enticing many of us to choose this discipline.

Although clinical excitement with obstetrics has been present since the millennium, medical practice has been greatly enhanced in recent years by impressive scientific advances. Methods of identifying pregnancies at high risk for complications have allowed various surveillance patterns to be initiated. Surveillance allows us to intervene in a more timely fashion than our predecessors could imagine. Moreover, obstetricians increasingly manage pregnant patients with medical complications, recognizing that the physiological changes during pregnancy result in disease manifestations different from that in the non-pregnant patient.

Yet the availability of scientific tools and understanding carries with it immense responsibilities. Each physician wants to do his or her best in managing each patient. However, keeping up with new advances is exhausting. Deciphering precisely which new advances are likely to become standard and, hence, immediately applicable is daunting. To this end there are many excellent and definite texts, especially for physicians in training. However, many of these are intimidating for the student or young physician. Alternatively, even experienced physicians need to refresh quickly their memory concerning a disease manifested by a patient in the next room. Although excellent and thorough, large tomes may also be unrealistic for the non-specialist.

The editors of *Clinical Manual of Obstetrics* have addressed these dilemmas in this crisp volume. All are practicing obstetricians or maternal fetal medicine specialists. In aggregate, the editors have applied their clinical prowess to define the key issues relating to modern obstetrics. They have carefully defined the core material in obstetrics and alerted the reader when more exhaustive considerations are appropriate. Like the companion volume, *Clinical Manual of Gynecology,* the contributors have throughout the volume provided the scientific underpinning for modern clinical application. This manual is easy to read, yet avoiding a "cookbook" approach. *Clinical Manual of Obstetrics* should find a place on the shelves of students, house officers, and attending physicians alike.

Joe Leigh Simpson, M.D.
Faculty Professor and Chairman
Memphis, Tennessee

Preface

This book is intended as a brief guide to the physician who is involved with the care of the obstetric patient. Each chapter attempts to approach an area of obstetrics in an up-to-date and comprehensive manner. The chapters do not go into great detail concerning etiology and differential diagnoses of different disease processes, nor were they intended to. Rather, the book is intended for the resident physician, whether in obstetrics, family medicine, or a related field, and the practicing physician who wishes to obtain quick and easy reference to varying disease processes in obstetric patients. Practical management reflecting current standards of care are presented in a format that is easy to use and succinct.

Numerous authors have been involved in the preparation of this work, and we are very thankful and appreciative of the many hours of work that went into preparing each chapter.

Part I

Normal Obstetrics

CHAPTER 1

History Taking and the Physical Examination

Charles R. B. Beckmann
Frank W. Ling
Barbara M. Barzansky
Barbara F. Sharf
Daniel L. Clarke-Pearson

I. **Introduction.** In addition to providing historical and physical information, the history and physical examination allow an opportunity to develop professional rapport with the patient, and to educate the patient about the importance of regular prenatal care and healthy living habits.

II. **Initial interaction with the patient**
   A. **The setting.** A private setting is important for history taking. Communication is aided by having the clinician seated at the same level as the patient.
   B. **Greetings and getting started.** Greeting the patient with a handshake is mannerly and demonstrates warmth. Using the surname is best, although some clinicians find it useful to ask the patient how she would like to be addressed. Taking notes while interviewing the patient is not distracting if preceded by an explanatory statement.
   C. **Personal or embarrassing topics.** Many issues (such as sexually transmitted diseases) may evoke strong emotional responses but are important parts of good prenatal care. Such responses can be avoided by an explanatory preamble such as "I must ask some personal questions to get information we need to help care for you during this pregnancy. I need to provide you with the best health care."
   D. **Husband.** Inclusion of the husband/partner in this and subsequent visits is helpful to patient and physician alike.

3

III. History
  A. Chief complaint. The chief complaint in the obstetric setting will focus on pregnancy-related issues. Complaints should be presented in chronological sequence.
  B. Menstrual history
    1. **Menarche** is the age at which menses began.
    2. **Menstrual history.** The menstrual history includes the duration, frequency of, and interval between menstrual periods. The **last menstrual period (LMP)** is dated from the first day of the last normal menses. Last contraceptive use should be documented, especially if an oral contraceptive pill was used, as this affects the calculated estimated date of confinement (EDC).
  C. Obstetric history. The obstetric history includes the number of pregnancies (gravidity) and the outcome of each (parity). The abbreviations used are as follows:

  Gravida (G) **a** Para (P) **b c d e**

  where a = number of pregnancies; b = number of term pregnancies; c = number of preterm pregnancies; d = number of spontaneous or induced abortions and ectopic pregnancies (including pregnancies ending before 20 weeks). e = number of living children.

  The antenatal course for each pregnancy should be reviewed, noting any obstetric or maternal problems (e.g., "small baby" or the onset of pregnancy-induced hypertension [PIH]), and should detail the events of delivery. These include onset of labor, any interventions and their indication (e.g., induction, cesarean section, forceps delivery), and any complications. When possible, the location, date, and physician's name are helpful should further detailed information need to be requested.
  D. Gynecologic history
    1. **Breast history.** The breast history should include previous or existing breast disease, history of and plans for breast-feeding, previous mammography or breast biopsy, and a family history of breast cancer.
    2. **Previous gynecologic surgery.** Questions should include what surgery took place, for what reason, when and where, by whom, and the results. Surgical records should be obtained.
    3. **Infectious diseases.** A history of sexually transmitted diseases, especially herpes (including recent recurrences), gonorrhea, chlamydia, HIV virus and risk factors associated with its acquisition, and condyloma should be documented. Symptomatic vaginitis should be reviewed.
    4. **A history of infertility** should include questions about previous diseases or surgery that have affected fertility evaluation and previous pregnancies.
    5. **Diethylstilbestrol (DES)** use, if any, by the patient's mother during her pregnancy should be noted.

E. **Sexual/contraceptive history**
 1. **Sexual history.** Information should include the patient's present sexual partner(s), types of sexual practices, and level of satisfaction with their sex lives. Issues related to sexuality and pregnancy should be discussed.
 2. **Contraceptive history.** The contraceptive history should include the contraceptive methods most recently used. Postpartum contraceptive plans may be discussed now but are more appropriate for later in pregnancy.
 3. **Child and adult sexual abuse and assault.** Inquiry about past or present sexual abuse or assault should be made.

IV. **Physical examination**
 A. **General principles.** The patient should empty her bladder prior to the examination.
  1. **Assistance.** An assistant is useful for the preparation of specimens and as a chaperone. Many patients are more comfortable with a chaperone present.
  2. **Explanation of procedures to the patient.** Procedures should be thoroughly explained to the patient before they are performed. Such explanation decreases anxiety and helps the patient to relax.
 B. **Generalized written report format.** Table 1.1 presents a format for the written report of physical examination findings. The note should be written clearly and legibly, with the date and time and a legible signature.

Table 1.1. Physical Examination Written Report Format

Breasts
Abdomen
  Shape
  Striae, status of umbilicus, and hernia(s), if any
  Fundal height
  Evaluation of the fetal lie by use of the maneuvers of Leopold, starting in the third trimester
  Fetal heart tones
Back
  Spinal contours
  Areas of tenderness
Pelvic examination
  Vulva
  Clitoris
  Bartholin's, urethral, and Skene glands
  Cervix (Pap smear or cultures performed should be noted)
  Uterus
  Adnexae
  Rectovaginal examination and results of stool guaiac if performed
Clinical pelvimetry

V. Breast examination (Fig. 1.1). Although patients in the obstetric age group are at relatively low risk for breast cancer, this examination is often avoided or is performed in a cursory manner. For their age group, these patients have a disproportionately large number of palpable findings (including carcinoma) missed on physical examination.

    A. Inspection is done first with the patient's arms at her sides and then raised over her head. Tumors may distort the relationships of the breast's support tissues, so that these movements disrupt the shape, contour, or symmetry of the breast.

    B. Palpation. The breasts are also palpated, first with the patient's arms at her sides and then raised over her head in the sitting and then supine positions. Palpation should be done using the flat of the fingers, not the tips. A spiral pattern is described over each breast so as to cover all of the breast tissue uniformly, including that of the axillary tail. If nodules are found, their size, shape, consistency, mobility, tenderness, and location should be noted.

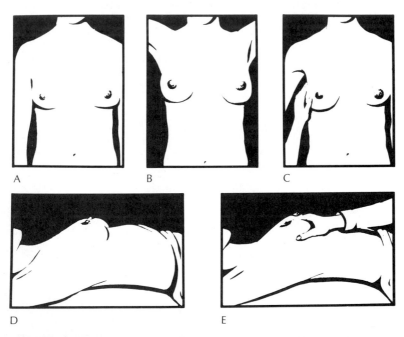

A   B   C

D   E

FIGURE 1.1. Breast examination. (A, B) Inspection of the breast with arms at rest and raised. (C) Palpation of the axilla with the arm in slight extension. (D, E) Positions for palpation of the outer and inner halves of the breast. (From Beckmann CRB, Ling FW, Barzansky BM, et al. History and physical examination. In: Stoval TG, Summitt RL, Beckmann CRB, et al, eds. Clinical Manual of Gynecology. 2nd ed. New York: McGraw-Hill; 1992:6. Reprinted with permission.)

VI. Examination of the back and abdomen

A. Examination of the back is accomplished with the patient sitting. The back is first examined for deviation of the spine, muscle spasm, or distorted posture. Gentle pressure over the costovertebral angles and over the sacrum will distinguish the muscle aches of anatomy strained by the change in center of gravity associated with pregnancy from pathologic situations.

B. Examination of the abdomen is accomplished with the patient supine. Late in pregnancy, care must be taken to have the patient lie slightly to one side, lest the pregnant uterus impede vena cava blood flow, leading to syncope (vena cava syndrome).

1. Determination of fundal height is made by palpation of the top of the fundus and measurement from that point to the top of the pubic bone. Although the main purpose of the determination is to note the growth pattern over several examinations (Fig. 1.2), the measurement in centimeters will roughly correspond to the number of weeks of gestation in the normal singleton pregnancy.

2. Determination of fetal presentation, lie, and, in the case of cephalic presentation, engagement is made by performance of the maneuvers of Leopold. (see Fig. 4.8).

3. Auscultation of the fetal heart rate is usually best performed over the fetal back. Fetal heart tones are heard at 10–12 weeks with modern Doppler instruments and usually by 18–20 weeks with an unenhanced stethoscope.

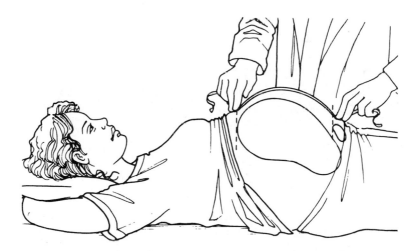

FIGURE 1.2. Measurement of fundal height—McDonald's technique. (From Martin LL, Reeder SJ. Essentials of Maternity Nursing. Philadelphia: JB Lippincott; 1991:167. Reprinted with permission.)

VII. Pelvic examination — procedure
A. Patient positioning
  1. **Helping the patient assume the lithotomy position.** Following the abdominal exam, the examining table's head may be raised 30 degress. The patient is asked to place her heels in the stirrups and move to the end of the table until her buttocks are at the edge of the table.
  2. **Draping.** The drape should cover the legs but should not obstruct the clinician's view. Some patients may prefer no drape.
  3. **Position of the examination light.** The lamp should be positioned in front of the clinician's chest at the level of the perineum so that the light is directed on the perineum (Fig. 1.3).
B. Gloving.
There should be minimal contact with equipment after gloves are donned. A clean glove should be used on the hand that performs the rectovaginal examination.
C. Inspection and examination of the external genitalia
  1. **Initial maneuvers and general principles.** After the patient is told that she is going to be touched, the examiner touches the patient's lower inner thighs with the backs of his hands, thereafter efficiently moving to sequential inspection and palpation of the external genitalia.
  2. **Examination of specific structures of the external genitalia**
     a. **Mons.** Inspect the mons for lesions, parasites, and evidence of irritation.

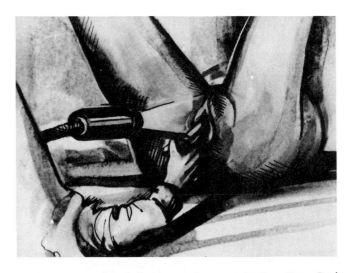

FIGURE 1.3. Position of the light for speculum examination. (From Beckmann CRB, Ling FW, Barzansky BM, et al. History and physical examination. In: Stoval TG, Summitt RL, Beckmann CRB, et al, eds. Clinical Manual of Gynecology. 2nd ed. New York: McGraw-Hill; 1992:7. Reprinted with permission.)

    b. **Clitoris**

    c. **Labium majus and minus.** Inspect the introitus, the urethral opening, and the areas of the urethral and Skene glands. Palpate the Bartholin's gland area between a finger in the vagina and the thumb.

    d. **Rectum and perirectal area**

D. Speculum examination

    1. Speculum selection and preparation. The narrow blades of the Pederson speculum work well for most nulliparous women, whereas parous women can accommodate a medium Graves speculum, which has wider blades (Fig. 1.4). Large specula are available for patients with pelvic relaxation. The speculum should be warmed before use.

    2. Insertion of the speculum and visualization of the cervix (Fig. 1.5)

        a. The speculum is held by the handle, with the blades completely closed. Moistening the speculum with water may facilitate insertion. Lubricants, which may contaminate specimens that are collected, should be avoided.

        b. The introitus is opened by gentle downward pressure on the perineum. The speculum is inserted at about a 45

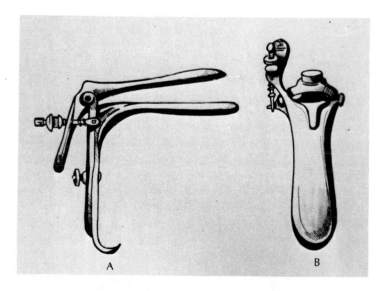

FIGURE 1.4. Adult-sized specula. (A) Medium Graves speculum. (B) Medium Pederson speculum. (From Beckmann CRB, Ling FW, Barzansky BM, et al. History and physical examination. In: Stoval TG, Summitt RL, Beckmann CRB, et al, eds. Clinical Manual of Gynecology. 2nd ed. New York: McGraw-Hill; 1992:8. Reprinted with permission.)

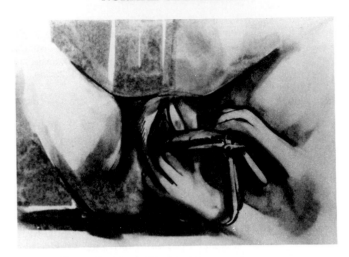

FIGURE 1.5. Speculum insertion. (From Beckmann CRB, Ling FW, Barzansky BM, et al. History and physical examination. In: Stoval TG, Summitt RL, Beckmann CRB, et al, eds. Clinical Manual of Gynecology. 2nd ed. New York: McGraw-Hill; 1992:9. Reprinted with permission.)

　　　degree angle from the horizontal. The speculum should pass the full length of the vagina, with little resistance. Care should be taken not to put pressure on the sensitive structures superior to the speculum.

c. The cervix will move into view between the blades of the speculum as it is opened. The speculum is then locked into the open position. The patient should be reassured that sensation of the need to urinate is due to the speculum. Failure to find the cervix may result from not having the speculum inserted far enough or from withdrawing the speculum slightly as it is opened.

d. For most patients, the speculum is opened sufficiently by using the upper thumb screw. More space may be obtained, if needed, by expanding the vertical distance between the blades by using the thumb screw on the speculum handle.

e. After speculum placement, the cervix and vaginal walls are inspected. A Pap smear and cultures for gonorrhea are obtained if it is the first prenatal visit. Chlamydia screen can also be done at this time if indicated. The cervix is often friable in pregnancy, and there may be some bleeding. The patient should be told that this is benign and self-limited.

3. **Speculum withdrawal and inspection of the vaginal walls.**
After the patient is told that the speculum is to be removed, the blades are opened slightly to avoid catching the cervix

between them. The speculum is withdrawn slowly to allow inspection of the vaginal walls. As the end of the speculum blades approach the introitus, there should be no pressure on the thumb hinge so that the speculum blades do not hit the sensitive vaginal, urethral, and clitoral tissues.

E. Bimanual examination
   1. **General procedures.** Two fingers are inserted into the vagina until they are in the posterior fornix behind and below the cervix. A lubricant is used to facilitate examination. Additional space may be created by downward distention of the perineum, but never upward pressure, which will cause pain by crushing tissue against the pubic arch.
   2. **Examination of the pelvic organs**
      a. **Cervix.** The cervix should be palpated to determine its size, length, shape, position, mobility, and the presence of tenderness or mass lesions.
      b. **Uterus.** The uterus is evaluated for its size, shape, consistency, configuration, and mobility, as well as for masses or tenderness and position (anteversion, midposition, retroversion, anteflexion, retroflexion). As pregnancy continues, this examination will not be possible as the uterus expands into the abdominal cavity.
      c. **Adnexae.** The adnexae are rarely palpable after the first trimester unless there is a clinically significant mass.
F. Clinical pelvimetry. An estimate of the size and shape of the pelvic midplane and outlet is made by manual examination. See Chapter 4 for details of the measurements.

VIII. The Pap Smear
   A. **Obtaining the Pap smear**
      1. **Specimens** are collected from both the exocervix and endocervix.
         a. The **exocervical sample** is obtained by rotating a wooden or plastic spatula around the exocervix (Fig. 1.6). The spatula is then lightly pressed onto a premarked slide.
         b. The **endocervical sample** is obtained in a similar manner, using the traditional moistened cotton swab. Care must be taken not to extend the swab too far into the cervix. The slide is then immediately fixed (Fig. 1.7).
         c. The **vaginal sample.** A vaginal lesion or the vaginal wall of a patient exposed to DES in utero is sampled by scraping the lesion with a second spatula and fixing the specimen immediately after it is obtained.
      2. **Fixing and handling the specimens.** Immediate fixation is important to avoid air-drying artifacts, which compromises cytopathologic evaluation. Lubricating gel and talcum powder should be avoided, as they cause distortion and reduce the quality of Pap smears. Slides left in air longer than 10 s demonstrate a very high incidence of such artifacts.

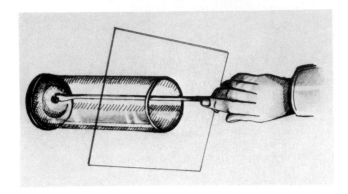

FIGURE 1.6. Obtaining the exocervical Pap smear specimen. The exocervical specimen is obtained by gently twirling a wooden spatula a few times on the outer portion of the cervix. (From Beckmann CRB, Ling FW, Barzansky BM, et al. History and physical examination. In: Stoval TG, Summitt RL, Beckmann CRB, et al, eds. Clinical Manual of Gynecology. 2nd ed. New York: McGraw-Hill; 1992:12. Reprinted with permission.)

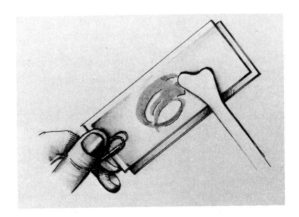

FIGURE 1.7. Placing the Pap specimen on the glass slide. The wooden spatula is gently pressed against the glass slide so that the material is transferred to the slide with minimal damage. (From Beckmann CRB, Ling FW, Barzansky BM, et al. History and physical examination. In: Stoval TG, Summitt RL, Beckmann CRB, et al, eds. Clinical Manual of Gynecology. 2nd ed. New York: McGraw-Hill; 1992:12. Reprinted with permission.)

IX. Concluding the initial evaluation of the obstetric patient
    A. After the evaluation is completed, the patient should be allowed to dress. The findings of the examination are then reviewed with the patient, including:

   1. The general status of the pregnancy.
   2. The EDC or, if uncertain, plans to better define the EDC.
   3. Tests that will be needed during the pregnancy, when, and for what reason.
   4. Medications recommended and their reasons.
   5. Dos and don'ts of pregnancy—primarily related to physical activity, sexual activity, diet, and drugs/tobacco use.
   B. An opportunity should be provided for the patient to ask questions, which should be answered clearly and completely.

CHAPTER 2

Care of the Patient

Roger P. Smith

The almost sacred trust placed in the physician by patients requires more than just caring for a specific disease process. It requires a total commitment to the well-being of the patient while under the physician's care. The physician must strive to improve patients by the effective treatment of their disease, while protecting them from further physical, emotional, and financial harm through the application of knowledge, skills, compassion, and understanding.

CARE OF THE AMBULATORY PATIENT

Obstetricians and gynecologists are the principal sources of medical care and advice for many women throughout their lives and may be their only regular medical contact. This contact grows even closer during the course of prenatal care. Because of the special nature of the problems that the obstetrician/gynecologist deals with, many women have very different feelings about their relationship with their doctor. The obstetrician/gynecologist provides continuity of care and referral that are uncommon in today's world of fragmented and specialized care.

The obstetrician/gynecologist should provide a continuum of health care that takes into consideration the need of the woman for information and education about health maintenance, developing and changing sexuality, family planning, and genetic risks of reproduction, as well as management of the specific medical and surgical conditions present. The physician should encourage breast self-examination and make the patient aware of common health risks to which she may be exposed. The physician must assist the patient in preparing for the physical and emotional changes brought about by her pregnancy, and support her preparation for and participation in the birth process. The need for the patient's participation in a "partnership" of health care should be stressed.

As part of a woman's overall health care, the physician should recognize the patient's sexual, psychological, and social needs, in addition to any demands made by pathologic processes. The physician should identify areas of difficulty above and beyond the presenting complaint and, when necessary, should involved other physicians and community resources available for the patient and her family.

The health history, physical examination, and laboratory evaluation of the patient have been covered in Chapter 1. The importance of a complete history, physical examination, and laboratory evaluation cannot be over-stressed. These elements are no less important for the patient receiving prenatal care than they are for the patient with acute abdominal pain.

Prenatal care is the ideal time for patient education and counseling. This opportunity for education need not be a stilted effort at impromptu seminars on today's health issues, but can often be as simple as anticipating a question that the patient has not yet asked. Simple thoughtfulness is often the key. For example, explaining how the uterus will grow and change, that mild contractions occur throughout pregnancy, or that a nipple discharge is normal late in pregnancy will not only save unnecessary phone calls but will give the patient peace of mind. Even the manner in which a prescription is given to the patient can affect the response to therapy. Confidence and reassurance can have many therapeutic effects. Ultimately, it is caring about the patient that leads to good care for the patient.

Today, as never before, the physician must also be conscious of the economic implications of the care that is provided. This is seen, for example, in the major institutional trend toward ambulatory (day) surgery, second opinions, and similar cost-containment measures. Since 1983, hospitals have been reimbursed a preset amount for patients within a specific diagnostic related category (DRG). Although the Prospective Payment System (PPS) for Medicare patients is directed at hospitals, it is critical to remember that it is the decisions of individual physicians that ultimately affect the cost of treatment. For example, 25 percent of a hospital bill comes from laboratory tests that are ordered by physicians for diagnosis and management. Cost effectiveness must now be judged along with the diagnostic yield of any test or procedure. Physicians have also had to become more aware of the necessity for accurate charting of relevant information (e.g., procedures, co-morbidities) that affect the final assignment of the patient to a diagnostic category. In some states, PPSs extend to all third-party payers, and it is likely that a similar system will eventually be applied to all physician charges. Therefore, it is imperative that physicians practice cost-effective as well as compassionate medicine.

CARE OF THE HOSPITALIZED PATIENT

In the hospital setting, the entire life of the patient is under the physician's control. Most of the time, care will be dictated by the condition that necessitated the hospital admission. This dictates much of the care the patient receives but does not relieve the obligation to provide care in the broader sense. Attention to detail and the needs of the patient in ways other than treating the disease at hand is constantly required.

I. Routine admitting orders

Admitting orders will vary according to the patient's condition, stage of pregnancy, presence of labor, bleeding, or rupture of the membranes, and any planned procedures. It is best to write orders in a specific sequence so that nothing is inadvertently omitted. One such sequence is as follows:

A. Vital signs. Vital signs (pulse, respirations, blood pressure, temperature, and weight) should be ordered based on the condition of the patient.

B. **Activity.** Unrestricted activity (up ad lib) may be appropriate for some patients early in labor after initial admitting procedures and fetal assessments have been carried out. Restrictions such as bed rest (with or without bathroom privileges) or instructions (e.g., "patient to remain on her left side") are specified in this section of the orders.

C. **Nursing.** This section contains special requests of the nursing staff regarding such matters as fetal monitoring, cleansing enemas, or special observations.

D. **Diet.** A regular (general) diet is appropriate for most patients who are not in active labor, except when the patient's condition dictates otherwise or when surgical procedures or specialized (radiographic) tests are planned. Patients should be restricted to nothing by mouth (NPO) for at least 8 to 12 h prior to scheduled surgical procedures. Special diets such as restricted-sodium, diabetic, or calorie-controlled diets may be required. Consultation with a dietitian should be considered when in doubt.

E. **Fluid intake and output.** The recording of fluid intake and output is very important to the management of the acutely ill or postoperative patient. The frequency of recording should be specified. Special instructions about notification in case of variance from expected output must be specific (e.g., "Notify service if urinary output is less than 25 mL/h," "Notify service if nasogastric suction >100 mL/h").

F. **Special medications.** In addition to therapeutic medications dictated by the patient's condition (e.g., oxytocin), any medications that the patient is taking at the time of admission to the hospital must be reordered if they are to be continued. Careful reevaluation of the need for these medications, the possible interactions with new medications, and the possible interference with labor, planned tests, and procedures is required. Even if the patient has brought medications with her (and the hospital allows her to keep bedside medications), each medication the patient will be taking must be written out in the orders, complete with dosage, route, and frequency.

G. **Sleep and other routine medications.** Medications for the comfort of the patient after delivery (analgesics, hypnotics, laxatives) should be specified.

H. **Examinations.** Radiographic or other special studies (e.g., proctoscopy, sonography, electrocardiogram [ECG], electroencephalogram [EEG], pulmonary function tests) planned for the antepartum patient should be specified. The sequence of these examinations should be considered and specified when necessary (e.g., an intravenous pyelogram (IVP) should not immediately follow an upper gastrointestinal (GI) study, but the reverse can often be done).

I. **Laboratory studies.** Both routine admission studies required by the individual hospital and laboratory studies mandated by the patient's status and condition must be written out. It is wise to list the studies that have been carried out during the process of admission to avoid duplication (e.g., "Complete blood count [CBC]—done").

II. **Preoperative considerations**
For patients in whom elective surgery is anticipated, several additional steps are necessary before the patient may safely be moved to the operating room. These steps may be carried out rapidly in cases of acute fetal or maternal distress, or may require several days of hospital care before all the necessary preparations are complete. In broad terms, these steps are as follows:

A. **Determining the appropriate procedure.** For elective surgery, such as repeat cesarean section or postpartum tubal ligation, the procedure usually has been determined in the outpatient setting before the patient's admission. Prior to the procedure, it is wise to reevaluate the plan with a view to the total care of the patient. Is the procedure necessary? (Consider other management options, such as vaginal birth after cesarean section.) Is it the best one for the patient? Are there alternative procedures that fit the patient's needs better (e.g., postpartum vs. interval tubal ligation)? Most often, these questions will not alter the planned course of operative management, but this reevaluation will ensure that the most efficient, appropriate, and safe care is given.

B. **Preoperative evaluations.** These evaluations can be broadly classified as follows:

1. **Laboratory data.** Most hospitals have policies that dictate the minimum laboratory studies acceptable at the time of labor admission or before surgery. These generally consist of a complete blood count and urinalysis. Some hospitals require screening chemical profiles including electrolytes, blood urea nitrogen (BUN), creatinine, direct and/or indirect bilirubin, alkaline phosphatase, serum glutamic-oxaloacetic transaminase (SGOT), serum glutamic-pyruvic transaminase (SGPT), or others. Additional tests such as prothrombin time (PT), partial thromboplastin time (PTT), platelet count, rapid plasma reagin (RPR) or Venereal Disease Research Laboratories (VDRL), and blood typing may be required or indicated based on the patient's condition. Even if these tests are not required, they should be strongly considered based on the patient's history (e.g., the use of diuretics that depress potassium, malnutrition, substance abuse) and condition (e.g., bleeding, toxemia, abruption). Additional tests may be indicated by the patient's general history (e.g., a history of thyroid disease might require such tests as triiodothyronine (T_3), thyronine (T_4), or thyroid-stimulating hormone).

2. **Imaging.** Hospitals may require a recent chest x-ray prior to surgery, depending on the patient's age and health status. Additional imaging with x-ray, tomography, ultrasound, or magnetic resonance imaging may be required for complete preoperative evaluation, though these studies may be

waived or modified because of concerns about exposing the fetus to radiation.

3. **Organ system function.** Evaluation of the cardiac and pulmonary systems is required for all patients undergoing repeat cesarean section or general anesthesia. Any patient over the age of 35 or one with a history of cardiopulmonary disease may require an electrocardiogram prior to surgery. All patients undergoing major procedures will benefit by being acquainted with incentive spirometry prior to surgery. The function of other organ systems (renal, hepatic) should be evaluated as indicated by the history and physical findings.

4. **Consultation(s).** Consultation with the anesthesiologist who will be responsible for the care of the patient in the operating room is required for elective cases and desirable when time permits during unanticipated procedures. This allows the anesthesiologist to become familiar with the patient and the procedure planned. Many anesthesiologists prefer to write their own preoperative medication orders. Additional consultations for evaluation or management should be dictated by the individual patient's needs.

C. **Informed consent.** Informed consent is required in most hospitals before deliver, surgery, and many invasive tests. This is not only a legal and moral obligation, but an important opportunity for patient education and improved rapport. Each institution will have its own consent form, but all embody the same basic information. The final consent should indicate that the physician has discussed the planned procedure in enough detail to allow an informed decision regarding the procedure. This discussion should be conducted using words that the patient can understand, and should include the alternatives available, the expected outcome, and the foreseeable complications. It should be balanced in its consideration of advantages and complications so as to neither frighten unnecessarily nor engender complacency. Adequate allowance for questions must be made and noted in the consent. In the case of emergency cesarean section, consent should be obtained from the patient if possible (if she is in a condition to provide it) or from her husband or family. Under these conditions, some aspects of the process will be truncated based on urgency.

Appropriate elements of informed consent include the following:

1. Indications for the procedure (including the condition being treated).
2. Risks and benefits of the procedure.
3. Alternative procedures or treatments, with their risks and benefits.
4. Expected outcome of treatment.
5. Anticipated length of treatment, hospitalization, or disability.

D. Preoperative notes. A preoperative note serves to organize and document the preparation for surgery. It should contain:
   1. Preoperative diagnosis
   2. Planned procedure
   3. Preoperative laboratory findings
   4. Preoperative imaging findings
   5. Status of blood and/or special equipment
   6. Statement of counseling for informed consent and the patient's agreement to the planned procedure

While a preoperative note is desirable even for acute procedures, the needs of the patient may take precedence. In such cases, a note after the fact may be permissible, but it should address the circumstances that lead to the decisions and procedures used.

E. Preoperative preparation and orders. Preoperative and intrapartum orders will vary with the type of surgery and the condition of the patient. They will usually contain the following elements:
   1. **Diet.** NPO after midnight or while in labor for all patients in whom surgery is planned (e.g., postpartum tubal ligation).
   2. **Patient preparation** (often known as *shave and prep*). This should include any preparations necessary for the following:
      a. **Operative area.** It is not generally recommended that the operative area be routinely shaved. If hair removal is necessary for the area of the incision, it should be done using a depilatory (when possible) or shaving immediately prior to surgery. Washing the surgical area with an antiseptic soap the night before surgery has been advocated, but its value is unproven. It probably does not cause harm.
      b. **Bowel.** For most mechanical cleansing of the colon, a tap water enema prior to surgery is all that is required and may have already been carried out in early labor.
      c. **Bladder.** For all procedures, have the patient void on call to the operating room. When a catheter is required, it may be placed in the operating room after the patient is asleep.
   3. **Preoperative medications.** Preoperative medication orders generally fall into the following categories:
      a. **Hypnotics.** A good night's sleep prior to elective surgery is desirable and should be ensured with the use of a hypnotic, if not ordered by the anesthesia consultant. Drugs such as flurazepam hydrochloride (Dalmane) 30 mg, or secobarbital (Seconal) 100 mg may be used. The order is best written for a specific time (e.g., "Give medication at 11 P.M.") rather than as a "p.r.n."
      b. **Sedatives.** Sedatives are generally not employed prior to elective cesarean section. They may be used prior to procedures carried out after delivery, such as tubal ligation. If not ordered by the anesthesiologist, sedation

with the combination of meperidine (Demerol) 50 mg, hydroxyzine (Vistaril) 25 mg, and atropine 0.4 mg given on call to the operating room is recommended.

c. **Prophylaxis.** Antibiotic prophylaxis is generally not required for elective cesarean sections or tubal ligation procedures. If indicated, it is given after the umbilical cord is clamped.

d. **Therapeutic medications.** Any therapeutic medication that may require maintenance during the operative procedure (e.g., insulin, dilantin, digitalis) must be specified, along with any alteration (e.g., $MgSO_4$) in the dose or route of administration.

4. **Preoperative laboratory and blood.** Any additional laboratory studies required prior to elective surgery should be specified, along with any special instructions about the time of the test or the disposition of results. For operative deliveries, a type and screen is generally indicated with a type and cross of blood done only if there is a high probability of a blood transfusion.

III. Postpartum and postoperative considerations

A. **Postoperative note.** Immediately following delivery or surgery, a postoperative note and orders are required. The postoperative note should include the following information:

1. Preoperative diagnosis
2. Postoperative diagnosis
3. Procedure
4. Assistant(s)
5. Anesthesia
6. Estimated blood loss
7. Fluids given during the case
8. Tubes and drains
9. Findings
10. Complications
11. Disposition and condition of the patient

With respect to the patient's long-term care, the parts of the note of greatest importance are the "procedure" and "findings" sections. Both need to be recorded in sufficient detail to provide all the information needed for future care. The "findings" section is often left out or is very incomplete, even though a complete statement of findings is one mark of the superior surgeon.

B. **Orders.** Following a surgical procedure or delivery, all previous orders are suspended. Therefore, postoperative or postpartum orders must include not only those orders specific to the immediate care required, but also any antepartum orders that are to be continued. The format of the orders will be very similar to that of the admitting orders, but with slight additions:

1. **Vital signs.** Vital signs (pulse, respirations, blood pressure [BP], temperature) should be ordered based on the condition of the patient. The frequency of these observations is gener-

ally decreased as the patient recovers (q15 min in recovery room, q30 min × 2, then q1 h × 2, then q4 h after the patient returns to the floor). If the physician is to be notified about abnormal findings, these should be specified here (e.g., "Notify physician if BP <100/60 or pulse >100").

2. **Activity.** After delivery, the activity allowed may be based on the duration of labor, the patient's strength, the amount of vaginal bleeding, and other considerations.

3. **Nursing.** Special orders regarding observation for vaginal bleeding, catheter or drain care, patient positioning, and the like must be specified. This is also where additional requests to be notified (e.g., excessive vaginal or wound drainage) should be made.

4. **Diet.** For patients who have delivered or undergone minor surgery, a return to a general diet when awake is generally appropriate.

5. **Fluid intake and output.** The frequency of recording should be specified. Special instructions about notification in case of variance from expected output must be specific (e.g., "Notify service if urinary output <25 mL/h," "Notify service if nasogastric (NG) suction >100 ml/h").

6. **Intravenous fluids.** The rate and character of the fluids must be modified based on the patient's ability to take oral liquids, blood loss, fluid loss from nasogastric suction, drains, or "third spacing" (ileus, edema), as well as the patient's cardiopulmonary and renal status.

7. **Pain medication.** Analgesics in appropriate amounts, routes, and frequencies must be provided to allow postoperative pain relief. Studies indicate improved analgesia when analgesics are given early in the postoperative period and continued on a regular basis to avoid the development of significant discomfort (meperidine [Demerol] 75 mg IM q3 h p.r.n., morphine sulfate 10 mg IM q3 h p.r.n.). Patient-controlled analgesia (PCA) systems meet these goals of providing optimal analgesia while reducing the total medication used. Strong analgesics should be used carefully in any patient who is breast-feeding.

8. **Sleep and other routine medications.** Hypnotics, laxatives, and any preoperative medications that are to be resumed after surgery must be ordered.

9. **Special medications.** Antibiotics, anticoagulants, sedatives, medications for nausea, or other specific medications

10. **Respiratory care.** For at least the first 24 h after major surgery, some form of respiratory care may be appropriate. This may range from encouragement (e.g., turn, cough, and deep-breathe q2 h, incentive spirometry q4 h) to supportive (e.g., intermittent positive-pressure breathing [IPPB] with ultrasonic nebulizer × 15 min q4 h).

11. **Laboratory studies.** Laboratory studies to monitor the patient's status and response to delivery or surgery should be

specified, along with the time the test is desired and any special instructions regarding the reporting of the results (e.g., "CBC in the morning — call results to floor").

C. **Postoperative rounds.** During the postpartum, daily rounds should be made, with appropriate notations in the medical record indicating attention to:

1. **Review of chart and objective data.**
2. **Patient complaints and observations.**
3. **Physical findings.** These could include pertinent negative findings, as well as any positive ones.
4. **Treatment plan.** Notations about planned management are not only important as an aid to formulating your thoughts, but serve as an alert to important changes in management for others who may care for the patient.

CHAPTER 3

Basic Prenatal Care and Childbirth Education

Sharon T. Phelan

Prenatal care allows detection of and intervention in problems relative to maternal and fetal well-being. This, in turn, allows prenatal care and labor management to be individualized to optimize the outcome of pregnancy while minimizing unnecessary intervention. Continued contact with the medical system allows education of the patient and involvement in her own health status.

I. Initial visit
A. Historical information
1. **Medical problems.** Emphasis is placed on those issues that may compromise or be exacerbated by a pregnancy (e.g., lupus, asthma, sickle cell disease, rheumatic heart disease, bleeding disorders).
2. **Gynecologic history**
   a. The issues of accuracy and normalcy of the last **menstrual period (LMP)** are crucial. Naegle's rule assumes 28-day cycles, so alterations due to the use of oral contraceptive pills are important. A *certain* LMP and a first-trimester pelvic exam may be as accurate as an ultrasound exam for clinical dating.
   b. Sexually transmitted disease (STD) history may increase the risk of ectopic pregnancy, transmission to the fetus or neonate, or preterm labor.
   c. Most recent form of contraception:
      (1) If it is an **intrauterine device (IUD)**, it is necessary to verify that it has been removed.
      (2) If it is in place and the strings are still visible, it needs to be removed.
      (3) If **oral contraceptive pills (OCPs)** have been used, assess how they may affect the accurate dating of pregnancy.
   d. History of infertility may possibly increase the risk of

ectopic pregnancy, miscarriage, or poor outcome of pregnancy.
3. **Surgical history**
   a. Uterine surgery may necessitate surgical delivery.
   b. Abdominal surgery may increase the risk of ectopic pregnancy or other complaints.
4. **Obstetric history**
   a. Include the dates and mode of delivery, length of the pregnancy and labor, weight and any complications involving the mother or infant.
   b. Previous complications of pregnancy may be repeated.
   c. When the infant is larger than 4000 g, the patient should be considered for a diabetes screen early in prenatal care, as well as at 24 to 28 weeks.
   d. Patients with prior cesarean section may be candidates for vaginal delivery.
   e. Prior congenital abnormality or fetal/neonatal death may indicate the need for special genetic counseling or antenatal fetal assessment.
5. **Family medical history**
   a. Congenital/chromosomal abnormalities may indicate the need for counseling or antenatal testing.
   b. Diseases that are familial may first be demonstrated during a pregnancy (e.g., diabetes, hypertension, blood dyscrasias).
   c. The patient may have an infectious disease such as tuberculosis (TB), hepatitis, acquired immunodeficiency syndrome (AIDS), or syphilis.
   d. Multiple gestations (non-identical) on the maternal side will increase the woman's risk of multiple gestation.
6. **History since the LMP**
   a. Febrile illnesses: especially viruslike rubella or fevers 38.8°C (>102°F) for possible central nervous system (CNS) concerns
   b. Drug or chemical exposure (prescription, recreational, or environmental)
   c. Radiation exposure
   d. Vaginal discharge
   e. Urinary symptoms
   f. Bleeding may represent threatened abortion, ectopic pregnancy, or actual menses
   g. Nausea/vomiting, especially if the patient shows signs of dehydration
7. **Pregnancy test(s):** when and type(s)
8. **Psychosocial and economic history**
   a. Nutrition: increased risk of preterm labor, growth retardation, and anemia if poor
   b. Lower socioeconomic class places the patient at increased risk of preterm labor, growth retardation, and compliance problems.

    c. Race and nationality may cause risk of glucose-6-phosphate dehydrogenase (G6PD), sickle cell disease, TB, hepatitis, malaria.

    d. Unplanned or undesired pregnancy: issues of family support/conflict

B. Physical exam

  1. General

    a. Record height, blood pressure, pulse, current weight, and prepregnant weight if known. If the weight was more than 10 percent under the ideal weight prior to pregnancy, the fetus is at increased risk of intrauterine growth retardation (IUGR). If the weight was more than 20 percent over the ideal weight prior to conception, the patient is at risk for diabetes (6.5 percent), hypertension, macrosomia (threefold increase), and increased operative and/or anesthesia risks.

    b. Perform a general physical exam, taking particular note of conditions that may worsen with pregnancy, such as scoliosis, varicose veins, obesity, dental hygiene, cardiac murmurs, and edema.

  2. Pelvic exam

    a. External genitalia and vagina: note lesions that may represent an STD, a vaginal discharge, or obstetric scars from a prior delivery.

    b. Cervix: Note evidence of old obstetric trauma, premature dilatation, premature effacement, abnormal discharge, or cyanosis.

    c. Uterus: Note size, consistency (soft = Hegar's sign), tenderness, fetal heart tones, fetal size and lie in an advanced pregnancy and abnormal shape (bicornuate/arcuate, fibroids).

    d. Examine adnexa for abnormal masses or tenderness.

    e. Perform clinical pelvimetry as indicated.

C. Initial laboratory tests

  1. For the recommended routine tests, see Table 3.1.

  2. Depending on the community, the patient's risk factors, and the laboratory resources, the following tests should be considered:

    a. TB skin test and possible chest x-ray (especially in Southeast Asians and Native Americans)

    b. Hepatitis screening: Studies have shown that 35 to 65 percent of hepatitis B surface antigen (HBsAg)-positive mothers would have been found by the following screening criteria (Southeast Asians, IV drug users, Native Alaskans, patients with a history of acute hepatitis before or during pregnancy). In 1988 the Centers for Disease Control recommended that all pregnant women be screened for HBsAg to allow identification of fetuses in need of treatment. This was supported by the American College of Obstetricians and Gynecologists'

Table 3.1. Prenatal Screening Laboratory Tests

A. Routine
  1. Initial Visit
      Pap smear
      Gonococcus culture
      Blood type
      Antibody screen (indirect Coombs' test)
      Urinanalysis (glucose, protein, nitrites vs. culture)
      Rubella
      Rapid plasma reagin (RPR)/Venereal Disease Research Laboratory (VDRL)
      Complete blood count (CBC)
  2. Every visit
      Urine dipstick for glucose, protein, with ketones, and nitrites done as indicated
  3. Interval
      Hct/Hmg at 32 to 34 weeks if patient is Rh negative
      RhoGAM evaluation for Rh at 28 weeks
      Glucose screening at 24 to 28 weeks

B. Recommended, depending on the population
    TB screen
    HBsAg
    Hmg electrophoresis
    HIV screen
    Chlamydia
    MSAFP

(ACOG's) Committee on Obstetrics in a committee opinion published in January 1990. Arguments are now being raised about whether this procedure is cost effective due to the low rate of HBeAg positivity in HBsAg-positive women with low-risk profiles.

  c. Screen for sickle cell disease and thalassemia.
  d. Screen for AIDS (IV drug users, patients in endemic areas such as Central Africa and Haiti, hemophiliacs, prostitutes, sexual partners of individuals at increased risk for human immunodeficiency virus [HIV] infection).
  e. A chlamydia evaluation.

  3. Ultrasound. Currently there is a great deal of controversy about routine versus indicated ultrasound screening. One issue in this debate is that patients with routine screening have two to three times as many scans as those patients who have scans only when indicated. However, the routinely screened group has half the rate of induction for postdates.

If scans are done only when indicated, one-third of fetal anomalies will be found prior to 22 weeks and two-thirds after 23 weeks. Since 3 percent of infants have congenital problems, some believe that ultrasound exams should be done to check for such anomalies while elective termination of pregnancy is still an option. Opponents inquire how many of these anomalies would be missed by a level I ultrasound exam or found by a maternal serum alpha fetoprotein (MSAFP) screening program or early prenatal care. Cost-effectiveness issues are pivotal in the controversy.

  D. Documentation

    1. All of the above information needs to be documented completely.

    2. To facilitate documentation of critical information and to allow development of a flow sheet to identify variations from normal, various forms have been designed by organizations such as the ACOG.

    3. In a busy obstetric service, detailed charting will reduce the likelihood of accidentally missing information that may have a major impact on the pregnancy and mode of delivery (e.g., a history of herpes).

    4. A current problem list should be maintained that is readily evident in the chart.

II. Subsequent routine prenatal care

  A. Timing of visits (Table 3.2)

  B. Issues to assess at each visit

    1. Subjective issues

      a. Quickening/maternal perception of fetal movement. Nulliparas note quickening by 20 weeks, whereas multiparas may note it from 16 weeks on. Fetal movement increases from 18 to 29 weeks, with a peak between 29 and 38 weeks. Then fetal movement decreases, especially in intensity, from 38 weeks until delivery.

      b. Uterine contractions or pain may represent possible preterm labor/contractions, or only Braxton-Hicks contractions.

      c. Vaginal discharge

        (1) Leukorrhea: Pregnant women are more at risk for monilia than nonpregnant ones.

        (2) Blood: One needs to assess for cervical disease (e.g., cervicitis, cancer), abruption, or previa (see Chapter 26).

        (3) Water: This may represent rupture of membranes (see Chapter 22).

Table 3.2. Timing of Routine Prenatal Care

1. Initial assessment as soon as feasible to allow patient education
2. Every 4 weeks until 28 weeks
3. Every 2 weeks until 36 weeks
4. Weekly until 41 weeks
5. Biweekly until delivery

    d.   Edema of the upper extremities and/or face requires active evaluation for pregnancy-induced hypertension (PIH) (see Chapter 29) or other causes of protein loss (see Chapter 30).

    e.   Headache, changes in vision, and/or abdominal pain should prompt evaluation for PIH, if the patient is at least 20 weeks' gestation.

    f.   Fever and chills raise the need to rule out pyelonephritis (Chapter 30) or chorioamnionitis.

    g.   Dysuria or suprapubic cramping requires evaluation for urinary tract infection (UTI).

2. Objective issues

    a.   Weight gain: See Section III for details.

    b.   Blood pressure: Slightly decreased in the second trimester is common. Failure of this to occur may be indicative of an increased risk of PIH in the third trimester. Diastolic pressure > 80 mm Hg or systolic pressure > 130 mm Hg is abnormal.

    c.   Fundal height: Measurements from the pubic symphysis to the top of the fundus is approximately 1 cm/week (from 18 to 34 weeks). Measurements are most important for verifying sequential growth patterns. Deviations from standard may be the first indication of a problem.

    d.   Fetal lie: This is determined by using Leopold maneuvers. A transverse or high floating vertex lie in the third trimester may indicate an abnormal placental location. The patient with a breech presentation at the end of the third trimester may be a candidate for an external version (see the discussion of abnormal lie in Chapter 12).

    e.   Estimated fetal weight:
          20 weeks: 250 to 350 g
          28 weeks: 1000 g
          34 weeks: 2000 g

    f.   Fetal heart tones
       (1)   They should be able to be heard with the fetoscope in an average-sized patient by 20 weeks and with a doptone by 12 weeks.
       (2)   The rate should be 120 to 180 beats per min.
       (3)   The location is variable, but by the third trimester it should be infraumbilical. If it is higher, one should consider an abnormal lie, macrosomia, or multiple gestations.

    g.   Assess for edema.

    h.   Perform cervical exams as indicated. It is not necessary as a routine.

C. Laboratory tests (see Table 3.1)

    1. Urine

       a.   Glucosuria may simply represent the lower renal threshold for glucose or may be the first indication of developing glucose intolerance.

    b. Proteinuria:
        (1) Trace of 1+ may represent a contaminated specimen if there are no other symptoms. This condition needs to be followed.
        (2) 2+ or more may represent developing PIH or significant renal disease and merits further evaluation promptly.
    c. Positive for nitrites: 87 percent of these patients will have positive cultures for UTI. Since 2 to 7 percent of pregnant women have asymptomatic bactiuria, with 25 to 50 percent of them progressing to symptomatic UTI including pyelonephritis, these women should be cultured and/or treated (see Chapter 30).

2. **Urine cultures** as indicated.

3. **Repeat hematocrit/hemoglobin (Hct/Hmg)**
    a. At 32 to 34 weeks. The physiologic anemia due to plasma volume expansion will bottom out at approximately 28 weeks, with up to a 3 to 5 percent drop in Hct. If the patient is anemic, therapy may be able to improve her status prior to delivery.
    b. Monthly if the patient is at high risk, such as one who
        (1) entered pregnancy with severe anemia
        (2) has multiple gestations
        (3) is a high nutritional risk

4. Antibody screening test for Rh– mothers
    a. At 28 weeks: If the antibody screening test (AST) is negative, antenatal rhoGAM (300 μg) is needed.
    b. At 36 weeks: If no antenatal rhoGAM was given, an AST test should be done. If an antenatal rhoGAM was given, the value of an AST test at this time is questionable.
    c. After a prophylactic rhoGAM, a titer $\leq 1:4$ should be interpreted as a passively acquired immunity.
    d. A positive AST test to Kell, Duffy, or Diego antigen should be followed carefully, since all of them cause mild to severe hemolytic disease of the newborn (see Chapter 19).

5. Depending on the risk factors in the community and the individual patient, do a third-trimester screen for
    a. Gonococcus, syphilis, and chlamydia
    b. Hepatitis (IV drug users, patients with a history of acute hepatitis before or during pregnancy, Southeast Asians or those from other endemic areas)

6. Diabetes screen: 50-g oral glucose challenge: A patient is given a 50-g oral dose of glucola, followed in 1 h by a glucose level test. A fasting state is not required, but is preferable that the patient not eat for 1 to 2 h prior to receiving the glucola. A serum level > 140 mg/dl merits further evaluation (e.g., a formal 3-h glucose tolerance test). Initial recommendations were to perform this screening at 24 to 28 weeks under the following conditions:

    a. A history of giving birth to an infant weighing > 4000 g
    b. Unexplained stillbirth or malformed infant
    c. First-degree relative with insulin-dependent diabetes
    d. Weight greater than 91 kg anticipated by delivery
    e. Glycosuria: more than a trace on two occasions
    f. A history of glucose tolerance in the past, but no current diabetes

    More researchers are recommending screening of all pregnant women at 24 to 28 weeks, with women with the above-listed risk factors receiving screening earlier in the pregnancy, as well as at 24 to 28 weeks.

  7. MSAFP: Draw at approximately 16 weeks of gestation (see Chapter 14).

D. High-risk pregnancies are those pregnancies that are at risk for a poor outcome and require closer supervision. Table 3.3 list some factors identifying a high-risk pregnancy.

Table 3.3. Factors Identifying High-Risk Pregnancies

A. Demographic criteria
  1. Age less than 16 or 35 or older
  2. Underweight — less than 20 percent of ideal body weight
  3. Overweight — more than 20 percent of ideal body weight
B. Prior obstetric history
  1. Grand multiparity
  2. Previous operative delivery
  3. Previous prolonged labor
  4. Previous fetal loss or infant death
  5. Previous premature delivery
  6. Traumatized infant or infant with congenital abnormalities
  7. Previous isoimmunization
  8. History of intrauterine growth retardation
C. Medical complications
  1. Hypertension
  2. Renal disease
  3. Diabetes
  4. Cancer
  5. Thyroid disease or other metabolic/endocrine disease
  6. Hereditary disorder
  7. Cardiovascular disease
  8. Isoimmunization to Rh
  9. Pulmonary disease
  10. History of infertility
D. Current pregnancy complications
  1. Fundal size small or large for dates
  2. PIH
  3. Bleeding
  4. Rubella exposure in a nonimmune patient
  5. Anemia
  6. Multiple pregnancy
  7. Abnormal presentation
  8. Use of drugs, alcohol, and/or tobacco

III. Patient education
   A. Early in pregnancy
      1. Normal fetal development
      2. Normal anticipated sequence of prenatal care
      3. Nutrition
         a. Energy needs
            (1) Not eating for two!
            (2) Calories required increase by 15 percent (or 300 calories/day) to a total of approximately 2,000 calories/day.
         b. Weight gain
            (1) Total of 11 kg, with 1 to 2 kg in the first trimester and 350 to 400 g/week in the second and third trimesters.
            (2) Prior to 28 weeks, the 6-kg weight gain is mainly in the maternal compartment: uterus, breast fat, blood, and extracellular fluid.
            (3) After 28 weeks, the 5-kg weight gain is mainly in the fetal compartment: fetus, placenta, and amniotic fluid.
            (4) Inadequate weight gain is < 1 kg/month in the second or third trimester.
            (5) There is a correlation between third-trimester weight gain and eventual birth weight.
         c. Protein: probably necessary to add approximately 25 to 30 g/d, with an overall intake of 78 g/d.
         d. Iron: necessary to increase the total by:
            (1) 500 mg for red blood cells (RBCs)
                 300 mg for the fetus and placenta
                 −100 mg for saving by amenorrhea
                 700 mg total per pregnancy
            (2) The normal diet has approximately 6 mg iron (Fe)/1000 calories or 10 to 15 mg/d, with only 10 percent absorbed. Thus, only 400 mg is absorbed throughout the entire pregnancy.
            (3) Supplement with 30 to 60 mg/day of ferrous salt:
                 300 mg ferrous sulfate = 60 mg Fe
                 320 mg ferrous gluconate = 36 mg Fe
                 200 mg ferrous fumarate = 67 mg Fe
         e. Folic acid
            (1) Recommended daily allowance (RDA) is 800 μg for pregnant women due to rapidly growing bone marrow and trophoblastic tissue.
            (2) A supplement is probably not needed in a normal pregnancy, but is necessary in
               (a) twin pregnancies
               (b) hemolytic anemia
               (c) anticonvulsant therapy, especially Dilantin
               (d) starvation
         f. Dietary recommendations for pregnant patients:

    (1) Four servings of dairy products
    (2) Three servings of meat/protein
    (3) Four or five servings of vegetable/fruits
    (4) Five servings of bread/cereals

4. Substance abuse
  a. Cigarettes
    (1) Increase perinatal mortality by 27 percent
    (2) Decrease birth weight by > 200 g
    (3) Increase the risk of placenta previa or abruption
    (4) Older gravids are at higher risk than younger ones
  b. Alcohol (teratogenic)
    (1) Increases the risk of spontaneous abortion
    (2) Causes growth retardation
    (3) Causes developmental delay
    (4) Causes fetal alcohol syndrome
  c. Heroin/methadone: Avoid going "cold turkey" but try to decrease gradually, at a maximum rate of 5 mg/week.
  d. Cocaine: Increases the risk of preterm delivery, abruption, low birth weight, preterm rupture of membranes, and potentially congenital anomalies.

5. Routine ultrasound exam
  a. No demonstrated adverse effect in humans after more than 20 years of experience.
  b. Older studies show little or no significant value of routine screening. However, more recent studies may refute this conclusion. Currently, routine screening is not recommended in the United States, but in Europe it is required by law (see I.C. 3).
  c. Indications for ultrasound
    (1) Evaluation for an ectopic pregnancy
    (2) Fundal size not consistent with dates
    (3) Second- or third-trimester bleeding to rule out previa
    (4) Prior to an amniocentesis
    (5) Part of evaluation of abnormal MSAFP result
    (6) Abnormal lie late in pregnancy

6. Genetic counseling/evaluation should be offered in the following situations:
  a. Mother age 35 or over at delivery
  b. History of/or compatible with a parent's having a chromosomal translocation
  c. Previous child with a chromosomal error or neural tube defect
  d. Family risk of a detectable autosomal or recessive X-linked trait
  e. Maternal exposure to a potential teratogenic agent

7. Exercise
  a. This should start prior to pregnancy.
  b. Avoid contact of balance sports such as skiing, skating, or biking; encourage swimming.

   c. Emphasize flexibility and strength exercises and avoidance of bouncing or Valsalva maneuvers.

   d. Position changes from lying to sitting or standing should be done slowly to avoid postural hypotension. The patient generally should avoid lying flat.

   e. The patient needs to appreciate the altered center of gravity and increase in weight that raise the probability of injury.

   f. Maternal considerations

     (1) Connective tissue is softer and more easily stretched. Joints are more susceptible to injury. Increased lordosis with increased strain on the back creates balance problems.

     (2) The cardiovascular system shows decreased cardiac reserve during increased physical activity. Maximum heart rate should not exceed 140 beats per min; strenuous exercise should not exceed 15 min. Postural hypotension becomes problematic.

     (3) The respiratory system has decreased pulmonary reserve and an inability to compensate effectively for aerobic exercise. Thus, there is an increased risk of lactic acidosis if high-intensity exercise is maintained for long periods.

     (4) Endocrine considerations include hypoglycemia, which may occur under conditions of prolonged or strenuous exercise.

   g. Contraindications

     (1) Absolute: a history of three or more spontaneous abortions, rupture of membranes, a history of premature labor, twin pregnancy, an incompetent cervix, third-trimester bleeding, known cardiac disease

     (2) Relative: hypertension, anemia or blood disorder, thyroid disease, diabetes, cardiac arrhythmias, a history of precipitous labors, a history of growth retardation, a history of bleeding during pregnancy, breech presentation in the third trimester, excessive obesity, extreme underweight

   h. Warning signs of possible problems

     (1) Abdominal pain

     (2) Bleeding

     (3) Dizziness

     (4) Shortness of breath

     (5) Palpitations

     (6) Faintness

     (7) Tachycardia

     (8) Pubic pain

     (9) Difficulty walking

8. Hygiene

   a. Tub bath or showers are fine as long as the patient

remembers the change in the center of gravity. Extremely hot temperatures should be avoided.
- b. Douching is not recommended unless needed for vaginitis. In this situation, the patient should administer a low-pressure douche.
9. Intercourse is permitted unless previa, threatened abortion, rupture of membranes, or premature labor occurs.
10. Work may continue as long as there is no exposure to environmental hazards. A woman can work up to the time of delivery as long as no complications occur.

B. Later in pregnancy (28+ weeks)
1. Fetal movement monitoring (fetal kick count [FKC]): evaluation for intrauterine hypoxia starting at 28 to 30 weeks; this should be explained to the patient (see Chapter 16).
2. The patient should come to the hospital if bleeding, rupture of membranes, or labor (immediately if less than 37 weeks, twin pregnancy, or abnormal lie) occurs.
3. PIH symptoms including headache, abdominal pain, visual disturbances, edema of the hands and face (especially for primagravids) should be reviewed.
4. Symptoms of UTI, especially fever, chills or recurrent vomiting should be given.
5. Prepared childbirth classes. Primagravids especially should be encouraged to enroll in classes.
6. Issue of postpartum contraception, especially if the patient desires a postpartum tubal ligation. A federal consent form must be signed 30 days prior to the procedure for patients receiving federal assistance.
7. Circumcision
8. Breast-feeding
9. Selection of a pediatrician

IV. Common problems
A. Nausea and/or vomiting
1. Small, frequent feedings, avoiding acidic foods, and separating solids from liquids may help. If not, the patient may use Phenergan suppositories, 25 mg q6 h p.r.n.
2. The patient should be hospitalized if she becomes dehydrated.
3. The patient may need to stop taking vitamins for a period of time.
4. If vomiting continues beyond 14 weeks, it is necessary to rule out other gastrointestinal causes (e.g., hiatal hernia or gallstones), major psychiatric disease, gestational trophoblastic disease (if there are no fetal heart tones), and multiple gestations.
B. Dependent edema
1. Frequent rests on the side during the day (1 h t.i.d.)
2. Use of support stockings
3. Decreasing the time spent sitting and standing

C. Hemorrhoids
   1. Stool softener, especially if the patient is on iron supplementation
   2. Sitz baths
   3. Topical suppositories or creams
D. Constipation
   1. Reevaluation of the need to continue iron supplementation
   2. Increased fluid intake
   3. Stool softener; avoid laxatives if possible
   4. Increased fiber and fruit in diet
E. Low backache
   1. Low-heeled shoes
   2. Specific exercises
   3. Firm mattress; place a pillow between the legs when sleeping on the side.
   4. Local heat and acetaminophen
F. Vaginitis. Treat as usual; although many recommend delaying the use of Flagyl (metronidazole) until after 14 weeks' gestation.
G. Varicose veins
   1. Same as for edema
   2. Be alert for signs of deep vein thrombosis
H. Headache. Acetaminophen, depending on the presentation and the response to analgesics; one may need to rule out sinusitis, PIH, or migraine.
I. Heartburn
   1. Elevating the head of the bed at night
   2. Antacid (30 mL pc)
   3. No laying down after meals
J. Urinary frequency, incontinence, and/or dysuria require ruling out UTI.
K. Breast tenderness: wear good support bra.
L. Syncope/dizziness: usually orthostatic, but it is necessary to rule out other causes such as cardiac, or vestibular
M. Travel: discourage long trips within the last month of pregnancy. If travel is necessary, the patient should have a 15-min walking break every 2 h. Most major airlines will not allow a woman who is 36 weeks pregnant or more to fly. Also, air travel in an unpressurized aircraft in the third trimester may not be wise at altitudes of over 10,000 m. Oversea travel may require immunizations. Also, foreign travel carries the risk of contracting endemic infectious diarrhea or other diseases.

V. Childbirth education
A. Methods
   1. **LaMaze method:** Psychoprophylaxis that is based on a conditioned response to pain
      a. Average of six sessions for the woman and her coach
      b. Emphasis on distraction from pain, with disciplined breathing techniques to allow decreased use of pain medications

2. **Bradley method:** eliminates all medication by using total relaxation and breathing, with the husband as coach. This method can be very dogmatic.

3. **Physician(s)-based courses:** often offered to familiarize the patient with the physician's style of practice and to ensure a less biased attitude toward medication or intervention as needed. Some LaMaze and Bradley instructors foster the feeling that the use of anything (even an IV) means that the woman is a failure as a mother.

B. **Effect.** Although there may be no significant difference in the duration of labor or mode of delivery, those in prepared groups have:
   1. A positive feeling about their pregnancy
   2. Decreased anxiety during pregnancy
   3. An increased incidence of breast-feeding

BIBLIOGRAPHY

American Academy of Pediatrics and American College of Obstretricians and Gynecologists. Guidelines for Perinatal Care. Washington, DC: AAP and ACOG; 1983.

American College of Obstetricians and Gynecologists. Prevention of Rho(D) Isoimmunization (Technical Bulletin 79). Washington, DC: ACOG; 1984.

American College of Obstetricians and Gynecologists. You and Your Baby: A Guide to Prenatal Care (Patient Education Booklet). Washington, DC: ACOG; 1984.

American College of Obstetricians and Gynecologists. Exercise during Pregnancy and the Postnatal Period (Home Exercise Programs). Washington, DC: ACOG; 1985.

American College of Obstetricians and Gynecologists. Management of Diabetes Mellitus in Pregnancy (Technical Bulletin 92). Washington, DC: ACOG; 1986.

American College of Obstetricians and Gynecologists. Ultrasound in Pregnancy (Technical Bulletin 116). Washington, DC: ACOG; 1988.

Bakketeig LS, Eik-Nes SH, Jacbobsen G, et al. Randomized controlled trial of ultrasonographic screening in pregnancy. Lancet 1984; 2:207.

Barry M, Bia F. Pregnancy and travel. JAMA 1989; 261:728.

Coustan DR, Nelson C, Carpenter MW, et al. Maternal age and screening for gestational diabetes: A population-based study. Obstet Gynecol 1989; 73:557.

Cruz AC, Frentzen BH, Behnke M. Hepatitis B: A case for prenatal screening of all patients. AJOG 1987; 156:1180.

Gabbe SG. Definition, detection and management of gestational diabetes. Obstet Gynecol 1986; 67:121.

Goldenberg RL, Davis RO, Cutter GR, et al. Prematurity, postdates and growth retardation: The influence of use of ultrasonography on reported gestational age. AJOG 1989; 169:462.

Hegge FN, Franklin RW. An evaluation of the time of discovery of fetal malformations by an indication-based system for ordering obstetric ultrasound. ACOG 1989; 74:21.

Jarrett J, Spellacy WN. Jogging during pregnancy: An improved outcome? Obstet Gynecol 1983; 61:705.

MacGregor SN, Keith LG, Bachicha JA, et al. Cocaine abuse during pregnancy: Correlation between prenatal care and perinatal outcome. Obstet Gynecol 1989; 74:882.

Moore TR, Piacquadio K. A prospective evaluation of fetal movement screening to reduce the incidence of antepartum fetal death. AJOG 1989; 160:1075.

Morbidity and Mortality Weekly Report. Prevention of perinatal transmission of hepatitis virus: Prenatal screening of all pregnant women for hepatitis B surface antigen. JAMA 1988; 260:165.

National Institute of Child Health and Human Development. Panel Issues Recommendations on Ultrasound Use during Pregnancy (Research Highlights and Topics of Interest) Bethesda, Md: NICHHD; 1984.

Rosendahl H, Kivinen S. Antenatal detection of congenital malformations by routine ultrasonography. Obstet Gynecol 1989; 73:947.

Rossavik IK, Fishburne JI. Conceptional age, menstrual age, and ultrasound age: A second-trimester comparison of pregnancies of known conception date with pregnancies dated from the last menstrual period. Obstet Gynecol 1989; 73:243.

Soisson A, Watson W, Benson B, et al. Value of a screening urinalysis in pregnancy. J Reprod Med 1985; 30:588.

CHAPTER 4

Normal Labor and Delivery

Susan Rice and Sharon T. Phelan

Normal labor and delivery is a physiologic process in which the attendant closely monitors the woman and fetus, with little medical intervention required.

I. **Determining labor**
   A. **Signs of impending labor**
      1. **Lightening** (dropping) is the descent of the presenting part into the true pelvis. In nulliparas, it typically occurs approximately two weeks before labor begins.
      2. An **energy spurt** ("nesting instinct") may occur 24 to 48 h before labor begins.
      3. An **exaggeration** of Braxton Hicks contractions (false labor) occurs.
      4. **Cervical changes** may begin to occur 3 to 4 weeks prior to labor.
      5. Increased **vaginal discharge,** loss of the **mucous plug,** and **bloody show** may indicate that labor is approaching in the next few days.
   B. **Differentiating true from false labor.** Labor is a physiologic process whereby contractions of the uterus and dilatation of the cervix enable the fetus to be expelled. When evaluating a woman who is experiencing contractions, false labor must be ruled out (Table 4.1). If doubt exists after cervical examination about whether or not a woman is in labor, she can be requested to ambulate for 2 h. Her cervix is reexamined after ambulation. If she is in true labor, a change should be noted on cervical examination.
   C. **Management of false or very early labor.** In the absence of ruptured membranes or complications and with assurance of fetal well-being, the woman in false or very early labor may be sent home. Before making this decision, however, the woman should be asked about her distance from and transportation back to the hospital when labor becomes active. She can be given a sedative such as secobarbitol, 100 mg p.o., if needed for sleep or relaxation.

Table 4.1. Characteristics of True Labor and False Labor

FACTORS	TRUE LABOR	FALSE LABOR
Contractions	Regular intervals	Irregular intervals
Interval between contractions	Gradually shortens	Remains long
Intensity of contractions	Gradually increases	Remains same
Location of pain	In back and abdomen	Mostly in lower abdomen
Effect of analgesia	Not terminated by sedation	Frequently abolished by sedation
Cervical change	Progressive effacement and dilatation	No change

Source: From Niswander KR. Manual of Obstetrics: Diagnosis and Therapy. 4th ed. Boston: Little, Brown and Company; 1991:390. Reprinted with permission.

II. Mechanics of labor

   A. **Powers.** Two forces are involved in effecting the descent and delivery of the infant.

   1. The myometrium contracts to force the presenting part through the cervix. Pacemakers near the uterotubal junctions cause active contraction of the upper segment of the uterus. The myometrium becomes thicker as labor advances and becomes fixed at a shorter length (brachystasis). This prevents the fetus from returning to its original position after each contraction. As the upper segment shortens, the fetus is forced farther down into the pelvis. This passive lower segment develops and becomes thin-walled as the cervix is "taken up."

   2. The patient voluntarily contracts the muscles of the abdomen and diaphragm to augment the force of uterine contractions in order to aid expulsion following complete cervical dilatation.

   B. **Passenger.** The head is the most important part of the fetus during labor, as it is the largest and least compressible. The shoulders also play an important role in fetal descent and rotation.

   1. **Sutures.** The sutures are membranous structures between the bones of the skull. Palpation of the sutures during labor, particularly the sagittal suture, is important in evaluating the fetal position. The sutures allow molding during labor (Fig. 4.1).

   2. **Fontanelles.** These are membrane-filled spaces where the sutures intersect. The anterior and posterior fontanelles aid in the diagnosis of fetal position (see Fig. 4.1).

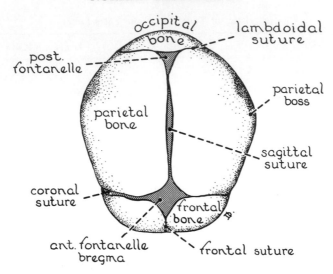

FIGURE 4.1. Landmarks of the fetal skull. (From Oxorn H, Foote WR. Human Labor and Birth. 5th ed. New York: Appleton-Century-Crofts; 1986:39. Reprinted with permission of H. Oxorn.)

3. **Diameters of the fetal skull.** These diameters represent effective parameters that must traverse the maternal pelvis during labor and delivery.
    a. **Anterior diameters** (Fig. 4.2)
       (1) The suboccipitobregmatic diameter is the shortest anterior/posterior diameter and is present when the head is well flexed. It is 9.5 cm long.
       (2) The verticomental diameter is the longest anterior/posterior diameter and is seen in brow presentations. It is 13.5 cm long.
       (3) The occipitofrontal diameter is present when the head is in the military attitude. It is 11 cm long.
       (4) The submentobregmatic diameter is seen in face presentations. It is 9.5 cm long.
    b. **Transverse diameters**
       (1) The biparietal diameter lies between the parietal bones and measures 9.5 cm.
       (2) The bitemporal diameter lies between the temporal bones and measures 8 cm.
C. **Passageway: Pelvis**
    1. **Pelvic planes and diameters**
       a. **Inlet**
          (1) Boundaries
             (a) Anteriorially: pubic crest and spine
             (b) Laterally: linea terminalis
             (c) Posteriorly: sacral promontory

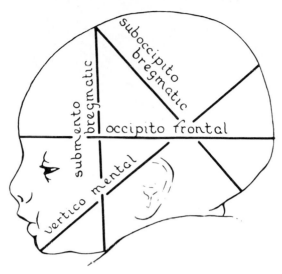

FIGURE 4.2. Anteroposterior diameters of the fetal skull. (From Oxorn H, Foote WR. Human Labor and Birth. 5th ed. New York: Appleton-Century-Crofts, 1986:43. Reprinted with permission of H. Oxorn.)

    (2)   Diameters

        (a)   Anterior/posterior (Fig. 4.3)

            (i) True conjugate: from the middle of the sacral promontory to the middle of the pubic crest. It has no obstetric significance.

           (ii) Obstetric conjugate: from the middle of the sacral promontory to the posterior superior margin of the pubic crest. This is the shortest distance through which the fetus must pass.

          (iii) Diagonal conjugate: from the subpubic angle to the middle of the sacral promontory. This can be measured when performing clinical pelvimetry. From this measurement the examiner subtracts 1.5 to 2 cm to estimate the obstetric conjugate.

        (b)   Transverse. This is the widest distance between the linea terminalis.

  b. **Midpelvis**

    (1)   Boundaries

        (a)   Anteriorially: posterior symphysis pubis

        (b)   Laterally: middle and upper obturator foramina, ischial spines, and sacrospinous ligaments

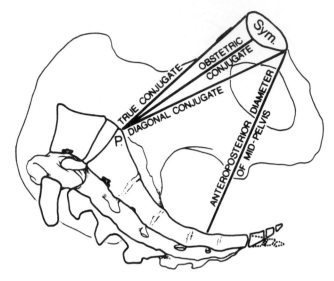

FIGURE 4.3. Various pelvic planes and diameters. Conjugata vera, true conjugate. (From Pritchard JA, MacDonald PC, Gant NF. Williams Obstetrics. 17th
ed. New York: Appleton-Century-Crofts; 1985:223.)

           (c) Posteriorally: junction of the second and third
               sacral vertebrae
      (2) Diameters
           (a) Anterior/posterior diameter is the distance
               from the lower margin of the symphysis pubis
               to the sacral tip.
           (b) Transverse diameter is the distance between
               the ischial spines. This is the smallest diameter
               of the gynecoid pelvis.
  c. **Outlet (composed of two triangular planes)**
      (1) Boundaries
           (a) Anterior triangle
               (i) Base: bituberous diameter
               (ii) Apex: subpubic angle
               (iii) Sides: pubic rami and ischial tuberosities
           (b) Posterior triangle
                (i) Base: bituberous diameter
               (ii) Apex: sacrococcygeal angle
      (2) Diameters
           (a) Anterior/posterior diameter is from the inferior
               symphysis to the coccyx.
           (b) Transverse diameter is between the inner sur-
               face of the ischial tuberosities.
  2. **Pelvic shapes.** Caldwell and Moley developed a classifica-

tion of pelvic shapes based on inlet and midpelvis characteristics. See Table 4.2 and Figure 4.4.
  3. **Fetopelvic relationships.** The fetus assumes a variety of pos-
tures during pregnancy and labor.
    a. **Lie.** This is the relationship of the long axis of the fetus to
the long axis of the mother. Types of lies include longitudinal, transverse, and oblique (or unstable).
    b. **Presentation.** This refers to the part of the fetus that first
enters the pelvic inlet.

Table 4.2. Pelvic Types

	GYNECOID	ANDROID	ANTHRO-POID	PLATYPEL-LOID
Incidence	50%	20%	25%	5%
Inlet shape	Round, transverse, oval	Rounded triangle, short posterior segment	Long, oval	Transverse oval, short posterior segment
Inlet				
Anteroposterior	Adequate	Adequate	Long	Shortened
Transverse	Adequate	Adequate	Adequate	Long
Midpelvis				
Anteroposterior	Adequate	Shortened	Long	Shortened
Transverse	Adequate	Shortened	Adequate	Long
Sacrum	Curved, average length	Straight, forward inclination	Curved, long	Curved
Sidewalls	Usually straight	Usually convergent	Straight	Straight
Sacrosciatic notch	Usually wide	Narrow	Wide	Narrow
Ischial spines	Not prominent	Prominent	Variable	Variable
Outlet				
Anteroposterior	Long	Short	Long	Short
Transverse	Adequate	Narrow	Adequate	Adequate
Subpubic angle	Wide	Narrow	Narrow	Wide

Source: Ellis JW, Beckmann CRB. A Clinical Manual of Obstetrics. New York:
Appleton-Century-Crofts; 1983:210.

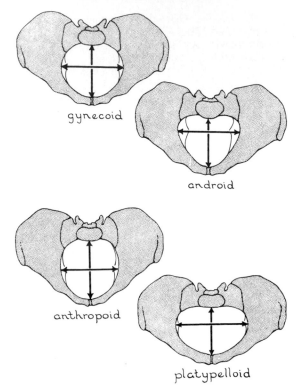

FIGURE 4.4. Pelvic inlet (Caldwell-Moloy classification). (From Oxorn H, Foote WR. Human Labor and Birth. 5th ed. New York: Appleton-Century-Crofts; 1986. Reprinted with permission of H. Oxorn.)

       (1) Cephalic, further divided into vertex, sincipital, brow, and face
       (2) Breech, further divided into frank, complete, and footling
       (3) Shoulder (acromian)
  c. **Attitude.** This describes the relation of fetal parts to one another.
       (1) Complete flexion: the fetal chin is near the chest. The vertex presents.
       (2) Complete extension: the occiput is near the back, with the neck extended. The face presents.
       (3) Intermediate degrees of flexion/extension result in sincipital and brow presentations.
  d. **Position.** This is an arbitrarily chosen point on the fetus in relation to the left or right side of the maternal pelvis (Fig. 4.5).

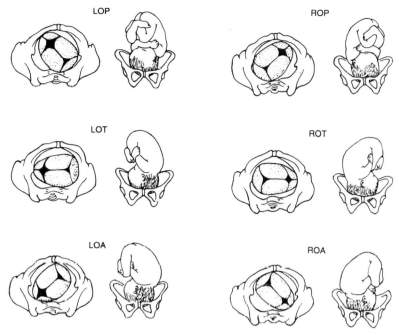

FIGURE 4.5. Vertex presentations. (From Beckmann CRB, Ling FW, Barzansky BM. Obstetrics and Gynecology for Medical Students. Baltimore, MD: Williams & Wilkins; 1992:162. Reprinted with permission.)

There are eight possible positions:
(1) Right and left anterior
(2) Right and left posterior
(3) Right and left transverse
(4) Direct anterior
(5) Direct posterior

4. **Fetal adaptations to the pelvis**
   a. **Molding.** As pressure from the pelvis is exerted on the fetal head, the soft skull bones overlap at the sutures.
   b. **Caput succedaneum.** This refers to edematous swelling over the most dependent part of the presenting head due to pressure from the cervix.
   c. **Synclitism/asynclitism.** These terms describe the relationship of sagittal sutures to the symphysis pubis and sacrum.
      (1) In synclitism the sagittal suture is midway between the symphysis and the sacral promontory.
      (2) Asynclitism describes the fetal head that is directed toward the symphysis pubis or sacrum.

(a) In anterior asynclitism the anterior parietal bone presents and the sagittal suture is more posterior.
(b) In posterior asynclitism the posterior parietal bone presents and the sagittal suture is more anterior. This is the most common manner in which the fetus engages.

III. Progress of labor

A. Stages of labor. Traditionally, three stages of labor have been identified, but recently some sources have added a fourth stage.

    1. First stage. The first stage begins with the onset of contractions and ends with complete dilatation of the cervix. It can be further divided into two phases (see Table 4.3).

        a. Latent phase. In this phase there is preparation of the cervix for active dilatation (0 to 3 cm). Contractions become established during this phase as they gradually increase in frequency, duration, and intensity.

        b. Active phase. This is the phase where most dilatation takes place. It can be further divided into three phases (Fig. 4.6). Contractions continue to increase in frequency, duration, and intensity, and by the end of the active phase, they are coming every 2 to 3 min, last for 60 to 90 s, and are strong. Intrauterine pressure reaches 50 to 70 mm Hg during the acme of the contraction, with the resting tone at 10 to 20 mm Hg.

Table 4.3. Mean Values of Various Components of Labor

	MEAN	STATISTICAL LIMIT (95%)
Nulliparous Labor		
Latent phase	8.6 h	20.6 h
Active phase	4.9 h	11.7 h
Deceleration	54 min	3.3 h
Maximum slope	3.0 cm/h	1.2 cm/h
Second state	57 min	2.5 h
Multiparous Labor		
Latent phase	5.3 h	13.6 h
Active phase	2.2 h	5.2 h
Deceleration	14 min	53 min
Maximum slope	5.7 cm/h	1.5 cm/h
Second stage	14 min	50 min

Source: Modified from Friedman EA. Labor: Clinical Evaluation and Management. 2nd ed. New York: Appleton-Century-Crofts; 1978:49.)

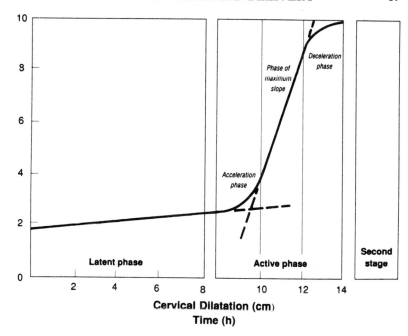

FIGURE 4.6. Composite of the average dilatation curve for nulliparous labor. (Reprinted with permission from Friedman EA. Labor: Clinical Evaluation and Management. 2nd ed. New York: Appleton-Century-Crofts; 1978.)

2. **Second stage.** The second stage begins with complete cervical dilatation and ends with the birth of the baby. Contractions during this stage are very intense, come every 2 min, and last 60 for 90 s. They are expulsive, and the woman usually feels an irresistible desire to bear down. Descent of the presenting part is more rapid during this stage than previously.

3. **Third stage.** The third stage begins with the birth of the baby and ends with the delivery of the placenta. Signs of placental separation are lengthening of the umbilical cord, change in the shape of the uterus from discoid to globular, and a sudden gush of blood.

4. **Fourth stage.** The fourth stage begins immediately after delivery of the placenta and lasts for 1 to 2 h. Near-tonic uterine contractions occur during this stage to effect hemostasis.

B. **Mechanisms of labor in vertex presentations.** The mechanisms of labor involve positional changes of the fetus as it adapts itself and moves through the maternal pelvis. The movements are listed separately, but several occur at once (Fig. 4.7).

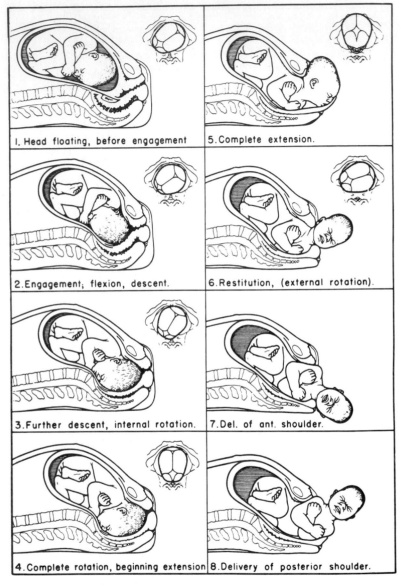

1. Head floating, before engagement
2. Engagement; flexion, descent.
3. Further descent, internal rotation.
4. Complete rotation, beginning extension
5. Complete extension.
6. Restitution, (external rotation).
7. Del. of ant. shoulder.
8. Delivery of posterior shoulder.

FIGURE 4.7. Principal movements in the mechanism of labor and delivery; left occipitoanterior position. (From Pritchard JA, MacDonald PC, Gant NF. Williams Obstetrics. 17th ed. New York: Appleton-Century-Crofts; 1985:324.)

1. **Engagement.** The biparietal diameter is level with the ischial spines.
2. **Descent.** The presenting part is pushed through the pelvis as a result of pressure of the fundus on the fetus and contraction of the abdominal muscles.
3. **Flexion.** The head is flexed as a result of resistance to descent and pressure from the cervix, pelvic walls, and pelvic floor.
4. **Internal rotation.** The fetal head rotates from an oblique to a direct anterior or posterior position. The shoulders remain oblique.
5. **Extension.** The occiput comes under the symphysis pubis, pivots under the symphysis pubis, and is born by extension.
6. **Restitution.** The head rotates 45° to realign with the shoulders.
7. **External rotation.** The head and shoulders rotate 45° to bring the shoulders into the anterior/posterior diameter and the head into the transverse diameter.
8. **Lateral flexion and expulsion.** The shoulders and body are born by lateral flexion following the curve of Carus.

IV. **Labor management**
   A. **Admission evaluation**
      1. **History.** If available, the prenatal record is reviewed. If no record is available, a history is taken that includes the current labor history, present pregnancy, past pregnancies, medical/surgical history, and family history.
      2. **Physical examination.** If time permits, a complete physical examination should be performed on admission, with careful evaluation of possible developing medical and/or obstetric complications. However, there may be time only for vital signs; auscultating the fetal heart; abdominal exam, with particular attention to determining fetal lie and estimated weight (Leopold maneuver); pelvic exam if delivery is imminent on admission to the labor and delivery area (Fig. 4.8).
      3. **Laboratory tests**
         a. Basic laboratory tests should include hematocrit, urinalysis for protein and glucose, and Venereal Disease Research Laboratory (VDRL).
         b. If no prenatal records are available, the following tests are also needed: type and Rh, rubella titer, sickle cell screen (as appropriate), and hepatitis screen.
         c. If the patient is at risk for surgical intervention, is severely anemic, or is at risk for significant postpartum hemorrhage, a type and screen or crossmatch is indicated.
   B. **First stage**
      1. **Maternal assessment.** This primarily involves vital signs for evidence of pregnancy-induced hypertension (PIH) or infection and evaluation for bladder distention.
      2. **Fetal assessment.** Fetal heart rate (FHR) monitoring is per-

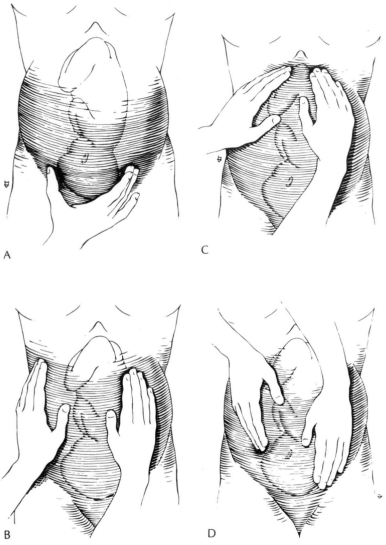

FIGURE 4.8. Leopold's maneuvers to diagnose fetal presentation and position of the fetus. (A) Palpation of the upper pole. (B) Determining the side of the small parts. (C) Palpation of the lower pole. The vertex is freely movable, and the breech moves with the body. (D) Is the prominence of the presenting part on the side opposite the small parts, as with the face presentation, or is it on the same side, as with vertex presentation? (From Oxorn H, Foote WR. Human Labor and Birth. 5th ed. New York: Appleton-Century-Crofts; 1986:20, 71. Reprinted with permission of H. Oxorn.)

formed to determine fetal well-being. Two methods are acceptable to monitor the FHR:

a. Intermittent auscultation every 30 min in a low-risk patient or every 15 min in a high-risk patient for at least 30 s after a contraction

b. Continuous electronic FHR monitoring via an external or internal monitor, with the tracing evaluated at the same time, as described for intermittent auscultation.

3. **Labor assessment**

a. Contractions. Assess their frequency, duration, and intensity. The intensity is determined by palpating the fundus during the acme of a contraction. If a finger can easily indent the fundus, the intensity is mild. If the fundus cannot be indented, the intensity is strong. An internal pressure catheter that registers 40 to 50 mm Hg above baseline with a resting tone of 10 mm Hg represents a strong contraction.

b. Vaginal exams. Assess the effacement, dilatation, descent (station), and position of the presenting part. Vaginal exams are used to determine the progress of labor.

4. **Maternal support**

a. Position/activity. The mother should determine the position most comfortable for her and assume it unless there are contraindications. Many women feel more comfortable ambulating in early labor. Walking may also stimulate contractions. Many women can void more easily on a toilet than on a bedpan and should be encouraged to do so. Some women are more comfortable sitting in a chair and can sit near the monitor.

Contraindications to ambulation during labor include the following:

(1) After analgesics are administered, causing drowsiness or dizziness.

(2) After membranes are ruptured in a nonvertex presentation or if the fetal head is not well applied to the cervix.

(3) Rapid labor in a multipara or second stage in a nullipara.

(4) Any complication that requires the woman to stay in bed.

While in bed, the woman should remain in the lateral or supine position, with the head of the bed elevated and a pillow under one hip.

b. Diet. During active labor, women can be given ice chips and/or clear liquid if this is acceptable to the anesthesiologist. Solid food should not be given at this time.

C. **Second stage**

1. **Maternal assessment.** This should be performed as in the first stage.

2. Fetal assessment
   a. Intermitted auscultation of FHR should be done at least every 15 min in low-risk patients and every 5 min in high-risk patients for at least 30 s after a contraction. Some practitioners monitor FHR after each contraction.
   b. Continuing FHR tracings need to be assessed at the same time intervals.

D. Spontaneous delivery
   1. Location of delivery. Many hospital policies and the physical layout of the hospital dictate the birth location. Many hospitals allow labor room deliveries or have special birthing rooms for delivery. The location for birth should be planned well before the second stage of labor. If maternal or neonatal complications are anticipated, the birth should take place in a room well equipped to handle the problem.
   2. Position of delivery. The birth attendant and the woman should decide on a delivery position prior to the second stage of labor. A traditional position is lithotomy, but safe alternatives include left lateral, knee-chest, dorsal with the head of the bed elevated, and squatting positions.
   3. Preparation for delivery. Due to the potential risks for both patient and provider, gowns, gloves, masks, and eye protection (universal precautions) are recommended for all deliveries, regardless of the location.
   4. Episiotomy. An episiotomy is a surgical incision into the vagina and perineum. There is no proof that routine episiotomy is beneficial.
      a. Types of episiotomy
         (1) Midline (central, median) episiotomy is cut in the center of the perineum, separating the bulbocavernosus and superficial transverse perineal muscles.
         (2) Mediolateral episiotomy is cut at a 45° angle from the midline toward the ischial tuberosity, avoiding the anal sphincter. It can be made to the left or right.
      b. Advantages of episiotomy potentially include:
         (1) Prevention of uncontrolled lacerations that are more difficult to repair
         (2) Preservation of the pelvic floor tissues and prevention of excess stretching
      c. Potential disadvantages of episiotomy include:
         (1) Increased changes of infection at the site
         (2) More discomfort postpartum
         (3) Increased incidence of dyspareunia
         (4) Increased risk of laceration into the rectum
      d. Considerations of the midline episiotomy (compared to the mediolateral) include:
         (1) The muscle is not cut

        (2)   Easier repair

        (3)   Less bleeding

        (4)   Rare dehiscense

        (5)   Easy extension into the rectum

   e. Indications for episiotomy

        (1)   Premature and small-for-gestational-age babies to protect the head from trauma

        (2)   Macrosomic babies to increase maneuverability in the event of shoulder dystocia

        (3)   Abnormal positions

        (4)   Fetal distress (to facilitate rapid delivery)

5. Delivery of a baby in the occiput anterior position

   a. Control the delivery of the head to prevent trauma to the head and to maternal tissues.

        (1)   Instruct the mother to perform controlled pushing. The delivery attendant may want to consider delivery between contractions when there is less force with pushing.

        (2)   Apply gentle pressure to the infant's head to prevent popping.

   b. "Supporting the perineum" is controversial and is considered by some to be unnecessary or detrimental. The modified Ritgen maneuver is designed to promote extension of the fetal head and thus expose the perineum to only minimal distention.

   c. When the head is born, slide the hands along the neck to check for a nuchal cord. If this is present:

        (1)   If it is loose, try to slip it over the baby's head.

        (2)   If it is tight, double clamp and cut it before delivery of the body.

   d. Wipe the baby's face and suction the mouth and nares with a bulb syringe.

   e. Watch for restitution and external rotation to occur. *(If the baby is at risk for shoulder dystocia, one may want to skip steps (d) and (e) and immediately deliver the anterior shoulders while they are still in an oblique position.)*

   f. Deliver the shoulders.

        (1)   Place the hands on either side of the baby's head.

        (2)   Exert downward and outward pressure on the head until the anterior shoulder is delivered.

        (3)   Exert upward and outward pressure on the head until the posterior shoulder is delivered.

   g. Deliver the body of the baby.

        (1)   Slide one hand along the baby's back to support the body during the birth.

        (2)   Keep the baby's head lower than the body to facilitate drainage of air passages.

6. Cord management

   a. Clamp the cord in two places and cut between the clamps.

      b. The timing for cutting of the cord is controversial. Some practitioners wait until it stops pulsating, while others clamp it as soon as possible. There are arguments supporting both views, but no consensus has been reached.

      c. Obtain cord blood from the placental end of the cord.

      d. If cord gases are to be obtained, double-clamp the cord again before obtaining the blood.

      e. Check for a three-vessel cord (two arteries, one vein).

E. Third stage

1. Observe for signs of placental separation.
2. When signs of separation occur, apply gentle, controlled traction on the cord with one hand while bracing the uterus with the other hand. The woman may push.
3. **Do not** yank or pull on the cord, as this could cause the cord to break off, leaving the placenta inside. It may also increase the risk of the uterus inversion.
4. If the membranes trail behind the placenta, they can be gently teased out with ring forceps or the placenta can be turned around and around, causing the membranes to twist.
5. The uterus should be checked for firmness and position immediately after delivery of the placenta.

F. Fourth stage

1. Oxytocics are generally administered routinely.

      a. Give pitocin, 10 U IM or 20 U in 1000 mL IV fluid. This drug stimulates intermittent contractions and is used most often prophylactically. It does not work well following a long induction. It should not be given via IV push.

      b. Give methergine, 0.2 mg IM and/or 0.2 mg p.o. This drug causes a sustained contraction and is used more often with patients who have had postpartum hemorrhage or when it is anticipated that the uterus may not contract well. Its use should be avoided in women with hypertension. The IM dose can be repeated in 2 to 4 h while the p.o. dose is every 6 h. With severe bleeding in a nonhypertensive patient, it can be given IV **slowly.**

      c. Prostaglandin F2α (Carbaprost, Hemabate) may be used, but this drug is usually reserved for severe postpartum hemorrhage. Prostaglandin F2α stimulates a sustained contraction. It is very costly and should be reserved for emergency situations.

2. The placenta is inspected for intactness, cord insertion, abnormalities, and accessory lobes.
3. The cervix, vagina, perineum, and vulva are inspected for lacerations.
4. Episiotomies and perineal lacerations are repaired. Most practitioners wait until the placenta is delivered to begin the episiotomy repair. This allows the practitioner to watch for signs of placental separation and to deliver the placenta in a timely manner. Episiotomies with third-degree extensions

and rectal wall involvement are repaired carefully to prevent rectovaginal fistulas. The rectal wall and fascia are closed with interrupted sutures, and the anal sphincter is reapproximated.

5. The mother is evaluated. The patient's blood pressure and pulse are taken every 15 min for 1 h. The fundus is palpated for firmness at least every 15 min. The lochia is checked every 15 min for amount and presence of clots. The bladder is assessed for fullness, and the mother is encouraged to void.

6. Breast-feeding and bonding are initiated. If the mother and baby are stable, the mother should be encouraged to begin breast-feeding if she has chosen this feeding method. If she is not breast-feeding, she should be encouraged to hold the infant to initiate bonding.

BIBLIOGRAPHY

Friedman EA. Labor: Clinical Evaluation and Management. 2nd ed. New York: Appleton-Century-Crofts; 1978.

Oxorn H, Foote WR. Human Labor and Birth. 5th ed. New York: Appleton-Century-Crofts; 1985.

Pritchard J, MacDonald PC, Grant NF. Williams' Obstetrics. 17th ed. New York: Appleton-Century-Crofts; 1985.

CHAPTER 5

Birthing Rooms: Alternative Styles of Labor and Delivery

Patrick J. Sweeney

I. **History of changing childbirth practices.** Early American obstetric care was provided almost exclusively in the parturient's home by midwives with varying degrees of skill. By the end of the colonial period, physician involvement in childbirth was becoming more frequent and a few hospitals had established lying-in wards. In 1935, 35 percent of all live births in the United States occurred in hospitals. The percentage of in-hospital births increased rapidly following World War II to 88 percent in 1950 and peaked in the early seventies, when more than 99 percent of births took place in the hospital setting. In the mid-seventies certain segments of the population began to opt once again for home delivery; consequently, the last decade has witnessed the proliferation of alternative types of childbirth facilities differing with respect to hospital affiliation, birth attendant, and degree of technological intervention. The purpose of these alternatives to traditional in-patient maternity care is to provide a family-centered birth experience in a setting that combines the natural atmosphere of the home with the safety of the hospital.

II. **Current options**
   A. **Traditional hospital labor and delivery.** In a traditional hospital labor and delivery experience, the patient is admitted to a labor room, restricted to bed rest, given nothing by mouth (NPO), started on intravenous fluids, and usually monitored electronically. At the time of delivery, the patient is transferred to a delivery room, where the delivery is conducted under surgically sterile conditions. Immediately postpartum, the mother is taken to a recovery room, where she can be closely monitored until she is stable enough to be transferred to a room in the maternity section of the hospital. The newborn is taken to the nursery for routine care and observation. The degree of maternal-infant interaction varies, depending on hospital policies, the mother's desires, and whether or not rooming in is available.

56

B. In-hospital birth room. An in-hospital birth room — also known as a *labor/delivery room (LDR)* — is usually located within the traditional labor and delivery area. The patient labors, delivers, and recovers in the same room, which represents a compromise between the traditional hospital labor and delivery facility and the birth center (see below). Equipment such as fetal monitors, resuscitation carts, and surgical supplies is available but is usually concealed unless needed. The room can be converted from a bedroomlike atmosphere to a nearly traditional delivery room by moving furniture, curtains, and room dividers. The newborn stays with the mother while she recovers in the birth room. Later, both are transferred to a postpartum room for rooming in.

C. In-hospital birth center. The birth center provides all inpatient care for the mother and her newborn. It is generally a large room or suite of rooms with a homelike atmosphere and may include bath and kitchen facilities. The center may be located within or adjacent to the labor and delivery suite, or it may be in a different area of the hospital. In either case, its location *within* the hospital permits ready access to emergency equipment and/or diagnostic laboratory tests. Following delivery, the new family remains together in the center until mother and baby are discharged, often within 12 to 24 h.

D. Free-standing birth center. The free-standing birth center is the same type of facility as the in-hospital birth center (see above) except that the free-standing center is not physically connected to a hospital, thus requiring patient transfer by ambulance for management of specific complications, including the need for operative delivery.

E. Home birth. Delivery occurs in the patient's home or some other residential facility.

III. The need for birthing alternatives

A. Home birth. Since the mid-seventies, the annual rate of out-of-hospital births in the United States has remained fairly constant at approximately 1 percent, with considerable variation among the states (Oregon's 3.5 percent was the highest rate in 1987). A 1981 survey by the American College of Obstetricians and Gynecologists (ACOG) of 90 responding birth centers reported that the birth centers managed 16.3 percent of the deliveries in the supporting hospitals. This indicated that a significant percentage of the people were dissatisfied with the traditional hospital experience, although an estimate of how many of these people would have attempted a home birth if a birth center were not available would be purely speculative. In addition, there are still many areas of the country (particularly rural areas) in which patients do not have access to a birthing room facility.

B. Increased consumer participation in health care. The health care industry has become very competitive, and hospital administrators are responding to patients' needs — in this case, the need for a safe alternative to a traditional hospital delivery.

C. **Cost.** Delivery in a birth center is generally less expensive than in a traditional hospital, particularly when early discharge is an option.

D. **Emphasis on family.** There has been a steady increase in family participation in the birth process since the late sixties. Initially, fathers were allowed to visit during labor. Later, they were encouraged to stay throughout labor and ultimately were permitted to observe the delivery. Many now attend childbirth classes and take a much more active role in the delivery of their child. Siblings who are old enough to understand may also be involved. Considerable research has attested to the benefits of early maternal-infant and paternal-infant bonding. Although the opportunities for the mother and father to bond with their newborn have improved markedly even in conservative institutions, participation of siblings or other family members in the birth process is generally not possible in a traditional hospital setting or LDR.

IV. **Special concerns.** Whenever a traditionally accepted therapy is questioned or changed, the proposed changes are generally the subject of considerable controversy.

A. **Patient's perspective**

1. **Use of technology.** Many patients consider childbirth to be a natural process and feel that the technical atmosphere of the modern labor and delivery area is dehumanizing. They believe that electronic fetal monitoring, analgesia and anesthesia, forceps delivery, and cesarean section are all over-utilized.

2. **Comfort.** Patients like to ambulate in early labor. It is uncomfortable to remain in bed for prolonged periods of time, particularly if one's movements are further restricted by intravenous lines or external monitors.

3. **Family support.** Since birth rooms are generally larger, more private, and less sterile than traditional labor rooms, they lend themselves to greater family participation. Family members can be present for the birth and not interfere with the care or privacy of other patients. Bathrooms and/or kitchenettes further help to minimize disruption of routine hospital services outside the birth room.

4. **Cost.** Patients with no third-party payer to help defray the cost of hospitalization are attracted by the optional early discharge program offered by most birth centers. Similarly, patients with health insurance based upon deductibles and copayments are also interested in decreasing the amount of out-of-pocket expenses.

5. **Special services.** In addition to the homelike atmosphere and the minimal regimentation, many birth centers offer unique services such as private nurses who stay with the family throughout labor, delivery, and the early postpartum period. These nurses provide direct nursing care plus one-on-one assistance with problems such as breast-feeding and care of

the newborn. In some cases, nurse practitioners or nurse midwives make home visits 1 to 3 days after discharge.

B. Provider's perspective

1. **Safety.** The ACOG bases its opposition to home birth on the potential hazards that labor and delivery present and states that babies should be delivered only in hospitals or birth centers equipped for emergencies.

   a. Reports from free-standing birth centers and private practices conclude that 23 to 33 percent of pregnant women initially considered to be at low risk will ultimately develop a significant prenatal or intrapartum complication. Eight percent of anticipated low-risk deliveries involve a serious, unpredicted complication that poses an immediate threat to the mother or baby.

   b. Well-organized out-of-hospital birth programs transfer an average of 15.8 percent of previously screened, low-risk intrapartum patients to hospitals.

   c. State vital statistics repeatedly report significantly higher perinatal mortality rates for out-of-hospital births. Although not many states specifically report home births, those states that subclassify out-of-hospital births into planned and unplanned categories report that as many as 94 percent of these births are **planned** out-of-hospital deliveries. Interestingly, births that occur en route to the hospital are classified as in-hospital.

2. **Medical liability.** With society's preoccupation with malpractice and the less than perfect outcome, it is not surprising that physicians are unwilling to take chances.

V. Establishment of in-hospital birth rooms. Those responsible for the establishment of the birth room/birth center should pay close attention to its functional organization and development of standards.

   A. Organization. The following questions must be addressed in considering the organization of in-hospital birth rooms. Who will use the facility? Who will be in charge? What will be the relationship between the birth room and the regular labor and delivery area? Who will staff the birth room? Have those professionals who will be using the facility been involved in its planning?

   B. Standards. Birth rooms should meet the standards for obstetric services published by the ACOG. These standards should not be confused with the guidelines for patient selection and management outlined below.

VI. Criteria for patient selection. The criteria for patient selection must be individualized based upon the level of perinatal care available at the institution, the staff support, the administration's desires, and the patient population. Criteria should be developed for each birth room or center and agreed upon by all professional departments involved — obstetric, neonatal, and nursing. Criteria should be considered as **guidelines,** allowing flexibility for individual patients and physicians, and should **not be interpreted as a standard** of care. The following are suggested guidelines that may be adjusted to fit the individual institution's needs.

A. **Basic patient eligibility requirements.** All patients who desire to deliver in the birth room/center should meet the following criteria:

1. **Adequate prenatal care** should be verifiable. Some arrangement should be made to have a copy of the patient's prenatal record available at the time of admission.
2. **The patient should have no significant risk factors,** past or present (see subsection B).
3. **Prenatal childbirth classes** should be attended by all those who plan to participate.
4. **At least one support person** should be identified.
5. **Plans for family participation** should be made before the birth. If children or other relatives or friends are to be present for the birth, this should be made known to the attending physician or midwife during the prenatal period and his or her consent obtained.
6. The patient should sign an **informed consent,** including a statement that she agrees to be transferred to the hospital's regular labor and delivery area if, in the opinion of her physician, such a transfer is considered necessary for optimal medical management.

B. **Risk factors** that might preclude patient participation include the following:

1. **Past medical history**
   a. Chronic hypertension
   b. Renal disease
   c. Cardiac impairment
   d. Diabetes mellitus (other than gestational)
   e. Anemia previously undiagnosed and/or unresponsive to therapy
   f. Pulmonary disease, symptomatic or potentially serious
2. **Past obstetric history**
   a. Previous eclampsia
   b. Previous stillbirth or neonatal loss
   c. Previous cesarean section
   d. Rh sensitization or other significant antibody identification
   e. Previous neurologically damaged infant
   f. Previous infant with a life-threatening genetic disorder
   g. Previous obstetric hemorrhage
3. **Current antepartum pregnancy complications**
   a. Preeclampsia
   b. Gestational age < 37 weeks or > 42 weeks
   c. Multiple pregnancy
   d. Abnormal presentation
   e. Third-trimester bleeding

    f. Predicted macrosomic infant
    g. Contracted maternal pelvis
    h. Substance abuse
    i. Intrauterine fetal demise
    j. Thrombophlebitis, receiving therapy or prophylaxis
    k. Polyhydramnios
    l. Suspected fetal growth retardation

  4. Current intrapartum pregnancy complications
    a. Maternal fever
    b. Meconium-stained amniotic fluid
    c. Abnormal fetal heart rate pattern
    d. Prolonged or arrested labor
    e. Significant vaginal bleeding
    f. Herpes — positive culture or suspicious lesion
    g. Need for forceps delivery or cesarean section

C. Participation of children or persons other than the principal support person
  1. All participants must remain in the center
  2. Participants should be screened for common communicable diseases.
  3. All who plan to be present for the birth should receive some formal childbirth instruction. It is particularly important that young children be adequately prepared concerning the effects labor might have on their mother, the amount of blood they might see, and the source of the bleeding.
  4. Each child must have his or her own support person who can attend to the child's needs and keep the child occupied during the mother's labor. This responsibility cannot be delegated to the hospital staff.

D. Early discharge guidelines (within 24 h following delivery). Patients who do not qualify for early discharge would be expected to remain in the hospital for a minimum of 48 h and may be transferred to a traditional postpartum hospital room for all or part of that time.
  1. Maternal guidelines
    a. Negative medical history
    b. No obstetric complications
    c. Uncomplicated episiotomy
    d. Full recovery from anesthesia (depends upon the method used)
    e. Acceptable postpartum hematocrit
    f. Fundus firm, with normal amount of bleeding
    g. Normal vital signs
    h. Able to ambulate
    i. Able to void
    j. RhoGAM eligibility determined
    k. Rubella immunization, if indicated
    l. Plan for assistance at home
  2. Infant guidelines
    a. Birth weight between 2500 and 4000 g

b. Normal vital signs
c. Normal newborn examination and laboratory values
d. Blood type determined; no evidence of incompatibility
e. At least one normal feeding, one stool, one voiding
f. Observed for a minimum of 6 h and one voiding following circumcision (if performed)
g. Birth certificate information obtained

VII. **Quality of care evaluation.** Implementation of a thorough plan for evaluation of patient care cannot be overemphasized. Since much of the controversy concerning birth rooms and centers is based on the question of safety, it is imperative that such facilities keep complete and accurate statistics. Many institutions that established birth centers in the late seventies have published the data on their first few years' experience. However, since patient selection criteria and patient populations vary widely from one center to the next, outcome data from different centers may not be comparable.

BIBLIOGRAPHY

Eakins PS. Free-standing birth centers in California — program and medical outcome. J Reprod Med 1989; 34(12):960–970.

Klaus MH, Kennell JH. Maternal–Infant Bonding. St Louis, Mo: CV Mosby; 1976.

Leonard CH, Irvin N, Ballard RA, et al. Preliminary observations on the behavior of children present at the birth of a sibling. Pediatrics 1979; 64(6):949–951.

Mehl LE, Peterson GH, Whitt M, et al. Outcomes of elective home births: A series of 1,146 cases. J Reprod Med 1977; 19(5):281–290.

Moawad AH. Some problems of professionally attended home births. J Reprod Med 1977; 19(5):298.

Moran JD, von Bargen N. Attitudinal and demographic factors influencing mother's choice of childbirth procedures. Am J Obstet Gynecol 1982; 142(7):846–850.

Moutquin J, Gagnon R, Rainville C, et al. Maternal and neonatal outcome in pregnancies with no risk factors. Can Med Assoc J 1987; 137:728–732.

National Center for Health Statistics. Advance report of final natality statistics, 1988. Monthly Vital Statistics Report 39(4, suppl). Hyattsville, Md: Public Health Service, 1990.

National Center for Health Statistics. Vital Statistics of the United States, 1987, Vol. 1 Natality. DHHS Pub. No. (PHS) 89–1100. Washington, DC: U.S. Government Printing Office, 1989.

Pearse WH. Trends in out-of-hospital births. Obstet Gynecol 1982; 60(3):267–270.

Rooks JP, Weatherby NL, Ernst EKM, et al. Outcomes of care in birth centers. The National Birth Center Study. N Engl J Med 1989; 321(26):1804–1811.

Sagov SE, Feinbloom RI, Spindel P, Brodsky A. Home Birth — A Practitioner's Guide to Birth Outside the Hospital. Rockville, Md: Aspen; 1984.

Speert H. Obstetrics and Gynecology in America. Baltimore: Waverly Press; 1980.

Standards for OB/GYN Services. 6th ed. Washington, DC: American College of Obstetricians and Gynecologists; 1985.

Sumner PE, Phillips, CR. Birthing Rooms: Concept and Reality. St. Louis, Mo: CV Mosby; 1981.

CHAPTER 6

Care of the Newborn

Charles Fitch

More than 80 percent of newborn infants are term and normal who are rapidly and successfully completing the transition to extrauterine existence. Such infants require a minimum of basic care. However, any infant is potentially susceptible to hypoxia, acidosis, and subsequent depression during labor, delivery, and the immediate postdelivery period; infants born of high-risk pregnancies are at even greater peril. Delivery room care of the newborn, therefore, includes not only provision of basic care for the normal neonate, but also the capacity to care for the distressed infant and to provide a prompt, organized, and skillful approach to emergencies.

CARE OF THE NORMAL NEWBORN

Responsibility for the initial postdelivery assessment and care of the neonate generally lies with the individual who delivers the infant until delegated to other personnel. Routine care of the normal infant may be provided by appropriately trained nurses and includes the following:

I. **Clearing of the airway**
   A. **Suctioning.** Initial clearing of the airway is done immediately upon delivery of the infant's head prior to delivery of the chest; fluid and secretions should be suctioned from the nose, mouth, and pharynx using a bulb syringe. If meconium is present in the amniotic fluid, suctioning the upper airway at this point is especially important, since it may prevent aspiration of meconium following delivery of the chest.

   After complete delivery, suctioning is again performed quickly, with the infant held head down at the level of the perineum.
   B. **Repeat suctioning.** If necessary, repeat suctioning is subsequently performed. Stimulation of the posterior pharynx by overly vigorous suctioning or the use of a nasal suction catheter in the first few minutes after delivery should be avoided, since vagal reflex apnea and/or bradycardia may result.

II. **Cord clamping.** Transfusion of blood from the placenta at birth may significantly alter the blood volume of the infant. Transfusion is influenced by the time that elapses between delivery and clamping of the cord and by the position of the infant after delivery in relation to the placenta. Normally, one-fourth of the potential transfusion occurs within 15 s of delivery and one-half by 1 min.

A. Factors influencing placental transfusion

　　1. Early clamping of the cord (< **30 to 40 s**) minimizes the blood volume transferred; this may be desirable for the erythroblastotic infant to minimize the transfer of sensitized red blood cells.

　　2. Late clamping of the cord (> **40 to 60 s**) may increase blood volume by 40 to 60 percent, resulting in a larger initial total blood volume. By about 3 days of age, differences in blood volume are insignificant, but the red blood cell mass remains higher during the first week of life.

　　3. Position of the infant in relation to the placenta affects the net transfer of blood between the infant and placenta. Constriction of the umbilical arteries shortly after birth minimizes arterial blood flow from the infant to the placenta, but the umbilical vein, which remains dilated, allows blood to flow between the placenta and infant by gravity. The infant held below the level of the placenta receives blood from it; if it is held above this level, blood loss may occur into the placenta.

B. Recommended procedure for cord clamping. There appears to be no consensus as to when the cord should be clamped, but approximately 30 to 40 s appears to be practical for the normal vaginal delivery with the infant held at the level of the introitus. Stripping the cord is not advised, except for specific emergency situations (e.g., signs of acute blood loss and shock at delivery), but even in these situations resuscitation should not be delayed.

III. Neonatal assessment: The Apgar score. Immediate assessment of the infant's status after delivery is essential and is best accomplished by use of the Apgar score. The Apgar score provides quantitative evaluation of five vital signs: heart rate, respiratory effort, muscle tone, reflex irritability, and color. Values of 0, 1, or 2 are assigned to each component at 1 min and at 5 min after delivery (Table 6.1).

A. Scoring system. The maximum score (a total of the score for each of the five vital signs) is 10, indicating an infant in the best possible condition. Apgar scores of 8 to 10 characterize a normal infant; 5 to 7, mild depression; 3 or 4, moderate depression; and 0 to 2, severe depression. One must be aware that because of immaturity, preterm infants may exhibit low Apgar scores in the absence of acid-base abnormalities.

　　1. The 1-min score coincides with the period of maximum depression and as an index of intrapartum stress identifies the neonate requiring resuscitation.

　　2. The 5-min score is more predictive of survival or later neurologic outcome and serves as an index of the rate of recovery from intrapartum stresses. If the 5-min score is < 7, assessment should be repeated at 5-min intervals for up to 20 min unless two successive scores ≥ 8 are obtained.

Table 6.1. Apgar Score

SIGN	0	1	2
Color	Pale, cyanotic	Body pink, extremities blue	Completely pink
Respirations	Absent	Weak, irregular	Vigorous crying
Heart rate	Absent	< 100 beats per min	> 100 beats per min
Muscle tone	Limp	Some flexion	Well-flexed, active motion
Reflex irritability (response to suctioning)	No response	Grimace	Cough or sneeze

    B. Advantages of the Apgar score
      1. Provides quantitative and reproducible evaluation of cardiopulmonary and neurologic status at birth
      2. Identifies the neonate requiring resuscitation and consequently at risk for mortality and morbidity
      3. Ensures close observation while monitoring the recovery rate during the critical early minutes after birth.

IV. Minimization of heat loss. Significant cold stress occurs in the neonate at delivery, and minimizing heat loss is an often neglected aspect of delivery room care. Without intervention, the skin temperature of the term infant may decrease as much as 4°C within 5 min; core temperature may decline ≥ 2°C within 30 min. Even greater heat loss may occur in the small premature infant. Physiologic responses to cold stress are active at birth, even in the premature infant. The neonate can increase oxygen consumption and metabolic heat production in response to cold stress, but to prevent a drop in body temperature in the delivery room, heat production must increase threefold or more in the first few minutes after delivery; even the healthy term infant cannot meet this metabolic demand without supportive measures.

    A. Factors that predispose neonates to heat loss include:
      1. A surface area disproportionately large for body weight.
      2. A relative paucity of tissue insulation (subcutaneous fat).
      3. Limited capacity for metabolic heat production in response to cold. This may be further impaired by hypoxia and acidosis.
      4. The wet skin of the neonate exposed to the air-conditioned environment of the delivery room, which contributes to tremendous evaporative and convective heat losses.
      5. Significant radiant heat loss.

    B. Supportive measures. Heat loss is reduced by quickly drying the neonate with prewarmed towels. A radiant warmer (prewarmed) in the delivery area is a most effective heat source and permits easy access to the infant during routine and resuscitative procedures. After initial management, the otherwise healthy term infant may be swaddled next to the mother for continued warmth while in the delivery room. Optimum temperature must also be maintained during transport from the delivery area to the nursery, and cribs or incubators should be prewarmed prior to use.

V. Eye care. Prophylaxis for prevention of gonococcal ophthalmia is required by law in most states. Silver nitrate, 1% solution in single-dose containers, is generally recommended, although antibiotic ophthalmic ointment (erythromycin 0.5% or tetracycline 1%) in single-use tubes may be acceptable. Topical prophylaxis has not been proven effective in prevention of chlamydial conjunctivitis. For penicillin resistant strains of Neisseria gonorrhea, silver nitrate solution 1% is preferred since the efficacy of erythromycin or tetracycline ointment prophylaxis for these strains has not been established. The agent should be instilled within 1 h of birth, dispersing it to all areas of the conjunctival sac. Irrigation afterward with sterile saline or distilled water may reduce its efficacy and is not recommended. Prophylactic eye care is also recommended for infants delivered by cesarean section although the risk of neonatal ophthalmia in such cases has not been defined. If gonorrheal infection is present in the mother at the time of delivery, the infant should receive a single dose of ceftriaxone, 125 mg intravenously or intramuscularly (25 to 50 mg/kg for low-birth-weight infants).

VI. Vitamin K. Hemorrhagic diathesis due to deficiency of vitamin K–dependent coagulation factors can be prevented by a single parenteral dose of 0.5 to 1.0 mg of natural vitamin K_1 (AquaMEPHYTON) within 1 h of birth.

VII. Identification procedures. Identification of the neonate while in the delivery room is essential. Usually this is the responsibility of the nurse in charge of the delivery room. Two identifying bands, noting the mother's admission number, date, and time of birth and the neonate's sex, should be applied to the wrist or ankle. These bands should be verified upon leaving the delivery room and again upon admission to the nursery. Footprinting and fingerprinting also may be performed, but require careful technique and are no longer recommended as universal practice.

VIII. Collection of cord blood. At the time of birth, a tube of cord blood should be collected, clearly labeled, and refrigerated in the event that tests such as blood type, Rh, and Coombs tests are needed. These tests should be routinely performed on cord blood at delivery if the mother is Rh (D) negative. In addition, serologic tests for syphilis should be performed if the mother's serology is uncertain.

IX. Bathing and circumcision

A. Bathing in the delivery room is not indicated and should be delayed until body temperature has been normal (> 36.5°C) and stable for at least 2 h.

B. Circumcision is considered an elective procedure and should not be performed in the delivery room or during the postdelivery period of stabilization. If performed, the procedure should be delayed for 12 to 24 h.

CARE OF THE DEPRESSED NEWBORN

I. **Incidence.** A relatively small percent (probably less than 1 percent) of infants born at term require vigorous resuscitation, and nearly all small premature infants require some form of resuscitative care at birth.

II. **Cause.** Perinatal asphyxia is a complex interaction of severe metabolic acidemia and hypoxia associated with injury to various organs including the brain, kidneys, heart, and gastrointestinal tract. While perinatal asphyxia is an etiologic factor of major concern in the depressed infant, many other factors may contribute to or be primarily responsible for a depressed infant and low Apgar scores. Since metabolic acidosis is a component of asphyxia, umbilical cord blood gas and pH analysis may be useful in separating asphyxia from other causes of neonatal depression. Asphyxia may be the result of:

A. **Interference with fetoplacental exchange** (e.g., cord compression, placental abruption, maternal hypotension)

B. **Failure at birth of the lungs to inflate** and establish adequate respiration (e.g., central nervous system depression, prematurity, obstructed airway)

Most neonates predisposed to depression as a result of hypoxia and acidosis may be identified by high-risk factors during pregnancy or labor, which include:

1. **Maternal disorders** such as preeclampsia, diabetes, infection, cardiopulmonary disease, renal disease, drug abuse, and uteroplacental complications.

2. **Fetal conditions** such as prematurity or postmaturity, deviant fetal growth, abnormal presentation, multiple births, hydrops, meconium passage, congenital anomalies, and intrapartum fetal distress.

III. Normal physiology and pathophysiology

A. The normal term neonate usually cries and breathes spontaneously within seconds after delivery. The onset of adequate respirations is a trigger event initiating certain physiologic changes that characterize the transition from fetal to neonatal life. These changes include rapid expansion and stabilization of alveoli and the development of effective gas exchange. The resulting prompt increase in arterial Po_2 and pH and the decrease in Pco_2 promote pulmonary arteriolar dilatation and initiate functional closure (constriction) of the ductus arteriosus. As pulmonary resistance decreases, pulmonary blood flow and venous return to the left atrium increase. Rising left atrial pressure functionally closes the foramen ovale, eliminating this fetal pathway of right-to-left shunting.

B. **Experimental total asphyxia** acutely induced in animal studies results in an initial phase of gasping respirations, thrashing movements, and peripheral vasoconstriction lasting for ~ 1 min. A period of apnea (primary apnea) ensues, lasting for ~ 1 min, during which blood pressure increases slightly and heart rate decreases. Primary apnea is followed by a 4- to 5-min period of gasping respirations, which gradually weaken and cease (last gasp), marking the onset of secondary or terminal apnea. Heart rate and blood pressure decrease and flaccidity develops. During primary apnea, gasping efforts can be restored by sensory stimuli; such stimuli are ineffective during secondary apnea, and vigorous resuscitation is necessary to initiate gasping at this time.

C. In the **asphyxiated neonate,** failure to establish adequate respirations promptly at delivery results in persistence of high pulmonary vascular resistance, lack of increase in pulmonary blood flow and venous return to the left atrium, failure of left atrial pressure to rise, and failure of the ductus arteriosus to constrict. Continued right-to-left shunting across the foramen ovale and ductus arteriosus may promote a cycle of progressive hypoxemia that is difficult to reverse. In response to asphyxia, the following physiologic abnormalities may occur to varying degrees: hypoxia; hypercarbia; mixed metabolic/respiratory acidosis; decreased cardiac rate, blood pressure, and cardiac output; increased pulmonary vascular resistance with persistence of fetal pathways of shunting across the ductus arteriosus and foramen ovale; and depletion of glycogen stores (hypoglycemia).

IV. **Resuscitation.** While certain basic information is presented here, completion of the neonatal resuscitation course jointly sponsored by the American Heart Association and the American Academy of Pediatrics is strongly recommended for those persons who potentially will be involved in neonatal resuscitation.

The Apgar score, although providing an objective assessment of the infant's condition at one and five minutes post delivery, is not useful as a basis for resuscitation decisions; valuable time is lost if resuscitative support is delayed for the first minute. The score is useful, however, in monitoring the efficacy and response to resuscitative efforts.

Successful management of the depressed infant involves coordination of anticipation, preparation, and assessment into an organized plan of response. This requires a collaborative team effort of the personnel involved — obstetrician, pediatrician (neonatologist), and nurses — each of whom should have a specific role in the resuscitation procedure. **Anticipation** should be triggered by awareness of risk factors, both maternal and fetal, that potentially may compel resuscitation. **Preparation** should ensure that appropriate personnel, equipment, and drugs are on hand. Personnel attending the high-risk delivery must be cognizant of problems peculiar to the neonate and must be competent in the technical skills required for neonatal resuscitation. Equipment (Table 6.2) should be carefully checked to ensure proper function (e.g., laryngoscope), and medications (Table 6.3) should be immediately available. **Assessment** of respiration, heart rate, and color (in that order) quickly identifies the depressed neonate and serves as a guide to the intensity of therapeutic intervention. The well-known ABC's of resuscitation should be followed in resuscitation of the neonate:

A—establish open Airway

B—initiate Breathing

C—maintain Circulation

A. **Respiratory support.** Although both respiratory and cardiovascular support may be necessary, effective respiratory support is of prime concern, since circulatory depression usually responds to adequate oxygenation. A clear airway is essential. Fluid and secretions should be suctioned from the nose and pharynx, using a bulb syringe or a catheter with regulated wall suction. Thick tracheal secretions or meconium are best removed under direct vision (larynogoscope) with a catheter connected to a regulated wall suction. This procedure should be repeated as necessary to remove as much material from the airway as possible before applying positive-pressure ventilation. Positive-pressure ventilation with supplemental oxygen can be provided with either a bag and face mask or by endotracheal intubation; with either technique, a manometer to monitor ventilatory pressure is desirable. Oxygen should always be warmed and humidified.

1. **Bag and mask ventilation.** This technique is usually effective in mild to moderately depressed infants. The infant's head is extended slightly, and the mask is firmly applied over the nose and mouth with the thumb and first two fingers of the left hand to ensure a tight seal. The fourth and fifth fingers should support the chin. Insufflations are provided in-

Table 6.2. Equipment for Resuscitation

Suction apparatus
Oxygen (warmed, humidified)
Infant resuscitation bag, assorted masks
Laryngoscope with sizes 0 and 1 straight blades
Assorted endotracheal tubes (2.5, 3.0, 3.5, 4.0 mm)
Blankets, prewarmed
Radiant warmer, prewarmed
Umbilical vessel catheterization tray and catheters (3.5 and 5.0 mm)
Blood pressure apparatus (Doppler)
Syringes, needles, three-way stopcocks
Medications

Table 6.3. Medications for Resuscitation

DRUG (PREPARATION)	DOSAGE AND ROUTE	INDICATION
Naloxone (0.4 mg/mL solution)	0.1 mg/kg IV, IM, SQ, or endotracheally	Narcotic depression
Sodium bicarbonate 0.5 mEq/mL (4.2% solution)	2.0 mEq/kg IV slowly	Metabolic acidosis
Epinephrine (1 : 10 0000 solution)	0.1 mg/kg IV or by endotracheal tube	Bradycardia, asystole
Dextrose (10% solution)	2 mL/kg IV	Hypoglycemia
Albumin (5% solution)	10 mL/kg IV	Hypovolemia
Dopamine	5–20 μg/kg/min IV	Bradycardia hypotension

Source: Adapted from Bloom RS, Cropley C, Drew CR. Textbook of Neonatal Resuscitation. Elk Grove, IL: American Heart Association; 1990.

termittently by the right hand to achieve an inflating pressure that produces good chest excursions and satisfactory bilateral air exchange by auscultation. The mask technique is more difficult to apply to the premature infant with poorly compliant lungs. Failure to achieve prompt improvement (30 to 60 s) in heart rate and color necessitates endotracheal intubation. If prolonged (>2 min) bag and mask ventilation is necessary, an orogastric catheter (#8 F feeding tube) should be inserted to prevent abdominal distention.

2. **Endotracheal intubation** and ventilation with 100 percent oxygen at a rate of 40 to 60 breaths per min is necessary in severely depressed infants. A manometer connected to the ventilatory apparatus to measure the inflating pressure is recommended. High initial pressures may be necessary to overcome the critical opening pressure of collapsed alveoli. An initial pressure of 40 to 50 cm H_2O is sometimes necessary for premature infants with hyaline membrane disease, but a pressure of 20 to 30 cm H_2O may be adequate for term infants. Thereafter, lower pressures should suffice.

   a. **Indications for intubation**
      (1) Severely depressed infants with an initial heart rate of ≤ 60 beats per min
      (2) Moderately depressed infants failing to respond quickly to suctioning, stimulation, and bag and mask ventilation with 100 percent oxygen (the heart rate fails to rise promptly above 80 to 100 beats per min or declines in spite of apparently adequate bag and mask ventilatory support)

    (3) Infants with meconium aspiration

    (4) Suspected diaphragmatic hernia

    (5) Prolonged ventilatory support is necessary.

b. **Technique for intubation**

    (1) Select an endotracheal tube of appropriate size. The infant's weight is a useful guide (Table 6.4). In general, a 3.0- to 3.5-mm tube is suitable for the term infant and a 2.5-mm tube for smaller premature neonates. In any case, the tube should easily pass through the cords without forcing. Tissue injury may result from the use of too large a tube.

    (2) Position the infant in the supine position with the head midline. Since the larynx of the neonate is in a more anterior position relative to that of the older patient, a neutral position of the head, neither extended nor flexed, is usually preferable.

    (3) While steadying the head with the right hand, the laryngoscope is held in the left hand between the thumb and first two fingers; the remaining fingers support the chin. The tip of the blade is inserted at the right corner of the mouth and rotated to a vertical midline position, displacing the tongue and permitting visualization of the epiglottis. Under direct vision, the blade tip is advanced gently into the vallecula, the space between the epiglottis and the base of the tongue. In this position, slight elevation of the tip lifts the epiglottis anteriorly, exposing the glottis. If difficulty is encountered in visualizing the glottis at this point, slight pressure over the hyoid bone with the little finger of the left hand (or by an assistant) will depress the glottis clearly into view.

    (4) The endotracheal tube is inserted from the right corner of the mouth along the blade to keep the tip of the tube in view as it enters the cords. Do not pass the tube down the groove of the laryngoscope blade, as this obstructs visualization of the glottis. Once through the vocal cords, the endotracheal

Table 6.4. Guide for Endotracheal Tube Size

BIRTH WEIGHT (g)	TUBE SIZE (mm)
< 1000	2.5
1000–2000	2.5 or 3.0
2000–3000	3.0 or 3.5
> 3000	3.0–4.0

tube should be advanced approximately 1.5 to 2.0 cm. A black line near the tip of the tube (vocal cord guide) identifies the proper level of insertion on most endotracheal tubes currently available.

(5) Temporarily hold the tube in position with the fingers of the left hand. The ventilating bag should be quickly attached and the lungs inflated while observing for symmetric chest excursion and auscultating for symmetric breath sounds. Adjust the tube position if necessary and tape it in place.

B. Cardiovascular support

1. **External cardiac massage.** A heart rate < 60 beats per min or failure of the rate to increase above 100 beats per min within 30 to 60 s following adequate ventilation with 100 percent oxygen denotes a need for external cardiac massage. Two techniques are available:

   a. **Two-finger technique.** Compressions are applied at lower third of the sternum, using the tips of the index and middle fingers, with the infant lying on a firm surface.

   b. **Two-handed technique.** Both hands encircle the infant's thorax, the fingers providing back support, while the thumbs compress the lower third of the sternum.

   c. **In either technique, the sternum is depressed** 1.5 to 2.0 cm at a rate of approximately 120 beats per min. **Coordinated with lung inflation** is not required if ventilation is by means of an endotracheal tube. Effectiveness should be monitored by palpation of the femoral or carotid pulse or by blood pressure determination.

2. **Volume expansion.** Hypovolemia is not necessarily present in asphyxiated neonates, although circulatory responses to both asphyxia and hypovolemia may be similar (e.g., vasoconstriction, tachycardia, poor perfusion); asphyxial myocardial impairment may also be a major factor contributing to these clinical features in the absence of hypovolemia. Intrauterine asphyxia in fact may promote transfer of blood from the placenta to the fetus, resulting in hypervolemia. Acute volume expansion in the absence of hypovolemia can be hazardous, particularly in the premature infant (e.g., intracranial hemorrhage). Hemorrhage from the fetoplacental unit (placental abruption, fetomaternal hemorrhage) and cord compression (prolapse, nuchal cord) can cause hypovolemia, but clinical signs of shock in the neonate may not be apparent until 20 percent or more of the blood volume has been lost. For acute losses, volume replacement with whole blood is preferred; if anticipated, O-negative blood crossmatched against the mother's blood can be on hand in the delivery room. Alternatively, a 5% albumin solution, normal saline or Ringer's lactate solution, may be used; transfusion with packed red blood cells may be needed later to raise the hematocrit. Volume replace-

ment is best accomplished by repeated small transfusions (5 to 10 mL/kg), assessing the infant's response until blood pressure and perfusion appear adequate.

C. **Drugs.** Since most depressed infants will respond to adequate ventilation and oxygenation, drugs are usually reserved for those neonates not responding appropriately to established ventilatory support. Drugs should never be given in lieu of such support. The most accessible route for drug administration is the umbilical vein. Asphyxia produces combined respiratory and metabolic acidosis. The only correction for respiratory acidosis is adequate ventilation. Metabolic acidosis results from hypoxemia and/or hypoperfusion and usually responds to correction of these factors. However, drugs may be beneficial if metabolic acidosis, bradycardia, and poor perfusion persist in spite of adequate respiratory support, cardiac message, and correction of hypovolemia. Only a limited number of drugs are currently recommended for neonatal resuscitation: naloxone, epinephrine, sodium bicarbonate, and dopamine. Of these, epinephrine and naloxone may be administered also via the endotracheal tube. Atropine and calcium are no longer considered useful in the acute situation.

1. **Narcotic-induced depression.** A specific indication for the initial use of drugs is the administration of a narcotic antagonist to the depressed infant of a mother given narcotics within 4 h of delivery. Naloxone hydrochloride (Narcan), 0.1 mg/kg IV, IM, SQ, or endotracheally, is a rapidly effective narcotic antagonist with a high therapeutic:toxic ratio. Awareness of maternal narcotic drug use is important, since naloxone in such cases may precipitate acute narcotic withdrawal in the infant.

2. **Metabolic acidosis.** Administer sodium bicarbonate, 2 mEq/kg, at a rate not exceeding 1 mEq/kg/min. **Caution:** This is a hypertonic solution; rapid infusion may elevate serum osmolality, with the risk of intracranial hemorrhage, particularly in premature infants. Since bicarbonate ultimately generates CO_2, administration in the presence of respiratory acidosis and inadequate ventilation may actually aggravate the acidemia. Subsequent doses of bicarbonate should be guided by blood gas determinations.

3. **Bradycardia and low cardiac output**
   a. **Epinephrine hydrochloride:** 0.1 to 0.3 mL/kg of a 1:10 000 dilution is given IV or instilled per the endotracheal tube after dilution 1:1 with saline.
   b. **Dopamine** can be administered if poor perfusion and hypotension continue despite the administration of epinephrine and volume expansion. The initial dose is 5 μg/kg/min to a maximum of 20 μg/kg/min. The flow rate must be carefully regulated by an infusion pump, and frequent assessment of heart rate and blood pressure is essential.

4. **Hypoglycemia.** Dextrose (10%) 2.0 mL/kg IV, is given as a

bolus infusion. Because of the inefficient and rapid utilization of glycogen during anerobic metabolism, hypoglycemia commonly occurs in asphyxiated neonates, especially premature infants with their limited glycogen reserves. Hypoglycemia can cause impaired cardiac contractility as well as seizures. Bolus infusions of concentrated glucose solutions (25% or 50%) are not recommended because of their hyperosmolality and the related potential risk of intracranial hemorrhage.

D. Errors in resuscitation
  1. Intubation technique
     a. Incorrect positioning
     b. Blindly advancing the laryngoscope blade (usually into the esophagus)
     c. Using an endotracheal tube of an improper size
     d. Insertion of the endotracheal tube too far (into the bronchus)
     e. Using the blade groove as a guide for tube insertion (thus blocking the view of the glottis)
     f. Failure to clear the airway of secretions
  2. Excessive inflation pressure
  3. Failure to maintain body warmth
  4. Overuse of drugs
  5. A "wait and see" attitude in the presence of inadequate respirations and bradycardia
E. Complications of resuscitation. These complications include pneumomediastinum or pneumothorax from excessive inflation pressure; and injury to the heart, lungs, or liver by overly vigorous cardiac compressions. They are generally preventable.
F. Postresuscitation management. Generally, neonates requiring vigorous resuscitation should have continued close observation in a neonatal intensive care unit and should not be admitted to a well-baby nursery.
G. Resuscitation sequelae. Asphyxia can produce multisystem sequelae, including the following:
  1. **Central nervous system hypoxic-ischemic injury** can result in coma, convulsions, the syndrome of inappropriate antidiuretic hormone secretion, or other neurologic sequelae. Especially in premature infants, intracranial hemorrhage may be associated with asphyxia.
  2. **Acute renal failure** may be a manifestation of acute tubular necrosis or renal cortical necrosis; occasionally, renal vein thrombosis is a complication of asphyxia.
  3. **Pulmonary vasoconstriction** may lead to the syndrome of persistent pulmonary hypertension or persistent fetal circulation, characterized by high pulmonary vascular resistance (pulmonary hypertension), failure of ductal constriction, right-to-left shunting at the ductus and foramen ovale, reduced pulmonary blood flow, and hypoxemia without hypercarbia.

4. **Asphyxial myocardial dysfunction** may result in impaired cardiac output, hypotension, continuing metabolic acidosis, cardiomegaly, and murmurs of tricuspid and/or mitral valvular insufficiency. Myocardial dysfunction can be demonstrated by echocardiography.

5. **Hepatic damage,** indicated by hyperbilirubinemia and other evidence of hepatic dysfunction, may occur.

6. **Metabolic complications** are common and include hypoglycemia, especially in premature neonates who have limited glycogen reserves and are more likely to suffer severe cold stress. Hypocalcemia occurs in about one-third of asphyxiated infants and may contribute to seizures or myocardial dysfunction. Metabolic acidosis and impairment of renal function may result in hyperkalemia.

BIBLIOGRAPHY

ACOG Technical Bulletin. Fetal and Neonatal Neurologic Injury. No. 163, January 1992.

American Academy of Pediatrics, Committee on Fetus and Newborn. Use and abuse of the Apgar score. Pediatrics 1986; 78:1148–1149.

Avery GB (ed). Neonatology: Pathology and Management of the Newborn. 3rd ed. Philadelphia: JB Lippincott; 1987.

Chameides L (ed). Textbook of Neonatal Resuscitation. Elk Grove Village, IL: American Heart Association/American Academy of Pediatrics; 1990.

Dijxhoorn MJ, Visser GHA, Fidler VJ, et al. Apgar score, meconium and acidaemia at birth in relation to neonatal neurologic morbidity in term infants. Br J Obstet Gynaecol 1986; 93:217–222.

Fanaroff AA, Martin RJ, eds. Neonatal–Perinatal Medicine: Diseases of the Fetus and Infant. 5th ed. St. Louis: Mosby Year Book; 1992.

Freeman RK, Poland RL (eds). Guidelines for Perinatal Care. 3rd ed. Elk Grove Village, IL and Washington, DC: American Academy of Pediatrics/American College of Obstetricians and Gynecologists; 1992.

Peter G, ed. Prevention of neonatal ophthalmia. Report of the Committee on Infections Diseases. 22nd ed. Elk Grove Village, IL: American Academy of Pediatrics; 1991.

Schoen EJ. The status of circumcision of newborns. N Engl J Med 1990; 322:1308–1312.

Taeusch HW, Ballard RA, Avery ME (eds). Diseases of the Newborn. 6th ed. Philadelphia: WB Saunders, 1991.

CHAPTER 7

The Puerperium

Sharon T. Phelan

I. **Definition.** Puerperium includes the first 6 weeks postpartum. By this time, the maternal physiology and anatomy have returned to their nonpregnant state. This includes the pituitary-ovarian axis in non-breast-feeding women.

II. **Physiology**
   A. **Cardiopulmonary.** There is an immediate *autotransfusion* after delivery of 500 to 750 mL of blood. This, along with the mobilization of extracellular fluid, can place a large load on the cardiac system for the first 2 weeks postpartum.
   B. **Renal**
      1. Anatomically, the ureteral dilation in an upright film resolves within a few days, but it may take up to 6 weeks to resolve on a supine film. Up to 11 percent of women may have persistent ureteral dilation postpartum. There may also be a persistent postvoid residual due to cystocele.
      2. Functionally, the kidneys are normal by 6 weeks, but the rate of recovery is variable. Thus, drugs with renal excretion should be given in decreasing doses during this time.
   C. **Reproductive**
      1. **Uterus.** The uterus involutes over the initial 6 weeks, changing from a 1-kg organ with a volume of over 5000 mL to a 60-g structure with a capacity of 5 mL. This decrease in size is due to autolysis of intracellular protein, causing a decrease in cell size but not in cell number. Over the first 7 to 10 days, the remaining decidua is sloughed. By the 16th to 18th day, a normal endometrium should be restored.
      2. **Cervix.** Within 2 weeks, the os is reduced to < 1 cm.
      3. **Hypothalamic–Pituitary–Ovarian Axis.** The period of postpartum amenorrhea is variable, with breast-feeding having the largest impact. In the non-breast-feeding woman, the first menses typically occurs at 55 to 60 days (range, 20 to 120 days), with over 75 percent of the initial menses being ovulatory. Ovulation rarely occurs prior to 45 days postpartum. In the exclusively breast-feeding woman, ovulation is commonly delayed until 84+ days postpartum.
      4. **Breasts** (see Chapter 8)

III. Clinical care

    A. Uterine involution

        1. The uterus should remain firm and demonstrate involution over the first few days postpartum. In multiparous women, the uterus will contract vigorously, causing pains that are known as *after pains*. These pains are triggered by breast-feeding with oxytocin release. They can be very uncomfortable for 48 to 72 h postpartum.

        2. Lochia generally represents shedding of the decidua and blood from the uterine cavity. Classically, there are three phases:

            a. Lochia rubra — a red, bloody discharge that typically lasts for 2 to 3 days. If it lasts for 2 weeks or longer, it may represent retained products, incomplete involution, and/or infection.

            b. Lochia serosa — a paler discharge from day 3 up to 10 days postpartum.

            c. Lochia alba — a white to yellow-white discharge, scanty in amount and containing numerous leukocytes.

        3. Intermittent uterine massage in the first 12 to 24 h after delivery may assist in promoting uterine contractions and allows evaluation for uterine atony.

    B. Perineal care. If there is no episiotomy or lacerations, simple cleansing after voiding or defecating is all that is required. If episiotomy or laceration occurred, care should include sitz baths two to three times a day for up to 1 week, cleansing after voiding or defecating, and inspection of the site at least daily during the hospital stay for hematoma formation, breakdown of repair, or infection (see Section IV.B).

    C. Breasts. Women often experience engorgement 24 to 72 h after delivery. In the non-breast-feeding woman, this condition can be treated with aspirin, ice packs, and the use of a tight supporting bra (see Chapter 8).

    D. Urinary tract. Due to edema around the urethra, a woman may have difficulty voiding postpartum. This problem can be compounded by regional anesthesia or a painful perineum from an episiotomy or lacerations. The patient should be monitored for retention and catheterization as needed. If catheterization is required more than twice, consider placing an indwelling catheter for 1 or 2 days. Also, evaluate for hematoma as a possible cause. A puerperal diuresis will occur usually from the second to the fifth day postpartum, with a loss of up to 2 L of fluid.

    E. Bowels. The use of narcotic analgesics may cause constipation. In addition, the perineal discomfort from a laceration or episiotomy may prompt a woman to delay defecating voluntarily. This rarely poses a problem except when a third-degree or greater midline episiotomy or laceration is present. In this situation, the stools must be kept soft with diet and medications.

    F. Immunizations

        1. If a woman has a nonimmune rubella status, vaccinate her postpartum.

      2. If the mother is Rh− (and Du−) and the infant is Rh+, give the mother RhoGAM.

      3. If the mother is HbsAg positive, the fetus must be immunized prior to discharge.

  G. **Discharge.** The timing of discharge has changed dramatically. Although for the past two decades it has been traditional to discharge women on the third postpartum day (for a vaginal delivery), economic pressures are prompting discharge at 24 h when the woman has had an uncomplicated vaginal delivery.

  H. **Diet.** The woman should be allowed to eat as soon as her appetite returns, although some recommend a delay of 2 h postpartum to make sure that there is no complication that requires anesthetic intervention (e.g., hemorrhage, inversion). At discharge, it is common to encourage the use of iron supplementation for 1 or 2 months and prenatal vitamins, especially if the woman is breast-feeding.

  I. **Activities.** Since the 1950s, progressively earlier ambulation has been encouraged, with women now up and walking (initially with assistance) within hours of a delivery. Resumption of normal activities at home should be encouraged, but most physicians recommend a 4- to 6-week maternity leave from employment or school. Part of the reason is to avoid physically taxing the mother, but the main purpose is to allow the mother to focus on the needs of her new infant. In the absence of extensive perineal lacerations or incisions, or excessive vaginal bleeding, coitus can resume in 2 or 3 weeks.

  J. **Follow-up clinic visits.** Traditionally, these visits occur 4 to 6 weeks postpartum. At the visit, the practitioner should assess for uterine involution, evidence of infection, breast status (especially if the woman is breast-feeding), and healing of any lacerations or episiotomy. At this time, it is common to obtain a Pap smear. One should also inquire about how well the mother is coping with the new baby (especially if it is the first), success in breast-feeding, difficulties with coitus, and comfort with the chosen contraceptive method.

IV. Complications

  A. **Delayed uterine bleeding.** Uterine bleeding occurring more than 48 h after delivery has a different group of differential diagnoses than a more acute bleed. One must consider retained products of conception that may be infected, endomyometritis (Chapter 25), placental site sloughing, and coagulation defects. Evaluation requires a complete blood count, cervical cultures for gonococcus and chlamydia, platelet count, prothrombin time, partial thromboplastin time, and possibly an ultrasound exam. Treatments such as antibiotics, methergine, and curettage are directed to the cause of the bleed. Rarely is this condition life-threatening, but in the rare cases of significant hemorrhage at 2 to 4 weeks postpartum, when other causes have been eliminated, the bleed may be a placental site slough. This can be resistant to curettage or methergine and requires uterine packing.

B. **Episiotomy**
1. **Hematoma.** This can occur if hemostatis is not adequately obtained prior to closure. These hematomas may become infected. It is best to evacuate any large, growing, or infected hematoma.
2. **Dehiscence.** Superficial dehiscence is usually due to infection or trauma such as early coitus. It can be managed by resuturing once there is healthy granulation tissue or by allowing healing by secondary intent. Deep breakdown (third or fourth degree) is due most commonly to infection or a large hematoma. There is no consensus as to the best management. A detailed review of the literature is included in an article by Owen and Hauth (see the Bibliography). Secondary suturing after the development of good granulation tissue appears to be the favored approach.
3. **Infection.** Episiotomy infection has a reported incidence of 0.05 to 3.0 percent. Shy and Eschenbach (see the Bibliography) divided episiotomy infections into the following four types:
   a. Simple infection is limited to the skin and superficial fascia along the incision line. No systemic symptoms should be present. Often broad-spectrum antibiotics will suffice. If the infection does not respond to antibiotics within 24 to 48 h, the episiotomy needs to be opened and debrided.
   b. Superficial fascial infection involves rudor and edema of the skin. Mild systemic symptoms may occur. Treatment is the same as for simple infection.
   c. Superficial fascial necrosis (necrotizing fasciitis) includes destruction of the superficial fascial layers. Overlying skin shows edema and eventually a gray discoloration, bulla, and ulceration as the superficial blood vessels thrombose. Eventually anesthesia may result from nerve necrosis. Treatment necessitates extensive, aggressive debridement until tissue is reached that bleeds, aggressive fluid management, cardiovascular monitoring, and broad-spectrum parenteral antibiotics. Without early recognition and aggressive management, maternal death can occur.
   d. Myonecrosis involves frank destruction of muscle tissue deeper than the superficial fascial layer. Treatment is the same as for superficial fascial necrosis.

C. **Mastitis** is a more delayed complication occurring after the patient has gone home. The patient returns with fever, a warm, tender breast, and often systemic symptoms. These need to be treated aggressively with oral antibiotics, continued drainage of milk by nursing or pumping, and surgical drainage of the abscess. Detailed are presented in Chapter 8.

D. **Urinary complications.** As previously mentioned, periurethral and trigone edema from blunt trauma and lacerations may cause dysfunction with resulting retention. This usually resolves within a few hours but may require an indwelling catheter for a few days. The use of a catheter, especially when there is inadequate emptying, may result in a urinary tract infection. This needs to be considered in the differential diagnosis of postpartum fever.

E. **Bowel complications.** The primary bowel complication is related to problems with fourth-degree episiotomy. (see Section IV.B for details).

F. **Deep venous thrombosis.** Due to the venous stasis occurring in pregnancy and the hypercoagulable state due to the estrogen effect on the liver, women are at an increased risk for deep venous thrombosis. Early ambulation and delay in oral contraceptive pill use until 2 or more weeks postpartum have decreased the occurrence of this complication. Assessment of the lower extremities for tenderness and increased warmth should be included in the routine postpartum assessment. In addition, any pelvic infection that does not clear with aggressive antibiotic therapy should prompt consideration of septic pelvic thrombophlebitis.

V. Postpartum contraception

A. **Resumption of ovulation** is variable, with the most important factor being breast-feeding. In the non-breast-feeding woman, ovulation can occur by 40 to 50 days postpartum. In the breast-feeding woman it is usually delayed until 70 to 80 days or longer. The first spontaneous menses in a breast-feeding woman is usually ovulatory.

B. **Barrier methods** (e.g., diaphragm, cervical cap) are not appropriate until approximately 6 weeks postpartum. At that time, the sizing should be verified.

C. **Spermicides and condoms** can be used as soon as coitus is initiated. Since many women, especially breast-feeding women, will have inadequate vaginal lubrication in the early puerperium, a spermicide is often very helpful.

D. **Intrauterine device (IUD).** Since the only IUDs currently available in the United States are chemically active (ParaGard and Progestesert), the primary reason for delaying insertion until complete involution occurs is to minimize the risk of malposition or expulsion. Traditionally, these IUDs can be inserted easily at 6 weeks postpartum.

E. **Oral contraceptive pills (OCPs).** Although the current low-dose pills have minimal thromboembolic risks, it is theoretically possible that these may precipitate a deep venous thrombosis during the heightened risk period (the first 2 weeks postpartum). Since the risk of pregnancy is very small until several weeks later, most women delay initiating OCP use until 2 to 4 weeks postpartum. The breast-feeding woman can initiate OCP use once lactation is well established (2 to 4 weeks postpartum).

F. Norplant. This subdermal mode of contraception has recently received U.S. Food and Drug Administration approval. Because of concern about interference with the quality or quantity of breast milk, the recommendation is to insert it 6 weeks postpartum in lactating women. Since the majority of the clinical trials were conducted in populations with a high percentage of breast-feeding, the Wyeth Pharmaceutical Company, which developed Norplant, has insufficient data regarding its insertion in the immediate postpartum period (1 to 3 days) for the nonlactating woman. At this time, Wyeth can neither encourage or discourage immediate postpartum placement. The primary theoretical concern is interference with involution, resulting in more postpartum bleeding.

G. Sterilization. Tubal sterilization is an increasingly popular form of contraception. Due to uterine enlargement, it is very easy to do an infraumbilical incision within the first 1 to 2 days postpartum. Prior to performing tubal sterilization, the physician should have evidence of patient counseling and of the patient's desire for the operation earlier in pregnancy. In fact, for procedures that are paid for with federal funds, a consent must be signed 30 days in advance of the procedure. One should be certain that this is a well-thought-out decision and not a potentially irrational response to an acute situation (e.g., a teenage pregnancy, divorce, a complicated pregnancy, or one with a bad outcome). Some physicians require the patient to be a certain age at the time of consent (e.g., age 21 for patients receiving federal support). The status of the infant should be ascertained. If it is unstable, interval tubal sterilization should be considered. The timing of tubal sterilization is traditionally 24 to 48 h postpartum. This allows evaluation of the newborn as well as stabilization of the mother. However, given the press of economics, in the stable, well-informed patient who has had an uncomplicated vaginal delivery under epidural anesthesia, tubal sterilization immediately after delivery is an option.

BIBLIOGRAPHY

Hankins GV, Hauth JC, Gilstrap LC, et al. Early repair of episiotomy dehiscence. Obstet Gynecol 1990; 75:48–51.

Owen J, Hauth JC. Episiotomy infection and dehiscence. In: Gilstrap LC, Faro S, eds. Infections in Pregnancy. New York: Alan R. Liss; 1990:61–74.

Rivera RR, Barrera M, Kennedy KI, et al. Breast-feeding and the return to ovulation in Durango, Mexico. Fertil Steril 1988; 49:780–787.

Shiono P, Klebanoff MA, Carey JC. Midline episiotomies: More harm than good? Obstet Gynecol 1990; 75:765–770.

Shy KK, Eschenback DA. Fatal perineal cellulitis from an episiotomy site. Obstet Gynecol 1979; 54:294–298.

CHAPTER 8

Lactation and Lactation Suppression

Truus Delfos-Broner
Nancee Neel
Sharon T. Phelan

The enthusiasm of the physician can influence the initial and continued success of breast-feeding mother. If the physician provides knowledgeable medical and psychological support, the desire to succeed increases. His or her comfort with the decision of the patient to breast-feed is directly related to the information provided. Not all physicians are informed about current knowledge on human lactation, nor do they provide the patient with local groups (e.g., LaLeche League contacts). Nevertheless, the physician can still be the most important link to successful breast-feeding.

The American Academy of Pediatrics has called breast-feeding the most appropriate method of feeding for infants. Further, perinatal guidelines of the American College of Obstetricians and Gynecologists state that breast-feeding alone provides the appropriate nutrition for most infants for the first 4 to 6 months of life. The American College of Nurse-Midwives actively supports breast-feeding as the best method of infant feeding.

I. Physiology of lactation

    A. During pregnancy the woman's breasts, body, and psyche are prepared for lactation, and at birth the human newborn is prepared to nurse at the breast.

    B. Three physiologic stages are involved in lactation.

        1. Mammary growth begins embryonically and culminates during pregnancy. A complex interaction of hormones affects breast development, causing breast growth, ductal growth, and globular formation. The initial development is at puberty, when increasing estrogen levels increase the size and pigmentation of the areola and stimulate growth of the ductal portion of the gland. The progesterone present influences the growth of the alveolar component. During pregnancy, the combination of estrogens with growth hormone, prolactin, and adrenal steroids results in proliferation of epithelial cells and alveolar development.

        2. Lactogenesis, the beginning of milk secretion, is initiated during pregnancy, with an increase at the time of birth. Particular hormones involved in lactogenesis include oxytocin and prolactin in the absence of estrogen and progesterone. When the infant suckles the breast, mechanoreceptors in the nipple and areola stimulate the posterior pituitary to release oxytocin. This oxytocin stimulates myoepithelial cells to contract, leading to milk ejection from the alveoli in the breast. Prolactin is secreted by the anterior pituitary in response to suckling and stimulates the production of milk in the alveoli.

3. Galactopoiesis, the maintenance of established lactation, begins a few days postpartum and continues as long as there is a stimulus. Galactopoiesis occurs through the same activation of hormonal pathways by the infant's suckling as occurs in lactogenesis.

C. Human milk is species specific for human infants and therefore is the perfect nutrient. Breast milk meets the protein, calorie, and fat requirements of the infant, and is easily and efficiently digested.

D. Breast milk contains a wide variety of agents active against bacteria and viruses. Factors with in vitro antibacterial properties identified in human milk include *Lactobacillus bifidus* growth factor, secretory IgA, lactoferrin, lactoperoxidase, lysozyme, lipids, and milk cells. Secretory IgA, lipids, nonimmunoglobulin macromolecules, and milk cells also have antiviral effects in vitro. Further, breast milk may play a role in preventing early childhood allergies.

II. Breast-feeding techniques

A. **Diet for successful lactation.** The two most important components in the mother's diet that can affect her milk production are fluids and calories. Insufficient intake of either will decrease milk volume, but milk quality generally remains unaffected. Energy requirements for lactation depend on the the amount of milk produced. Maternal fat stores of 2 kg laid down during a normal pregnancy provide 200 to 300 kcal per day for the first 3 months of milk production. This amounts to one-third of the cost of producing 850 mL of milk each day. The remaining calories must be supplied by increased food intake. The Food and Nutrition Board of the National Research Council recommends that a nursing mother increase her energy intake by 500 calories per day for the first 3 months of lactation.

B. **Nipple care.** Wash the nipples with water only. Expose the nipples to air for 15 to 20 min after each feeding. Additional heat from either sunshine or a 25-watt light bulb may be helpful. After exposure, a water-based cream such as lanolin or vitamin A and D ointment may be applied.

C. **Initiating nursing.** Successful lactation depends on learned feeding techniques, not on instinct. An unstressful emotional environment is essential in this period of adaptation, since anxiety in the mother inhibits oxytocin release and milk letdown.

Breast-feeding should begin as soon as possible after delivery and should occur frequently and on demand, usually every 2 to 3 h.

D. Let-down reflex. A cycle of events, initiated by infant sucking and triggered by the release of oxytocin, leads to milk availability. Poor let-down or absence of it is most often caused by maternal stress or anxiety. Reinforcing her ability to breast-feed successfully can be done by assistance from a lactation consultant or nurse experienced with or supportive of breast-feeding. A trial of synthetic oxytocin, available as a nasal spray, is very useful in some women.

E. Milk supply maintenance. The amount of milk available to the infant depends on several factors:

    a. Supply and demand (the milk supply is best stimulated by suckling). The more frequently the infant nurses, the faster and larger the supply of milk.

    b. No missed feedings. Nighttime feedings should not be skipped in a misguided concern for the mother's rest.

    c. Minimize supplementary feedings, especially the first few weeks after delivery.

    d. Rotation of breasts as starting and ending breasts to provide for complete emptying of both breasts.

    e. Relaxation and comfort of the mother, with a supportive environment.

    f. Proper positioning of the baby on the breast.

F. Positioning. The mother's position during a feeding can vary as long as the infant has access to the breasts. She may be on her side or sit upright, in a position that will be comfortable for about 20 min. The baby should be positioned so that he or she will not be doubled up or have a twisted neck when sucking and so that the head and body are supported (Fig. 8.1).

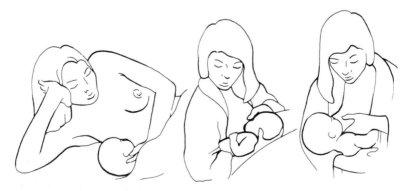

FIGURE 8.1. Common positions used for breast-feeding.

III. Potential problems

A. Nipple soreness.
Sore nipples can be a problem for some women. Mothers need to know that this is a self-limiting problem that usually improves rapidly, provided that the infant is properly positioned for nursing.

1. Measures that will help sore nipples include:
   a. Exposing the nipples to air for 15 to 20 min following each feeding.
   b. Light applications of lanolin or vitamin A and D ointment or cream.
   c. Prevention of engorgement with short, frequent feedings (every 2 to 3 h) and hand expression to initiate flow of milk.
   d. Position change with each feeding.
   e. Application of ice to the breast in case of cracked nipples and application of ice to the affected area may be helpful.
   f. Manual expression. In rare cases, soreness may be so severe that nursing is impossible, and manual expression by hand pump may be necessary until the nipples heal.
2. Reassurance that in most cases sore nipples respond to exposure to air, short, frequent nursings, and support to continue breast-feeding are important.

B. Engorgement
1. This is usually caused by a blocked excretory duct, with a swollen, tender, firm breast segment.
2. It is differentiated from mastitis by lack of signs of infection; there are no fever and chills and no focal redness in the affected breast (Table 8.1).
3. Recommended treatment is continued nursing (or expression of milk by breast pump or manually), application of hot compresses locally, a hot shower or prone soaking in hot water to help relieve the obstruction, and maternal rest.

C. Mastitis
1. This problem occurs in 2 to 3 percent of nursing women as the result of pathogenic bacteria from the infant's mouth or the mother's skin entering breast tissue through a cracked or possibly normal nipple.
2. The most common pathogen is *Staphylococcus aureus* (cultured in about 50 percent of cases). Other common pathogens are beta-hemolytic streptococci, *Hemophilus influenzae*, *H. parainfluenza*, *Escherichia coli*, and *Klebsiella pneunomiae*.
3. Clinical signs include chills and flulike aching, temperatures of 38.8°C to 40°C, and focal redness in the affected breast.
4. Treatment is with dicloxacillin, 250 mg q.i.d., for at least 1 week. In patients allergic to penicillin, use cephalothin, 250 mg q.i.d., or clindamycin, 300 mg q.i.d. In addition to

Table 8.1. Comparison of Findings of Engorgement, Plugged Duct, and Mastitis

CHARAC- TERISTICS	ENGORGEMENT	PLUGGED DUCT	MASTITIS
Onset	Gradual, im- mediately post- partum	Gradual, after feedings	Sudden, after 10 days
Site	Bilateral	Unilateral	Usually unilateral
Swelling and heat	Generalized	May shift/little or no heat	Localized, red, hot, and swollen
Pain	Generalized	Mild but local- ized	Intense but localized
Body temperature	$< 38.4°C$	$< 38.4°C$	$> 38.4°C$
Systemic symp- toms	Feels well	Feels well	Flulike sym- ptoms

Source: Lawrence RA. Breastfeeding: A Guide for the Medical Profession. 3rd ed. St. Louis: CV Mosby; 1989:596. Reproduced by permission of Mosby-Year Books, Inc.

            antibiotics, treatment should include measures recommended for engorgement.

5.   Nursing should be continued to prevent breast engorgement. Cessation of nursing increases the risk of prolonged infection and abscess formation. Finally, no ill effects are seen in infants who continue to nurse.

D. **Pharmacologic agents in lactation**

1.   Treatment of the lactating woman for a medical illness must consider both the mother and the child. Several questions must be answered: (a) Is drug therapy really necessary? (b) What is the safest drug that can be successfully used? (c) In long-term maternal therapy, where there is the possibility that the drug may present a problem for the infant, should the infant's blood level of the drug be measured? (d) Can the mother take the prescribed medication just after completion of breast-feeding to minimize drug exposure of the infant? (Table 8.2).

2.   In 1989 the American Academy of Pediatrics published a comprehensive list of drugs transferred in human milk. In this publication, drugs were listed in seven separate groupings, depending on their impact on the neonate. Tables 8.3 and 8.4 list the drugs that are contraindicated during breast-feeding.

Table 8.2. Drugs with Zero or Negligible Oral Bioavailability

ANTIMICROBIALS	OTHERS
Amikacin	ACTH
Amphotericin B	Epinephrine
Carbenicillin	Heparin
Cefamandole	Insulin
Cefazolin	Trimethaphan
Cefonicid	Vasopressin
Cefoperazone	
Cefoxitin	
Ceftizoxime	
Cephalothin	
Cisplatin	
Doxorubicin	
Gentamycin	
Kanamycin	
Methicillin	
Moxalactam	
Neomycin	
Streptomycin	
Tricarcillin	

Some of these drugs were documented to be excreted into breast milk, but should not pose any risk to the infant because of lack of oral bioavailability.

Source: Rivera-Calimlin L. The significance of drugs in breast milk. Clin Perinatol 1987; 14:57.

E.   Infection

   1.   Human immunodeficiency virus (HIV)

      a.   Although the extent of transmission of the virus through breast milk is unclear, HIV has been isolated in breast milk from infected women, and several reports implicate breast-feeding as a mode for vertical transmission.

      b.   The U.S. Public Health Service currently recommends that women who are HIV positive not breast-feed.

   2.   Hepatitis B

      a.   Although the hepatitis B virus has been isolated in breast milk, studies in England and Taiwan do not show that hepatitis B surface antigen (HbsAg)-positive breast-feeding mothers increase the risk of hepatitis B infection in their infants.

      b.   Infants of mothers known to be HbsAg positive at delivery should receive hepatitis B immune globulin (HBIG), 0.5 mL IM, and human hepatitis vaccine immediately after birth. Human hepatitis vaccine should be repeated at 1 and 6 months of age.

      c.   If the infant receives immune globulin and hepatitis vaccine as recommended, breast-feeding can occur without harm to the infant.

Table 8.3. Drugs That Are Contraindicated During Breast-Feeding

DRUG	REPORTED SIGN OR SYMPTOM IN INFANT OR EFFECT ON LACTATION
Bromocriptine	Suppresses lactation
Cocaine	Cocaine intoxication
Cyclophosphamide	Possible immune suppression; unknown effect on growth or association with carcinogenesis; neutropenia
Cyclosporine	Possible immune suppression; unknown effect on growth or association with carcinogenesis
Doxorubicin*	Possible immune suppression; unknown effect on growth or association with carcinogenesis
Ergotamine	Vomiting, diarrhea, convulsions (doses used in migraine medications)
Lithium	⅓ to ½ therapeutic blood concentration in infants
Methotrexate	Possible immune suppression; unknown effect on growth or association with carcinogenesis; neutropenia
Phencyclidine (PCP)	Potent hallucinogen
Phenindione	Anticoagulant; increased prothrombin and partial thromboplastin time in 1 infant (not used in USA)

*Drug is concentrated in human milk.

Source: Committee on Drugs, 1988–1989. Transfer of drugs and other chemicals into human milk. Pediatrics 1989; 84(5):925. Reproduced by permission of Pediatrics.

    d.   If hepatitis B is diagnosed in the mother weeks or months postpartum, the baby should receive immune globulin and hepatitis vaccine, and breast-feeding can continue.

3. Herpes simplex virus
    a.   It is not necessary to separate the breast-feeding infant from the mother, but rather from the mother's lesions. Thus, if lesions are present on the breast, the baby should not breast-feed.

4. Varicella zoster virus
    a.   Infants whose mothers develop chickenpox within 5 days before delivery or within 48 h after delivery are given varicella zoster immune globulin.
    b.   Antibodies appear in the milk within 48 h of disease onset in the mother, so breast-feeding can continue.

IV. Working mothers. Common concerns of mothers returning to work and planning to continue breast-feeding involve expression of breast milk and storage of expressed milk.

  A. Breast pumping
    1.   Milk is most easily and completely expressed using a handheld or electric pump. Hand-held pumps are inexpensive and easy to carry. The schedule for pumping of breast milk at

Table 8.4. Drugs of Abuse That Are Contraindicated During Breast-Feeding*

DRUG	EFFECT
Amphetamine	Irritability, poor sleep pattern
Cocaine	Cocaine intoxication
Heroin	
Marijuana	Only one report in literature; no effect mentioned
Nicotine (smoking)	Shock, vomiting, diarrhea, rapid heart rate, restlessness; decreased milk production
Phencyclidine	Potent hallucinogen

*The Committee on Drugs believes strongly that nursing mothers should not ingest any of these compounds. Not only are they hazardous to the nursing infant but they are detrimental to the physical and emotional health of the mother.

Source: Committee on Drugs, 1988–1989. Transfer of drugs and other chemicals into human milk. Pediatrics 1989; 84(5):925. Reproduced by permission of Pediatrics.

    work should be similar to the feeding schedule the mother and infant have established.
2. Relaxation and drinking of liquids aid let-down and successful milk expression. A quiet, private room at work should be used, if available.
3. Each breast should be completely emptied at each pumping.

B. **Milk collection and storage**
1. Containers used for collecting and storing milk should be sterile.
2. Breast milk can be safely stored in a refrigerator for 24 to 48 h. When breast milk is expressed at work, it should be refrigerated until the woman goes home.
3. If breast milk is not to be fed within 48 h, it should be frozen as soon as possible. Each freezer container should be labeled with the date and filled about three-fourths full to allow for expansion.
4. Breast milk may be frozen for up to several months if the freezer temperature is consistent.
5. Frozen milk should be thawed under lukewarm water. Thawed milk should be fed right away or refrigerated and fed within 3 h.
6. Breast milk should not be refrozen. A microwave oven should not be used to thaw or warm breast milk.

V. **Psychological issues related to breast-feeding.** Benefits associated with breast-feeding are numerous; the health benefits for the infant were discussed earlier in this chapter. Another important benefit of breast-feeding is the reduced cost. The minimum amount of money necessary for artificial feeding is more than the minimum amount needed to purchase extra food to supplement lactation. This fact is especially significant in low-income groups. It is not necessary for lactating mothers to eat expensive foods to produce an adequate milk supply. Since breast-fed babies are less prone to infections, medical care costs may also be reduced.

Convenience is also a significant factor for new mothers to consider. While breast-feeding, no extra time is spent preparing and buying artificial milk or washing feeding equipment. The breast-feeding mother can travel with the baby and is always sure of a milk supply, as well as the right time, place, and amount. Once a feeding pattern is established, the mother can take some time away from her baby while her infant is bottle-fed with breast milk. Another benefit — the most difficult one to measure — is the emotional bond between mother and child. In unrestricted breast-feeding, the breast not only satisfies hunger, but also relieves many other discomforts and fears. The psychophysiologic experience of breast-feeding is expressed in phrases such as "emotionally charged" and "a precious and unique relationship." The psychological communication between mother and child is often filled with a sense of trust of well-being, comfort, and rest.

VI. **Weaning/suppression.** The process of weaning the human infant is defined by the transfer of the infant from dependence on the mother's milk to other sources of nourishment. The appropriate time for this to take place depends on the age and nutritional needs of the infant and the needs of the mother.

   A. **Suppression.** Women who decide not to breast-feed currently have certain options to prevent lactation. Lactation suppression can be obtained either by nonpharmaceutical (natural) means or by the use of drugs.

   1. **Natural suppression.** The natural method requires patience and a binder. Many products can function as a binder: a draw/regular sheet, a bath towel, or any strip of absorbent material. The term *Breast binder* is a misnomer since the product does not bind, but rather firmly supports and lifts the breasts up and in. The patient must be instructed *not* to milk breasts. Ice packs and analgesics, such as aspirin or acetaminophen, will help with the 1 to 3 days of discomfort.

   2. **Pharmaceutical suppression.** In the last few years, lactation suppressants have become more popular.

      a. Initially, hormonal substances (Deladumone, Tace) were used, with an increased risk of thromboembolic disease. Side effects included nausea, flushing and headaches, rebound breast congestion, engorgement, and secretion.

      b. Bromocriptine, an ergot alkaloid, has recently been demonstrated to be effective for lactation suppression. Bromocriptine is a dopamine receptor agonist, and thus suppresses prolactin release by the anterior pituitary. Bromocriptine mesylate, 2.5 μg b.i.d. with meals for 14 days, should be initiated within 8 h after a vaginal delivery or as soon as oral intake is tolerated after an operative delivery. If rebound engorgement and/or secretions occur, an additional 7-day treatment may be needed. The nonpharmaceutical approach can be used in conjunction with the medication. Bromocriptine has been associated with a severe form of postpartum hypertension, so it should not be used in patients who had hypertension complicate their pregnancy. In addition, it may be wise to record a blood pressure 1 to 2 days after initiating therapy. Given the cost, occurrence of rebound, and potential risks, many practices use the pharmaceutical suppression only in extreme cases (a term stillbirth) and use binders for the remainder of their nonbreast-feeding patients.

B. Weaning is done by gradually eliminating alternate feedings and providing a bottle or cup. This prevents or minimizes physical engorgement for the woman.

BIBLIOGRAPHY

Committee on Infectious Disease Report. 20th ed. Elk Grove Village, IL: American Academy of Pediatrics; 1986.

Common problems of initiating breastfeeding. The physician's role in encouraging success for the "nursing couple." Postgrad Med 1987; 82(6):159–167.

Duchesne C, Lake R. Bromocriptine mesylate for prevention of postpartum lactation. Obstet Gynecol 1981; 57(4):464–467.

Guidelines for Perinatal Care. Washington, DC: American College of Obstetricians and Gynecologists; 1992.

Hager WD. Puerperal mastitis. Contemp Ob/Gyn 1989; 33:27–31.

Lawrence R. Breastfeeding, A Guide for the Medical Profession. 2nd ed. St Louis: CV Mosby; 1985.

Lawrence RA. Breastfeeding and medical disease. Med Clin North Am 1989; 73:583–603.

Lifson AR. Do alternate modes for transmission of human immunodeficiency virus exist? JAMA 1988; 259:1353–1356.

Lissauer T. Impact of AIDS on neonatal care. Arch Dis Child 1989; 64:4–7.

Michel FB, Bousquet J, Dannaeus A, et al. Preventive measures in early childhood allergy. J Allergy Clin Immunol 1986; 78:1022–1027.

Niebyl JR. When the nursing mother has mastitis. Contemp Ob/Gyn 1985; 26:31–32.

Roberts RJ, Blumer JL, Gorman RL, et al. Transfer of drugs and other chemicals into human milk. Pediatrics 1989; 84:924–936.

Valman HB. Jaundice in the newborn. BMJ 1989; 299:1272–1274.

Varney H. Nurse Midwifery. 2nd ed. Boston: Blackwell Scientific; 1987.

Welsh JK, May JT. Anti-infective properties of breast milk. J Pediatr 1979; 94:672–675.

Part II

Obstetric Intervention

CHAPTER 9

Obstetric Analgesia and Anesthesia

Michael N. Skaredoff

GENERAL CONSIDERATIONS

All anesthetics may cause neurologic, pulmonary, or cardiovascular compromise. In general, **no anesthetic should ever be administered in the absence of**:

1. Personnel trained in anesthesia and its complications; certain regional blocks that are traditionally performed by the obstetrician alone are the exception to the rule.
2. Modern anesthesia equipment equal in quality to that used in the operating room.
3. Resuscitation equipment and drugs as required for management of possible anesthetic complications. Table 9.1 lists the necessary drugs and equipment. It is, therefore, incumbent on the physician to have resuscitative skills and have **at hand or within easy reach** those drugs and materials needed to manage complications resulting from either the local anesthetic used or the nerve block itself.

I. **Physiologic changes during pregnancy.** The pregnant female is different from the nonpregnant one. During pregnancy, significant physiologic changes occur in almost every organ system. Of particular note are the changes in the cardiovascular, pulmonary, gastrointestinal, endocrine, and renal systems.

   A. **Cardiovascular changes.** During gestation cardiac output increases by about 50 percent. This is due to:

      1. Decrease in systemic vascular resistance secondary to placental hormone effects.
      2. Increased venous return resulting from the functional arteriovenous shunt of the placenta. Recent evidence shows that this increase is evident up to the time of parturition. In the past it, was believed that a decrease in venous return occurred at about 35 weeks' gestation, but the supposed decrease has been found to be an artifact secondary to coincident aortocaval compression. Many pregnant women instinctively lie on their left sides during the last trimester to avoid dizziness or a feeling of sickness. It is critical to ensure that the parturient is afforded every means to avoid aortocaval compression. In most cases, this will consist of a blanket

Table 9.1. Resuscitation Drugs and Equipment

DRUGS

Aminophylline, 500-mg syringe
Atropine, 0.4 mg/mL vials
Bretylium tosylate, 500 mg/10 mL ampule
Calcium chloride 10%, 10 mL
Dextrose, 50% syringe
Digoxin, 0.5 mg/2 mL ampules
Dopamine, 250-mg vials
Dobutamine, 200-mg ampules
Ephedrine, 50-mg ampules
Epinephrine, 1:1000 (1-mL) ampules
Epinephrine, 1:10 000 syringe
Furosemide, 20 mg/2 2 mL ampules
Heparin, 1000 U/mL, 10-ml vial
Hydrocortisone, 100-mg vial
Isoproterenol, 1 mg/5 ml ampules
Lidocaine, 100-mg syringes
Lidocaine, 2-g vial
Naloxone, 0.4 mg ampules
Nitroglycerine, 50-mg vial
Nitroprusside sodium, 50-mg vial
Norepinephrine, 1 mg/mL, 4-mL amps
Phenylephrine, 1% 1 mL ampule
Physostigmine 1 mg/mL, 2-mL amps
Sodium bicarbonate, 50-mL syringes
Sodium chloride, 10-mL vials
Succinylcholine, 20 mg/mL, 10-mL vials*
Terbutaline, 1-mL ampules
Verapamil, 5 mg/2 mL vial
Water, sterile, 10-mL vials

SOLUTIONS

0.9% saline (normal saline), 250-, 500-, 1000-mL bottles
Lactated Ringer's solution, 1000-mL bottles
Dextrose 5% (D5) in lactated Ringer's solution, 1000-mL bottles

EQUIPMENT

IV sets (both regular and "mini-drip"), IV solutions
Ambu or other similar ventilation bag with mask
Oxygen tubing
Laryngoscope battery handle (at least two)
Set of spare batteries (preferably alkaline)
No. 3 and no. 4 MacIntosh blade with spare light bulbs
No. 2, no. 3, and no. 4 Miller blade with spare light bulbs
No. 6.0 to no. 8.0 soft nasal airways
Oral airways (small, medium, large)
No. 6 to no. 8 endotracheal (ET) tubes with soft cuff
Malleable stylette for ET tubes (at least two)
McGill forceps
Yankauer (tonsil) suction tips with suction tubing
Stethoscope
Paper tape (for hyperallergenic patients)
Silk tape
Tuberculin, 3-, 5-, and 10-mL syringes
18-, 20-, 22-, and 25-gauge needles

*To be kept in refrigerator.

roll under the right hip both in the labor bed and on the delivery or cesarean section table.

3. Engorgement of vessels of the venous plexus in the epidural space. The net effect of this engorgement is that both the subarachnoid and epidural spaces will be smaller. As a consequence, the **volume of anesthetic** needed for an epidural or subarachnoid block is less than that needed for a nonpregnant patient.

B. **Pulmonary changes.** The primary changes in pulmonary physiology are:

1. **Increased minute ventilation** (secondary to increased tidal volume and frequency), probably due to hormonal effects.

2. **Decrease in functional residual capacity resulting from elevation of the diaphragm.**

These two pulmonary changes **increase the rate at which anesthesia is induced by inhalation methods.** Parturients will enter the anesthetic state with lower concentrations of the volatile anesthetics (halothane, enflurane, isoflurane) or nitrous oxide. Although increased cardiac output slows anesthetic uptake, this effect is counteracted by the overwhelming pulmonary forces.

C. **Gastrointestinal changes.** At the gastroesophageal junction there exists a "physiologic" rather than an anatomic sphincter. In the normal nonpregnant patient, this usually prevents regurgitation. However, in the pregnant patient, this physiologic sphincter becomes compromised in function due to the effect of placental hormones; that is, less gastric pressure is required for the sphincter to open and allow passage of gastric contents into the esophagus. In addition, gastrointestinal motility is adversely affected when a parturient goes into labor. It is for these reasons that **every parturient should be considered to have a full stomach when anesthetized.**

D. **Endocrine changes.** Circulating levels of plasma cholinesterase (pseudocholinesterase) are decreased in pregnancy, and this decreased level **may prolong the effect of the muscle relaxant succinylcholine** (Anectine, Quelicin, Sucostrin). For such patients, the nondepolarizing relaxant atracurium (Tracrium) might be selected. This drug undergoes spontaneous, inorganic decomposition and is also eliminated by nonspecific cholinesterases. Vecuronium (Norcuron), another medium-duration, nondepolarizing muscle relaxant, may also be chosen. Pseudocholinesterase deficiency is quite rare (< 1:10,000), and specific tests for this enzyme deficiency are expensive. A good history will uncover this problem in many instances. In the case in which there has been no previous surgery, it is simply not feasible to tell beforehand. There is concern as to the advisability of administering ester-type local anesthetics to patients deficient in pseudocholinesterase. Available evidence suggests that these drugs are also decomposed by nonspecific cholinesterases, but the time for elimination is significantly increased. Final judgments as to the use of these local anesthetics should be made on a case-by-case basis.

E. **Renal changes.** The glomerular filtration rate and renal plasma flow increase during pregnancy. These measurements reach 150 percent of normal by the fourth month of gestation, with a consequent 40 percent reduction in measured serum creatinine and blood urea nitrogen (BUN). Normal values for a parturient are 8 to 9 mg/dL (BUN) and 0.46 mg/dL (creatinine). It is important to remember that normal hospital laboratory (i.e., nonpregnant) values (BUN = 15–22 mg/dL and creatinine = 1.0 to 1.2 mg/dL) in a parturient mean that significant renal excretion problems are present.

II. **Effect of anesthesia on labor and delivery**
   A. **Transplacental passage of anesthetic/analgetic agents**
      1. All anesthetics and analgesics cross the placental barrier. However, both depolarizing and nondepolarizing muscle relaxants, with the exception of the older agent gallamine (Flaxedil), do not cross the placenta in clinically significant quantities.
      2. Anesthetics and analgesics pass through the placenta by simple diffusion.
         a. Features of the anesthetic agent influencing transplacental passage (in order of importance):
            (1) Lipid solubility
            (2) Degree of ionization
            (3) Molecular weight. As a rule of thumb, those substances having a weight of > 1000 pass with great difficulty.
         b. Changes in maternal physiology and acid/base status also may play a role in the transplacental passage of anesthetic-analgesic agents.
      3. Effects of anesthetics and analgesics on labor
         a. **Inhalation anesthetics.** All the potent inhalation anesthetic agents are myometrial depressants. They can arrest uterine contractions and in the third stage of labor may lead to postpartum hemorrhage as a result of low myometrial tone.
         b. **Local anesthetics.** Local anesthetics act indirectly. Laboratory evidence definitely demonstrates that direct application of local anesthetic to myometrium strips in vitro shows a definite alteration of contractions. However, local anesthetics as clinically applied generally are in concentrations too weak to affect the labor process significantly — **provided that it is well established.** In the latent phase of labor contractions are not yet coordinated and small amounts of an analgesic (such as meperidine [Demero]) or a local anesthetic (such as the induction of an epidural anesthetic) may significantly slow the process and result in a prolonged latent phase.

However, if the labor is well established, then any effect of local anesthetic will be temporary (Table 9.2).

c. **Regional blocks**
   (1) All blocks relax the pelvic musculature. They can interfere with internal rotation and flexion and may thus prolong the second stage of labor.
   (2) **Bearing down.** Major conduction blocks induced during labor will anesthetize the perineum and **deprive the parturient of the urge to bear down.** In patients with cardiovascular or pulmonary compromise, this may be a desired side effect. The Valsalva maneuver (the bearing down) is effected by closing the glottis and using the diaphragm and, secondarily, the medial recti muscles. Unless the patient is absolutely blocked up to about T4 with a surgical anesthetic dose of agent, **it is doubtful that the patient has been deprived of the ability to bear down.** It is important to provide effective labor coaching, which has been shown to be an adequate substitute.

d. **Epinephrine.** Epinephrine is frequently added to local anesthetics to prolong the anesthetic effect. Uterine tone, and the intensity as well as the frequency of uterine contractions, may be diminished secondary to the beta-2 effect of epinephrine.

III. **Regional anesthesia**
   A. **General principles.** Regional anesthetic techniques have become the **preferred method of anesthesia and/or analgesia during labor, vaginal delivery, and cesarean section.** They are popular for a variety of reasons, not the least of which is that the physiologic functions of both the mother and the fetus or newborn are less perceptibly affected than with other techniques; pain relief can be extended over prolonged periods of time. The mother is conscious at parturition and is thus able to participate more fully in the birthing process. Since the mother is relieved of pain and discomfort, participation by the father is now more appropriate and feasible.
   B. **Neurophysiology of labor**
      1. **First stage.** During this period, pain is secondary to both myometrial contractions and stretching of the uterine cervix. Nerve endings in these structures are stimulated, and pain sensations at the end of the first stage of labor may become sufficiently severe to cause pain to spread from T10 to L1–2.
      2. **Second stage.** Pain and pressure sensations during this stage are mediated by fibers originating in the lower vagina, vulva, and perineum and reach the spinal cord via the anterior primary divisions of roots S2–4.
   C. **Problems and complications common to all regional blocks**
      1. **Local anesthetic intoxication.** This complication generally

Table 9.2. Local Anesthetics Commonly Used in Obstetrics

LOCAL ANESTHETIC	MOLECULAR WEIGHT DURATION	% PROTEIN BINDING	pK_a	MATERNAL: FETAL RATIO AT BIRTH	NEONATAL ELIMINATION HALF-LIFE (H)	IN VIVO	POTENCY	LATENCY
2-Chlorprocaine (Nesacaine)	307	—	8.7	—	43 s	1	Fast	Short
Tetracaine (Pontocaine)	264	75	8.2	—	—	8	Slow	Long
Lidocaine (Xylocaine)	271	50	7.9	2:1	1.6	2	Fast	Moderate
Bupivicaine (Marcaine, Sensorcaine)	325	95	8.1	4:1	3.5	8	Moderate	Long
Etidocaine (Duranest)	276	94	7.7	5:1	2.6	6	Moderate	Long

Note: Procaine (Novocaine) is not commonly used in obstetrics, having been superseded by more advanced drugs. Mepivicaine (Carbocaine), although used in surgery, is not recommended for obstetric use, as a landmark study by Scanlon et al. (see Bibliography) found that various neotatal reflexes are depressed.

results from an accidental intravenous dose of local anesthetic, causing a transient but potentially lethal overdose. Accidental intravenous injection is associated with but not limited to paracervical and conduction blocks.

a. **Signs and symptoms.** Prodromal symptoms and signs include **tinnitus, a metallic taste in the mouth, dizziness, twitching, and inappropriate behavior.** A grand mal seizure and cardiovascular collapse may occur.

b. **Treatment**

(1) Oxygen must be **immediately** administered by mask, as cerebral oxygen consumption is increased several times.

(2) Thiopental sodium (50 mg) is given IV to abort the seizure. Thiopental is superior to diazepam, as it redistributes quickly and its effects on the fetus are more transient. If the patient cannot be easily ventilated or is in danger of aspiration, intubation using succinylcholine is recommended. **If this is done, it must be by experienced personnel.** The parturient should be placed in the left lateral decubitus position, and as soon as possible the fetal heart tones must be auscultated or the fetal monitor read and, if indicated and feasible, a fetal scalp pH done. If there are signs of fetal distress or serious acidosis, emergency cesarean section should be considered.

2. **Allergic reactions.** True allergic reactions are limited to the ester-type local anesthetics (2-chlorprocaine, tetracaine). This is because these compounds are derivatives of para-aminobenzoic acid, which acts as an allergen. True allergy to the amide-type compounds (lidocaine, bupivicaine) is rare. Often a patient who is "allergic to Novocaine" will relate an incident that took place in a dental office: A local block was given, and the patient had a headache, a "feeling of doom," and so on. This is usually due to accidental intravenous injection of a local anesthetic with epinephrine. Since most dentists use either mepivicaine (Carbocaine) or lidocaine (Xylocaine), both of which are amide drugs, a true allergic reaction is doubtful. (It ought to be kept in mind that in most lay people's minds *Novocaine* is simply a synonym for *local anesthetic,* rather than the brand name for procaine, which is now rarely used.) True allergic reactions occasionally do indeed occur. They are manifested as generalized erythema, edema, respiratory wheezing and/or dyspnea, hypotension, tachycardia, headache, or loss of consciousness. Treatment includes maintenance of the airway, administration of oxygen, controlled/assisted ventilation as indicated, circulatory support by proper positioning, intravenous fluids, and, if necessary, vasopressors. Antihistamines and corticosteroids may also be given to control the effects of systemic histamine release.

ANESTHETIC TECHNIQUES DURING LABOR

I. **Psychological analgesia.** Psychological support for the laboring parturient is a traditional part of obstetric management. The following methods of psychological analgesia employ no exogenously administered drugs that can cross the placenta and affect the fetus.

   A. **Natural childbirth.** This method was introduced by Grantly Dick-Read in 1933, and is dedicated to encouraging and supporting natural childbirth (without anesthetics or other drugs) by breaking the vicious cycle of fear/tension/pain through a series of prenatal lectures and exercises.

   B. **Psychoprophylactic method (Lamaze method).** In 1947, a Russian physician, Velvovski, introduced this concept, which is based on Pavlov's conditioned reflex theory. Lamaze introduced the method in France; it was introduced in the United States by Karmel. This is the most popular method of psychological anesthesia used in the United States today.

   C. **Hypnosis.** Used for centuries, hypnosis is employed for pain relief in labor and delivery. In certain very controlled situations, it has even been used for cesarean section. However, it is unpredictable and is seldom used.

   D. **Acupuncture.** This method uses needle placement according to precepts of oriental medicine. It has had very limited success in the West.

   E. **Disadvantages**
      1. Each method requires that the parturient be motivated and willing to spend time working with the method **before labor begins.** In addition, the patient must truly believe that the method will work. Finally, the parturient must understand that these methods produce a reduction of pain **to manageable levels,** rather than total analgesia.
      2. Because these are natural methods, they may be inadvisedly proselytized and used to the exclusion of other methods even when other methods are desirable or even necessary.
      3. In the absence of medication, labor may lead to hyperventilation with a resulting drop in P_aCO_2, maternal respiratory alkalosis, vasoconstriction of the uterine bed, diminished intervillous space perfusion, altered maternal-fetal gas exchanges, fetal hypoxia, and fetal metabolic acidosis.

II. **Systemic medication provided by the obstetrician**

   A. **Analgesia during labor** may be effected with:
      1. Morphine, 5 to 7 mg IM every 3 to 4 h or 2 to 4 mg IV every 3 to 4 h
      2. Meperidine (Demerol), 50 to 100 mg IM every 3 to 4 h or 10 to 25 mg IV every 1.5 to 3 h
      Parenteral narcotics cross the placenta and may cause fetal depression. This is recognized by a loss of beat-to-beat variability in the fetal monitor tracing. A depressed fetus will have difficulty breathing and will be less able to effect appro-

priate temperature regulation at birth. **Narcotics should be avoided if it is felt that their peak maternal concentration will not have been dissipated by the time delivery occurs. The time of delivery is quite variable; thus the narcotic antagonist naloxone (Narcan)** should be immediately available. The dosage of naloxone is O.4 mg/mL IV or IM, and the neonatal dosage is 0.01 mg/kg IM.

3. Tranquilization during labor is achieved by administration of one of the following sedatives:
   a. Hydroxizine (Vistaril), 50 to 100 mg IM
   2. Promethazine (Phenergan), 25 mg IM
   3. Promazine (Sparine), 25 mg IM
4. Diazepam (Valium) is **contraindicated during labor.** Diazepam has a long elimination half-life (up to 40 h), and its active metabolite, desmethyldiazepam, has an elimination half-life of up to 140 h. This drug causes flaccidity in the newborn and may derange its temperature-regulating mechanisms. It is also known to compete for bilirubin binding sites. Diazepam is useful in the obstetric suite for sedating the fetus to minimize fetal movement during percutaneous umbilical blood sampling (PUBS) procedures. In this context, about 6 to 7 mg of diazepam is given to the mother IV.
5. Scopolomine is also contraindicated during labor. This drug is primarily a sedative and amnesic. It apparently affects areas in the brain that have to do with emotions. Parturients who have been given this drug have had hallucinations and have been wildly uncontrollable, with absolutely no memory of any incident after the birthing experience.
6. Midazolam (Versed) is a relatively new water-soluble benzodiazopine with a shorter half-life than diazepam. However, in the context of labor and delivery, this drug is contraindicated for the same reasons as diazepam.

B. **Paracervical block (routinely performed by the obstetrician)**
   1. **Indications**
      a. Absence of anesthesia personnel
      b. Uncomplicated, well-progressing labor
      c. Spontaneous vaginal delivery
      d. Straightforward forceps delivery
      e. Repair of low vaginal or perineal lacerations and episiotomies
      f. Minor vaginal/perineal surgical repairs
   2. **Contraindications**
      a. Lack of knowledge of the pertinent anatomy, technique, and local anesthetic pharmacology
      b. Lack of knowledge and/or skill in managing systemic toxic reactions
      c. Intrauterine manipulations
      d. Complex and difficult forceps maneuvers
      e. Infection of the perineum or of the perianal, labial, or ischiorectal space.

3. **Physiology.** Paracervical blocks interrupt the sensory pathways that come from the uterus and cervix. Therefore, they are useful only in the management of pain generated by the first stage of labor.

4. **Technique.** The block consists of the injection of local anesthetic into the nerve-rich zones at the base of the broad ligament. Specifically, the technique involves the transvaginal administration of local anesthetic into the fornices on either side of the cervix. Traditionally the sites are 3 and 9 o'clock, but these particular points also contain arteries and veins. Therefore, it is preferable to inject at 4 and 8 o'clock, respectively.

5. **Advantages.** There is a simplicity of instrumentation and a relative ease of administration. In addition, it is readily accepted by the patient in labor and, when successful, gives excellent analgesia during the first stage of labor.

6. **Disadvantages and complications**

   a. Postparacervical block fetal bradycardia: The administration of a local anesthetic in the paracervical areas can result in a 10 to 90 percent incidence of postparacervical block fetal bradycardia. This has been attributed to:

      (1) Large quantities of local anesthetic passing the placental barrier secondary to intravenous injection (Fig. 9.1);

      (2) Reflex increase in uterine tone; or

      (3) Decrease in intervillous space perfusion due to increased uterine artery vasoconstriction.

   b. Failure to produce analgesia in 10 to 50 percent of parturients.

   c. Retroperitoneal infections.

   d. Hematomas.

   e. Maternal local anesthetic intoxication.

C. **Lumbar/caudal epidural block.** These blocks have been occasionally performed by the obstetrician in certain situations, but present standards of care mandate that they be done only by an anesthesiologist or nurse anesthetist. The complications of any of these techniques are so disastrous that it is a serious breach of judgment for any practitioner to consider administering a major conduction anesthetic and have the patient either unmonitored or monitored by untrained people.

An epidural block affords the greatest flexibility in both extent and quality of blockage. By injecting appropriate volumes and/or concentrations, a variety of anesthesias tailored to the clinical situation can be effected. Small volumes will block specific nerve roots, and low concentrations will avoid or at least minimize motor blockade. By limiting the volume of local anesthetic given during the first stage of labor to about 4 to 5 mL, it is possible to achieve a "segmental" block involving the dermatomes T10 to T12. This spares the sacral segments and there-

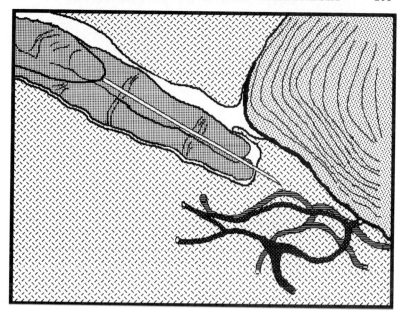

FIGURE 9.1. Proximity of vessels in a paracervical block.

fore should not interfere with the parturient's reflex bearing-down efforts. In practice, after several "top-up" doses, the cumulative effect of the anesthetic results in an area of analgesia considerably greater than the original segments, usually extending from T10 to S5.

1. **Indications**
   a. When general anesthesia is contraindicated or undesirable.
   b. When it is desirable to spare the fetus the potential systemic effects of general anesthesia.
2. **Contraindications**
   a. Hypovolemia from any cause.
   b. Hypotension.
   c. Infections at the site of contemplated skin puncture.
   d. Anticoagulation therapy. When full-dose heparin or coumadin is used, conduction block is contraindicated. At the time of this writing, most anesthesiologists feel that it is **not safe to use conduction block with low-dose heparin if the results of coagulation tests are abnormal.**
   e. Active central nervous system disease.
   f. Patient refusal.
   g. Lack of availability of an anesthesiologist or nurse anesthetist and equipment/medications necessary for the

management of complications arising from these procedures, including emergency life support measures.

h. Absence of monitoring equipment and nursing personnel for the continuous evaluation for the duration of the block.

i. Absence of guaranteed IV access to the systemic circulation.

3. **Advantages**

a. Segmental blockade of T10 to L2 is feasible.

b. Repeated injections or a continuous infusion can be made through a catheter placed in the epidural space. This results in an anesthetic that may be prolonged at will and requring only one needle puncture.

c. Muscle relaxation can be avoided.

4. **Disadvantages**

a. Sympathetic blockade increases the incidence of hypotension.

b. Large quantities of local anesthetic are needed, increasing the potential for a systemic toxic reaction.

c. Accidental dural puncture with the epidural needle (typically, 17 gauge) can cause a high incidence of postpuncture headache.

5. **Complications**

a. **Hypotension.** Hypotension is caused primarily by two factors.

(1) **Aortocaval compression.** The gravid uterus has been shown to obstruct the inferior vena cava mechanically and thereby cause impedence of venous return, resulting in circulatory compromise. This effect is resisted by a resting level of sympathetic tone of the blood vessels. When a conduction block is effected, this tone is lost and compression is completely unopposed.

(2) **Sympathetic blockade.** Besides offering opposition to uterine compression, sympathetic activity regulates the capacity of the venous circulation. With sympathetic blockade there is a sudden large increase in venous capacity with venous pooling, also resulting in compromised circulation.

(3) **Hypotension management.** The parturient suffers insensible losses of fluid and is often dehydrated. One should administer at least 1 L of a replacement crystalloid solution in order to increase rapidly the circulatory volume. The parturient should be placed in a partial or complete left lateral decubitus position. The right hip can be elevated using a variety of measures; a blanket roll is cheapest. After the block is initiated, blood pressure and other vital signs should be frequently monitored. If the systolic blood pressure falls below 100 mm Hg, more crys-

talloid should be administered; if little improvement is seen, 5 to 10 mg of the vasopressor **ephedrine** should be given IV. Some clinicians advocate giving 50 mg ephedrine IM before the block, but this issue is controversial.

Ephedrine is the only appropriate vasopressor. It causes the least amount of uterine vasoconstriction and fetal compromise.

Note: Sequential or simultaneous use of ergotrate derivatives with ephedrine has been responsible for reported maternal deaths secondary to acute hypertensive crisis, with resulting heart failure and cerebrovascular accidents.

b. **Postpuncture of "spinal" headache.** After a subarachnoid puncture, cerebrospinal fluid leaks until the puncture site heals. If enough fluid leaks out, the brain is no longer bouyantly suspended in the skull and exerts traction on pain-sensitive meninges. The incidence of headache after puncture with a 17-gauge epidural needle is about 50 percent compared to only 1 percent after the use of a 26-gauge needle. The headache is occipital or circumferential and usually appears the day after the block; it can last a week or longer. It is worsened by assuming an upright position and alleviated by lying flat.

(1) **Conservative management.** Milder forms of this headache are treated by bed rest, generous amounts of fluids, and analgesics.

(2) **Management of refractory headache.** For headaches refractory to conservative management, an epidural blood patch should be considered. This consists of placing 10 to 15 mL of the patient's own aseptically drawn blood in the epidural space at the site of the original needle puncture.

6. **Caudal epidural block**
   a. Advantages. The advantages are the same as those for lumbar epidural block.
   b. Disadvantages. The disadvantages are the same as those for lumbar epidural block. In addition, the reliability (success rate) in experienced hands is lower than for a lumbar epidural block (approximately 85 percent vs. 95+ percent for lumbar epidural block).

ANESTHETIC TECHNIQUES FOR DELIVERY

I. **Pudendal block**
   A. **Indications.** The same as for paracervical block, but now specifically for delivery.
   B. **Contraindications.** The same as for paracervical block.
   C. **Physiology/anatomy.** The pudendal nerve, which consists of the anterior primary division of S2, S3, and S4, is blocked. The

pudendal nerve divides into three major branches: the inferior hemorrhoidal nerve, the perineal nerve, and the dorsal nerve of the clitoris. It is evident that this block is suited for second-stage labor and episiotomy repair. However, it is not at all appropriate for complicated maneuvers such as midforceps rotations.

D. **Technique.** The block involves the administration of local anesthetic into Alcock's canal as it courses under the ischial spine. A pudendal block may be given through the perineum or, more frequently, transvaginally.

E. **Advantages**
   1. Instrumentation is simple.
   2. Easily identifiable landmarks necessary for performing the block exist.
   3. Excellent pain relief is provided during second-stage labor.
   4. Progress of labor is usually not altered.
   5. It is readily accepted by parturients.
   6. It provides sufficient anesthesia for low forceps deliveries and possibly low midforceps deliveries.
   7. Specialized postanesthetic care is usually not necessary.

F. **Disadvantages**
   1. The area of anesthesia may not be as predictable as one treated with a conduction anesthetic.
   2. The pudendal artery and veins are in close proximity to the pudendal nerve.
   3. Failure to obtain satisfactory analgesia may lead to repeated injections, which can result in local anesthetic toxicity.
   4. It does not relieve the pain sensations emanating from the uterus and cervix (T10 to T12).

G. **Complications**
   1. Vaginal and ischiorectal hematomas
   2. Retroperitoneal infections
   3. Infections of the acetabulum or femoral head
   4. Local anesthetic toxicity

II. **Subarachnoid block**
   A. **Indications.** The same as for lumbar epidural block.
   B. **Contraindications.** The same as for lumbar epidural block. In addition, the nature of subarachnoid block reserves it for vaginal delivery or cesarean section.
   C. **Advantages**
      1. It is simple to perform.
      2. A clear endpoint (cerebrospinal fluid) exists.
      3. Direct effects on the fetus are minimal, and indirect effects are usually avoidable and treatable and are predominantly secondary to induced changes in maternal physiology.
      4. The patient is allowed to remain awake at delivery.
      5. Excellent muscle relaxation — both perineal, as for forceps delivery of the premature baby, and abdominal, as for cesarean section — is afforded.

6. Local anesthetic intoxication is virtually impossible because of the small amounts (1 to 2 mL) injected.
D. **Disadvantages**
1. Frequent hypotension occurs due to loss of sympathetic tone (20 to 90 percent, depending on the series).
2. Spinal headache may occur (see Section II.C.5).
3. Direct neurologic damage may occur.
4. It is poorly accepted by some patients.
5. Segmental blocks, as achieved with a lumbar epidural block, cannot be performed.
6. Generally, a spinal block may be performed only once.

III. **Lumbar/caudal epidural block.** The indications, contraindications, physiology, and complications of this block have been discussed in Section II.C. Because of the usually greater strength of the anesthetic solution (since true anesthesia rather than analgesia is sought) administered, greater caution and mindfulness of a toxic reaction are needed.

IV. **General anesthesia**
A. **Indications.** General anesthesia is reserved for the following situations:
1. Refusal of a regional technique when an anesthetic is otherwise indicated or requested. However, the elective use of general anesthesia for vaginal delivery, especially by mask, puts the patient at high risk for aspiration of gastric contents.
2. **When minor blocks are insufficient** and the patient's **cardiovascular status precludes major regional anesthesia.**
3. Unmanageable, retarded, or psychotic patients.
4. Intrauterine manipulations.
5. Any surgical or obstetric situation when administration of anesthesia is immediately necessary and the administration of regional anesthesia would be too time-consuming.
6. Congenital or anatomic anomalies that make regional anesthesia impractical or impossible.
B. **Contraindications**
1. Lack of trained personnel.
2. Lack of adequate equipment.
3. Refusal by the patient.
4. Asthma.
5. Known anatomic anomalies that would make intubation extremely difficult or impossible. This category includes the patient with a high or "anterior" larynx and the patient with significant anatomic distortion of the head or neck. It should be noted that with enough time (especially if the patient is, for example, having an elective cesarean section), intubation while the patient is awake can usually be done if the clinical situation demands it.
C. **Preoperative antacids.** In view of the potentially lethal effects of aspiration of acid gastric juices of pH < 2.5 (mortality for acid

aspiration, despite the best intensive care, exceeds 50 percent), the administration of **a clear antacid 30 min before induction of anesthesia is highly recommended.** The common particulate antacids (Riopan, Gelusil, Maalox) can cause chemical burns of the lung that equal the severity of an acid aspiration. It is presently recommended that 15 to 30 mL of sodium citrate 0.3 M (Bicitra) be given.

D. **Myometrial depressant effects of drugs used for general anesthesia.** Halothane, enflurane, isoflurane, and methoxyflurane all depress the myometrium. Nitrous oxide, ketamine, barbiturates, narcotics, and muscle relaxants do not.

E. **Complications.** The most common and serious complications are:
1. Aspiration of gastric contents
   a. Particulate matter (food or antacid)
   b. Gastric juices (pH ≤ 2.5)
2. Cardiovascular complications, up to and including circulatory collapse
3. Pulmonary complications (hypercarbia, hypoxia, respiratory acidosis) either from anesthetic overdose or from poor airway management

POSTOPERATIVE PAIN MANAGEMENT

I. **Traditional methods**
   A. **The pain cycle** (Fig. 9.2), a diagrammatic representation of a typical pain-patient-nursing interaction
   B. **Doses**
      1. 5 to 10 mg morphine IM
      2. 50 to 100 mg meperidine IM
   C. **Advantages**
      1. Simplicity
      2. No mechanical devices needed
   D. **Disadvantages**
      1. Time between patient's perception of pain and relief is very long
      2. Great variability in potential absorption of pain medications

II. **Patient-controlled analgesia (PCA)**
   A. **PCA devices**
      1. **General description.** A PCA device usually consists of a syringe pump interfaced with a microprocessor timing unit linked to a switch or button activated by the patient. When the switch is activated, a predetermined bolus dose of a narcotic analgesic (morphine sulfate, 1 to 2 mg/mL) is provided for the patient. The timing unit prohibits the patient from receiving bolus injections continuously by imposing a delay of 5 to 10 min between doses. The amount of the bolus and the period of delay can be manipulated to provide improved analgesia.

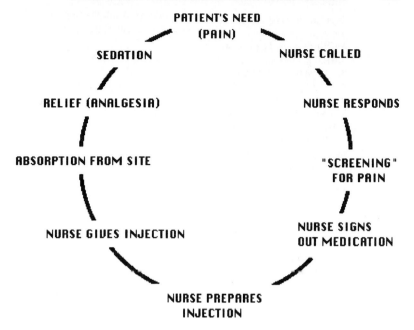

FIGURE 9.2.   The rain cycle. (Reproduced with permission from Graves DA, Foster TS, Batenhorst RL. Patient-controlled analgesia. Ann Intern Med 1983; 99:361.)

2. **Advantages**
   a. Permits the patient to control the amount and timing of pharmaco-therapy
   b. Links the sensory neurophysiology of pain management with the psychology of the pain process
   c. Reduces anxiety
   d. Minimizes physical delay between pain perception and analgesic administration
   e. Ability to carefully titrate the dose of medication needed to maintain a desired level of analgesia while avoiding the undesirable side effects (Fig. 9.3)
3. **Disadvantages**
   a. Mechanical device needed
   b. Initial capital expense
   c. Possible clumsiness of the mechanism
4. **Abbot Lifecare** 4100 PCA Infusor (Abbot Laboratories, North Chicago, IL 60064)
   a. Cost — about $3000 to $5000
   b. Bulky — 7 kg
   c. Moderately complex programming
5. **Pancretec Provider** 5500 Infusor (Pancretec, Inc., San Diego, CA 92128-0968)

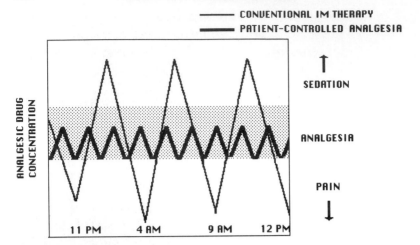

FIGURE 9.3. Dose–analgesia–time relationship. (Adapted from White PF. Use of a patient-controlled analgesia infusor for the management of postoperative pain. In: Harmer M, Rosen M, Vickers MD, eds. Patient Controlled Analgesia. Cambridge, MA: Blackwell Scientific Publications; 1985:147.)

      a. Cost — about $3000 to $5000
      b. Small, battery-operated, linear peristaltic pump
      c. Moderately complex programming
      d. Very lightweight
   6. **Bard** Ambulatory PCA Pump (Bard MedSystems Division, C.R. Bard, Inc., North Reading, MA 01864-2601)
      a. Cost — about $3000
      b. Small, battery-operated, linear peristaltic pump
      c. Simplified programming
      d. Very lightweight
   7. **Baxter Travenol Infusor** with Patient Control Module (Baxter Healthcare Corporation, Deerfield, IL 60015)
      a. Cost — $35
      b. Nonelectronic (totally mechanical)
      c. Simple to operate
      d. Disposable
B. **Effects.** Perceived reduction in pain potentially improves postoperative function.
   1. Coughing
   2. Deep breathing
   3. Postoperative ambulation significantly improved
C. **Safety/efficacy**
   1. It has been shown to be safe in cesarean section patients.
   2. Patients prefer PCA over traditional systems.

III. Epidural opioids. The direct application of narcotics into the epidural space has opened up a new field of anesthetic endeavor, providing regional analgesia without autonomic or motor blockade.

A. **Advantages**
1. Dense analgesia with low-dose narcotics
2. Continuous pain relief for up to 24 h
3. Minimal sedation
4. No peripheral nerves blocked (sympathetic, sensory, motor)
5. Parturient can interact effectively with family
6. Early ambulation, decreasing the hospital stay
7. Improved pulmonary function
8. Stable cardiovascular status, especially in compromised patients

B. **Morphine sulfate.** A preservative-free morphine sulfate (Duramorph) is available for epidural injection by the anesthesiologist. Side effects of this method of analgesia include pruritus and urinary retention, as well as significant nausea and vomiting. Respiratory depression may also appear. Such patients must be closely monitored for 24 h.

C. **Fentanyl and analogs.** At the time of this writing, fentanyl (Sublimaze) and sufantanil (Sufenta), with or without ultra-low-dose local anesthetics, are also being used epidurally. Many anesthesia services offer post-cesarean section patients the option of epidurally delivered fentanyl or sufentanil. The doses are given in Table 9.3.

D. **Side effects**
1. **Respiratory depression.** This problem is found almost exclusively with **morphine or meperidine.** Since fentanyl and sufentanyl are, respectively, 700 and 1700 times more soluble, the peak effect is seen within about 10 to 15 min of epidural administration. In addition, studies with fentanyl and sufentanil show that the amount of plasma opioid is undetectable after the first hour (i.e., well below 0.1 ng/mL, which itself is an order of magnitude below the level needed for respiratory depression. Clinically, this means that 2 h after epidural administration of either fentanyl or sufentanyl, the probability of respiratory depression, while not zero, is vanishingly small.

   a. **Mechanism.** This is a biphasic phenomenon, with the initial respiratory depression due to systemic absorption from the epidural depot of narcotic, often within the first hour or so of injection, and a much later (6- to 18-h)

Table 9.3. Narcotics Used in Epidural Infusions

Morphine, 0.1 mg/mL, ± bupivicaine, 1 mg/mL, @ 3–7 mL/h
Fentanyl, 10 μg/mL, ± bupivicaine, 1 mg/mL, @ 5–10 mL/h
Sufentanil, 1 μg/mL, ± bupivicaine, 0.5 mg/mL, @ 8–10 mL/h

depression due to cerebral migration of the drug. In the postoperative patient, the residual systemically administered narcotics and residual anesthetic agents may well summate with a lack of tolerance to the opioid drugs to produce this complication.

    b. Factors that predispose to respiratory depression
- (1) Advanced age
- (2) Water-soluble opioid
- (3) High doses
- (4) Narcotic-naive subjects
- (5) Artificial ventilation
- (6) Coincident administration of narcotics by other routes

    c. **Incidence.** A large study has shown it to be 0.33 percent in 6000 patients given epidural morphine. No incidence with epidural fentanyl (100 μg) has been reported.

    d. **Precautions and treatment**
- (1) **Precautions**
  - (a) The patient should be monitored with a pulse oximeter.
  - (b) If morphine was given, the patient must be in a monitored bed for 24 h.
  - (c) If fentanyl was given, then 2 to 4 h is sufficient.
  - (d) Have naloxone (Narcan), 0.4 mg, drawn up at the bedside.
  - (e) Observe for respiratory depression (defined as < 10 breaths per min).
- (2) **Treatment.** If respiratory depression or SaO_2 < 90 percent occurs, the nurse should give naloxone, 0.4 mg IV, then call the pain service for definitive action.

2. Conclusion. It seems that the risk of respiratory depression is less than was initially feared when these drugs are given by the epidural route. Nevertheless, vigilant monitoring is warranted to detect the small percentage of patients at risk.

    a. **Nausea and vomiting.** The incidence of nausea and vomiting following epidural administration is significant but not excessively more than that occurring with systemic administration. The symptoms are readily reversible by administering 0.4 mg IV naloxone, and this does **not** alter the analgesia.

    b. **Urinary retention.** Like respiratory depression, this condition seems to occur more frequently (22 percent of cases) when epidural opioids are administered postoperatively.

    c. **Itching.** Like retention and respiratory depression, itching is more of a problem postoperatively than with the use of epidural narcotics for chronic pain. Pruritis is commonly mentioned when patients are questioned.

Severe itching probably occurs much less often and is reversible by naloxone, 0.4 mg IV or nalbuphine (Nubaine) 3 to 5 mg IV. Reports indicate that prior use of epidural bupivicaine reduces the incidence of subsequent pruritus with epidural opioids.

BIBLIOGRAPHY

American College of Obstetricians and Gynecologists. Obstetric anesthesia and analgesia. ACOG Technical Bulletin January 1988; 112:1–6.

American College of Obstetricians and Gynecologists. Anesthesia for emergency deliveries. ACOG Committee Opinion, March 1992; 104:1–2.

Clark RB, Seifen AB. Complications of obsterical anesthesia. Semin Anesth 1982; 155–167.

Kotelko DM, Dailey PA, Shnider SM, et al. Epidural morphine analgesia after cesarean delivery. Obstet Gynecol 1984; 63:409–413.

Malinow MD, Ostheimer GW. Anesthesia for the high-risk parturient. Obstet Gynecol 1987; 69:951–964.

Mazze, RI, Källén B. Reproductive outcome after anesthesia and operation during pregnancy: A registry study of 5405 cases. Am J Obstet Gynecol 1989; 161:1178–1185.

Rayburn WF, Geranis BJ, Ramadei CA, et al. Patient controlled analgesia for post-cesarean section pain. Obstet Gynecol 1988; 72:136–139.

Scanlon JW, Brown WV, Weiss JB, et al. Neurobehavioral responses on newborn infants after maternal epidural anesthesia. Anesthesiology 1974; 40:121–128.

Scanlon JW, Ostheimer GW, Lurie AO, et al. Neurobehavioral responses and drug concentrations in newborns after maternal epidural anesthesia with bupivicaine. Anesthesiology 1976; 45:400–405.

Sinatra RS, Lodge K, Sibert K, et al. A comparison of morphine, meperidine, and oxymorphone as utilized in patient-controlled analgesia following cesarean section. Anesthesiology 1989; 70:585–590.

Viscomi CM, Hood DD, Melone PJ, et al. Fetal heart rate variability after epidural fentanyl during labor. Anesth Analg 1990; 71:679–683.

CHAPTER 10

Operative Obstetrics

David C. Shaver

Operative procedures in obstetrics have changed considerably in recent years. In the past, most procedures were devised to facilitate delivery of the fetus, with the primary consideration being maternal welfare. For various reasons, concern for fetal well-being has increased, and many techniques, such as fetal destructive procedures, are seldom employed.

I. **Cesarean section.** Cesarean section has increasingly become a more common operative procedure in obstetrics. As recently as 30 or 40 years ago, most hospitals reported cesarean section rates of well below 5 percent. This rate increased dramatically during the late 1960s and early 1970s; currently, rates of 25 to 30 percent are common. Many reasons have been cited for this increase, including improved anesthetic techniques, better management of maternal complications, electronic fetal monitoring, and the current medicolegal atmosphere. Although many would argue that the current cesarean section rate is too high, and although many approaches to decrease the rate have been advocated, it will continue to be a frequently used method of delivery. The major concern, then, should be to determine, in the individual case, the safest method of delivery for both mother and baby.

   A. **Classification.** Cesarean section involves delivery of the fetus through a uterine incision, usually made through a cut in the abdominal wall. This can be accomplished in several ways, and classification is based on the type or location of the uterine incision.

      1. **Transverse incision.** The most common uterine incision is a transverse incision in the lower uterine segment (Kerr technique). This incision is associated with less blood loss, as a general rule, and is less prone to rupture in subsequent pregnancies.

      2. **Vertical incision.** The second most common uterine incision is the lower uterine segment vertical (Kronig technique). This incision has the advantage that it can be extended up in case of difficulty in delivery; for this reason, it is often recommended in cases of fetal malpresentation. Disadvantages include a greater chance of extension either up to the uterine fundus or down into the cervix, and a greater chance of

rupture in subsequent pregnancies, especially if extension into the upper segment occurs.

3. **Classical cesarean section,** a vertical incision through the upper segment, was the standard incision until earlier in this century. Because it is associated with greater blood loss, an increased risk of infection, and an increased risk of rupture in future pregnancies, it is performed less commonly now. However, it is still indicated for women in whom the lower uterine segment is poorly developed or inaccessible, or if the bladder cannot be dissected off the cervix. In addition, it should be considered in cases of transverse fetal lie or anterior placenta previa.

4. **Extraperitoneal cesarean section.** Several techniques for extraperitoneal cesarean section have been devised (by Waters and Latzo). Developed for the purpose of limiting intraperitoneal contamination and subsequent infection, they are now rarely performed. Technical difficulty, as well as availability of effective antimicrobial agents, outweigh any advantages of these procedures.

B. **Indications.** Cesarean delivery is indicated in situations in which prompt delivery is believed to be advantageous for the mother or fetus, or both, and in which vaginal delivery is impossible or unsafe. Some of the common indications are as follows:

1. **Fetal indications.** Fetal indications for cesarean section are varied and are now more frequently considered than in the past.

   a. **Fetal distress** constitutes a major reason for abdominal delivery. Widespread use of electronic fetal monitoring has given the obstetrician a valuable tool for assessing fetal well-being and offers advantages over purely clinical assessment of the fetal condition.

   b. **Abnormal presentations** are usually regarded as valid reasons for cesarean section. Babies with **transverse lie** and most babies with **breech presentation** are delivered abdominally. Many would question the need for cesarean section in all cases of breech presentation, but until this issue is resolved, most breech babies will continue to be delivered abdominally.

   c. **Ultrasound-diagnosed fetal conditions,** such as hydrocephalus or large fetal tumors, are considered to be a justification for cesarean section rather than vaginal delivery.

2. **Maternal indications.** There are **few "pure" maternal indications** for cesarean section, since fetal well-being is usually considered in the decision.

   a. **Dystocia** is the most commonly cited reason for cesarean section. Most commonly it is a clinical diagnosis made for failure to progress in labor, usually with findings consistent with cephalopelvic disproportion. Unless there is marked contracture, cesarean section without a trial of labor in patients with suspected pelvic contraction is not indicated.

b. **Hemorrhage** continues to be a frequent indication for abdominal delivery. Most cases of placenta previa and abruptio placentae with a live fetus are best managed by cesarean section.

c. **Previous cesarean section** has become a prominent reason for cesarean section in most institutions. Current recommendations include allowing a trial of labor in patients with a previous single low transverse incision. The safety of labor in these patients has been well established, and success in most series has been quite good.

d. **Many intercurrent illnesses** in the mother, such as pre-eclampsia and diabetes mellitus, often require delivery prior to onset of spontaneous labor. As a result, cesarean section is often required to effect delivery in a timely fashion.

C. **Contraindications.** There are very few absolute contraindications to cesarean section.

1. **Fetal death** removes all fetal indications for abdominal delivery. However, cesarean section may still be indicated for maternal reasons.

2. **Maternal illnesses or conditions** may make surgery extremely unsafe for the mother. Therefore, surgery is contraindicated until maternal stability is attained. Examples are pulmonary edema and severe asthmatic attack.

D. **Procedure.** The procedure for low transverse cesarean section, the most commonly performed surgery, is as follows:

1. **Preoperative preparation** is important in ensuring the safest procedure possible.

   a. Either a **crossmatch or a screen of the mother's blood** should be performed so that blood replacement can be expedited if necessary.

   b. **Preparation of the stomach** by antacids or other means is important, especially if general anesthesia is contemplated.

   c. An **indwelling Foley catheter** should be placed.

2. Following surgical preparation of the abdomen and induction of adequate anesthesia, the abdomen is entered through a lower abdominal transverse or vertical incision.

3. The abdominal cavity is entered, and a retractor is placed on the abdominal wall to provide exposure of the bladder and the lower uterine segment.

4. The uterus is examined to assess rotation.

5. The vesicouterine fold is identified next and is incised transversely. The bladder is then dissected off the lower uterus in the midline and is retracted inferiorly.

6. Using a scalpel, an incision is made transversely in the lower segment in the midline. This incision is then extended, either

bluntly, using the forefingers and forcing them up and out, or using blunt scissors and incising the uterus in a crescentic manner.

7. The fetal membranes are ruptured if this has not already occurred, and a hand is introduced into the uterine cavity below the fetal head. The head is lifted up and out through the incision, aided by fundal pressure. Forceps can be applied if difficulty with manual delivery occurs.

8. Following delivery of the infant, the placenta is removed manually and the endometrial cavity carefully inspected to remove all placenta and membrane fragments.

9. The edges of the uterine incision are grasped with Allis or ring forceps. Classically, the incision is closed in two layers, although recent studies indicate that one layer may be adequate.

10. The vesicouterine fold is then reapproximated, effectively covering the uterine incision.

E. **Complications.** Although the safety of cesarean section has increased markedly over the last several years, significant morbidity continues to be associated with it.

1. **Postoperative infection** remains the most common complication, although its severity has been reduced and medical therapy is much more successful than in the past. A prime contributor to the decrease in morbidity associated with cesarean section is the increasing use of **prophylactic antibiotics.** It is generally agreed that those patients undergoing cesarean section who are at high risk of infection (e.g., in labor with ruptured membranes) will benefit from prophylactic antibiotics. **Irrigation of the uterine cavity with an antibiotic solution or intravenous administration of antibiotic are probably equally effective.**

   a. **Administration of the antibiotic** should be deferred until after clamping of the umbilical cord and should not be continued for more than three doses.

   b. The **choice of antibiotic** is not critical; therefore an inexpensive, broad-spectrum agent such as ampicillin or a first-generation cephalosporin (e.g., **cefazolin**) is recommended. Specifically, there appears to be no benefit from using any of the more expensive newer antibiotics.

   c. The **dosage of antibiotics** is 1 to 2 g of ampicillin or cefazolin for one to three doses.

2. **Hemorrhage** also occurs more frequently following cesarean section than vaginal delivery.

   a. **Drug therapy.** Traditional uterotonic agents such as pitocin and methylergonovine (Methergine) can be used to help control bleeding believed to be secondary to uterine atony. Newer drugs, such as the 15-methyl derivative of prostaglandin $F2\alpha$, are also helpful.

   b. **Surgical therapy.** Hemorrhage not controlled by medical therapy may requiire **ligation of the uterine or hypogastric arteries, or occasionally hysterectomy.**

3. **Operative injury to other pelvic viscera,** notably the urinary tract, can occur. Avoidance of significant morbidity requires prompt recognition and appropriate repair.

II. Cerclage. Cervical cerclage is a procedure that involves placement of a suture to prevent premature dilatation and effacement of the cervix in those patients who are believed to have an incompetent cervical os.

A. **Classification.** Several procedures are performed in patients with an incompetent cervical os. Choice of the cerclage procedure depends on several factors, such as the surgeon's familiarity with each operation, the timing of suture placement (i.e., before or after conception), and the findings on examination of the cervix at the time of operation. No single procedure offers a distinct advantage in terms of success rate.

1. The **Shirodkar operation** involves dissection of the bladder and posterior fornix with placement of a suture, usually a Mersilene strip, at the level of the internal os. It is often done as a planned procedure before conception, when bleeding from the dissection is less, although it may be performed in early pregnancy.

2. The **McDonald procedure** is the simplest of the cerclage procedures, performed without dissection or advancement of tissues. In this operation, a nonabsorbable suture is placed around the cervix in a purse-string fashion, usually at 14 to 16 weeks if done electively.

3. **Several other procedures** have been described for use primarily when significant dilatation and effacement have already occurred. An example is the **Worm procedure,** which involves suturing across the cervix to prevent further dilatation.

4. A **transabdominal procedure** is rarely performed when a contraindication to the vaginal approach (e.g., a severely hypoplastic cervix) exists.

B. **Indications.** Cerclage is indicated in patients with an incompetent cervical os. Correct diagnosis and identification of the patient at risk is much more important than the choice of procedure.

1. **History.** Historically, a patient is believed to have an incompetent cervix if she has had two or more pregnancy losses in the midtrimester characterized by premature, usually painless, dilatation and effacement of the cervix. Watery discharge, low abdominal pain, or slight vaginal bleeding may be the only premonitory signs.

2. **Diagnostic studies.** Tests can aid in the diagnosis so that repetitive losses are not required before therapy is initiated.

   a. **Passage of a no. 6 or 8 Hegar dilator** through the cervix in the nonpregnant state is consistent with the diagnosis.

    b. **Hysterosalpingography or hysteroscopy** may reveal funneling of the internal os.

    c. **Ultrasonography** early in pregnancy can be helpful if characteristic changes in the cervix or lower segment are seen.

    d. If the diagnosis cannot be firmly established prior to pregnancy, **frequent digital examination of the cervix early in gestation** may reveal changes early enough so that surgery can be performed.

C. Contraindications. Careful selection of patients for cerclage is necessary to ensure success.

    1. **Advanced dilatation of the cervix** makes the operation very difficult and decreases the likelihood of a successful outcome.

    2. **Rupture of the membranes or heavy vaginal bleeding** contraindicates the procedure.

    3. There is no place for cerclage operations in patients with conditions other than incompetent cervical os that are associated with **premature dilatation.** For example, it has been documented that cerclage has no effect on premature labor in twin gestations.

D. Procedure. The Shirodkar procedure, which is the most complicated to perform, is as follows:

    1. With the patient in the dorsal lithotomy position, adequate anesthesia is induced and the operating table is placed in the deep Trendelenburg position.

    2. The cervix is grasped with two or three ring forceps.

    3. Incisions are then made anteriorly and posteriorly in the cervical muscosa, and gentle dissection of these tissues is performed.

    4. A Mersilene strip is then passed around the cervix, using an aneurysm needle. The strip can be tied either anteriorly or posteriorly.

    5. The cut edges of mucosa are than reapproximated with fine catgut.

E. Complications. Serious complications from cerclage are unusual, although they are more common when dilatation of the cervix has already begun.

    1. **Bleeding** may occur, especially when significant dissection is performed during pregnancy.

    2. **Infection,** although uncommon, may occur. The role of prophylactic antibiotics is unresolved.

    3. **Rupture of the membranes** may result, primarily when dilatation of the cervix has occurred.

    4. **Premature labor** may be precipitated by manipulation of the cervix.

III. Forceps delivery

    A. Types and design of forceps. Virtually all obstetric forceps in use today are used as a paired instrument and are articulated by crossing of their shanks. Although sometimes markedly different in size and shape, they have several common components.

1. The **blades** of forceps have two basic curves. The **cephalic curve** is designed to fit the lateral aspects of the fetal head. A second curve, the **pelvic curve,** corresponds to the curve of the maternal pelvis. Depending on the function of the forcep (i.e., traction or rotation), the pelvic curve may vary in degree.

2. The **shanks** of forceps are also variable and are generally classified as either **parallel** (e.g., Simpson) or **overlapping** (e.g., Elliot) (Figs. 10.1 and 10.2).

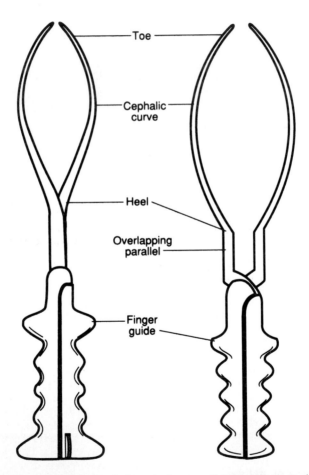

FIGURE 10.1. Components of obstetric forceps. (From Laufe LE, Berkus MD. Assisted Vaginal Delivery: Obstetric Forceps and Vacuum Extraction Techniques. New York: McGraw-Hill; 1992:30. Reprinted with permission.)

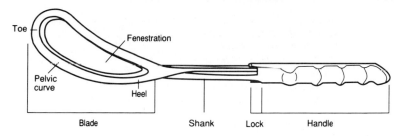

FIGURE 10.2. Anatomy of obstetric forceps (lateral view). (From Laufe LE, Berkus MD. Assisted Vaginal Delivery: Obstetric Forceps and Vacuum Extraction Techniques. New York: McGraw-Hill; 1992:30. Reprinted with permission.)

3. The **locks** are the point of articulation of the forceps, and are named either after the school of teaching where they originated or by function. Most forceps today employ the **English** (Elliot and Simpson types) or the **sliding** (Kielland) lock (Fig. 10.3).

4. The **handles** make up the final division and frequently employ finger grips for added traction.

B. **Operative classification.** As a rule, the type of forcep operation is **classified by the station of the presenting part** at the time of forcep application.

1. **Outlet forceps** require that the fetal scalp be visible without separating the labia, the fetal head positioned on the perineum, the skull reaching the pelvic floor, and rotation (either in the occiput anterior or posterior position) of less than 45°.

2. **Low forceps** deliveries indicate that the fetal head is at +2 station or more, and are classified as rotation of ≤ 45° or > 45°.

3. **Midforceps** deliveries apply to applications to an engaged fetal head above +2 station.

Note: High forceps operations were once used for delivery of the fetus with an unengaged head. Because of the significant risk of this procedure to both mother and infant, they are never indicated in modern obstetric practice.

C. **Indications.** There are two broad indications for use of obstetric forceps—maternal and fetal.

1. **Maternal indications** for use of forceps are primarily those in which there are insufficient labor contractions. Most forceps operations today are prophylactic or elective. DeLee was the first to introduce this concept, with the purpose of sparing both the mother and fetus and effects of prolonged fetal pressure on the perineum. Forceps operations are also frequently performed in cases of maternal exhaustion or in

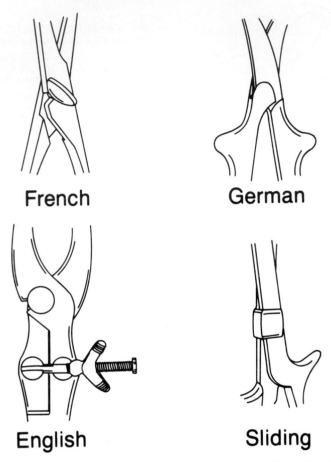

French   German

English   Sliding

FIGURE 10.3. Four types of locks. (From Laufe LE, Berkus MD. Assisted Vaginal Delivery: Obstetric Forceps and Vacuum Extraction Techniques. New York: McGraw-Hill; 1992:31. Reprinted with permission.)

other situations in which maternal expulsive efforts are inadequate for delivery.

2. **Fetal indications**
   a. Provided that delivery can be safely accomplished, **fetal distress** is a valid indication for forceps delivery.
   b. **Disorders of fetal descent and rotation** are the most difficult, and potentially dangerous, situations in which forceps are currently used. Because delivery in these circumstances is potentially dangerous, considerable operator experience is mandatory. Clinical judgment is also extremely important in this circumstance because

of the possibility of cephalopelvic disproportion. Careful clinical assessment is mandatory, and **if a safe and atraumatic forceps delivery is not probable, cesarean section should be used.**

3. **Prerequisites for use of forceps.** Several prerequisite exist for safe forceps delivery.

   a. Above all, the attendant must be familiar and comfortable with the instrument that is being used. This is especially true in difficult deliveries.

   b. The fetus must be presenting either by the vertex or by the face, with the mentum anterior.

   c. The fetal head must be well engaged.

   d. The fetal position must be known. This can usually be accomplished by palpation of the sutures; if this is unsuccessful, palpation of the ear is helpful.

   e. The cervix must be fully dilated. Failure to observe this cardinal rule can result in severe trauma.

   f. The membranes must be ruptured to ensure good application.

   g. The bladder should be empty to decrease the chance of maternal trauma, especially in deliveries requiring rotation. However, routine catheterization prior to all forceps deliveries is not necessary.

D. **Contraindications.** Obviously, forceps delivery is contraindicated if all of the above prerequisites cannot be met. Several additional points should be made, however.

   1. In situations in which there is significant molding of the fetal head and caput formation, vaginal examination may suggest engagement of the fetal head when this does not exist. Careful abdominal palpation is critical to confirm that engagement has occurred.

   2. There should be no likelihood that cephalopelvic disproportion exists prior to attempted delivery.

   3. If the forceps cannot be successfully applied, or if undue trauma is anticipated once traction or rotation is attempted, the procedure should be terminated and cesarean section performed.

      a. **Trial forceps** is defined as an attempt at forceps delivery in which the operator recognizes the possibility that the attempt may be unsuccessful. If the attempt is unsuccessful, a prompt cesarean section is performed.

      b. **Failed forceps** occurs when a vigorous attempt is made to perform vaginal delivery without success, often with resultant maternal and fetal trauma. Operator inexperience contributes significantly to the problem.

E. **Procedure.** The technique for low forceps delivery in the left occipitoanterior position is as follows:

   1. Adequate anesthesia is necessary to ensure cooperation and prevent injury to the mother.

   2. The patient is prepared in the usual manner for vaginal

delivery, with the dorsal lithotomy position preferred and the legs held in stirrups.

3. The fetal position is confirmed.

4. The left branch of the forceps is inserted. This is accomplished by inserting the middle and index fingers of the right hand between the fetal head and the left vaginal sidewall, and using the left thumb and forefinger to hold the handle much like a pencil. The blade is introduced between the head and the vaginal fingers. At this point, the handle should be almost perpendicular to the floor. With the thumb of the right hand facilitating introduction of the blade, the handle is swept gently down in an arc alongside the mother's right leg. The blade should enter without difficulty; if force is required, then the application is not proper.

5. Examination is then performed to determine if the blade is well applied. Some adjustment can be made without removing the blade.

6. The right blade of the forceps is then inserted in an identical fashion, except that all maneuvers are reversed.

7. Next, the blades are articulated. It is sometimes necessary to make minor corrections in the position of the forceps before articulation can be easily accomplished.

8. The correct position is then confirmed by determining that the sagittal suture is equidistant between the forcep blades.

9. Downward traction is then carried out along the pelvic curve, taking care not to squeeze the handles of the forceps. This is most easily done using the Satorph-Pajot maneuver: traction is applied with the right hand on the underside of the handles while the index and middle fingers of the left hand are placed across the shanks and provide downward pressure.

10. An episiotomy is performed as the perineum is stretched, and downward pull is continued until the occiput passes the pubic arch.

11. At this point the fetal head is delivered by extension, maintaining even traction and slowly raising the position of the handles. Once the biparietal diameter has cleared the vulvar ring, the forceps can be removed and the head delivered by the modified Ritgen maneuver.

F. **Complications.** Due to associated factors that are frequently present in forceps deliveries (fetal distress, prolonged labor, etc.), it is difficult to assess accurately the impact of forceps deliveries on obstetric morbidity. Several generalizations can be made.

1. Excluding high forceps, there should be virtually no maternal mortality from forceps deliveries.

2. Maternal morbidity (trauma, blood loss) attributed to forceps is negligible with low forceps and increases to 10 to 20 percent with midforceps.

3. Any increase in fetal morbidity or mortality can be ascribed to **difficult** midforceps deliveries.

IV. **Vacuum extractor**
   A. **Classification.** Until recently, there has been very little experience with the vacuum extractor in the United States, although it has been popular in Europe for some time. There are two types in common use.
   1. The **Malmstrom extractor** is a device consisting of a rigid metallic cup attached to a traction handle by a chain, which is covered by rubber tubing. This apparatus, in turn, is connected to a device for establishing a vacuum. The metal cup is available in several sizes.
   2. The **soft cup (Silastic or Mityvac)** vacuum extractor is the second type available in the United States. Both the Silastic and the Mityvac extractor are made of soft material and are available in only one size.
   B. **Indications.** The indications for use of the vacuum extractor are essentially the same as for forceps. However, several differences do exist.
   1. The vacuum extractor can only be used in **vertex presentations.** Specifically, they cannot be used in face presentations.
   2. **Full cervical dilatation** is strongly recommended, although it is not required prior to use.
   3. Many authors, primarily European, advocate use of the Malmstrom extractor in situations in which there is **malrotation of the fetal head.**
   C. **Contraindications.** Contraindications to the use of vacuum extractors are similar to those for forceps, although there are several exceptions.
   1. The vacuum extractor cannot be used for any **presentation other than vertex.**
   2. Because of an increased risk to the fetus, its use is precluded in the **premature infant.**
   3. Excessive fetal blood loss may occur when the vacuum is applied over **puncture sites used for scalp blood sampling;** therefore its use is contraindicated when this procedure has been performed. The presence of a scalp electrode, however, does not preclude its use.
   4. **Suspected cephalopelvic disproportion** contraindicates vacuum extraction.
   5. **High fetal position,** that is, above O station, also contraindicates vacuum extraction.
   D. **Procedure.** Although their use is similar, differences do exist in the application of the two types of vacuum extractors.
   1. **Malmstrom extractor.** This extractor requires several minutes for correct application.
      a. Although regional anesthesia may be used, local or pudendal anesthesia is usually adequate.
      b. The largest cup possible should be used.
      c. To aid in flexion, the cup should be placed as far posteriorly on the fetal head as possible.

    d.   A vacuum is next established, to a negative pressure of 0.2 kg/cm^2 (150 mm Hg).

    e.   The vacuum is increased every 2 min by the same degree until a pressure of 0.8 kg/cm^2 is obtained (approximately 6 min). This will result in a chignon, or artificial caput, which aids in maintaining suction and traction.

    f.   Traction should then be applied perpendicular to the cup during each contraction. No attempt at fetal rotation should be made or fetal trauma may result; if rotation is needed, it should occur spontaneously as fetal descent takes place.

2. Soft cup vacuum extractor (Silastic or Mityvac). The procedure for using the soft cup is similar, although simpler and less time-consuming.

    a.   The cup is applied to the fetal scalp in a manner similar to that for the Malmstrom extractor (see Section 1.c above).

    b.   The pressure of the vacuum device is set to 100 mm Hg.

    c.   During a contraction, the pressure is increased to 380 to 580 mm Hg (not to exceed 600 mm Hg) and traction is applied).

    d.   The pressure is decreased to 100 mm Hg between contractions.

3. Several general points about the safe use of all vacuum extractors should be made:

    a.   When applying the cup to the fetal scalp, care should be taken that no maternal tissue is caught in the cup.

    b.   If efforts at delivery are unsuccessful after 30 min or if no descent occurs after attempts during three contractions, the procedure should be terminated and cesarean section performed.

E. Complications

1. Maternal complications are unusual and are usually limited to **lacerations of the birth canal** secondary to poor application of the cup.

2. Fetal complications are more common but fortunately are generally minor.

    a.   The most serious complication is **intracranial bleeding,** which is rare and occurs more often in premature infants.

    b.   **Abrasions and lacerations of the scalp** can occur but are usually minor if proper technique is followed.

    c.   **Cephalohematomas** are occasionally seen.

    d.   The chignon that develops resolves rapidly and should be of no consequence.

BIBLIOGRAPHY

Branch DW. Operations for cervical incompetence. Clin Obstet Gynecol 1986; 29(2):240–254.

Druzin ML, Berkeley AS. A simplified approach to Shirodkar cerclage procedure. Surg Gynecol Obstet 1986; 162:375–376.

Harger JH. Comparison for success and morbidity in cervical cerclage procedures. Obstet Gynecol 1980; 56:543–548.

Interim report of the medical research council/Royal College of Obstetricians and Gynaecologists multicentre randomized trial of cervical cerclage. Br J Obstet Gynaecol 1988; 95:437–445.

Scheerer LJ, Lam F, Bartolucci L, et al. A new technique for reduction of prolapsed fetal membranes for emergency cervical cerclage. Obstet Gynecol 1989; 74:408–410.

Shortle B, Jewelewicz R. Cervical incompetence. Fertil Steril 1989; 52:181–188.

Witter FR. Soft-cup vacuum extractors safely assist normal deliveries. Contemp Ob/Gyn 1986; 26(suppl):109–118.

CHAPTER 11

Abnormal Labor

Aldo D. Khoury
Sharon T. Phelan

I. Definitions

A. **Normal labor** (see Chapter 4) is the timely and consistent progression of dilatation of the cervix and the descent of the presenting part, propelled by uterine contractions and eventually maternal effort through the bony pelvis. This can be summarized graphically by a Friedman curve (Fig. 11.1)

B. **Dystocia** is difficult labor or childbirth. Abnormalities of the fetus, the maternal pelvis, or uterine contractions can cause dystocia. According to a National Center for Health Statistics Report, dystocia accounted for 28 percent of all cesarean sections performed in 1987.

   1. **Cephalopelvic disproportion (CPD)** is stated to be:
      a. **Absolute** when the size of the fetal head, whether or not it presents optimally, is disparate from the size of the maternal pelvis.
      a. **Relative** when asynclitism, or extension of the fetal head, causes a bony diameter too great to pass through the maternal pelvis.

   2. First-stage abnormalities of labor complicate 8 to 11 percent of all cephalic deliveries.
      a. **Prolonged latent phase** is one > 20 h in a nullipara and > 14 h in a multipara.
      b. **Protracted active phase** dilatation (protracted dilatation) is one that demonstrates a slope of dilatation < 1.2 cm/h in a nullipara and < 1.5 cm/h in a multipara after achieving at least 4 cm dilation.
      c. **Secondary arrest** of **dilatation** is diagnosed when the cervix is dilated ≥ 4 cm and there is no further cervical dilatation after 2 h of adequately intense contractions.

   3. Second-stage abnormalities complicate 8 to 10 percent of all cephalic deliveries.
      a. **Protracted descent** is a slope of descent < 1 cm/h in a nullipara and < 2 cm/h in a multipara.
      b. **Secondary arrest** of **descent** is diagnosed when there is no descent after 1 h.

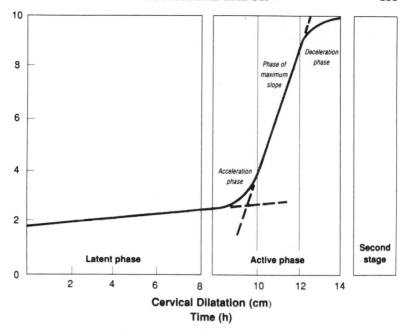

FIGURE 11.1. Composite of the average dilatation curve for nulliparous labor. (From Friedman EA. Labor: Clinical Evaluation and Management. 2nd ed. New York: Appleton-Century-Crofts; 1978.)

II. Power abnormalities of labor

A. Normal contractions in active labor should occur every 2 to 5 min and should be of sufficient intensity that the uterus cannot be indented when palpated. If there is normal progression of labor, it is assumed that the contractions are of adequate intensity. If there is a disorder of dilatation, the adequacy of intensity of the contractions must be verified.

While the frequency and duration of the contractions can be determined by palpation or external tocodynamometry, the intensity of contractions can be accurately measured only by an intrauterine pressure monitor. In spontaneous labor, the amplitude of the contractions will range from 25 to 75 mm Hg, with a frequency of 2 to 5 min. These will achieve Montevideo units of 100 to 400 (Fig. 11.2).

During the second stage of labor, maternal effort assists the uterine contractions in prompting fetal descent. Since the pressure generated by good maternal effort will exceed 100 mm Hg, the intensity of the contractions is not a major issue during the second stage. However, the frequency of the contractions is critical, ideally occurring every 2 to 3 min.

B. **Cause**

1. **Prolonged latent phase** is not associated with CPD or an adverse perinatal outcome and is not predictive of subse-

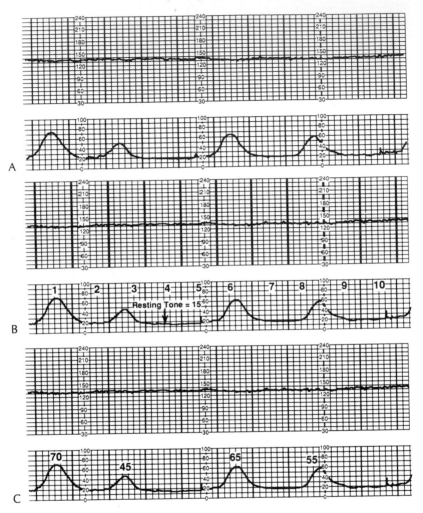

FIGURE 11.2. Quantification of uterine activity by Montevideo units (MVUs). (A) A segment of the fetal monitor strip with an internal pressure catheter in place is utilized. (B) A 10-min segment is identified, and the uterine resting tone is quantitated. (C) The peak pressure of each contraction is noted, and the MVUs are calculated as the sum of net pressures during the 10-min period. In the above example, the MVU = (70-15) + (45-15) + (65-15) + (55-15) = 175.

quent abnormalities of labor. A definite cause is usually not determined, but it may be associated with maternal sedation or anesthesia. Distinction from false labor may be possible only in retrospect.

2. Protracted active phase may also be associated with excessive maternal sedation or anesthesia. An increased incidence of CPD is seen in this condition, accounting for approximately 30 percent of cases. Minor degrees of fetal malpresentation are also increased.

3. **Secondary arrest** of **dilatation** occurs with increased frequency in patients with protracted labor patterns. CPD occurs in about 50 percent of severe cases, and fetal malpresentations are common.

4. **Descent disorders** are frequently associated with abnormal dilatation patterns and have the same causes. Maternal expulsive efforts are also important, and inability to cooperate may be secondary to excessive regional anesthesia or neuromuscular disease.

C. **Treatment**

1. Uterine hypotonia may be a response to CPD and thus should be assessed when abnormalities of labor occur.

Assuming that there is no fetal intolerance of labor and that the only identified cause for the dystocia is uterine hypotonia, the primary mode of therapy is augmentation of labor with intravenous (IV) pitocin. Since pitocin administration can cause overstimulation of the uterus, with resulting fetal compromise and potential uterine rupture, it is imperative that during administration the fetus and the mother are closely monitored. Continuous fetal monitoring is recommended. If the diagnosis of inadequate contractions has been made based on inadequate frequency of contractions, an intrauterine pressure monitor need not be in place. It may be acceptable to augment labor without an intrauterine monitor in these situations. However, in most cases, an intrauterine pressure catheter will allow one to determine the intensity of the uterine contractions in response to the pitocin dose given. Ideally, one should strive for 200 to 250 Montevideo units.

2. Pitocin administration has risks, as noted above. Each labor and delivery unit should have written guidelines for pitocin augmentation/induction. Basic requirements include the following:

a. A primary IV line should be established.

b. The pitocin solution should be piggybacked into the main line as close to the IV line as possible.

c. Intrapartum pitocin should be administered only through an infusion pump.

d. Continuous fetal and uterine monitoring is necessary.

3. Usually 10 or 20 U of pitocin is mixed in 1000 mL of isotonic crystalloid solution. The rate of infusion will vary among institutions and according to whether it is for augmentation or induction. For augmentation the usual starting dose is 0.5 to 1.0 mU/min, with increases of 1 to 2 mU/min at regular intervals until adequate labor is achieved, fetal intolerance occurs, or a maximum dose (approximately 30

mU/min) is reached. The rate of the increase will vary from every 15 minutes (aggressive therapy or active management) to every 60 minutes (conservative or low-dose approach). For induction the initial dose is commonly 1.0 mU/min, with increases of 1 to 4 mU/min at regular intervals. The potential advantages of low-dose infusion include lower total dosage, less hyperstimulation, and the same duration of labor as with the aggressive approach. Proponents of active management cite a lower number of cesarean sections. The ideal approach is unresolved.

4. If hyperstimulation or "camelbacking" of the contractions (frequency of contractions is so rapid that there is no return to baseline between them) occurs, the pitocin must be stopped immediately. If fetal intolerance is marked, a tocolytic such as $MgSO_4$ or terbutaline can be given to encourage uterine relaxation. Once the fetus has recovered, pitocin administration may be resumed at a lower level.

5. Specific recommendations regarding therapy for the various abnormalities of labor are outlined in Table 11.1. Prolonged latent phase is unique in that pitocin augmentation or maternal sedation can be used for therapy. The effect of amniotomy on the conduct of spontaneous labor is controversial and unresolved.

6. If adequate contractions cannot be achieved with pitocin administration or if, despite the stimulation of adequate contractions, labor as defined above fails to progress, then delivery by cesarean section may be warranted.

Table 11.1. Abnormal Labor Patterns, Diagnostic Criteria, and Treatment

LABOR PATTERN	NULLI-GRAVIDA	MULTIPARA	TREATMENT
Prolonged latent phase	> 20 h	> 14 h	Rest or oxytocin
Protraction disorders Dilation	< 1.2 cm/h	< 1.5 cm/h	Oxytocin if contractions are inadequate
Descent	< 1.0 cm/h	< 2.0 cm/h	
Arrest disorders Dilation	> 2 h	> 2 h	Oxytocin if contractions are inadequate
Descent	> 1 h	> 1 h	Forceps, vacuum, or cesarean delivery

Source: American College of Obstetricians and Gynecologists. Dystocia. ACOG Technical Bulletin No. 137. Washington, DC: ACOG © December 1989.

7. For second-stage protracted or arrested descent in the absence of fetal distress, the treatment needs to be directed to the cause of insufficient expulsive forces.
   a. If the **frequency** of the contractions has become inadequate (e.g., after the birth of the first twin), then gentle pitocin augmentation may be useful.
   b. **Maternal exhaustion** can be addressed by either rest (especially if an epidural block is in place) or assistance with forceps or vacuum.
   c. If an **excessive anesthetic block** is interfering with the urge to push, allowing it to wear off will often be effective.
   d. In cases where **pushing is** contraindicated or not possible (cardiac or neuromuscular diseases), uterine contractions should gradually cause fetal descent to a level where forceps or vacuum can be used to effect delivery.

III. **Passenger abnormalities**
   A. **Definition.** Any problem with fetal presentation, size, or anatomy may prevent the fetus from negotiating the maternal pelvis despite adequate contractions.
   B. **Cause**
      1. Abnormal presentations or positions may result in dystocia.
         a. **Nonlongitudinal fetal presentations,** including the transverse/shoulder presentation, occur in 1/320 deliveries.
         b. **Nonvertex cephalic presentations** will cause a larger fetal diameter to present to the maternal pelvis, possibly resulting in relative CPD. Examples include a face (1/600 deliveries) or brow presentation.
         c. An **occiput posterior** position may cause difficulty in the fetal head's negotiation of the maternal pelvic curve.
         d. A **compound presentation** occurs when the hand or arm prolapses alongside the vertex (1/700 deliveries). This makes the relative diameter larger and may interfere with descent.
         e. **Asynclitism** of the presenting part will cause a larger bony diameter to present. Predisposing factors are inductions when the vertex is not engaged and/or a pelvic architectural abnormality is missed. They result in over-expression of one side of the head compared to the other during descent. The sagittal suture is not in the midplane of descent. This may also present as a protracted labor pattern.
      2. **Fetal macrosomia** will cause dystocia not only because of the larger and less moldable head with increasing weight but also because of entrapment of the larger shoulders at the pelvic brim or outlet. Factors that increase the likelihood of fetal macrosomia include large size of the mother, multiparity, maternal diabetes, maternal obesity, excessive maternal

weight gain, prolonged gestation, and a history of a prior macrosomic infant. Estimations of fetal macrosomia even by ultrasound are frequently very inaccurate. If clinically macrosomia appears to be present, one should monitor the labor pattern closely for evidence of dystocia.

3. **Anomalies of fetal anatomy** can also cause dystocia. These can include hydrocephalus (1/2000 fetuses), as well as a large fetal abdomen from tumor, ascites or distended bladder, or conjoined twins. Due to the increased use of ultrasound antenatally, this has become a rare cause of undiagnosed dystocia. Still, ultrasound evaluation should be considered in labor when the examination results are unusual or when there is a persistently high (floating) presentation.

C. **Treatment**

1. In the cases of malpresentation, one must determine if vaginal delivery is possible. In the cases of transverse lie and face with mentum posterior, vaginal delivery cannot occur. The other vertex positions or asynclitism may cause relative CPD that requires rotation of the fetal presentation either manually or with forceps. If this is unsuccessful or if the attendant does not possess these skills, a cesarean section is indicated. For example, an occiput posterior position will prolong the second stage by 1 to 2 h and may eventually result in arrest of descent. If the head can be rotated to an occiput anterior position, delivery may proceed normally. Compound presentations in particular will usually resolve if the presenting extremity is causing labor dysfunction. However, occasionally one may need to try to replace the extremity.

2. The presence of macrosomia requires careful clinical pelvimetry to assess the probability of a successful vaginal delivery. One suggested method for determining if CPD is the cause for a labor arrest is the Muller-Hills maneuver. The impression of easy downward movement of the presenting part in response to fundal pressure suggests that CPD is not the cause of the dystocia. Due to the fear of shoulder dystocia, some advocate elective cesarean section in cases of macrosomia, especially if estimated fetal weight is > 4500 g in diabetic mothers.

3. In many cases, particularly in the primigravida, the active management of labor, which includes amniotomy, oxytocin, and aggressive treatment of arrest or protraction disorders, may be helpful in preventing cesarean section deliveries previously labeled as CPD (see Section II). However, once CPD is diagnosed, further pitocin administration or attempted forceps delivery is unwarranted and a cesarean section should be done.

4. The presence of conjoined twins or fetal tumor may necessitate a cesarean section. Fetal hydrocephalus, if associated with macrosomia, also is usually managed by cesarean sec-

tion. Needle aspiration (cephalocentesis) may be indicated in severe cases, but may result in fetal death and should be done only in extreme cases after careful counseling of the parents. Dystocia caused by fetal ascites, bladder distention, or other cystic masses may be avoided by needle aspiration of the cystic structure. The fetal risk in this procedure must be balanced against the risk of abdominal delivery.

5. The risks of mismanagement of dystocia are great. Fetal risks include injury from malpositioned forceps or inappropriate attempts at forceps delivery, infection, intracranial hemorrhage, fractures of the skull, and shoulder dystocia, resulting in injury or death. Maternal risks include abnormal thinning of the lower uterine segment with possible uterine rupture, pressure necrosis of the bladder, pelvic lacerations, postpartum hemorrhage due to uterine atony, and increased risk of postpartum infection.

IV. Passageway abnormalities

A. **Definition.** Passageway abnormalities include any soft tissue mass or bony abnormality that causes a distortion or blockage of the pelvic curve and prevents fetal descent. Only 1 percent of pregnant women will have a clearly inadequate pelvis, and an additional 13 to 14 percent will have a borderline pelvis.

B. **Cause**
1. Most bony pelvic abnormalities are due to contractions from the normal gynecoid pelvis (see Chapter 4). These can be determined clinically or radiographically. The following factors indicate a possible contracted pelvis:
   a. The ability to touch the sacral promontory with the index finger
   b. Significant convergence of the pelvic side walls
   c. Forward inclination of a straight sacrum
   d. Sharp ischial spines with a narrow interspinous diameter
   e. Narrow pubic arch
   d. Adolescent pregnancy
2. Pelvic contracture may occur at the level of inlet, at the midpelvis, or at the pelvic outlet.
   a. Contracted pelvic inlet: at this level the two most important diameters are the anteroposterior and transverse diameters. A diagonal conjugate < 11.5 cm or an obstetric conjugate < 10 cm plus a transverse diameter < 12 cm (by x-ray pelvimetry) are considered to be evidence of a contracted pelvic inlet. Pelvic inlet disproportion can be diagnosed by radiologic pelvimetry and clinically when adequate labor fails to result in engagement of the fetal head.
   b. Midpelvic contracture is more an impression of decreased size or a nongynecoid shape than of actual measurement. It may be suspected when the ischial spines are prominent, with an interspinous diameter

< 10 cm, the anteroposterior diameter is short, the pelvic side walls are converging, and the sacrosciatic notch is narrow. This type of pelvic contracture is the most common cause of deep transverse arrest.

c. Pelvic outlet contractures occur when the intertuberous diameter is < 8 cm, with a narrow pubic arch leading to a decrease in the anterior triangle area, pushing the fetal head posteriorly during descent and increasing the possibility of significant perineal injury. Pelvic outlet contractures usually coexist with a contracture in the midpelvis. Therefore, it is important to assess both entities, especially before a forceps delivery is attempted.

3. Pelvic abnormalities and maternal diseases include kyphosis, scoliosis, childhood diseases such as rickets and poliomyelitis, and pelvic fractures due to trauma.

a. **Kyphosis** affects the pelvis mainly when the curvature is in the lumbar region; the pelvis is typically funnel-shaped, so that the arrest of labor invariably occurs late.

b. **Scoliosis,** like kyphosis, depends on the region affected. Lower vertebral column lesions will move the sacral promontory to one side, giving the pelvic brim an irregular shape.

c. **Childhood rickets** is always associated with a true conjugate between 9 and 10 cm, frequently causing CPD.

d. Motor vehicle accidents are responsible for the majority of **pelvic fractures;** however, in many cases where healing takes place in an appropriate and satisfactory fashion, no significant change occurs in either the size or the shape of the pelvis and the probability of vaginal delivery is high. Assessment of such pelves may be done prior to conception by x-ray pelvimetry. Otherwise, thorough pelvic assessment is mandatory and a trial of labor, unless absolutely contraindicated, should be the ultimate test of pelvic capacity.

4. Soft tissue problems can be organized by the structure of origin.

a. Vaginal scarring following injury or surgery, extreme vulvar edema, vaginal septum, or vaginal neoplasm may cause protracted or arrested descent. A tetanic contraction of the levator ani may interfere with descent.

b. The only cervical processes that tend to cause difficulty are cervical stenosis from prior cone/cauterization or extensive cervical carcinoma or condyloma.

c. Pelvic tumors, especially if they are positioned in the posterior cul-de-sac, may block the pelvic inlet. These include myomas (especially cervical or lower uterine), ovarian tumors, pelvic kidney, sacral teratoma, and spinal tumors including fibromas, osteomas, chondromas, and sacromas.

    d. Pelvic adipose tissue in morbidly obese women (> 135 kg) can be excessive, and CPD can occur despite adequate bony structure and uterine contractions. This should be suspected when CPD is diagnosed in the absence of significant molding.

    5. Finally, epidural analgesia may increase midpelvic arrest disorders from failure of rotation from a transverse position to an occiput anterior (or posterior) position due to decreased tone of the pelvic floor muscles.

C. Treatment. Treatment requires identification of the abnormality. With degrees of pelvic contractions incompatible with vaginal delivery, the cervix seldom dilates satisfactorily. Thus, the behavior of the cervix has prognostic value in regard to the outcome of labor in women with inlet contraction.

In the management of a labor complicated by a midpelvic contraction, the main approach is to allow the natural forces of labor to push the biparietal diameter beyond the potential interspinous obstruction. Forceps delivery, if attempted prior to the passage of the biparietal diameter through the midpelvis, will be difficult. Problems will occur because (1) pulling on the fetal head with forceps destroys flexion, whereas pressure from above increases it, and (2) although the forceps occupy only a few millimeters, this may be enough to prevent descent. In most cases, delivery is accomplished by cesarean section. Timely operative delivery is critical since neglected labor with pelvic contracture may result in uterine rupture.

V. Overview of the management of dystocia. During the management of labor, the practitioner should keep in mind the normal labor curve described by Friedman. Deviations from this curve should be actively and aggressively evaluated. Obvious CPD needs to be identified first. If it is present, operative delivery should be undertaken. If the fetal presentation is compatible with the maternal pelvis and there is no evidence of fetal compromise, then the quality of the contractions should be assessed. If they are found to be inadequate in frequency or intensity, pitocin augmentation should be initiated. If contractions cannot be made adequate or if, despite adequate labor, progression does not occur, then operative delivery should be undertaken.

BIBLIOGRAPHY

Akoury HA, MacDonald FJ, Brodie G, et al. Oxytocin augmentation of labor and perinatal outcome in nulliparas. Ob Gyn 1991; 78:227–230.

Friedman E. Labor: Clinical Evaluation and Management. 2nd edition. New York: Appleton-Century-Crofts; 1978.

Hauth JC, Hankins GDV, Gilstrap LC. Uterine contraction pressures achieved in parturients with active phase arrest. Ob Gyn 1991; 78:344–347.

Hayashi R. Induction and augmentation of labor. ACOG Technical Bulletin No. 110; November 1987.

Mercer B, Pilgrim P, Sibai B. Labor induction with continuous low-dose oxytocin infusion: A random trial. Ob Gyn 1991; 77:659–663.

O'Driscoll K, Foley M, MacDonald D. Active management of labor as an alternative to cesarean section for dystocia. Ob Gyn 1984; 63:485–490.

Perkins R. Dystocia. ACOG Technical Bulletin No. 137; December 1989.

Schifrin BS, Cohen WR. Labor's dysfunctional lexicon. Ob Gyn 1989; 74:121–124.

CHAPTER 12

Abnormal Fetal Lie, Including the Breech

Stanley Gall

I. **Fetal accommodation to the maternal pelvis**
   A. **Mechanisms of labor.** The fetus must accommodate itself to the configuration of the maternal pelvis in order to pass through the birth canal during labor. These postural adjustments made by the fetus are called the *mechanisms of labor.*
   B. **Lie.** An important event that will determine the mechanisms of labor is the manner in which the fetus presents itself to the pelvis. The term *lie* describes the spatial relationship of the fetal spine to the maternal spine. If the two spines are parallel, the lie is longitudinal; if they are perpendicular, the lie is transverse. Intermediate relationships are called *oblique lies.*
   C. **Presentation** describes the most dependant part of the fetus lying closest to the pelvic inlet. Therefore, the part of the fetus felt by the examiner on vaginal examination is the presenting part. More than 95 percent of term infants present cephalically.
   D. **Position** describes the relationship between a fetal reference point and the maternal pelvis. The fetal reference points are the occiput for vertex presentation, the chin for face presentation, the sacrum for breech presentation, and the scapula for the transverse lie.
   E. **Attitude** refers to the relationship of the fetal parts to each other, particularly that of the fetal head to the spine. Flexion of the head so that the chin is against the chest wall is the most common attitude. The arms are usually folded in front of the body, the body curves forward, and the legs are flexed at the hips and knees.
   F. **Abnormal presentations** refer to all presentations other than vertex. The frank breech presentation has been thought to be a variant of normal, but in today's obstetrics, the breech presentation must be considered abnormal and as demanding special care.
      1. **Breech presentation** refers to the fetal buttocks, and the engagement of the fetal buttocks at the maternal pelvic inlet is referred to as a *breech presentation.* The sacrum is the arbitrarily chosen part of the fetus used to describe the fetal

orientation to the maternal pelvis. Breech presentations are classified as frank breech, complete breech, and incomplete breech. Of all breech births, the frank breech is present in 67 percent, the complete breech in 3 percent, and the incomplete breech in 30 percent.

   a. Frank breech is present when the legs are flexed at the hip and extended at the knees.

   b. Complete breech is present when one or both knees are flexed rather than both extended.

   c. Incomplete breech is present when one or both hips are not flexed and one or both feet or knees lie below the breech. (Also called footling breech.)

2. **Transverse lie** is a presentation in which the long axis of the fetus is approximately perpendicular to that of the mother, while the shoulder is usually presenting over the pelvic inlet.

3. **Face presentation** involves hyperextension of the head so that the occiput is in contact with the fetal back and the chin is the presenting part. In the brow presentation, the portion of the fetal head between the anterior fontanel and the orbital ridge presents at the pelvic inlet, with the fetal head occupying a middle position between full flexion (cephalic) and extension (face).

4. **Compound presentation** is a presentation in which an extremity is present alongside the presenting part and both are entering the pelvis simultaneously.

II. **Incidence of abnormal presentation.** The incidence of abnormal presentation is related to gestational age, as shown in Table 12.1. As term approaches, the incidence of cephalic presentation increases, while that of other presentations decreases. For example, at the beginning of the third trimester, the incidence of breech presentation is about 20 percent, a situation that complicates the management of

Table 12.1. Fetal Presentation at Various Gestational Ages Determined Sonographically

GESTATION (WEEKS INCLUSIVE)	TOTAL NO.	CEPHALIC (%)	BREECH (%)	OTHER (%)
21–24	264	54.6	33.3	12.1
25–28	367	61.9	27.8	10.4
29–32	443	78.1	14.0	7.9
33–36	638	88.7	8.8	2.5
37–40	463	91.5	6.7	1.7

Source: Modified from Scheer K, Nobar J. Variation of fetal presentation with gestational age. Am J Obstet Gynecol 1976; 125:269.

obstetric problems such as preterm premature rupture of membranes (PROM). Although a study by Scheer and Nubar lists the incidence of breech presentation at 6.7 percent, the gestational age is listed as 37 to 40 weeks. It is recognized that the incidence of breech presentation in labor at 40 weeks is 3 to 4 percent. The incidence of other abnormal presentations at 40 weeks gestation is as follows: face presentation, 0.2 percent; brow presentation, 0.05 percent; shoulder presentation, 0.3 percent; compound presentation, 0.14 percent.

III. **Morbidity and mortality.** The morbidity and mortality of the fetus for abnormal presentations are higher than for vertex presentations.
   A. **Breech presentation**
      1. **Maternal effects.** The maternal morbidity in breech presentations is greater than for vertex presentations because (a) the effacements and dilatation of the cervix are less predictable, (b) vaginal and perineal lacerations are more common, and (c) aberrations in the mechanisms of labor occur more often and require operative interference. Labor is usually not prolonged in breech presentations.
      2. **Fetal effects.** The prognosis for the fetus in a breech presentation is considerably worse than that for a vertex presentation.
         a. **Mortality.** It is important to stress that contrary to popular belief among some physicians, multigravid patients experience breech mortality far in excess of primigravid women (Table 12.2). At every stage of gestation — antepartum, intrapartum, and neonatal — deaths are significantly greater in breech births.
         b. **Apgar scores.** For infants surviving breech delivery by any means, the average Apgar score is lower than for those who are delivered from a cephalic presentation.
         c. **Birth anoxia and cord accidents.** Birth anoxia, characterized by metabolic acidosis in the immediate neonatal period and a depressed 5-min Apgar score of 6 or less, occurs more frequently in breech than cephalic pre-

Table 12.2. Maternal Parity and Breech Perinatal Mortality

MATERNAL PARITY	NO. OF CASES	PERINATAL DEATHS	PERINATAL MORTALITY RATE
Primigravida	109	13	123
Multigravida	118	16	136

Source: Adapted from Mansani FE, Cerutti M. The risk in breech delivery. In: Contribution to Gynecology and Obstetrics, Vol 3. Basel: Karger; 1977:86–90.

sentations, owing largely to the increased incidence of umbilical cord prolapse and difficulty in delivering the aftercoming head. The incidence of cord prolapse in cephalic presentation is approximately 0.5 percent; it is significantly higher in breech presentations (Table 12.3).

    d. **Traumatic injury.** A fundamental difference exists between delivery in cephalic and breech presentations. With the cephalic presentation, the largest structure, the head, is delivered first, with the remainder of the body following without difficulty, whereas with the breech presentation, successively larger and less compressible parts of the fetus are delivered. Therefore, an assessment of the size of the infant and the size of the pelvis must be made prior to labor. The efficiency of the laboring process is not predictable in advance. It is appreciated that the fetus may not be deliverable via the vaginal route and, in fact, may become impacted in the pelvis. This has led to traumatic injuries of the fetus, including the brain, spinal cord, liver, adrenal glands, and spleen, in decreasing order of frequency of injury.

    e. **Birth weight.** During the second half of pregnancy, the birth weight at any gestational age is less for breech infants than for nonbreech infants.

    f. **Congenital abnormalities** occur more frequently in breech deliveries (6.3 percent) than in nonbreech deliveries (2.4 percent).

B. **Shoulder, brow, or face presentations.** The morbidity and mortality in unattended labor of fetuses with either a shoulder presentation or a brow presentation is 100 percent since neither can successfully be delivered vaginally and cesarean section is required. A similar statement could be made for the face presentation when the mentum is posterior.

C. **Compound presentation.** The morbidity of the compound presentation is almost entirely related to associated cord prolapse or compression, causing fetal distress. Therefore, with signs of fetal intolerance of labor, cesarean delivery should be done.

Table 12.3. Incidence of Cord Prolapse in Breech Presentation

STUDY	OVERALL INCIDENCE (%)	TYPE OF BREECH PRESENTATION		
		FRANK (%)	INCOMPLETE (%)	COMPLETE (%)
Moore & Steptoe (1943)	4.4	0.9	10.9	4.4
Hall et al. (1965)	3.7	1.2	10.3	5.3
Morley (1967)	4.1	4.1	0.0	5.1

IV. Cause. The cause of abnormal presentations, especially breech presentations, has been discussed for decades. With any abnormal presentation, one must always conclude that something has prevented the fetus from assuming a vertex presentation. The vertex position results from the accommodation of the fetal ovoid head to the inlet of the pelvis, as the compact fetal head fits into the pelvis better than the more diffuse buttocks. Abnormal presentations may be due to the following conditions:

A. Uterine aberrations of abnormal shape (especially bicornuate uterus), presence of tumors, polyhydramnios, and great multiparity, causing laxness of the anterior wall of the uterus

B. Fetal factors such as premature, multiple fetuses or an anomalous fetus

C. Pelvic factors such as a severely contracted pelvis or fetopelvic disproportion

D. Placental factors such as cornual-fundal implantations, as well as placental previa.

V. Diagnosis
   A. Breech presentation
      1. Abdominal examination. Inspection of the abdomen rarely allows the diagnosis of a breech presentation, but on occasion a rounded mass will be visible through a very thin abdominal wall. **Leopold's maneuvers** will demonstrate a hard spherical mass present in the fundus, and gentle ballottement of the head will confirm the initial impression. The second maneuver should reveal the location of the fetal back, and the third maneuver allows the examiner to palpate the breech if engagement has not occurred. Auscultation of the fetal heart usually reveals the heart tones to be loudest in the upper abdomen.

      2. Pelvic examination. The fetal anal orifice is usually distinguishable on vaginal examination. Both ischial tuberosities and the sacrum are easily palpable. The external genitalia of the fetus can usually be recognized. The examiner must be particularly careful if labor has been prolonged, as the buttocks may be markedly edematous, making differentiation of the face and breech difficult. The anus may be mistaken for the mouth and the ischial tuberosities for the malar prominences. Another common error is to mistake the anus for a closed fingertip cervix when in reality the cervix is fully effaced and dilated. The most accurate information is based on the location of the sacrum and its spinous processes, which establishes the diagnosis of position and variety.

      3. Ultrasound exam. The clinical finding of a breech presentation may be confirmed with ultrasonography. The location and size of the head, the degree of flexion of the fetus, and the position of the lower limbs may be viewed. Fetal anomalies that may be the cause of the breech presentation can be detected, as well as the amount of amniotic fluid, uterine abnormalities, or abnormal position of the placenta.

    4. Radiography. Radiographic confirmation of the diagnosis of breech presentation is used less often but may be combined with pelvimetry if vaginal delivery is contemplated.

B. Transverse lie (shoulder presentation). The early diagnosis of transverse lie may be the most important factor in reducing morbidity. In one study, 16.1 percent of patients with a transverse lie presented with a prolapse of either the cord or an extremity.

    1. Abdominal examination. The diagnosis of a transverse lie is usually made by visual inspection of the width from side to side and a diminished fundal height. On palpation with the first maneuver of Leopold, no fetal pole is felt in the fundus; on the second maneuver, a ballottable head is found in one iliac fossa and the buttocks in the other. The third and fourth maneuvers are negative unless labor is far advanced, with the shoulder impacted in the pelvis.

    2. Vaginal examination. The findings on vaginal examination are variable. If the patient is in early labor with intact membranes, the pelvis may be empty or the side of the fetal thorax may be recognized by palpation. With more advanced labor, the fetal scapula and the clavicle are distinguishable on opposite sides of the thorax. The shoulder may become tightly impacted and wedged into the pelvis, frequently with a hand and arm prolapsed.

C. Face presentation

    1. Physical examination. The diagnosis of face presentation is rarely if ever made on abdominal examination, but rather depends on vaginal examination. The most important finding by the examiner is that the usual features expected in a vertex presentation are absent and numerous "bumps" are palpated. Once this is realized, the distinctive features of the face, nose, molar bones, and orbital ridges can be discerned.

    2. Radiography. The radiographic demonstration of the hyperextended head at the pelvic inlet is characteristic.

D. Brow presentation. The diagnosis of brow presentation can be made on abdominal examination when both the occiput and the chin can be palpated. However, in reality, vaginal examination is required. Since neither the mouth nor the chin is palpated, the frontal sutures, large anterior frontanel, orbital ridges of the eyes, and bridge of the nose will present.

E. Compound presentation. The diagnosis is made by vaginal examination when an extremity or part of an extremity presents alongside the presenting part and both are entering the pelvis simultaneously.

VI. Management. The presence of congenital malformations should be sought in any patient with breech presentation.

A. General considerations. Safe vaginal delivery may be possible for selected fetuses with weights of 2500 to 3800 g in the breech position, but for all abnormal presentations, cesarean section is generally preferable.

  1. Cesarean delivery of abnormal presentations. Once the diagnosis of abnormal presentation is made, the appropriate course of action in most situations is delivery by cesarean section. In fact, because of the potential for increased morbidity and mortality as well as for litigation, one should plan to deliver all patients with abnormal lies by cesarean section. An occasional delivery by the vaginal route may be preferred (see Bibliography).

  2. Version as prophylaxis. When abnormal presentations are recognized during the third trimester, some obstetricians believe that external version should be attempted. External version, if properly and gently performed, carries little danger. The procedure is performed in the hospital, with tocolytics given as indicated. The optimal time for successful external version has been debated. The earlier in gestation the procedure is performed, the higher the success rate. However, version prior to 37 weeks is associated with a high rate of reversion to breech, and the spontaneous version rate prior to this time is high. Success rates of 60 to 70 percent after 37 weeks of gestation are widely reported. Ranney (1973) decreased the overall frequency of breech delivery to 0.6 percent, which is one-sixth the expected incidence, but it is unlikely that anyone can duplicate his results. Enthusiasm for external version is not shared by all clinicians. **Various complications** have been described and include **antepartum hemorrhage, abruptio placenta, premature labor, fetal death,** and **premature rupture of membranes.** Significant **fetal-maternal hemorrhage** has also been identified. Therefore immunoprophylaxis with anti-D globulin should be considered for the unsensitized Rh⁻ patient on whom external version is to be attempted.

B. Management for specific abnormal presentations

  1. Breech presentation

    a. Cesarean section. Because of the significant increase in perinatal mortality with vaginal delivery in breech presentation, the role of mortality in cesarean delivery must be reviewed. As Table 12.4 shows, despite a significantly increased cesarean delivery rate for breeches, the perinatal mortality rate is still approximately four times that of the general population. Analysis of the breech perinatal deaths in the series from which Table 12.4 is taken shows 15 antepartum stillbirths and 21 neonatal deaths. Six of twenty-one neonatal deaths were due to congenital malformations incompatible with life, and six neonates weighed less than 1000 g. Nine neonatal deaths occurred with birth weights between 1000 and

Table 12.4. Role of Cesarean Section in Management of Breech Presentations

		CESAREAN RATE	PERINATAL MORTALITY
Total births	11,585	9.3%	21
Breech deliveries	375	67.5%	96

Source: Adapted from Collea JV, Weghorst GR, Paul RH, et al. Singleton breech presentation: One year's experience. In Contribution to Gynecology and Obstetrics, Vol 3. Basel: Karger; 1977:91–98.

1840 g, with four of the nine infants delivered by cesarean section.

b. **Breech vaginal delivery.** Vaginal delivery may be considered for a frank breech at the discretion of the attending physician and with the informed consent of the mother if the following conditions are present:

(1) The pelvis is judged to be adequate to large, as confirmed by x-ray pelvimetry.

(2) The fetus is judged to be of average size or smaller.

(3) The fetal head is flexed.

(4) Spontaneous labor has occurred, and there is normal progress in labor with regard to dilation and effacement of the cervix and descent of the breech in the pelvis.

(5) Appropriate anesthesia is present.

Note: Techniques for effecting breech delivery may be obtained from any standard obstetric textbook or from ACOG Technical Bulletin No. 95 (see the Bibliography).

2. **Transverse lie (shoulder presentation).** The management of the patient in active labor with a transverse lie is cesarean delivery. The lower uterine segment may not be developed because of the lack of a presenting part. In addition, with neither the feet nor the vertex of the fetus present in the lower uterine segment, it becomes difficult to extract the fetus through a low transverse uterine incision. Therefore, a vertical uterine incision is usually indicated for delivery of a transverse lie, often called a *classic cesarean section.*

3. **Face presentation.** The management of the face presentation in the absence of a contracted pelvis and with normal uterine contractions without fetal distress will result in successful vaginal delivery. However, face presentation in term infants is frequently accompanied by pelvic contraction, and in these cases cesarean section is the best route of delivery. The presence of a persistent mentum posterior position is also an indication for cesarean delivery.

4. **Brow presentation.** The patient with a brow presentation

may be treated expectantly, anticipating a change to either a vertex or face presentation. If progress in labor is not being made or fetal intolerance of labor occurs, prompt cesarean delivery is indicated.

5. **Compound presentation.** In most cases, the prolapsed part will not interfere with labor. Fetal monitoring is essential, since cord prolapse, either overt or occult, is increased. If the prolapsed limb does not move out of the way with descent of the presenting part, it may be gently pushed out of the way. If fetal compromise is detected, prompt cesarean delivery should be accomplished.

BIBLIOGRAPHY

American College of Obstetricians and Gynecologists. Management of the breech presentation. ACOG Technical Bulletin No. 95, August 1986.

Bradley-Watson PJ. The decreasing value of external cephalic version in modern obstetrics. Am J Obstet Gynecol 1975; 123:237.

Brenner WE, Bruce RD, Hendricks CH. The characteristics and perils of breech presentation. Am J Obstet Gynecol 1974; 118:700.

Collea JV, Weghorst GR, Paul RH, et al. Singleton breech presentation: One year's experience. In: Manduzzato GP, ed. Contribution to Gynecology and Obstetrics, Vol 3. Basel: Karger; 1977:91–98.

Flanagan TA, Mulchahey KM, Korenbrot CC, et al. Management of term breech presentation. Am J Obstet Gynecol 1987; 156:1492.

Hall JE, Kohl SG, O'Brien F, et al. Breech presentation and perinatal mortality. Am J Obstet Gynecol 1965; 91:665.

Marcus RG, Crewe-Brown H, Kravits S, et al. Feto-maternal hemorrhage following successful and unsuccessful attempts at external cephalic version. Br J Obstet Gynecol 1975; 82:578.

Morley GW. Breech presentation: A 15-year review. Obstet Gynecol 1967; 30:745–751.

Moore WT, Steptoe PP. The experience of the Johns Hospkins Hospital with breech presentation. South Med J 1943; 36:295.

Ranney B. The gentle art of external cephalic version. Am J Obstet Gynecol 1973; 116:239.

Scheer K, Nubar J. Variation of fetal presentation with gestational age. Am J Obstet Gynecol 1976; 125:269–270.

Watson WJ, Benson WL. Vaginal delivery for the selected frank breech at term. Obstet Gynecol 1984; 64:638.

Part III

Fetal Assessment and Management

CHAPTER 13

Drugs and Toxic Substances

Sandra Ann Carson

The pregnant woman today has many concerns and questions regarding exposure to pharmaceutical and environmental agents. In one study, the average antenatal patient ingested 34 drugs during her pregnancy. Fortunately, most drugs cause no harmful effects to the fetus; drug causes have been documented in relatively few instances of adverse effects. Nonetheless, no drug can be considered absolutely safe. Drugs that alter embryonic development and result in congenital anomalies are called *teratogens*. It is the responsibility of the obstetrician to be familiar with known teratogens in order to counsel the pregnant female.[1-5]

I. Principles of teratology
    A. Teratogenic effects. The teratogenic effects of any agent depend on several factors:
        1. The agent itself. Some agents cause abnormal fetal development in all cases, whereas other agents are less consistently, if at all, teratogenic.
        2. The pharmacogenetics of the mother and fetus. Not all embryos exposed to a teratogen will be affected. The effect will be influenced by the relative rate of absorption, maternal metabolism, placental transfer, and fetal metabolism.
        3. Time of exposure during gestation. The time during embryogenesis when cells of a given organ system divide most rapidly is the period of greatest teratogenic susceptibility. Once developed, the system becomes relatively resistant to teratogens. Table 13.1 lists the embryonic periods during which major organ systems develop.
        4. Dose. Low doses of teratogens may have no effect; intermediate doses cause a specific malformation pattern; high doses may lead to death of the embryo. Moreover, doses that produce malformation may differ, depending on gestational age.

Table 13.1. Development of Fetal Organ Systems

EMBRYONIC AGE (WEEKS FROM CONCEPTION)	EMBRYONIC DEVELOPMENT
1	Implantation; embryo relatively resistant to teratogenic effects, except for those of embryocides
2–3	Craniofacial development; musculoskeletal and CNS differentiation
4	Limb buds; cardiovascular system enlarges
5	Limb buds segment; nose, eyes, and ears become prominent
6	Fingers and toes formed
7–8	Maxilla fused; eyelids formed
9–10	External and internal genitalia differentiate; most other major organ systems formed; embryo relatively resistant to teratogens
11	Genitourinary system completed

II. **Drugs.** The principles of teratology should be considered when assessing the potential effects of a drug to be given during pregnancy.[6–8] Unfortunately, such considerations have not always been raised. Even formal studies often show flaws in experimental design. Not surprisingly, the literature consists of many confusing and incomplete reports condemning certain agents. Often only one or two cases exist to illustrate a teratogenic effect, and negative evidence is unlikely to be reported. Frequently, it is difficult to differentiate an anomaly that occurs as a result of a chronic disease process (e.g., epilepsy) from a result of the drug used to treat that disease (e.g., diphenylhydantoin). Many drugs are used in combination, and their teratogenic effects may be additive and individually indistinguishable (e.g., antineoplastic drugs). Teratogenicity of an agent is thus difficult to prove or disprove. Decisions based on less than ideal scientific evidence were necessary in order to construct Table 13.2, which lists commonly used drugs and their purported teratogenic effects. Inclusion of a drug in Table 13.2 is somewhat arbitrary, and the table includes only agents in general use. Exclusion of a drug from this list does not confirm its safety. For example, thalidomide, a well-known confirmed teratogen, is not included because of its market unavailability. For each drug in Table 13.2, evidence is categorized as confirmed, strong, suggestive, or poor. There are few confirmed teratogens. However, in advising patients, it is wise to emphasize that no drug can be verified as absolutely safe to all fetuses. Thus, drugs should be administered only if the benefit to the mother or fetus outweighs the potential risk. When counseling a patient about the

Table 13.2. **Teratogenic (T)/Neonatal (N) Effects of Various Agents**

AGENT	EFFECT	EVIDENCE	REF.
	ANTICOAGULANTS		
Heparin	N: increased intrauterine death	Poor	11
Warfarin	T: nasal hypoplasia, retardation, chondrodysplasia punctata in first trimester; retardation, optic atrophy, microcephaly in second trimester	Confirmed Strong	11, 12 11
	ANTICONVULSANTS		
Diphenylhydantoin	T: digital hypoplasia; nail dysplasia; intrauterine growth retardation; ptosis; microcephaly, broad, depressed nasal bridge; hernias	Confirmed	14, 15
Magnesium sulfate	N: respiratory and motor depression	Strong	16
Phenobarbital	T: no known effects N: withdrawal not usual at anticonvulsant doses		16
Trimethadione	T: developmental delay; V-shaped eyebrows; epicanthal folds; low-set ears; irregular teeth; cardiovascular and visceral anomalies	Confirmed	17, 18
Valproic acid	T: Neural tube defects	Confirmed	19
	ANTIEMETICS		
Chlorpromazine	N: respiratory depression	Suggestive	20, 21
Meclizine	T, N: no known effects		22
Prochlorperazine	T, N: no known effects		22
	ANTIHYPERTENSIVES		
Alpha methyldopa	T, N: no known effects		23
Hexamethonium	N: fetal ganglionic blockade resulting in paralytic ileus	Confirmed	24
Hydralazine	T, N: no known effect in humans T: possible skeletal defects in animals		25

Table 13.2. *(Continued)*

AGENT	EFFECT	EVIDENCE	REF.
Propranolol	N; hypoglycemia, brady-cardia	Suggestive	26
	T: intrauterine growth retardation, intrauterine death	Poor	27–29
Reserpine	N: nasal discharge	Confirmed	30
	T: no known effects		
	ANTIMICROBIALS		
Cephalosporins	T, N: no known effects		20
Chloramphenicol	T: no known effects	Confirmed	16
	N: bone marrow depression; abdominal distention; cyanosis; vascular collapse (gray baby syndrome)	Confirmed	
Chloroquine	T: sensorineural deafness in two case reports	Poor	31
Erythromycin	T, N: no known effects		23
Ethambutol	T, N: no known effects		32, 33
Ethionamide	T: CNS defects	Strong	34
Gentamicin	T, N: no known effects		23
Isoniazid	T, N: no known effects		35
Kanamycin	T: hearing deficit	Suggestive	36
Lincomycin	T, N: no known effects		37
Metronidazole	T, N: no known effect in humans		
	T: mutagenic in bacteria	Poor	20, 38
Neomycin	T, N: no known effects		23
Nitrofurantoin	N: hemolytic anemia in G6PD-deficient fetus	Confirmed	16
Para-aminosalicylic acid (PAS)	T, N: no known effects		35
Penicillin	T, N: no known effects		20, 37
Primaquine	N: hemolytic anemia in G6PD-deficient fetus	Confirmed	16
Pyrimethamine	T: cleft lip and cleft palate	Suggestive	20, 39
Quinacrine	T: one case of multiple anomalies reported	Poor	40
Rifampin	T, N: no known effects		32
Streptomycin	T: hearing deficit	Strong	41, 42

Table 13.2. *(Continued)*

AGENT	EFFECT	EVIDENCE	REF.
Sulfonamides	T: no known effects N: hemolytic anemia in G6PD-deficient fetus; displaces bilirubin from albumin-binding sites, possibly leading to kernicterus	Confirmed Strong	43
Tetracycline	T: incorporated in deciduous teeth and bones in second to fifth months of gestation	Confirmed	44
Tobramycin	T, N: no known effects		20
Trimethoprin and sulfamethoxazole	T: limb defects, cleft palate, and microagnathia in rats	Poor	20, 45
	ANTINEOPLASTICS		
Actinomycin D	T: cranial anomalies in rats	Suggestive	20
Aminopterin	T: triangular facies; intrauterine growth retardation; arched palate; abortifacient		46–48
Azathioprine	T; adrenal insufficiency; intrauterine growth retardation; leukopenia	Poor	20, 49
Busulfan	T: intrauterine growth retardation; gonadal dysgenesis; various malformations	Strong	50, 51
Chlorambucil	T: one reported case of unilateral renal agenesis	Poor	52
Cyclophosphamide	T: limb defects; craniofacial anomalies; germ cell aplasia	Confirmed	53, 54
5-Fluorouracil	T: radial aplasia, absent digits, hypoplastic aorta, gastrointestinal aplasias, urinary tract dysplasia in one case report	Poor	55
6-Mercaptopurine	T, N: no known effects		21
Methotrexate	T: skeletal defects	Confirmed	56
Nitrogen mustard	N: intrauterine death T: spontaneous abortion	Suggestive Suggestive	57, 58
Procarbazine	T: possible renal anomalies	Poor	59, 60
Triethylenemelamine	T, N: no known effects		61
Thiotepa	T: growth retardation and skeletal defects in rats T, N: no known effect in humans		20 61

Table 13.2. *(Continued)*

AGENT	EFFECT	EVIDENCE	REF.
Vinblastine Vincristine	T, N: no known effects in humans; ocular and facial anomalies in rats		62, 63
	DIURETICS		
Furosemide	T, N: no known effects		
Spironolactone	T, N: no known effects		20
Thiazides	N: thrombocytopenia	Confirmed	64
Androgens	T: masculinization of female fetus; little effect in male fetus	Confirmed	37
Bromocryptine	T, N: no known effects		65, 66
Clomiphene citrate	T, N: no known effects		67
	HORMONES AND ANTAGONISTS		
Corticosteroids	T: no known effects in humans; cleft palate in rodents N: acute adrenal insufficiency	Strong	68, 69
Cyproterone acetate	T: feminization of male fetus	Strong	70
Danazol	T: masculinization of female fetus	Strong	71, 72
Diethylstilbestrol (DES)	T: anomalies of the genital tract; vaginal adenosis and adenocarcinoma in females; epididymal cysts, hypotrophic testes, abnormal semen analysis in males	Strong	73, 74
Estrogens (other than DES)	T: no known effects in humans; feminization of male rats		75
Human menopausal gonadotropin (Pergonal)	T: aneuploidy	Poor	76
Iodine-131 Millicurie dose	T: cretinism	Confirmed	20
Microcurie dose	T: no known effect		
Iodides (inorganic)	T: fetal goiter; cretinism	Confirmed	77
Insulin (and oral hypoglycemics)	T: unable to differentiate teratogenic effects from those related to diabetes mellitus		

Table 13.2. *(Continued)*

AGENT	EFFECT	EVIDENCE	REF.
Methimazole	T: ulcerlike midline scalp defect	Suggestive	78
Oxytocin	N: hyperbilirubinemia	Suggestive	79
Prednisolone	N: thymic dysplasia, adrenal insufficiency	Suggestive	80
Progestins	T: masculinization of female fetus (large doses of 19-nor derivatives except norethyndrel)	Confirmed	81–83
	N: vertebral, anal, tracheoesophageal, renal, limb, cardiovascular anomalies	Suggestive	84, 85
Thiourea agents (other than methimazole)	T: hypothydroidism; compensatory hypertrophic goiter; no cretinism	Confirmed	86
Thyroid hormone	T, N: no known effects		
	PSYCHOTROPIC DRUGS		
Alcohol	T: intrauterine growth retardation; ocular, joint, and cardiac anomalies (strongly dose related)	Confirmed	87, 88
	N: alcohol withdrawal		
Amphetamines	T: biliary atresia, oral clefts	Poor / Poor	89 / 90
Cocaine	T: Prune belly syndrome	Poor	91
	N: depressed interactive behavior		
Chlordiazepoxide	T; sporadic cases with no pattern of anomalies	Poor	22, 92
Diazepam	T: no known effects	Strong	93
Haloperidol	T: two case reports of limb malformations	Poor	94
Lithium	T: Ebstein's anomaly and other cardiovascular defects	Strong	95, 96
Lysergic acid diethylamide (LSD)	T: limb bud defects; CNS anomalies	Suggestive	97, 98
Marijuana	T: sporadic cases with no pattern of anomalies	Poor	99
Meprobamate	T: sporadic cases with no pattern of anomalies	Poor	22

Table 13.2. *(Continued)*

AGENT	EFFECT	EVIDENCE	REF.
Narcotic addiction	T: intrauterine growth retardation	Strong	16
	N: withdrawal; premature labor	Confirmed	
Phenothiazines	T: cardiovascular anomalies	Poor	100
Tricyclic anti-depressants	T: no known effects		101
	VAGINAL PREPARATIONS		
Miconazole	T: no known effects		20
Nonoxynol-9	T: no known effects		37, 102, 103
Providine-iodine	T, N: iodine may be absorbed (see sulfonamides)		
	MISCELLANEOUS		
Aspirin	T, N: no known effects		104, 105
Aminophylline	T, N: no known effects		37
Caffeine	T, N: no known effects		106
Cyclosporine	T, N: no known effects		107
Dextromethorphan	T, N: no known effects		37
Digitalis	T, N: no known effects		108
D-Penicillinamine	T: generalized connective tissue defects	Poor	109, 110
Diphenhydramine	T: cleft palate	Poor	111
Expectorants	T, N: no known effects		37
Isotretinoin	T: skeletal deformities	Confirmed	112, 113
Smoking (nicotine)	T: intrauterine growth retardation	Strong	114, 115
	N: intrauterine death		
Sulfasalazine	T, N: no known effects		116, 117
Theophyline	T, N: no known effects		37
Vitamin A (pharmacologic doses)	T: CNS, urinary tract, and ocular anomalies	Strong	118–120
Vitamin D (pharmacologic doses)	N: infantile hypercalcemia T: supravalvular aortic stenosis	Strong	121

teratogenic risk of drugs, one must also remember the overall incidence of congenital anomalies in an unexposed population (i.e., 2 to 3 percent).

III. **Environmental agents.** Environmental agents often concern the pregnant women because of their ubiquity and insidiousness. However, like drugs, few environmental substances are confirmed teratogens. Table 13.3 lists environmental substances suspected of causing congenital malformations. However, only **mercury** and **naphtalene** are confirmed teratogens.[6] Mercury causes neurologic abnormalities that include cerebral palsy chorea, ataxia, seizures, and mental retardation. Naphthalene causes hemolytic anemia in the glucose-6-phosphate dehydrogenase (G6PD)-deficient fetus.

IV. **Physical agents.** Physical agents can also be teratogenic.[9] Such agents include radiation, ultrasound, hyperthermia, and microwaves. Exposure may occur in the home, workplace, medical or dental facility, or general environment. Effects on the fetus vary with the dose, exposure rate, and stage of gestation, in accordance with the principles of teratology noted above. Microwaves, hyperthermia, and ultrasound have not been shown to exert deleterious effects on humans in the doses normally incurred. However, ionizing radiation is a well-established cause of congenital anomalies in humans.

Radiation received by the average American equals 1.25 Gy per year of background radiation and another .55 Gy from medical x-rays.[10] Only if exposure is much higher does the potential for a teratogenic effect exist. In addition to the dose, several other major considerations are apparent:

A. Ionizing radiation **early in gestation** (1 or 2 weeks after conception) usually results in a all-or-none phenomenon, that is, the embryo is either killed or the radition damage is corrected by cell repair. During this stage the embryo consists of undifferentiated

Table 13.3. Environmental Agents

Anesthetic gases
Cadmium
Cyclamates
Dioxin
Food colorings
Hair dyes
Hexachlorophene
Lead
Mercury*
Monosodium glutamate
Naphthalene*
Nitrates
Nitrates
Organic solvents
Saccharin

*Only confirmed environmental teratogens.

Table 13.4. Effects of Radiation

DOSE	EFFECT
Less than .05 Gy	No evidence of induced malformations
Greater than .10 Gy	Fetus considered to be at significant risk
Greater than .25 Gy	Microcephaly, mental retardation; CNS most sensitive
Greater than 1 Gy	Radiation sickness; growth retardation
4.50 Gy	Fifty percent of exposed persons die; survivors may be predisposed to malignancy

1 Gy = 100 rad.

cells, all of which have the potential to develop into many different organ systems.

B. Exposure during the **3rd to 10th embryonic weeks,** the period of major organogenesis, may result in gross malformations.

C. The central nervous system (CNS) is particularly sensitive throughout the **first trimester,** because radiation preferentially affects the CNS. Claims that malformations of other systems were caused by irradiation can be dismissed if such defects are not accompanied by a CNS defect.

D. The human fetus becomes more resistant to radiation damage each gestational week.

E. Radiation given over a period of time (chronic) is less likely to produce damage than a comparable dose given acutely.

F. **Fetal germ cell** exposure may result in genetic mutations that become manifest only in offspring of the fetus.

G. Radiation exposure may predispose to later development of malignancy, presumably also as result of mutations.

H. It is evident that accurate **counseling following exposure** during pregnancy requires knowledge of many factors: nature of the radiation, dose, exposure time, and, of course, the stage of gestation in which exposure occurred. Consultation with a radiation physicist may be necessary to calculate the exact radiation exposure. Table 13.4 summarizes current opinions concerning the relationship of exposure to teratogenic effects.

REFERENCES

1. Forfar J, Nelson M. Epidemiology of drugs taken by pregnant women: Drugs that may affect the fetus adversely. Clin Pharmacol Ther 1973; 14:633.
2. Simpson JL, Golbus MS, Martin A, et al. Genetics in Obstetrics and Gynecology. New York: Grune & Stratton; 1982.
3. Wilson JG, Fraser FC, eds. Handbook of Teratology. New York: Plenum Press; 1977.

4. Kalter H, Warkany J. Congenital malformations — etiologic factors and their role in prevention. N Engl J Med 1983; 308:424.
5. Nelson MM, Forfar JO. Association between drugs administered during pregnancy and congenital abnormalities of the fetus. Br Med J 1971; 1:523.
6. Anzieulewics JA, Dick HJ, Chairulli EE. Transplacental naphthalene poisoning. Am J Obstet Gynecol 1959; 78:518.
7. Brent RL. Radiation and other physical agents. In: Wilson JG, Fraser FC, eds. Handbook of Teratology. New York: Plenum Press; 1977:153.
8. Edwards MJ, Wanner RA. Extremes of temperature. General principles and etiology. In: Wilson JN, Fraser FC, eds. Handbook of Teratology. New York: Plenum Press, 1977:421.
9. United Nations. A report of the United Nations' Scientific Committee on the Effects of Atomic Radiation to the General Assembly, with Annexes. United Nations Publication No. E. 77; 1977.
10. Harvey EB, Boice JD, Honeyman M, et al. Prenatal x-ray exposure and childhood cancer in twins. N Engl J Med 1985; 312:541.
11. Hall JG, Pauli RM, Wilson KM. Maternal and fetal sequelae of anticoagulation during pregnancy. Am J Med 1980; 68:122.
12. Holzgreve W, Cary JC, Hall BD. Warfarin-induced fetal abnormalities. Lancet 1976; 2:914.
13. Von Sydow G. Hypoprothrombinemia and cerebral injury in a newborn infant after dicoumarin treatment of the mother. Nord Med 1947; 34:1171.
14. Barr M Jr, Poznanski AK, Schmickel RD. Digital hypoplasia and anticonvulsants during gestation: A teratogenic syndrome? J Pediatr 1974; 84:254.
15. Hanson JW, Smith DW. The fetal hydantoin syndrome. J Pediatr 1975; 87: 285.
16. Stevenson RE. The Fetus and Newly Born Infant. 2nd ed. St Louis: CV Mosby; 1977.
17. Zackai FH, Mellman WJ, Neiderer B, et al. The fetal trimethadione syndrome. J Pediatr 1975; 87:280.
18. Feldman GL, Weaver DD, Lovrien FW. The fetal trimethadione syndrome. The American Society of Human Genetics 28th Annual Meeting, Program and Abstracts. San Diego, Cal; 1977:41A.
19. Gomez MR. Possible teratogenicity of valproic acid. J Pediatr 1981; 98:808.
20. Shepard TH: Catalog of Teratogenic Agents. 3rd ed. Baltimore: Johns Hopkins University Press; 1980.
21. Sokal JE, Lessmans EM. Effects of cancer chemotherapeutic agents on the human fetus. JAMA 1960; 172:1765.
22. Milkovich L, Van Den Berg BJ. Effects of prenatal meprobamate and chlordiazepoxide hydrochloride on human embryonic and fetal development. N Engl J Med 1974; 291:1268.
23. Berkowitz R, Coustan D, Mochizuki T. Handbook for Prescribing Medications during Pregnancy. Boston: Little, Brown; 1981.
24. Morris N. Hexamethonium compounds in the treatment of preeclampsia and essential hypertension during pregnancy. Lancet 1953; 1:322.
25. Rapalea RS, Parr RN, Lin TZ, et al. Biochemical basis of skeletal defects induced by hydralazine. Teratology 1977; 15:185.
26. Habib A, McCarthy JS. Effects on the neonate of propranolol administered during pregnancy. J Pediatr 1977; 91:808.
27. Gladstone GC, Hordof A, Gersony WM. Propranolol administration during pregnancy; effects on the fetus. J Pediatr 1974; 86:962.
28. Featherstone HJ. Fetal demise in a migraine patient on propranolol. Headache 1983; 23:213.

29. Redmond GP. Propranolol and fetal growth retardation. Semin Perinatol 1982; 6:142.
30. Desmond MM, Rogers SF, Lindley JE, et al. Management of toxemia of pregnancy with reserpine. Obstet Gynecol 1957; 10:140.
31. Wyler DJ. Malaria resurgence, resistance, and research. N Engl J Med 1983; 308:875.
32. Jentgens H. Antituberculise chemotherapre und Schwagerschaftsabbusch. Prax Pneumol 1973; 27:479.
33. Bobrowitz ID. Ethambutol in pregnancy. Chest 1974; 66:20.
34. Potwprpwslo M, Sianozecka E, Szufladowicz R. Ethionamide treatment and pregnancy. Pol Med J 1966; 5:1152.
35. Marynowski A, Sianoazecka E. Comparison of the incidence of congenital malformations in neonates from healthy mothers and from patients treated for tuberculosis. Ginekol Pol 1972; 43:713.
36. Fujimori H. Influence of kanamycin on hearing acuity in the neonate and suckling. Presented at the 10th Anniversary of the Kanamycin Conference, Tokyo; 1967.
37. Heinonen OP, Slone D, Shapiro S. Birth Defects and Drugs in Pregnancy. Littleton, Mass: Publishing Sciences Group; 1977.
38. Roe FJ. Toxicologic evaluation of metronidazole with particular reference to carcinogenic, mutagenic, and teratogenic potential. Surgery 1983; 93:158.
39. Sullivan GE, Takacs E. Comparative teratogenicity of pyrimethamine in rats and hamsters. Teratology 1971; 4:205.
40. Vevera J, Zatloukal F. Pfipad urozenych malformaet zpusobenyck pravdepodobne atetrinem, podavan-ym uranem tehotenstvi. Cs Pediatr 1964; 19:211.
41. Rasmussen F. The oto-toxic effect of streptomycin and dihydrostreptomycin on the foetus. Scand J Respir Dis 1969; 50(1):61–67.
42. Ganguin G, Rempt E. Streptomycinbehandlung in der schwangerschaft und ihre ansirkung auf des gehor des kindes. Z Laryngol Rhinol Otol Ihre Grenzgeb 1970; 49:496.
43. Richards IDG. A retrospective inquiry into possible teratogenic effects of drugs in pregnancy. In: Klingberg MA, Abramovici A, Chenuke J, eds. Drugs and Fetal Development. New York: Plenum Press; 1972:441.
44. Zbella EA, Gleicher N. The oral cavity. In: Gleicher N, ed. Principles of Medical Therapy in Pregnancy. New York: Plenum Press; 1985:811–812.
45. Udall V: Toxicology of sulphonamide-trimethoprim combinations. Postgrad Med J 1969; 45:42.
46. Thiersch JB. Therapeutic abortions with a folic acid antagonist, 4-aminopteroyglutamic acid (4-amino P.G.A.) administered by the oral route. Am J Obstet Gynecol 1952; 63:1298.
47. Thiersch JB. The control of reproduction in rats with the aid of antimetabolites. Early experience with antimetabolites as abortifacient agents in man. Acta Endocrinol 1956; 28(suppl):37.
48. Goetsch C. An evaluation of aminopterin as an abortifacient. Am J Obstet Gynecol 1962; 83:1474.
49. Nolan GH, Sweet RL, Laros RK, et al. Renal cadaver transplantation followed by successful pregnancies. Obstet Gynecol 1974; 43:732.
50. Diamond I. Anderson MM, McCreadie SR. Transplacental transmission of busulfan (Myleran) in a mother with leukemia. Pediatrics 1960; 25:85.
51. De Rezende J, Coslovsky S, De Aguiar PB. Leucemia et gravidez. Rev Ginecol Obstet 1965; 117:46.
52. Shotton D, Monie IW. Possible teratogenic effect of chlorambucil on a human fetus. JAMA 1963; 186:74.
53. Greenberg LH, Tanaka KR. Cogenital anomalies probably induced by cyclophosphamide. JAMA 1964; 188:423.

54. Toledo TM, Harper RC, Moses RH. Fetal effects during cyclophosphamide and irradiation therapy. Ann Intern Med 1971; 74:87.
55. Stephens JD, Golbus MS, Miller TR, et al. Multiple congenital anomalies in a fetus exposed to 5-fluorouracil during the first trimester. Am J Obstet Gynecol 1980; 137:747.
56. Milunsky A, Graef JW, Gaynor MF Jr. Methotrexate-induced congenital malformations, with a review of the literature. J Pediatr 1968; 72:790.
57. Nicholson HO. Cytotoxic drugs in pregnancy. Review of reported cases. J Obstet Gynecol Br Commonw 1968; 75:307.
58. Garrett MJ. Teratogenic effects of combination chemotherapy. Ann Intern Med 1974; 80:667.
59. Mennuti MT, Sheppard TH, Mellman WJ. Fetal renal malformation following treatment of Hodgkin's disease during pregnancy. Obstet Gynecol 1975; 46:194.
60. Wells JH, Marshall JR, Carbone PP. Procarbazine therapy for Hodgkin's disease in early pregnancy. JAMA 1968; 205:935.
61. Nishimura H, Tanimura T. Information in prenatal hazards of drugs. In: Clinical Aspects of the Teratogenicity of Drugs. Amsterdam: Excerpta Medica; 1976:106.
62. Armstrong JG, Dyke RW, Fonts PJ. Vinblastine sulfate treatment of Hodgkin's disease during pregnancy. Science 1964; 143:703.
63. Demyer W. Cleft lip and jaw induced in fetal rats by vincristine. Arch Anat 1965; 48:181.
64. Rodrigues SU, Leiken SL, Hiller MC. Neonatal thrombocytopenia associated with antepartum administration of thiazide drugs. N Engl J Med 1964; 270:881.
65. Molitch ME. Pregnancy and the hyperprolactinemic women. N Engl J Med 1985; 312:1364.
66. Turkals I, Braun P, Krupp P. Surveillance of bromocriptine in pregnancy. JAMA 1982; 247:1589.
67. Kurachi K, Toshihiro A, Junnosuke M, et al. Congenital malformations of newborn infants after clomiphene-induced ovulation. Fertil Steril 1983; 40:1187.
68. Bongiovanni AM, McPaddan AJ. Steroids during pregnancy and possible fetal consequences. Fertil Steril 1960; 11:181.
69. Serment H, Ruf H. Les dangers pour le produit de conception de medicaments administrés à la femme enceinte. Bull Fed Soc Gynecol Obstet Lang Fr 1968; 20:69.
70. Steinbeck H, Neuman F. Aspects of steroidal influence on fetal development. In: Klingberg MA, Abramovici A, Chemke J, eds. Drugs and Fetal Development. New York: Plenum Press; 1972:227.
71. Shaw RW, Farquhar JW. Female pseudohermaphoditism associated with danazol exposure in utero — case report. Br J Obstet Gynecol 1984; 91:386.
72. Schwartz R. Ambiguous genitalia in a term female infant due to exposure to danazol in utero. Am J Dis Child 1982; 136:474.
73. Herbst AL, Ulfelder H, Psokanzer DC. Adenocarcinoma of the vagina. Association of maternal stilbestrol therapy with tumor appearance in young women. N Engl J Med 1971; 284:878.
74. Gill WB, Schumacher GFB, Bibbo M. Pathological semen and anatomical abnormalities of the genital tract in human male subjects exposed to diethylstilbestrol in utero. J Urol 1977; 117–477.
75. Greene RR, Burrill MW, Ivy AC. Experimental intersexuality: The effects of estrogen on the antenatal sexual development of the rat. Am J Anat 1940; 67:305.
76. Boue J, Boue A, Lazar P. Retrospective and prospective epidemiological

studies of 1500 karyotyped spontaneous human abortions. Teratology 1975; 12:11.

77. Wolff J. Iodide goiter and the pharmacologic effects of excess iodide. Am J Med 1969; 47:101.

78. Milham S Jr, Elledge W. Maternal methimazole and congenital defects in children. Teratology 1972; 5:125.

79. Davies DP, Gomersall R, Robertson R, et al. Neonatal jaundice and maternal oxytocin infusion. Br Med J 1973; 3:476.

80. Hou S. Pregnancy in women with chronic renal disease. N Engl J Med 1985; 313:836.

81. Jacobson BD. Hazards of norethindrone therapy during pregnancy. Am J Obstet Gynecol 1962; 84:962.

82. Nora JJ, Nora AH, Perinchief AG, et al. Congenital abnormalities and first-trimester exposure to progestaten/oestrogen. Lancet 1976; 1:313.

83. Heinonen OP, Slone D, Monson RR, et al. Cardiovascular birth defects and antenatal exposure to female sex hormones. N Engl J Med 1977; 296:67.

84. Nora JJ, Nora AH. Birth defects and oral contraceptives. Lancet 1973; 1:941.

85. Nora AH, Nora JJ. A syndrome of multiple congenital anomalies associated with teratogenic exposure. Arch Environ Health 1975; 30:17.

86. Burrow GN, Bartsocas C, Klatskin EH, et al. Children exposed in utero to propylthiouracil. Am J Dis Child 1968; 116:161.

87. Jones KL, Smith DW, Ulleland CN, et al. Pattern of malformation in offspring of chronic alcoholic mothers. Lancet 1973; 1:1267.

88. Jones KL, Smith DW, Streissguth AP, et al. Outcome in offspring of chronic alcoholic women. Lancet 1974; 1:1076.

89. Levin JN. Amphetamine ingestion with biliary atresia. J Pediatr 1971; 79:130.

90. Milkovich L, Van Den Berg BJ. Effects of antenatal exposure to anorectic drugs. Am J Obstet Gynecol 1977; 129:637.

91. Chasnoff IJ, Burns WJ, Schnoll SH, et al. Cocaine use in pregnancy. N Engl J Med 1985; 313:666.

92. Hartz SC, Heinonen OP, Shapiro S, et al. Antenatal exposure to meprobamate and chlordiazepoxide in relation to malformations, mental development and childhood mortality. N Engl J Med 1975; 292:726.

93. Rosenberg L, Mitchell AA, Parsells JL, et al. Lack of relation of oral clefts to diazepam use during pregnancy. N Engl J Med 1983; 309:1282.

94. Kopelman AE, McCullar FW, Heggeness L. Limb malformations following maternal use of haloperidol. JAMA 1975; 231:62.

95. Weller RO. Lithium, Ebstein's anomaly, and other congenital heart defects. Lancet 1974; 2:594.

96. Linden S, Rich C. The use of lithium during pregnancy and lactation. J Clin Psychiatry 1983; 44:358.

97. Jacobson CB, Berlin CM. Possible reproductive detriment in LSD users. JAMA 1972; 222:1367.

98. Eller JL, Morton JM. Bizarre deformities in offspring of users of lysergic acid diethylamide. N Engl J Med 1970; 283:395.

99. Greenland S, Staisch KJ, Brown N, et al. The effects of marijuana use during pregnancy. A preliminary epidemiologic study. Am J Obstet Gynecol 1982; 143:408.

100. Zbella EA, Vermesh M, Tiemstra J, et al. Phenothiazines in pregnancy. Neonatol Perinatol. In press.

101. Banister P, Dafoe C, Smith ESO, et al. Possible teratogenicity of tricyclic antidepressants. Lancet 1972; 1:838.

102. Shapiro S, Slone D, Heidonen O, et al. Birth defects and spermicides. JAMA 1982; 247:2381.

103. Bracken MB. Spermicidal contraceptives and poor reproductive outcome:

The epidemiologic evidence against an association. Am J Obstet Gynecol 1985; 151:552.
104. Bleyer WA, Breckenridge RT. Studies on the detection of adverse drug reactions in the newborn. II. The effect of prenatal aspirin on newborn hemostasis. JAMA 1970; 213:2049.
105. Corby DG. Aspirin in pregnancy: maternal and fetal effects. Pediatrics 1978; 62:930.
106. Kurppa K, Holmberg P, Kuosma E, et al. Coffee consumption during pregnancy and selected congenital malformations: A nationwide case control study. Am J Public Health 1985; 73:1397.
107. Davison JM, Lindheimer MD. Pregnancy in women with renal allografts. Semin Nephrol 1984; 4:240.
108. Laros RK, Hage ML, Hayashi RH. Pregnancy and heart valve prosthesis. Obstet Gynecol 1970; 35:241.
109. Solomon L, Abrams G, Dinner M, et al. Neonatal abnormalities associated with D-penicillamine treatment during pregnancy. N Engl J Med 1977; 296:54.
110. Zbella EA, Gleicher N. Metals and metalloproteins. In: Gleicher N, ed. Principles of Medical Therapy in Pregnancy. New York: Plenum Press; 1985:295–300.
111. Saxen I. Cleft palate and maternal dephenhydramine intake. Lancet 1974; 1:407.
112. Benke PJ. The isotretinoin teratogen syndrome. JAMA 1984; 25:3267.
113. dela Cruz E, Sun S, Vanguanichtakorn K. Multiple congenital malformations associated with maternal isotretinoin therapy. Pediatrics 1984; 74:428.
114. Simpson WJA. A preliminary report on cigarette smoking and the incidence of prematurity. Am J Obstet Gynecol 1957; 73:808.
115. Rush D, Kass EH. Maternal smoking: A reassessment of the association with perinatal mortality. Am J Epidemiol 1972; 96:183.
116. Khosla R, Willoughby CP, Jewell DP. Crohn's disease and pregnancy. Gut 1984; 25:52.
117. Donaldson RM. Management of medical problems in pregnancy — inflammatory bowel disease. N Engl J Med 1985; 25:1616.
118. Bernhardt IB, Dorsey DJ. Hypervitaminosis A and congenital renal anomalies in a human infant. Obstet Gynecol 1974; 43:750.
119. Gal I, Sharman IM, Pryse-Davies J. Vitamin A in relation to human congenital malformations. Adv Teratol 1972; 5:143.
120. Lamba PA, Sood NN. Congenital microphthalmus and colobomata in maternal vitamin A deficiency. J Pediatr Ophthalmol 1968; 5:115.
121. Friedman WF. Vitamin D and the supravalvular aortic stenosis syndrome. Adv Teratol 1968; 3:85.

CHAPTER 14

Reproductive Genetics and Prenatal Diagnosis

Lee P. Shulman

Over the past two decades, human genetics has become an integral part of the practice of obstetrics and gynecology. As such, an understanding of genetic principles and practices is essential for obstetricians and gynecologists. This chapter will serve as a brief introduction to and outline of selected topics in genetics that pertain to the practice of obstetrics and gynecology.

I. **Genetic Principles.** Deoxyribonucleic acid, or DNA, is the molecule that serves as the basis for human biological function. DNA serves as the template for the formation of proteins and enzymes necessary for human life.

   A. **Structure**
      1. DNA is a long molecule composed of two intertwining chains of nucleotides; purines (adenine [A] or guanine [G]) or pyrimidines (cytosine [C] or thymine [T]) variably arranged in an alpha-helix configuration. Each strand has a sugar (deoxyribose)-phosphate-sugar (deoxyribose) "backbone" (Fig. 14.1).
      2. Nucleotides of one strand are bound by hydrogen bonds to nucleotides on the other strand. Guanine invariably binds to cytosine by three hydrogen bonds, whereas adenine invariably binds to thymine by two hydrogen bonds. Thus, the two strands of DNA are complementary. For example, if the nucleotide sequence on one strand is ATCGATT, the sequence on the opposite strand will be TAGCTAA.
      3. In humans, chromosomes are composed of DNA. DNA is also found in the mitochondria of each cell.
      4. The nucleotide sequence determines the genetic information. A codon, composed of three consecutive nucleotides, encodes for a specific amino acid. Since there are four different nucleotides, a maximum of 64 amino acids (4^3) could be encoded; however, only 20 amino acids exist. Several amino acids have multiple codons that encode for

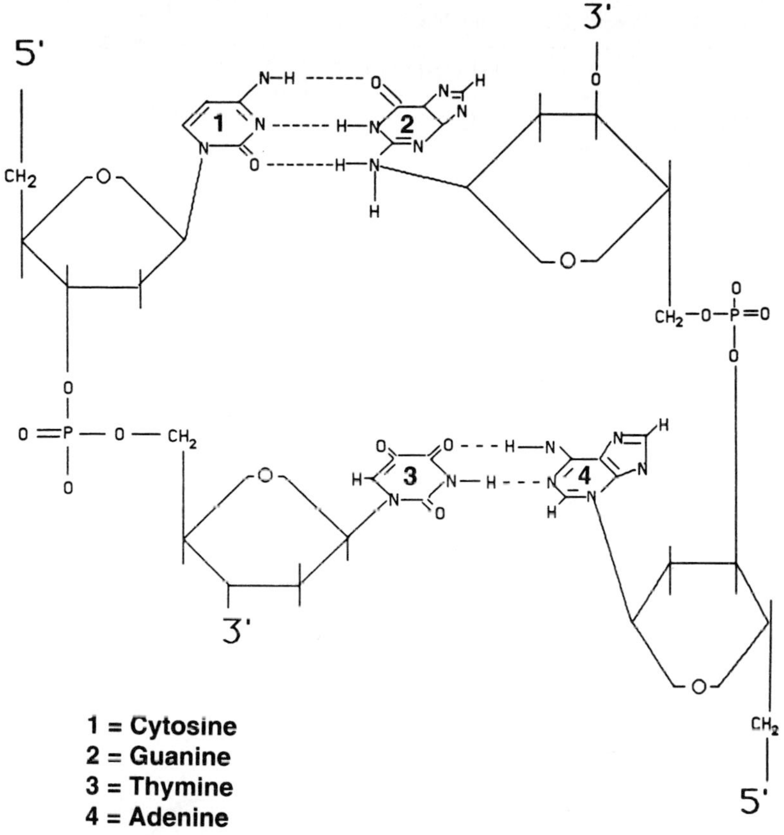

1 = Cytosine
2 = Guanine
3 = Thymine
4 = Adenine

FIGURE 14.1. DNA. Purine nucleotides are adenine (A) and guanine (G), and pyrimidine nucleotides are cytosine (C) and thymine (T). Note that cytosine binds to guanine (1 to 2) by three hydrogen bonds, whereas adenine binds to thymine (3 to 4) by two hydrogen bonds.

their production, and certain codons serve to initiate and stop transcription (Table 14.1). This is known as the *degeneracy* of the genetic code.

B. **Transcription.** DNA does not serve as a direct template for protein synthesis. This function is left to ribonucleic acid (RNA), a single-stranded molecule structurally similar to a single strand of DNA except that the backbone of RNA is composed of ribose sugar molecules instead of deoxyribose sugar molecules. In addition, the pyrimidine base thymine is replaced by uracil (U) in RNA. Transcription, which occurs in the nucleus, involves the generation of a single-stranded RNA molecule from a double-stranded DNA molecule (Fig. 14.2). It is this RNA molecule,

Table 14.1. Genetic Code of mRNA Codons

FIRST POSITION	SECOND POSITION				THIRD POSITION
	G	C	A	U	
G	Glycine	Alanine	Glutamine	Valine	G
	Glycine	Alanine	Aspartic acid	Valine	C
	Glycine	Alanine	Glutamine	Valine	A
	Glycine	Alanine	Aspartic acid	Valine	U
C	Arginine	Proline	Glutamine	Leucine	G
	Arginine	Proline	Histidine	Leucine	C
	Arginine	Proline	Glutamine	Leucine	A
	Arginine	Proline	Histidine	Leucine	U
A	Arginine	Threonine	Lysine	Methionine	G
	Serine	Threonine	Asparagine	Isoleucine	C
	Arginine	Threonine	Lysine	Isoleucine	A
	Serine	Threonine	Asparagine	Isoleucine	U
U	Tryptophan	Serine	Nonsense/stop	Leucine	G
	Cysteine	Serine	Tyrosine	Phenylala-nine	C
	Nonsense/stop	Serine	Nonsense/stop	Leucine	A
	Cysteine	Serine	Tyrosine	Phenylala-nine	U

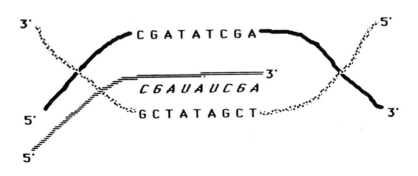

■■■ sense strand of DNA

░░░ anti-sense strand of DNA

≡≡≡ mRNA

FIGURE 14.2. Transcription results in the formation of mRNA from the DNA template; it occurs in a 5' to 3' direction.

known as *messenger RNA (mRNA)*, that serves as the direct template for protein synthesis.

1. The formation of RNA is catalyzed by the enzyme RNA polymerase. Certain sequences are present in DNA that serve to signal the start of transcription (promoters); other sequences serve to halt transcription.

2. Two other forms of RNA, namely, transfer RNA (tRNA) and ribosomal RNA (rRNA), are found in cytoplasm. These two molecules are integral to the formation of protein from the mRNA template (translation).

C. **Translation.** Proteins are produced as a result of translation. Although the entire sequence between the start and stop codons is transcribed, not all mRNA is translated. After transcription, portions of most mRNA sequences are excised prior to transport to cytoplasm. Once this process of *maturation* is complete, mRNA is ready to serve as the template for protein synthesis.

1. Protein synthesis occurs on ribosomes located in the cytoplasm.

2. Most human DNA does not encode for protein synthesis. Approximately 10 percent of human DNA is employed for protein formation; this type of DNA is termed *unique-sequence* DNA. The remaining portion of DNA is composed of *repetitive-sequence* DNA, which serves no known function.

D. **Cell division.** Two types of cell division occur in human cells: mitosis and meiosis (Table 14.2).

1. Mitosis is the process by which daughter cells receive identical copies of DNA from the parent cell; therefore, daughter

Table 14.2. Comparison of Mitosis and Meiosis

	MEIOSIS	MITOSIS
Location	Gonads	All cells
Timing	After puberty in males; suspended until after puberty in females	Anytime
DNA synthesis	One cycle per two divisions	One cycle per division
Length of prophase	Short	Long
Homologous pairs	Yes	No
Crossing-over	Frequent	Rare
Cellular result	Haploid gametes	Diploid daughter cells

Source: Adapted from "Medical Genetics Syllabus," University of Tennessee, Memphis; Marian L. Rivas, Ph.D., director.

cells have the same chromosome number, or diploid complement, as the parent cells. The human diploid number is 46. Mitosis occurs after DNA has been duplicated in a "semiconservative" fashion; that is, parent cell DNA separates, with each strand serving as both the template for a new strand and the second strand in a new DNA molecule. Prior to DNA synthesis, the cell destined to divide enters the G1 phase. Following DNA synthesis, the cell enters a second gap phase, or G2, prior to mitosis (Fig. 14.3). Mitosis is further divided into four stages: prophase, metaphase, anaphase, and telophase.

2. Meiosis is the process by which gametes are formed with a haploid number of chromosomes, which for humans is 23. Meiosis is actually two different processes. Meiosis I is a reductional division that results in a haploid complement, whereas meiosis II is similar to mitosis following DNA synthesis.

3. An important feature of meiosis I is that homologous chromosomes pair prior to reduction and *crossing-over* occurs. For example, this permits DNA from one number 22 chromosome to transfer to the other (homologous) number 22 chromosome prior to gamete formation. As such, each chromosome contributed by a parent will not be an exact copy (i.e., daughter cell) of one of the parental chromosomes. Crossing-over has major implications for gene mapping and DNA analysis. Pairing of homologous chromosomes and crossing-over occur during prophase of meiosis I.

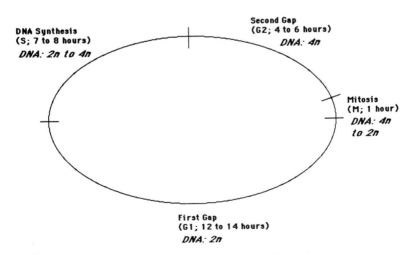

DNA Synthesis
(S; 7 to 8 hours)
DNA: 2n to 4n

Second Gap
(G2; 4 to 6 hours)
DNA: 4n

Mitosis
(M; 1 hour)
DNA: 4n
to 2n

First Gap
(G1; 12 to 14 hours)
DNA: 2n

FIGURE 14.3. The cell cycle, which results in formation of identical daughter cells.

E. Chromosomes

1. **Cytogenetic analysis.** Chromosome analysis can be performed on any cell that has an intact nucleus; as such, chromosome analysis cannot be performed on mature red blood cells. Karyotypes of cells are obtained when the cell is in metaphase (Fig. 14.4). It is necessary to stimulate the cells artificially into cell division, thereby increasing the percentage of cells in metaphase at any specific time. Mitogens are substances that induce cell growth and permit cytogenetic evaluation. Two commonly used mitogens are phytohemagglutinin (PHA) and pokeweed (Therman).

One example of a cell type that has an increased proportion of cells in rapid and spontaneous division and therefore has a relatively high percentage of cells in metaphase is the cytotrophoblast, found in chorionic villi. As such, cytogenetic evaluation of cytotrophoblasts can be achieved without mitogen stimulation. This is known as *direct* cytogenetic analysis and allows results to be available in a shorter period of time than is possible from analyses of cells that require mitogen stimulation. Cytogenetic analysis of cells that re-

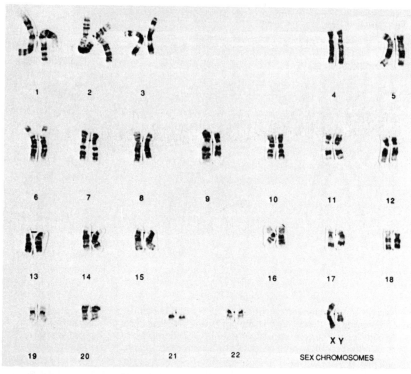

FIGURE 14.4. Normal human male karyotype.

quire mitogen stimulation to obtain an appropriate percentage of cells in metaphase is known as *cultured* cell analysis.

Other substances required for cytogenetic analysis of all cells are: (a) colchicine or vinblastine, a substance that preferentially arrests cell development in metaphase, (b) hypotonic solution, which serves to swell the cells and cause them to burst, thereby releasing the chromosomes, (c) a methanol-acetic acid fixative, and (d) a dye to enhance visualization of the chromosomes. Most laboratories routinely employ Giemsa stain for routine cytogenetic analyses; other methods (e.g., quinacrine, Diamidine-2-phenyl indole-2 HCl, silver) that preferentially stain specific regions of the chromosome are used when clinically indicated.

2. **Structure.** Chromosomes are numbered according to their size and centromeric position. The centromere divides the chromosome into a short arm, denoted p, and a long arm, denoted q. Based on the position of the centromere, one can classify chromosomes as metacentric ($p = q$), submetacentric (p, q), or acrocentric ($p << q$) (Fig. 14.5). In addition to chromosome size and centromere location, chromosomes can be identified by bands, or horizontal stripes, that are produced by certain dyes (usually Giemsa).

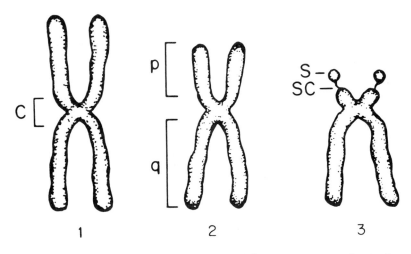

FIGURE 14.5. Denver classification of human chromosomes according to size and shape: (1) a metacentric chromosome (the centromere is equidistant from the ends of the chromosome arms), (2) submetacentric chromosome, (3) acrocentric chromosome. C indicates centromere; p, short arm (from "petite"); q, long arm; SC, secondary constriction; and S, satellite. (From Kelly TE. Clinical Genetics and Genetic Counseling. 2nd ed. Chicago: Year Book Medical Publishers; 1986:11.)

3. **Nomenclature.** Chromosome complements are always expressed by the following nomenclature rules:
    a. The total number of chromosomes present, followed by a comma
    b. the sex chromosomes present
        If no other structural or numerical autosomal abnormalities are present, this information is sufficient to describe the chromosome complement. For example, 46,XY represents a normal cytogenetic male complement and 46,XX represents a normal cytogenetic female complement; 45,X represents an aneuploid complement consistent with Turner syndrome (note that 45,XO is *not* correct; there is no O sex chromosome!).

        If, however, there are structural chromosome or autosomal numerical abnormalities, a second comma follows the sex chromosome complement and the abnormality is denoted. For example, 47,XY,+21 represents a male with an extra number 21 chromosome (Down syndrome), and 46,X,Xdel(X)(q26) denotes a terminal deletion of the long arm distal to band 26 of one of the two X chromosomes. Current rules for cytogenetic nomenclature can be found in the most recently published International System for Human Cytogenetic Nomenclature guidelines.

II. **Genetic heritability.** Traits or disorders that are inherited on the basis of Mendel's laws are known as *Mendelian disorders*. In order to understand Mendelian inheritance, several terms require definition (Table 14.3).

Table 14.3. Terms Describing Genetic Inheritance.

Genotype: the genetic constitution of an individual

Phenotype: the observed physical characteristics of an individual, usually as a result of the individual's genotype and environment

Locus: specific location on a chromosome

Gene: a DNA sequence at a specified locus that encodes for a protein product. Not all protein products have been identified from known genes (e.g., Huntington's chorea)

Allele: alternate forms of a gene at a given locus

Homozygote: an individual with two identical alleles at the specified locus

Heterozygote: an individual with two different alleles at the specified locus

Mutation: a change in DNA, RNA, or protein that results in abnormal expression of a gene's product

Mutant allele: an allele that does not result in the proper quality or quantity of protein product

Wild-type allele: the normal gene; that which occurs most commonly in the population

A. **Autosomal dominant.** Disorders that occur when an individual is heterozygous for a mutant allele are known as *autosomal dominant* disorders. Individuals who possess such an allele have a 50 percent chance of passing on the allele, and therefore the disorder, to their children. Examples of autosomal dominant disorders are found in Table 14.4. These disorders have certain unique features:

1. Since only one mutant allele is needed for phenotypic expression of the disorder, sporadic cases of autosomal dominant disorders can arise as a result of new mutations. For severe autosomal dominant disorders that restrict the reproductive capability of an individual, almost all new cases of such lethal disorders arise as a result of new mutations (e.g., osteogenesis imperfecta).

2. Autosomal dominant disorders tend to exhibit penetrance; that is, the disorder is not expressed by all individuals who possess the mutant allele. Penetrance is an all-or-nothing condition.

3. Autosomal dominant disorders also are variably expressed; that is, the phenotypic expression of the mutant allele can differ from one individual to another. For example, a father with Marfan syndrome may enhibit ectopia lentis and arachnodactyly, whereas his affected offspring may exhibit only the cardiac manifestations (e.g., aortic valve dilation or rupture of large vessels) of the disorder.

B. **Autosomal recessive.** Autosomal recessive disorders (Table 14.5) are those that are exhibited only when an individual is homozygous for a mutant allele. Most affected individuals are born to phenotypically normal parents who are heterozygous for the responsible mutant allele. The lower the frequency of the mutant allele, the higher the likelihood that the affected individual is the result of a consanguineous mating.

1. Matings between two heterozygous individuals (carriers) result in a 25 percent chance that their children will be affected; that is, 75 percent of their children will be phenotypically normal. However, 50 percent of their children, or two-thirds of the unaffected children, will be carriers (Fig. 14.6).

Table 14.4. Autosomal Dominant Disorders

Adult polycystic kidney disease	Huntington disease
Achondroplasia	Marfan syndrome
Ehlers-Danlos syndrome, type I	Myotonic dystrophy
Familial hypercholesterolemia	Neurofibromatosis
Familial colonic polyposis	Noonan syndrome

Table 14.5. Autosomal Recessive Disorders

Alpha-1-antitrypsin deficiency	Phenylketonuria
Congenital adrenal hyperplasia (21-hydroxylase deficiency)	Refsum's disease
Cystic fibrosis	Sickle cell anemia
Homocystinuria	Tay-Sachs disease
Meckel-Gruber syndrome	Wilson's disease (hepatolenticular degeneration)

2. Frequencies of heterozygotes and homozygotes can be estimated by the Hardy-Weinberg law. According to this law, p represents the frequency of the mutant allele and q represents the frequency of the normal, or *wild-type*, allele. $p + q = 1$; $p^2 + 2pq + q^2 = 1$. 2pq represents the frequency of heterozygotes (carriers), p^2 represents the frequency of affected individuals, and q^2 represents the frequency of nor-

Parent
Carrier-Normal

Parent
Carrier-Normal

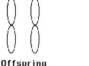 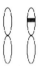 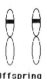

Offspring
Homozygous-Normal

Offspring
Carrier-Normal

Offspring
Carrier-Normal

Offspring
Homozygous
Affected

Affected: 1 of 4 (25%)

Unaffected: 3 of 4 (75%)

Of Unaffected: 2 of 3 (66%) are Carriers

FIGURE 14.6. Potential results of the mating of two individuals heterozygous for a mutant gene (bar) that can result in an autosomal recessive disorder. The risk of having an affected child (homozygous for the mutant gene) is 25 percent. In children who are phenotypically normal, two-thirds will be carriers of the mutant gene.

mal homozygotes. $2pq + q^2$ represents the frequency of phenotypically normal individuals in the study population.

C. **X-linked.** X-linked disorders are caused by mutant genes found on the X chromosome (Table 14.6). Like autosomal disorders, X-linked diseases can be recessive or dominant; however, since males have only one X chromosome, males will express an X-linked recessive disorder with only a single mutant allele present. Affected males are therefore said to be *hemizygous* for X-linked recessive disorders. Since males inherit their X chromosomes from their mothers and their chromosomes from their fathers, male-to-male inheritance of X-linked disorders is impossible.

1. **Recessive disorders**
   a. Many individuals affected with X-linked recessive disorders are born to phenotypically normal parents, with the mother being a carrier of the mutant allele. However, since an X-linked recessive disorder in males is the result of a single mutant allele, new mutations are responsible for many sporadic cases.
   b. Females will rarely exhibit X-linked recessive disorders. Such disorders can result from (1) mating between an affected male and a carrier woman, or (2) 45,X chromosome complement with the mutant allele present on the sole X chromosome, or (3) X chromosome inactivation that inactivates the portion of the X chromosome that has the wild-type allele.
   c. The concept of X inactivation, or the Lyon hypothesis, states that all X chromosomes in excess of **one** are genetically inactive. If both X chromosomes are structurally normal, this inactivation is usually random. However, structural changes such as deletion or translocation may predispose either the normal or the altered chromosome to inactivation, depending on the type of alteration. Cytogenetic representation of the inactivated X chromosome is the Barr body, or X-chromatin mass. The number of Barr bodies is equal to the number of X chromosomes minus one.

Table 14.6. X-Linked Diseases, Recessive (REC) or Dominant (DOM)

Duchenne muscular dystrophy (REC)	Hemophilia B (REC)
Ehlers-Danlos syndrome, type V (REC)	Hunter's syndrome (Mucopolysaccharidosis II) (REC)
Glucose-6-phosphate deficiency (REC)	Hypophosphatemic (vitamin D-resistant) rickets (DOM)
Hemophilia A (REC)	Nephrogenic diabetes insipidus (REC)

d. For males affected with X-linked recessive disorders who are able to reproduce, all daughters will be obligate carriers since they will receive their father's only X chromosome that has the mutant allele. Sons of fathers with X-linked recessive disorders will not inherit the abnormal gene and, therefore, will not express the disorder because they will inherit only the Y chromosome from their fathers. In conclusion, X-linked recessive disorders are most commonly inherited through maternal transmission of genes located on the X chromosome but are expressed almost exclusively in males.

2. **Dominant disorders.** Several X-linked disorders are expressed in a dominant fashion; that is, the disease phenotype is expressed when only a single mutant allele is present. Because women possess twice as many X chromosomes as men, the ratio of affected women to men is $2:1$. There is a 50 percent chance that the children (irrespective of sex) of an affected mother will inherit the mutant allele and exhibit the disease. If the father is affected with an X-linked disorder, all of his daughters but none of his sons will inherit the mutant allele.

D. **Mitochondrial inheritance.** As stated earlier, DNA is found in the mitochondria of cells. Mitochondrial DNA is maternally inherited; only maternal mitochondria are incorporated into the zygote. Several diseases have been attributed to mitochondrial DNA mutations and are inherited through maternal transmission. All children (irrespective of sex) of a mother with abnormal mitochondrial DNA will inherit the disorder, whereas no children (irrespective of sex) of an affected father will inherit the disorder.

E. **Techniques of DNA analysis.** It is estimated that there are approximately 10 000 to 100 000 genes in the human genome. The size of these genes ranges from a few hundred to over 1 million base pairs. Evaluation of these genes and their functions is termed *recombinant DNA analysis*. Recombinant DNA technology permits investigation of DNA sequences and mutations.

1. **Southern blotting.** Named for Dr. E. M. Southern, this technique has been the mainstay for DNA analysis over the past decade (Fig. 14.7). Certain terms require definition prior to describing the technique.

Restriction endonuclease: bacterial enzyme that cleaves DNA at a specific sequence.

Genomic DNA: complete DNA sequence of an individual restriction fragment length polymorphism (RFLP): differences between individuals in the nucleotide sequence of DNA fragments obtained by restriction endonuclease cleavage. A given DNA sequence must be present in at least 1 percent of the population to be defined as an RFLP.

a. Genomic DNA is cleaved using specific restriction en-

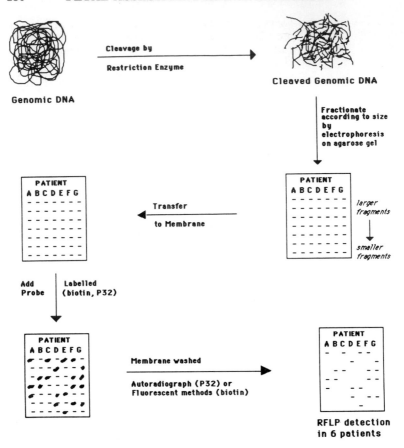

FIGURE 14.7. Southern blotting. Genomic DNA is first denatured into single-stranded DNA and cleaved into various-sized pieces by restriction endonuclease. These fragments are separated by size and hybridized with labeled probes.

    donucleases. The resulting fragments are then denatured
    into single-stranded fragments. These fragments are sep-
    arated by gel electrophoresis according to size; larger
    fragments move a shorter distance on the gel than small-
    er fragments.
b. Southern blotting can be used to detect differences in
    DNA sequences. These differences may be the cause of
    disease, as in sickle cell disease, or more frequently
    represent an RFLP that may be associated with a disease
    state, such as Huntington's chorea. It is important to
    understand that RFLPs are not directly representative of
    or responsible for the disease in question; they merely

serve as a marker for the chromosome that has the purported mutant gene.

   c. Because RFLPs are not the actual mutant genes involved in a disease state, errors in diagnosis can occur as a result of crossing-over between the actual gene locus and the site of the RFLP.

2. **Northern blotting.** This is similar to Southern blotting except that probes are used to analyze mRNA fragments instead of DNA fragments. Evaluation of RNA fragments is useful in verifying gene expression.

3. **Western blotting.** Western blotting employs antibodies to identify specific proteins. It is used to identify proteins associated with the human immunodeficiency virus (HIV) and to evaluate further patients with positive HIV screening tests.

4. **Polymerase chain reaction.** Polymerase chain reaction (PCR) permits the amplification of short sequences of DNA, thereby allowing analysis of DNA sequences without having to clone them.

F. **Polygenic/multifactorial inheritance**

1. In addition to Mendelian inheritance, certain traits and disorders are inherited in a polygenic or multifactorial fashion. Polygenic traits are those caused by the interaction of multiple genes, whereas multifactorial traits are those caused by the interaction of environmental factors with numerous genes. Many of these traits exhibit a Gaussian, or normal, distribution in the population.

2. The risk of inheriting a polygenic or multifactorial trait depends not on the presence or absence of a single gene but rather on the presence or absence of numerous genes and their interaction with environmental factors. For example, if a couple are both carriers of the Tay-Sachs gene, their risk of having a child with Tay-Sachs disease is 25 percent, irrespective of the number of relatives with the disorder. However, the risk of having a child with cleft lip and palate increases with the number of relatives affected with cleft lip and palate. Also, the risk of cleft lip and palate is increased if relatives have severe clefting (e.g., bilateral clefting) compared to the risk if relatives have milder forms (e.g., unilateral) of the disorder.

3. If the sex ratio of a polygenic/multifactorial trait differs greatly from unity, the risk is greatest for offspring of the less affected sex. For example, pyloric stenosis is far more common in males than in females; the risk of pyloric stenosis is therefore highest for sons of affected mothers.

4. These differences from Mendelian inheritance can be related to the concepts of liability and threshold. *Liability* refers to the sum total of genetic and environmental factors that influence the presence or absence of a trait or disorder, and

threshold refers to a level above which an individual develops a trait or disease. If a trait or disease is relatively severely expressed, this may be indicative that the affected individual possesses more genes or is more susceptible to environmental stimuli and, therefore, that his or her relatives are at a higher risk for developing the trait. In the case of pyloric stenosis, a higher level of genetic liability (more genes and greater environmental susceptibility) exists for affected females. Therefore, the son of such a female is at the greatest risk for developing pyloric stenosis since he does not require the same high level of liability for expression of the disorder but is inheriting one-half of his mother's genes as well as sharing her environment.

III. **Chromosome abnormalities.** Chromosome abnormalities are relatively common; approximately 0.6 percent of newborn infants have an abnormal chromosome complement (Nora and Fraser, 1989). In addition, up to 50 percent of spontaneous miscarriages are associated with abnormal chromosome complements. This chapter will focus on several common autosomal and sex chromosome abnormalities. Certain phrases require definition prior to a review of cytogenetic abnormalities (Table 14.7).

A. **Autosomes**

1. **Numerical abnormalities.** The most common autosomal numerical abnormality involves an extra single chromosome; this is known as *trisomy*. Autosomal monosomy, or a deficiency of a single chromosome, is extremely rare. The most common autosomal trisomies in newborns involve chromosomes 21, 18, and 13. A strong maternal age effect is noted with the incidence of trisomic disorders; that is, the frequency increases as maternal age at the time of delivery in-

Table 14.7. Terms Describing Chromosome Abnormalities

Nondisjunction: the failure of two homologous chromosomes to separate, or "disjoin," during meiosis, resulting in one daughter cell with an extra chromosome and one daughter cell with one less chromosome

Balanced translocation: an exchange of material between chromosomes without resulting loss or gain of genetic material

Unbalanced translocation: translocation with resulting loss or gain of genetic material

Robertsonian translocation: translocation involving two acrocentric chromosomes at their centromeres and subsequent loss of their short arms

Polyploidy: increase in the number of haploid sets of chromosomes. Triploidy = $3n$, or 69 chromosomes; tetraploidy = $4n$, or 92 chromosomes

Mosaicism: the presence of two or more distinct cell lines derived from a single zygote. Although abnormalities in meiosis can lead to mosaicism, mitotic abnormalities are most frequently responsible for this condition

creases. In approximately 80 percent of the cases, maternal nondisjunction is the source of the extra chromosomes in the trisomies described below.

a. **Trisomy 21 (Down syndrome)**
   (1) **Incidence.** The most common and least severe autosomal numerical abnormality, with an incidence of 1/800 liveborns.
   (2) **Cause.** Ninety-five percent of affected patients have an extra chromosome 21; 3 percent have an unbalanced translocation, resulting in a "triple dose" of DNA found at band q22 of chromosome 21, and 2 percent are mosaic for a normal and trisomy 21 cell line.
   (3) **Findings.** Characteristic faces—a "mongoloid" slant of the eyes with epicanthal folds, low nasal bridge, protruding fissured tongue; Brushfield spots in the iris; flat occiput, occasional webbed neck (pterygium coli), diastasis recti, and umbilical hernias. Sixty percent have a congenital heart defect: Ventricular septal defect and endocardial cushion defects are most common. Hypotonia and mild to severe psychomotor retardation. Cryptochidism male infertility. Increased incidence of leukemia and thyroid disorders. Characteristic changes in dermatoglyphics (simian crease, ulnar loops, distal axial triradius, hallucal loop).
   (4) **Prognosis.** Decreased life span; survival depends on the presence of somatic (cardiac disease, leukemia) manifestations of Down syndrome.

b. **Trisomy 18**
   (1) **Incidence.** 1/6000.
   (2) **Cause.** Approximately 80 percent of affected patients are trisomic for chromosome 18; 10 percent are unbalanced translocation carriers and 10 percent are mosaics.
   (3) **Findings.** Severe failure to thrive, severe psychomotor retardation, hypertonia, prominent occiput, low-set ears, micrognathia, microstomia. Characteristic clenched fist, "rocker-bottom" feet. Almost all have congenital heart defects, most commonly ventricular septal defect (VSD) or patent ductus arteriosis (PDA).
   (4) **Prognosis.** Only 10 percent are alive after 1 year.

c. **Trisomy 13**
   (1) **Incidence.** 1/15 000.
   (2) **Cause.** Eighty percent of patients with complete trisomy, 15 percent unbalanced translocation carriers (frequently involving chromosomes 13 and 14), and 5 percent mosaics.
   (3) **Findings.** Severe psychomotor retardation, holo-

prosencephaly, iris colobomata, cleft lip and palate, postaxial polydactyly of the hands and feet, micropthalmia. Congenital heart disease in 90 percent of patients, most commonly VSD, PDA, and cardiac rotational abnormalities. Renal anomalies.

(4) **Prognosis.** Only 10 percent are alive at 6 months.

2. **Structural chromosome abnormalities**

a. The most common structural defects, such as chromosome inversions and balanced translocations (i.e., reciprocal, Robertsonian), exist in phenotypically normal individuals. These structureal defects can result in an increased risk of spontaneous abortion or chromosome abnormalities in the offspring of affected individuals (e.g., balanced or unbalanced translocation between chromosomes 14 and 21) or can be benign (e.g., paracentric inversion of chromosome 9). In addition to being inherited from parents, structural abnormalities can arise de novo; that is, the abnormality is new in the affected individual and is not present in either parent or as a result of abnormal crossing-over of translocated parental chromosomes.

b. With improvement in our ability to detect small chromosome abnormalities, structural chromosome defects have been implicated in several disorders (e.g., Prader-Willi syndrome, Langer-Gideon syndrome, Beckwith-Wiedemann syndrome) as well as in familial cancer syndromes (e.g., retinoblastoma, Wilms' tumor-aniridia syndrome).

c. del(tp): Cri-du-chat syndrome

(1) **Incidence.** Probably the best-known and best-described chromosome structural defect.

(2) **Cause.** Involves the loss of the distal portion of the short arm of chromosome 5; loss of the region involving bands p14–p15 is usually responsible for clinical symptoms (Fig. 14.8) Most cases are sporadic, although cases of this syndrome as a result of familial translocations have been reported.

(3) **Findings.** Microcephaly, moderate to severe psychomotor retardation. Anti-mongoloid slant of the eyes, occasional (25 percent) cardiac defects. Characteristic "cat-cry" sound similar to a kitten's mew, hence the name *cri-du-chat.*

(4) **Prognosis.** Survival to adulthood is relatively common.

B. **Sex chromosomes.** Sex chromosome abnormalities have a higher likelihood of viability than autosomal abnormalities. This is probably due to the fact that very few genes reside on the Y chromosome and that all but one X chromosome are inactivated (Lyon hypothesis), forming X-chromatin bodies (Barr bodies) within the nuclei. Mosaicism is also far more common with sex chromosome abnormalities than with autosomal abnormalities.

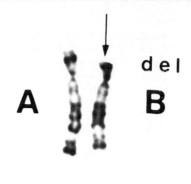

FIGURE 14.8. (A) Normal chromosome 5. (B) Deleted chromosome 5 [del(5p14) associated with cri-du-chat syndrome].

1. **Numerical abnormalities.** As a group, numerical sex chromosome abnormalities are far more common in liveborns than autosomal numerical abnormalities. In addition, monosomy X is the most frequently found abnormal complement in spontaneously aborted fetuses. Generally, the greater the number of X or Y chromosomes found, the lower the IQ and the higher the risk of somatic abnormalities.

   a. **45,X (Turner syndrome)**
      (1) **Incidence.** 1/5000 liveborns. It is the most common chromosome abnormality found in spontaneously aborted fetuses.
      (2) **Cause.** No maternal age effect noted. The paternal X chromosome is most commonly missing; mosaicism involving a 45,X cell line is relatively common. Certain structural defects (e.g., del(Xp), the isochromosome for the long arm of the X chromosome) can mimic the 45,X phenotype.
      (3) **Findings.** Short stature, normal IQ with deficiencies in three-dimensional problem-solving capabilities (space-form blindness). Distinctive faces, numerous pigmented nevi, low posterior hairline, webbed neck, shield chest, widely spaced, hypoplastic nipples. One-third have cardiac defects, most commonly coarctation of the aorta. Lymphedema of distal extremities during infancy, short fourth and fifth fingers with clinodactyly of the fifth finger, cubitus valgus. Ovarian dysgenesis with subsequent primary amenorrhea and infertility. No Barr bodies present.
      (4) **Prognosis.** Normal life span.

b. **47,XXX**
   (1) **Incidence.** 1/800 females.
   (2) **Cause.** Maternal age effect noted.
   (3) **Findings.** Normal female phenotype with normal puberty and fertility. Intellectual ability may be slightly impaired. Two Barr bodies present.
   (4) **Prognosis.** Normal life span
c. **47,XXY (Klinefelter syndrome)**
   (1) **Incidence.** 1/800 males.
   (2) **Cause.** Maternal age effect noted.
   (3) **Findings.** Tall, eunuchoid habitus with good intellectual development that frequently lags behind that of siblings. Gynecomastia, partial virilization, small penis and testes, infertility. One Barr body present.
   (4) **Prognosis.** Normal life span.
d. **47,XYY**
   (1) **Incidence.** 1/800 males
   (2) **Cause.** Maternal age effect noted despite the fact that a nondisjunctional event must occur during paternal meiosis.
   (3) **Findings.** Tall stature with normal male habitus. Slightly impaired intellectual ability with antisocial behavior. Severe acne during adolescence. Normal puberty and fertility. No Barr bodies present.
   (4) **Prognosis.** Normal life span.
2. **Structural abnormalities.** A wide variety of X and Y chromosome structural defects have been observed. The resulting phenotype depends on the portion of the X or Y chromosome that is deleted or duplicated. Phenotypic abnormalities can range from none [e.g., del(Yq)] to Turner syndrome [e.g., isoX(q)]. However, structural defects tend not to result in the severe phenotypic changes found with complete absence or duplication of entire sex chromosomes.

IV. **Prenatal diagnosis.** Obstetricians will will have their greatest exposure to the field of genetics as it pertains to prenatal diagnosis. They need to understand not only the techniques of prenatal diagnosis but also what is required prior to and after procedures.
   A. **Indications for prenatal diagnosis.** The following are the most common indications for offering invasive prenatal diagnosis to a couple. This testing is offered to couples who are at increased risk of producing children with chromosome abnormalities; Mendelian disorders detectable by DNA, enzyme, or abnormal substrate analysis; neural tube defects; or any fetal structural defect detected by abnormal substrate levels in amniotic fluid, chorionic villi, or fetal blood.
      1. Advanced maternal age (≥ 35 years at the estimated time of delivery)

2. Previous child with a chromosome abnormality
3. Parental chromosome translocation or abnormality (aneuploidy, structural abnormalities)
4. Increased risk of neural tube defect (i.e., affected first- or second-degree relatives of the current pregnancy)
5. Abnormal genetic screening test
6. Two or more spontaneous miscarriages
7. Family history of a Mendelian disorder detectable by DNA analysis
8. Determination of fetal sex when fetus is at increased risk for an X-linked disorder and no DNA analysis is available
9. Exposure to certain teratogenic agents

B. **Genetic/environmental history**
1. Obtaining an accurate family history is an essential part of prenatal diagnosis. Health information of first-degree (parents, siblings, and offsprings) and second-degree (grandparents, uncles, aunts, nephews, and nieces) relatives should be routinely obtained. Any history of miscarriages should also be obtained.
2. The ethnic origin of families should be ascertained since certain disorders are more prevalent in certain ethnic groups (e.g., sickle cell disease in African-Americans, Tay-Sachs disease in Ashkenazic Jews, beta thalassemia in Italians and other Mediterranean peoples), and screening tests can be offered to specific patients who may be increased risk for being carriers of certain Mendelian disorders.
3. In addition to the aforementioned information, the obstetrician must obtain information concerning exposure to potential teratogens. This can occur as a result of drug (both legal and illicit) ingestion, as well as exposure to environmental toxins at home or work.

C. **Genetic screening**
1. In addition to identifying individuals at risk for certain disorders based on family history, tests are available that identify individuals at increased risk for certain disorders. These tests can be applied to either specific ethnic groups or the population at large.
   a. **Specific ethnic groups**
      (1) Sickle cell testing to identify carriers (hemoglobin AS) of sickle cell disease among African-Americans
      (2) Hexosaminidase A to identify Tay-Sachs disease carriers among Ashkenazic (Eastern or Northern European) Jews
      (3) Mean corpuscular volume (MCV) to identify beta thalassemia minor in Italians and other ethnic groups from the Mediterranean area
      (4) Eventual use of gene mutations (e.g., $\Delta F508$) to identify carriers of genes associated with Mendelian disorders

　　　b. **The population at large**

　　　　　(1) Maternal serum alpha fetoprotein (MSAFP) screening for neural tube defects

　　　　　(2) MSAFP, maternal serum human chorionic gonadotropin (hCG), and unconjugated estriol (uE3) in aggregate (multiplex screening or triple test) for Down syndrome

　　　　　(3) Determination of Rh and indirect Coombs' test status to determine the risk of hydrops fetalis

　2. It is important to understand that screening tests are not diagnostic; they serve to identify individuals at increased risk for having children with specific disorders so that those individuals can be offered specific diagnostic tests (e.g., amniocentesis to detect fetal neural tube defects). Patients should only be offered screening tests that apply to them; patients should never be forced to undergo screening tests; and patients who test positive for a specific assay should never be forced to undergo further diagnostic tests. As with other obstetric and gynecologic decisions, it is essential to discuss with patients all the risks, benefits, limitations, and expectations of a particular screening test.

D. Obstetricians should offer MSAFP screening to all eligible, low-risk patients. Women at low risk for fetal neural tube defects are those carrying a fetus without first- or second-degree relatives (to the fetus) affected with neural tube defects and not exposed to teratogens commonly associated with neural tube defects (e.g., valproic acid); women at increased risk for fetal neural tube defects should be offered amniocentesis to evaluate their pregnancy further. Multiplex screening involving MSAFP, hCG, and uE3 assays is now available to screen patients at low risk for having offspring affected with Down syndrome; as with MSAFP screening for Down syndrome, women at increased risk for fetal Down syndrome (e.g., advanced maternal age, prior pregnancy affected with Down syndrome) should be offered prenatal cytogenetic analysis. A calculation of assay results and maternal age results in an adjusted risk for fetal Down syndrome (Wald et al., 1989). The multiplex screen is currently considered investigational. The similarities between the MSAFP and multiplex screening tests are as follows:

　1. Performed between 15 and 20 weeks' gestation (will vary according to the laboratory)

　2. Performed on serum obtained from 5 to 10 mL clotted peripheral maternal blood

　3. Results rapidly available

　4. Ultrasonography and invasive prenatal diagnostic techniques required to evaluate further most abnormal results

E. Diagnostic techniques. Although several diagnostic tests are available to diagnose disorders prenatally, amniocentesis and chorionic villus sampling are the procedures most commonly used for fetal evaluation. As noted earlier, a detailed discussion of the indications for invasive prenatal diagnosis, as well as the risks, benefits, and limitations of the test, must precede all procedures.

1. Amniocentesis
    a. Typically performed between 14 and 20 weeks' gestation under ultrasound guidance; early amniocentesis prior to 14 weeks' gestation is currently investigational and is performed in a fashion similar to midtrimester amniocentesis (Fig. 14.9).
    b. Chromosome and alpha fetoprotein analysis usually performed irrespective of the specific reason for amniocentesis
    c. Risks
        (1) Increase in the miscarriage rate of 0.5 percent or less
        (2) Minor complications such as minimal fluid leakage, self-limited spotting per vagina
        (3) Safety and accuracy of early amniocentesis still uncertain
    d. Diagnostic accuracy: greater than 99 percent accurate

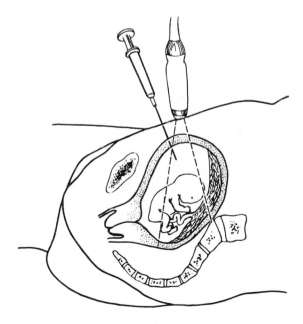

FIGURE 14.9. Amniocentesis performed by passage of a 22-gauge spinal needle, under continuous ultrasound guidance, into the amniotic cavity. (Reprinted with permission from Simpson JL, Elias S. Prenatal diagnosis of genetic disorders. In: Creasy RK, Resnick R, eds. Maternal-Fetal Medicine: Principles and Practice. Philadelphia: WB Saunders; 1989:83.)

2. **Chorionic villus sampling (CVS)**
   a. Typically performed between 10 and 12.5 weeks' gestation, either transvaginally (TC-CVS) or transabdominally (TA-CVS), under ultrasound guidance. It is necessary to remove at least 10 mg of chorionic tissue. The placental location as well as certain conditions (e.g., vaginal herpes will preclude TC-CVS) guide the obstetrician's choice as to which approach to utilize (Figs. 14.10 and 14.11).
   b. The major benefit of CVS is early diagnosis of fetal abnormalities; it permits first-trimester pregnancy termination, which is both physically and emotionally beneficial to the patient.
   c. Risks
      (1) Canadian and American trials both showed that the risk of miscarriage with TC-CVS is not significantly different from that with second-trimester amniocentesis.
      (2) Minor complications such as spotting per vagina

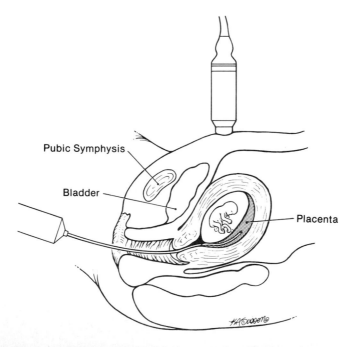

Pubic Symphysis

Bladder

Placenta

FIGURE 14.10. TC-CVS performed by passage of a catheter, under continuous ultrasound guidance, through the cervix into the placenta. (Reprinted with permission from Shulman LP, Elias S. Chorionic villus sampling. Semin Perinatol 1990; 14(6):447.)

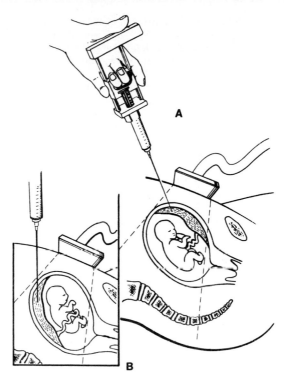

FIGURE 14.11. TA-CVS performed by passage of a spinal needle, under continuous ultrasound guidance, into the placenta. (A) TA-CVS performed on the anterior placenta. (B) TA-CVS performed on the posterior placenta. (Reprinted with permission from Elias S, Simpson JL, Shulman LP, et al. Transabdominal chorionic villus sampling for first-trimester prenatal diagnosis. Am J Obstet Gynecol 1989; 160:881.)

       are more common with TC-CVS than with TA-CVS. Remote obstetric complications such as intrauterine growth retardation, premature delivery, preeclampsia, and placental abruption are not increased by TC-CVS.

(3) The relative safety of TA-CVS is yet to be determined, although reports from several centers indicate risks to be comparable to that of TC-CVS.

d. Diagnostic testing. In addition to cytogenetic analysis of cultured villus cells, rapidly dividing cytotrophoblasts can be used to perform so-called direct cytogenetic analysis. Results from direct analyses are usually available within 48 h but carry disadvantages (e.g., poorer-quality metaphases) that must be balanced with the information obtained from analysis of cultured cells. Although cytogenetic and DNA analyses can be performed on chorionic villi, fetal neural tube defects and some enzymatic defects cannot be diagnosed by chorionic villus analysis.

   e. Diagnostic accuracy. Both amniotic fluid cell analysis and chorionic villus analysis carry diagnostic pitfalls that need to be recognized by obstetricians. Inadvertent inclusion of maternal cells is of particular concern with chorionic villus specimens but is rare. One advantage of direct analysis is that decidua rarely contributes metaphases to direct cytogenetic preparations because decidual cell growth is so much slower than that of cytotrophoblasts. The accuracy of CVS approximates that of amniocentesis; however, diagnosis of chromosome abnormalities in chorionic villus specimens does not always signify fetal chromosome abnormalities. Discrepancies also occur between cytotrophoblasts (direct), mesenchymal core (culture), and fetal tissue. Because of these potential discrepancies, interpretation of the cytogenetic results of CVS requires expertise. Amniocentesis may be required in the 1 percent or so of ambiguous CVS cytogenetic results.

3. Percutaneous umbilical blood sampling (PUBS). PUBS has been employed for physiologic, infectious, and cytogenetic evaluation of the second- and third-trimester fetus. Originally performed with a fetoscope, PUBS is currently performed by transabdominal passage of a 22- or 25-gauge spinal needle preferentially into the placental insertion site of the umbilical cord (Fig. 14.12) or into a free loop of umbilical cord; both techniques are performed under continuous ultrasound guidance. PUBS is not only useful for the recovery of fetal blood and serum but also provides access to fetal circulation for the introduction of therapeutic agents.

   Although PUBS has been shown to be relatively safe, a rigorous assessment of its safety and accuracy has yet to be reported. It appears appropriate to counsel patients that PUBS may increase the risk of fetal demise 2 to 3 percent over baseline, although this risk may be substantially higher if the indication for PUBS is fetal anomaly. This increased risk may reflect the additional stress on an already compromised fetus. As a rule, one should not perform PUBS when a less invasive procedure such as amniocentesis would suffice.

4. Fetal skin sampling. Biopsy of fetal skin is required to diagnose certain genetic skin disorders, or genodermatoses. Amniotic fluid for chromosome analysis should be collected prior to biopsy of fetal skin. Too few fetal skin sampling procedures have been performed to assess their safety and

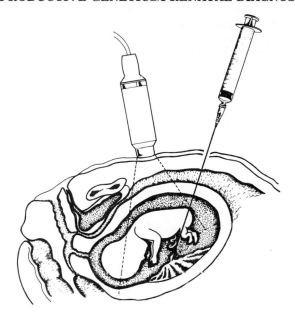

FIGURE 14.12. PUBS performed by passage of a 22-gauge spinal needle, under continuous ultrasound guidance, into the placental insertion site of the umbilical cord. (Reprinted with permission from Shulman LP, Elias S. Percutaneous umbilical cord blood sampling, fetal skin sampling and fetal liver biopsy. Semin Perinatol 1990; 14(6):457.)

accuracy; however, loss rates have been estimated to be 2 to 3 percent over background.

F. **Communicating prenatal diagnostic test results.** Test results should be communicated as soon as they are available. In most cases, they should be discussed directly with the patient unless the patient has selected another person.

The ability to provide counseling services to individuals with either abnormal screening or diagnostic test results is essential. Although the obstetrician should provide information and support to such patients, referral to personnel skilled in counseling and support services (e.g., geneticists, genetic counselors, nurses, social workers) may be required in certain situations (Simpson et al., 1982).

REFERENCES AND SUGGESTED READINGS

Canadian Collaborative CVS-Amniocentesis Clinical Trial Group. Multicentre randomized clinical trial of chorion villus sampling and amniocentesis. First report. Lancet 1989; 1:1.

Elias S, Simpson JL. Amniocentesis. In: Milunsky A, ed. Genetic Disorders and the Fetus. New York: Plenum Press; 1986:31–52.

Elias S, Simpson JL, Shulman LP, et al. Transabdominal chorionic villus sampling for first trimester prenatal diagnosis. Am J Obstet Gynecol 1989; 160:879.

Gelehrter TD, Collins FS. Principles of Medical Genetics. Baltimore: Williams and Wilkins; 1990.

Ledbetter DH, Martin AO, Verlinsky Y, et al. Cytogenetic results of chorionic villus sampling: High success rate and diagnostic accuracy in the U.S. Collaborative Study. Am J Obstet Gynecol 1990; 162:495.

NICHD National Registry for Amniocentesis Study Group. Midtrimester amniocentesis for prenatal diagnosis; safety and accuracy. JAMA 1976; 236:1471.

Nora JJ, Fraser FC. Medical Genetics—Principles and Practice. Philadelphia: Lea and Febiger; 1989.

Report of the Standing Committee on Human Cytogenetic Nomenclature. An International System for Human Cytogenetic Nomenclature (ISCN: 1985). Basel: Karger; 1985.

Rhoads GG, Jackson LG, Schlesselman SE, et al. The safety and efficacy of chorionic villus sampling for early prenatal diagnosis of cytogenetic abnormalities. N Engl J Med 1989; 320;609.

Schochetman G, Ou C-Y, Jones WK. Polymerase chain reaction. J Infect Dis 1988; 158:1154.

Shepard TH. Catalogue of Teratogenic Agents. 6th ed. Baltimore: Johns Hopkins University Press; 1989.

Shulman LP, Elias S. Chorionic villus sampling. Pediatri Ann 1989; 18:714.

Shulman LP, Meyers CM, Simpson JL, et al. Fetomaternal transfusion depends upon the amount of chorionic villa aspirated but not upon method of chorionic villus sampling. Am J Obstet Gynecol 1990; 162:1185.

Simpson JL. General principles of teratology and embryology. In: Simpson JL, Golbus MS, eds. Genetics in Obstetrics and Gynecology. 2nd ed. Philadelphia: WB Saunders; 1992.

Simpson JL, Elias S. Prenatal diagnosis of genetic disorders. In: Creasy RK, Resnick R, eds. Maternal-Fetal Medicine. Philadelphia: WB Saunders; 1989:78–107.

Simpson JL, Golbus MS, Martin AO, et al. Genetics in Obstetrics and Gynecology. Orlando, Fla: Grune and Stratton; 1982.

Southern EM. Detection of specific sequences among DNA fragments separated by gel electrophoresis. J Mol Biol 1975; 98:503.

Tipton RE, Tharapel AT, Chang HT, et al. Rapid chromosome analysis using spontaneously dividing cells derived from umbilical cord blood (fetal and neonatal). Am J Obstet Gynecol 1989; 161:1546.

USNICHD Collaborative CVS Study Group. Transcervical and transabdominal chorionic villus sampling are comparably safe procedures for first trimester prenatal diagnosis: Preliminary analysis, abstracted. Am J Hum Genet 1990; 47:A278.

Wald NJ, Cuckle HS, Densem JW, et al. Maternal serum screening for Down's syndrome in early pregnancy. Br Med J 1988; 297:883.

Watson JD, Tooze J, Kurtz DT. Recombinant DNA—A Short Course. New York: Freeman; 1983.

CHAPTER 15

Management of Congenital Anomalies

Joseph A. Spinnato

The availability of high-resolution ultrasonographic imaging and bio-chemical and chromosomal markers for fetal disease has dramatically increased the potential for the antenatal diagnosis of fetal abnormalities. This capability imposes upon us new responsibilities to both our obstetric and fetal patients to (1) provide accurate and timely information; (2) describe all treatment options; (3) counsel accurately regarding the relative merits of each option; (4) select options that balance the moral, ethical, and legal issues that, not infrequently, accompany antenatal diagnosis; and (5) design clinical therapeutic strategies that optimize the fetomaternal outcome, including, but not limited to, the route, timing, and location of delivery. This requires the practitioner to update continually information regarding new therapy, technology, and diagnostic modalities or to seek the assistance of those who do.

I. General considerations
   A. Most fetal abnormalities are discovered during Level I ultrasound examination performed for that or other purposes. An additional group of fetuses are identified during primary Level II examination prompted by the prior obstetric history. The identification or suspicion of fetal anomaly, in most cases, should prompt referral for **Level II ultrasound evaluation** and perinatal/genetic consultation. Table 15.1 lists the situations that warrant Level II ultrasound examination.
   B. **Perinatal consultation** begins a process that includes a diligent investigation of the latest diagnostic and treatment modalities to enable proper counseling and care.
   1. As this task often exceeds the boundaries of any one specialty, many centers have generated multispecialty groups whose tasks are to:
   a. Ensure the accuracy of diagnoses
   b. Provide accurate prognostic information
   c. Support and counsel patients
   d. Determine management
   2. **Management** decisions include:
   a. Evaluation for possible pregnancy termination

Table 15.1. Indications for Level II Ultrasound in Fetuses with Known or at Risk for Congenital Anomaly

Cranial abnormalities
   Anencephaly
   Hydrocephaly
   Microcephaly
   Encephalocele
   Cystic hygroma

Thoracic abnormalities
   Lung masses
   Diaphragmatic hernia
   Tracheoesophageal fistula

Cardiac abnormalities

Spinal abnormalities
   Spina bifida cystica
   Sacral agenesis
   Sacrococcygeal teratoma

Gastrointestinal abnormalities
   Omphalocele/gastroschisis (ventral wall defect)
   Duodenal/esophageal atresia
   Bowel obstruction (cystic fibrosis, etc.)

Genitourinary abnormalities
   Hydronephrosis/hydroureter
   Multicystic kidney
   Infantile polycystic kidney disease
   Renal agenesis
   Grossly enlarged bladder
   Abdominal masses

Skeletal abnormalities

Miscellaneous
   Abnormal umbilical cord
   Severely polyhydramnios
   Oligohydramnios
   Insulin dependent diabetes mellitus
   Maternal hydantoin therapy

---

     b.   Ethical considerations and legal constraints
     c.   Prenatal versus postnatal therapy
     d.   Timing and execution of selected therapy
     e.   Timing and mode of delivery

C. When congenital abnormalities are diagnosed, the care providers must understand the influence of the grief responses of both parents (which are often different from each other) and even the care provider's emotional response to the discovery, birth, or anticipated birth of an anomalous fetus. Anxiety, sorrow, guilt, anger, denial, shock, and ambivalence at times hamper and even preclude sound decision making. Multispecialty involvement may protect the parents, physicians, fetus, and/or infant from emotion-based decisions that later may be regretted.

D. In the situation of the prenatally diagnosed anomaly, counseling is predominantly negative. It describes the physical and mental prognoses, short- and long-term requirements for care, and long-term consequences. Carefully balanced counseling that offers encouragement, limits overestimates of the disability, enlarges the family's scope of values, and fosters noncomparative evaluation of the child is crucial to long-term family therapy.

II. Termination of pregnancy before 24 weeks' gestation

A. Before viability (before 24 weeks' gestation in most areas), **abortion** is a legally available option for pregnancy management independent of fetal health. This option should be presented to couples whose fetus is diagnosed as anomalous.

B. **Counseling** must accurately reflect the certainty of the diagnosis and the likely extent of the handicap. Further, diagnostic options (e.g., karyotyping, fetal blood studies, follow-up examination) that improve the accuracy of counseling should be completely explored (if not performed) before termination is offered. Frequently, the time available for such investigations is limited.

C. Every attempt should be made to expedite an evaluation so that the option of termination is preserved for those who consider it. For example, certain genetic laboratories offer rapid karyotyping from amniotic fluid samples (1- week turnaround). Fetal blood karyotyping (from umbilical vein sampling) can be accomplished in 2 to 3 days.

D. Regardless of the best efforts, in some cases it is necessary to consider termination of pregnancy without a firm diagnosis. Some couples would rather terminate the pregnancy than risk the delivery of a handicapped child. As this is their right, every effort to provide the best information to the couple should be made.

E. The legal constraints to termination of pregnancy vary from locale to locale. It is important for those who counsel patients with identified fetal anomalies to be aware of these constraints and, for selected patients, to be knowledgeable about alternative sites for termination in less restrictive legal jurisdictions. Counseling that conceals legally available options to the patients by deception, delay, or deliberate omission is ethically flawed.

III. Termination or nonaggressive management of pregnancy after fetal viability

A. Chervenak and colleagues, in a series of articles, have focused on the ethical dilemmas of caring for the pregnant patient with an anomalous fetus after fetal viability. These articles provide a firm footing for difficult decisions in such cases, and their review is encouraged. The guidelines are based upon the accuracy of the diagnosis, the severity of the anomaly, the potential for postnatal cognitive function, and the postnatal life expectancy.

Decisions are directed, in large part, by the beneficence-based obligations to the fetus — in other words, by whether the fetus benefits by its own birth. These concerns are then balanced by concerns for maternal autonomy. In general, when there is more than a minimal beneficence-based obligation to the fetus, maternal autonomy concerns rarely justify other than aggressive fetal management. Interventions such as antenatal testing, inhibition of preterm labor, amniocentesis (to time delivery or for bilirubin studies), and indicated cesarean section, for example, are less hazardous to the mother than are the consequences to the fetus if they are not performed.

B. **Termination of pregnancy in the third trimester** is deemed morally justifiable when:
1. The fetus is afflicted with a condition that is either:
   a. Incompatible with postnatal survival for more than a few weeks or
   b. Characterized by the total or virtual absence of cognitive function and
2. Highly reliable diagnostic procedures are available for determining prenatally that the fetus fulfills either condition 1a or 1b.
3. The list of anomalies fulfilling both criteria is small and, unequivocally, includes only anencephaly and triploidy. In these cases (Category A), there is virtually no cognitive function and the diagnosis can be made with certainty. There is no beneficence-based obligation to the fetus.

C. Chervenak and colleagues describe a second group (Category B) of anomalies wherein there is (1) certainty or a very high probability of accurate prenatal diagnosis and (2) either certainty or a very high probability of death or absence of cognitive developmental capacity. However, the certainty of either condition 1 or condition 2 is not present simultaneously. Third-trimester termination is not offered to this group because the certainty of diagnosis and of death or absence of cognitive function cannot be completely assured. Hence, there exists a minimal beneficence-based obligation to the fetus. Examples in this group include trisomy 18, renal agenesis, and thanatophoric dysplasia. In this group, however, the obligations to the fetus do not necessarily override concerns for maternal safety and well-being. Recommendations to the couple include a choice between aggressive (standard obstetric interventions intended to optimize the fetal outcome) and nonaggressive management (no interventions on behalf of the fetus, including no cesarean section for fetal distress or abnormal lie). The rationale for offering nonaggressive management is that the minimal beneficence-based obligations to the fetus ethically neither permit third-trimester termination nor compel interventions that might increase maternal risk (i.e., cesarean section).

D. A third category (Category C) includes situations where the probability of accurate diagnosis is less than very high or the probability of death or absence of cognitive function is less than very high. In these situations there is more than minimal beneficence-based obligation to the fetus. The recommendations in these cases are for aggressive management and against nonaggressive management or termination of pregnancy. Such cases include Down's syndrome and achondroplasia. Withholding care intended to maximize fetal outcome is ethically unjustified.

IV. **In utero therapy: General considerations.** Fetal therapy began in the early 1960s when intrauterine fetal transfusions were first attempted. Initially, exchange transfusion was performed via an open technique involving laparotomy and uterine incision. The resultant maternal morbidity and increased hazard to the pregnancy itself (infection, labor, etc.) prompted a switch to fluoroscopy-guided intraperitoneal fetal transfusion, which dramatically improved fetal salvage. Ultrasound-guided transfusion replaced fluoroscopy in the 1970s. Recently, direct intravascular transfusion of the fetus via percutaneous ultrasound-directed needle puncture of the umbilical vein has been employed. Each change in management has not only improved the outcome and reduced morbidity, but has also increased the number of candidates for therapy. Experience with fetal hemolytic disease began the formulation of strategies for fetal therapy.

When a potentially treatable or correctable fetal anomaly is diagnosed, several factors determine clinical decisions: (1) Is therapy **necessary?** Is the natural history of the lesion such that in utero therapy is unnecessary and can be delayed until birth? (2) Will **delay** in therapy until birth worsen the prognosis? (3) Is it possible to **correct** an anomaly or **treat** an abnormality to lessen the consequences to the fetus? (4) What **risks** to the mother or fetus do in utero therapies create? (5) When are the **advantages** of in utero therapy exceeded by delivery and postnatal therapy?

In utero medical and surgical therapy of the fetus should be considered when (1) the consequences of the untreated anomaly or abnormality can be predicted to result in severe handicap or death, (2) the selected therapy has been demonstrated to improve the fetal/neonatal outcome, and (3) the risk to the fetus or mother is clearly outweighed by the potential benefit.

V. **Route of delivery**
    A. For several of the anomalies to be discussed, the route of delivery is controversial. This is particularly true for neural tube defects, omphalocele, gastroschisis, sacrococcygeal teratoma, and diaphragmatic hernia.
    B. The essence of the problem is as follows:
        1. Few, if any, prospective, randomized studies exist that compare vaginal with abdominal delivery (with or without labor) when these anomalies are present.
        2. In general, the available studies compare prospectively managed patients whose fetal defect is identified antenatally (who are very likely to have been delivered by cesarean section) to patients whose fetal defect is unsuspected and

whose abdominal delivery is performed only for obstetric indications. The latter group is more likely to deliver outside a tertiary center, with antenatal surveillance being less frequently performed. These factors delay definitive therapy, allow less expert management of acute stabilization, and may bias care decisions in the tertiary center.

3. In general, studies of this type are apt to suggest a benefit for abdominal delivery when what is really demonstrated is the benefit of aggressive antenatal therapy that is potentially independent of the delivery route. Until better studies are available, we are guided largely by theory and conjecture.

C. The potential benefits of cesarean section (timed delivery, logistical problems for patients living far from the tertiary center, staffing problems at the center) must be weighed against the short- and long-term increased maternal risks and the potential that no fetal benefit will be gained.

VI. Specific anomalies
A. Fetal hydrocephalus
1. **Incidence.** Fetal hydrocephalus occurs in approximately 1/2000 pregnancies. From 25 to 30 percent of cases are associated with coexistent spina bifida.
2. **Cause.** Idiopathic aqueductal stenosis (43 percent) and the communicating type (38 percent) are the most common causes of congenital hydrocephalus.
3. **Diagnosis**
   a. Thirty percent of cases (most with spina bifida) are associated with polyhydramnios. The remainder are without symptoms and are found incidentally at ultrasound examination for other indication.
   b. In early gestation (before 24 weeks) the circumference of the head often is not excessive, and serial examinations are necessary, at times, to confirm the diagnosis.
   c. The diagnosis is suggested when, after 20 weeks' gestation, the ratio of the lateral ventricular width to the lateral hemispheric width (LVW:HW) exceeds 33 percent (Fig. 15.1). Prior to 20 weeks' gestation, the diagnosis is difficult to make with confidence since the normal range for the LVW:HW ratio is broad. Serial examinations are often necessary.
4. **Prognosis.** The outcome of fetal hydrocephalus is closely linked to the presence or absence of associated anomalies. Chromosomal aneuploidy is present in 20 to 25 percent of cases. From 55 to 60 percent coexist with non–central nervous system (non-CNS) anomalies. The total anomaly rate, including CNS anomalies, ranges from 70 to 85 percent. Despite careful antenatal evaluation, in one series 40 to 60 percent of these anomalies were missed ultrasonographically. The overall mortality rate is as high at 67 percent, com-

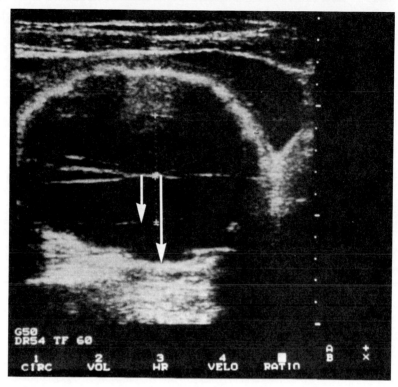

FIGURE 15.1. Increased ventriculohemispheric ratio of 51 percent (normal <
33 percent) at term in a fetus with hydrocephalus.

pared to 23 percent for isolated hydrocephalus. Mental
retardation and developmental delay occur in as many as 70
to 80 percent. However, the prognosis of isolated hydrocephalus or hydrocephalus associated with spina bifida cystica is considerably better, with upward of 70 percent of
survivors having intelligence quotients in the normal range.
Several reports have documented spontaneous resolution of
hydrocephalus in utero.

5. **Management**
   a. The multiple causes of prenatally diagnosed hydro-
      cephaly, coupled with the limitations of prenatal assess-
      ment for coexistent cranial and extracranial anomalies,
      as well as the wide range of postnatal mental and motor
      performance observed for the various causes, require
      caution when selecting among management options.
   b. For most cases, delivery at a fully staffed perinatal center
      is necessary to optimize the neonatal outcome.

    c. Amniocentesis for karyotype, alpha fetoprotein, and acetylcholinesterase, in addition to serial evaluations for coexistent anomalies and progression of ventriculomegaly, is necessary. Selected patients may benefit from umbilical vein blood sampling for assessment of a possible viral cause.

    d. Therapeutic options include termination of pregnancy before viability, nonaggressive management including cephalaocentesis, and aggressive management including cesarean section for obstetric indications including macrocephaly.

      (1) Nonaggressive management is probably justifiable when hydrocephalus is associated with trisomy 13 or 18, alobar holoprosencephaly, thanatophoric dysplasia, and renal diseases associated with prolonged oligohydramnios. Cephalocentesis (when necessary), draining cerebrospinal fluid to facilitate vaginal delivery, is justifiable in these cases. Fetal or neonatal death follows cephalocentesis in most cases.

      (2) The beneficence-based obligations to the fetus with isolated hydrocephalus or hydrocephalus associated with less severe anomalies preclude nonaggressive management with or without cephalocentesis.

    e. While cesarean section is frequently necessary for macrocephaly (head size greater than two standard deviations above the mean for gestational age), standard indications are otherwise appropriate.

    f. The management of progressive hydrocephalus remote from term is uncertain. There currently exists a de facto (no catheters available) moratorium for in utero ventriculoamniotic shunting. Outcomes of reported cases suggest questionable, if any, benefit from this procedure. Most perinatal centers appear to endorse delivery by cesarean section for progressive ventriculomegaly once fetal pulmonary maturity has been demonstrated. The largely unproven benefit of early delivery must be weighed against neonatal management problems associated with prematurity, including a possibly increased risk of ventriculoperitoneal shunt complications in smaller babies.

B. Neural tube defects. Neural tube defects (NTDs) are among the most common serious congenital anomalies. In 90 percent of cases there are no antecedent identifiable risk factors.

  1. The overall **incidence** is 1–2/1000 births in the United States.

    a. The incidence increases to 2 percent following one affected pregnancy and to 5 to 6 percent after two affected pregnancies.

    b. Insulin-dependent diabetics are at increased risk for NTDs, with as many as 2 percent of pregnancies affected.

2. The cause is unknown. Periconceptional euglycemia has been demonstrated to eliminate most of the increased risk for diabetics in comparison to the general population. The neural tube closes at 21 to 23 days postconception, and attempts to reduce the risk of NTDs after that time are futile. Valproic acid ingestion has been associated with a 2 percent risk of NTDs and is contraindicated in pregnancy.

3. Diagnosis

    a. Ninety percent of NTDs are "open" (not skin covered) and therefore elevate amniotic fluid and maternal serum levels of alpha fetoprotein (AFP) (Fig. 15.2). Maternal serum alpha fetoprotein (MSAFP) is adequate to screen the general population and should be offered to all patients.

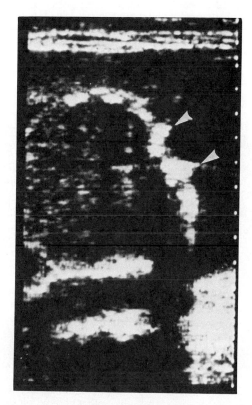

FIGURE 15.2. Splayed lumbar spine of spina bifida.

b. Individuals with an increased risk of NTDs should be evaluated ultrasonographically.

 (1) From 80 to 90 percent of NTDs can be identified ultrasonographically.

 (2) Cranial abnormalities are present in a high percentage of patients with spina bifida. A misshapen fetal head (lemon sign) (Fig. 15.3) and/or a misshapen (banana sign) or absent fetal cerebellum (Figs. 15.4 and 15.5) are present in more than 95 percent of spina bifida cases evaluated before 24 weeks' gestation. More than 75 percent have associated ventriculomegaly. The absence of these associated anomalies dramatically reduces the probability that an NTD is present.

 (3) Most patients' residual risk of fetal NTDs (initial risk estimate reduced by the detection rate of ultrasound) can be lowered to the point where the risk of amniocentesis for amniotic fluid AFP is substantially greater than the residual risk. For example, the estimated risk of spina bifida with an MSAFP of 2.5 multiples of the median is approx-

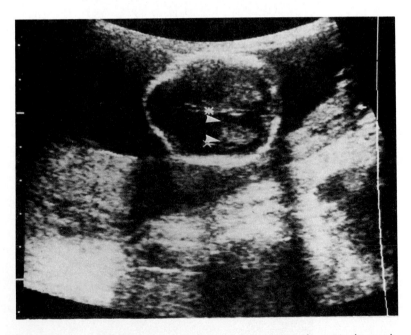

FIGURE 15.3. Abnormally shaped skull (lemon sign) and ventriculomegaly associated with lumbar spina bifida. Note that choroid plexus fails to fill the lateral dimension of the ventricle (arrows).

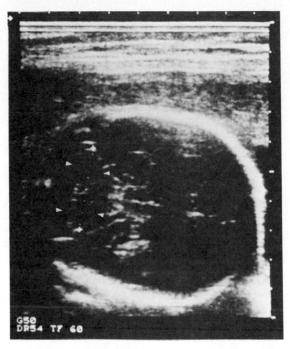

FIGURE 15.4. Normal transcerebellar diameter (calipers) and cerebellum (arrows) at 28 weeks.

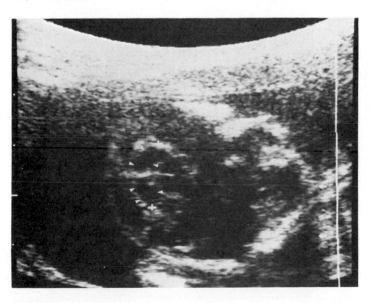

FIGURE 15.5. Abnormally shaped cerebellum (banana sign) at 15 weeks' gestation associated with lumbar spina bifida.

imately 1/140. A normal Level II ultrasound examination reduces that risk by 80 percent, leaving a
residual risk of 1/700, substantially less than the
often quoted 1/200 risk of amniocentesis. Most
couples will be reassured enough to decline
amniocentesis in this case.

4. **Prognosis.** There is a nearly 50–50 distribution of NTDs as
either anencephaly (Fig. 15.6) or spina bifida cystica, with
approximately 5 percent of cases involving encephalocele.

   a. **Anencephaly** is uniformly lethal. Fifty percent of infants
      with this anomaly are stillborn, and only 5 percent sur-
      vive for more than 1 week.

      (1) As previously mentioned, termination of pregnancy
          is appropriate whenever anencephaly is diagnosed.
      (2) Patients declining termination should be aware of
          the potential for prolonged pregnancy and excess

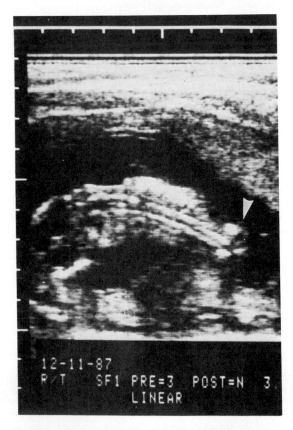

FIGURE 15.6 Absent fetal calvarium (arrow) of anencephaly.

fetal growth as potential complications. In continuing pregnancies, nonaggressive management is appropriate.

b. **Encephalocele** represents approximately 5 percent of the cases of NTDs. It is most commonly located in the occipital region (Fig. 15.7) but occurs in the frontal and parietal regions as well.

    (1) Its occurrence is sporadic in most cases, with an increased incidence in families with a history of NTDs. There is a lethal autosomal recessive cause (Meckel's syndrome) that is associated with polydactyl and polycystic kidneys. Amniotic band syndrome is a nongenetic cause. Hydrocephalus is

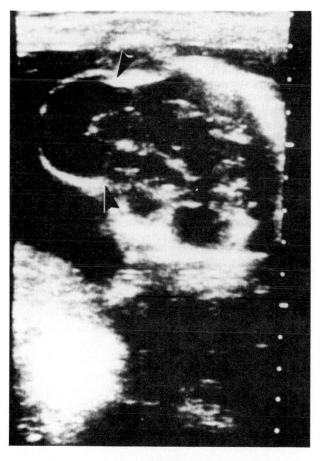

FIGURE 15.7 Occipital encephalocele.

present in 65 percent of occipital encephaloceles. Spina bifida coexists in 7 to 15 percent, and microcephaly is present in 20 percent. The presence of brain tissue in the herniated sac is associated with a 44 percent mortality rate, and only 9 percent of these infants are intellectually normal. Microcephaly is particularly ominous, with 40 percent mortality and 100 percent intellectual impairment among survivors.

(2) Nonaggressive management after viability (Chervenak Category B) is appropriate in the presence of well-documented microcephaly, iniencephaly, aneuploidy, or encephalocele with Meckel's syndrome. It likewise appears appropriate when large amounts of brain tissue are herniated into the sac.

(3) In the absence of the above qualifiers, the isolated small encephalocele (Category C) is managed aggressively in a tertiary center. No clear evidence of advantage exists for elective abdominal delivery in these cases. Larger lesions may require abdominal delivery.

c. The prognosis for spina bifida is variable and is related to the level and extent of the lesion and, to a lesser and less predictable degree, to the severity of hydrocephalus.

(1) Approximately 70 to 75 percent of individuals will have some degree of lower limb dysfunction, ranging from total paralysis to minimal motor defect (with intensive therapy).

(2) Nonaggressive management is not appropriate for isolated spina bifida with secondary hydrocephalus.

(3) Nonaggressive management may be appropriate when severe anomalies (aneuploidy, renal agenesis, etc.) or severe forms of spina bifida (craniospinal rachischisis, iniencephaly) are present.

(4) As mentioned before, the route of delivery for spina bifida is controversial. In the absence of macrocephaly (from hydrocephalus), the benefit, if any, of abdominal delivery, especially for small lesions (< 4 cm), is largely unproven and has recently been challenged. The practice of delivering these patients as soon as pulmonary maturity is demonstrated (35 to 37 weeks) to protect the fetal brain from prolonged or worsening hydrocephalus has become popular, but in the absence of distinct macrocephaly or signs of other fetal jeopardy, the benefit is unknown and the probability of cesarean section (elective or failed induction) is increased. Delivery in a tertiary center with appropriate sur-

gical staff and facilities, preceded by careful assessment for coexistent anomalies and aneuploidy, is
strongly suggested.
C. **Ventral wall defects.** Defects of closure of the anterior abdominal wall include omphalocele, gastroschisis, the body stalk
anomaly, and defects associated with amniotic band syndrome.
Such defects are associated with elevated MSAFP. The body stalk
anomaly is a lethal, near-total defect of the abdominal wall, with
virtually all abdominal organs lying outside the cavity, associated with absence of the umbilical cord, fetal fixation to the
placenta, and additional anomalies. Amniotic band syndrome is
a broad group of anomalies caused by mechanical damage to the
fetus by compression/amputation from intrauterine amniotic
bands. One of its consequences is disruption of the ventral wall.
The syndrome can cause minor to lethal damage, and management must be individualized.
D. **Omphalocele** (Fig. 15.8) is a ventral wall defect with herniation
of intraabdominal contents into the base of the umbilical cord.
The defect is covered by an amnioperitoneal membrane that
distinguishes it from gastroschisis. However, should in utero
rupture of that membrane occur (frequency unknown, but probably rare), differentiation from gastroschisis may be difficult.
1. The **incidence** is 2–4/10 000 births.
2. **Cause**
a. Most cases are sporadic. However, nearly half of the
cases are associated with trisomy (13, 18). Cardiac (47
percent), genitourinary (40 percent), and NTDs (39 percent) frequently accompany omphalocele, particularly
when the fetus is chromosomally abnormal.
b. Two syndromic causes of omphalocele deserve note.
(1) The pentalogy of Cantrell includes a midline supra
umbilical abdominal defect, intracardiac abnormalities, and defects of the lower sternum, diaphragmatic pericardium, and anterior diaphragm.
Survival with this condition is 20 percent.
(2) Beckwith-Wiedemann syndrome includes macro-
glossia and viseromegaly (gigantism).
3. **Prognosis.** The overall mortality rate from omphalocele
ranges from 30 to 40 percent in the literature and is closely
correlated with the presence of other anomalies and trisomy.
Clearly, a careful search for other anomalies and fetal
karyotype is necessary.
4. **Management** decisions are largely influenced by the size of
the defect and the presence of associated anomalies.
a. Nonaggressive management is appropriate with trisomy.
b. For aggressively managed cases, vaginal delivery is considered appropriate for small defects without liver
herniation. The largely theoretical risk of injury or
laceration of the liver with larger lesions has prompted a
recommendation for cesarean section for such cases.

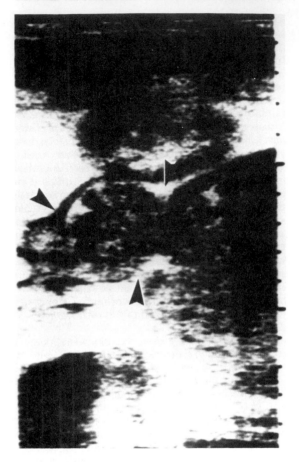

FIGURE 15.8 Omphalocele with hepatic herniation.

Data supporting this position is lacking, though, and recent authors have questioned its value.

E. **Gastroschisis** is a full-thickness periumbilical defect of the anterior abdominal wall associated with evisceration of the abdominal organs.

1. The **incidence** of gastroschisis is approximately 1/15 000 births.

2. Gastroschisis is an isolated defect of unknown **cause,** and other anomalies occur no more frequently than in the general population.

3. The defect is not covered and, in general, free loops of bowel in the amniotic fluid are noted ultrasonographically.

The defect is located to the right of the midline, and hepatic herniation occurs infrequently.

   a. Intrauterine growth retardation occurs in 77 percent of cases, and it may be hazardous to assume that the small size of the abdominal circumference is merely due to evisceration. Among affected fetuses, there is an increased risk of associated gastrointestinal problems including malrotation, atresia, and stenosis.

   b. Polyhydramnios is frequently observed and may complicate management (preterm labor).

4. **Diagnosis.** Gastroschisis must be differentiated from omphalocele. If doubt exists, follow-up ultrasound examination and fetal karyotyping may be necessary. When the defect is clearly gastroschisis and there are no associated anomalies, the likelihood of chromosomal abnormality probably does not justify the risk of amniocentesis.

5. **Prognosis.** The perinatal mortality rate for gastroschisis is 13.5 percent.

6. **Management**

   a. The management of gastroschisis is straightforward. When diagnosed prior to viability, termination of pregnancy is available. However, the good prognosis for fetuses with this condition should be clearly understood by the couple.

   b. After viability, serial ultrasound evaluation for growth monitoring is necessary. Not infrequently, dilatation of the gut is noted and may represent obstruction. No clear recommendations can be made when dilated bowel loops are noted, and observation alone is probably appropriate. Polyhydramnios may prompt preterm labor. Indomethacin has been used in such cases for both its tocolytic effect and pharmacologically to reduce fetal urination and amniotic fluid volume. Great caution is necessary to avoid oligohydramnios and its consequences if indomethacin is used.

   c. While cesarean section has been used to time delivery, recent authors have suggested that it is not beneficial to the fetus and should be reserved for obstetric indications. Delivery in a center capable of neonatal surgery and support is mandatory.

F. **Diaphragmatic hernia**

1. **Incidence.** Diaphragmatic hernia (DH) occurs in approximately 1/2000 pregnancies.

2. **Cause.** Generally, DH has a multifactorial cause, and the recurrence risk is low. The defect represents a failure of embryonic fusion of the leaflets of the developing diaphragm.

3. **Diagnosis.** Ninety percent of hernias are left-sided through the foramen of Bochdalek. Right anterior herniation through

the foramen of Monroe is a less frequent site and carries with it an increased risk of liver herniation and a worsened prognosis. Antenatally detected cases are almost invariably discovered during ultrasound examination for other purposes. Frequently, ultrasound findings include discontinuity of the diaphragm coupled with evidence of herniated bowel within the fetal chest, with or without displacement of the mediastinal contents to the right. The differential diagnosis includes primary pulmonary lesions that simulate a bowel pattern and eventration of the diaphragm.

4. **Prognosis.** DH carries a high risk (50 to 75 percent) of perinatal mortality.

   a. Herniation of fetal abdominal contents into the chest, with or without a mediastinal shift, markedly reduces the area available for pulmonary growth. Most of the deaths are associated with pulmonary hypoplasia and failure of neonatal oxygenation.

   b. Polyhydramnios occurs in as many as 76 percent of patients and is the result of outlet obstruction of the herniated fetal stomach. This increases the risk of prematurity and decreases the survival rate.

5. **Management.** Care of the patient with fetal DH requires planned delivery in a tertiary center.

   a. Since survival with DH is thought to be improved by postnatal extracorporeal membrane oxygenation (ECMO), high-frequency ventilation techniques, and possible artificial surfactant, antenatal transport to select tertiary centers with those facilities is recommended.

   b. No specific benefit of cesarean section, other than timing of delivery, has been demonstrated. Since a variable period of preoperative neonatal stabilization with or without ECMO is necessary, no particular benefit is obtained by timed delivery (in most cases). Cesarean section should be reserved for standard obstetric indications.

   c. Recently, the Fetal Treatment Program at the University of California at San Francisco has reported the successful in utero repair of a DH, with subsequent neonatal survival after six unsuccessful attempts. This case was the culmination of 10 years of animal research and surgery. The success of this one case has to be balanced against the maternal morbidity, the expense, and the possibility that an improvement in survival will not be demonstrated. This procedure is and will continue for some time to be experimental.

G. **Bilateral renal agenesis (BRA)**

   1. **Incidence.** BRA is a lethal anomaly that occurs 1–3/10 000 births.

   2. **Etiology.** It can occur as a sporadic multifactorial lesion or associated with chromosomal aneuploidy, or it can be syn-

dromic, with autosomal dominant and recessive forms reported.

3. **Diagnosis.** Careful perinatal autopsy, chromosome analysis, and a thorough family history are necessary to counsel appropriately regarding recurrence risks, which range from 2 to 50 percent. Care must be taken to diagnose this condition accurately.

   a. Severe oligohydramnios associated with trisomy 13 or 18 or with triploidy can mimic BRA.

   b. In the second and third trimesters, severe intrauterine growth retardation with oligohydramnios may be difficult to distinguish from BRA. With oligohydramnios, decreased ultrasound visualization is common and a confident statement that the kidneys and bladder are absent is, at times, difficult.

4. **Prognosis.** The prognosis is lethal.

5. **Management.** Identification prior to 24 weeks' gestation permits a recommendation for termination of pregnancy. Later in gestation, nonaggressive management, as recommended by Chervenak and colleagues (Category B), is appropriate. However, it might be argued that if the diagnosis is made with a high degree of certainty, BRA may be a justification for third-trimester termination.

H. **Other lethal urinary tract anomalies**

1. Several obstructive and nonobstructive urinary tract anomalies share with BRA the potential to be lethal. The mechanism of death for BRA and these anomalies is pulmonary hypoplasia. Prolonged absence of amniotic fluid volume induces pulmonary hypoplasia and an inability of the neonate to oxygenate successfully. Common to each of these conditions, when lethal, is the prolonged, marked or absolute oligohydramnios. When the process is something other than BRA, the duration and severity of oligohydramnios are, in most cases, unknown. The resultant uncertainty regarding the prognosis requires reasonably aggressive management even when, in most cases, the outcome is fatal. When severe oligohydramnios is present from before 20 weeks' gestation, the outcome is usually lethal.

2. Several authors have described criteria from analysis of fetal urine (collected by amniocentesis) that indicate nonfunctional fetal kidneys. These criteria have been used to select nonaggressive management. Hypertonic fetal urine (sodium > 100 mEq/mL, chlorine > 90 mEq/mL, and osmolarity > 210 mOsm) implies nonfunctional kidneys.

3. Among the obstructive causes of oligohydramnios, the most common is posterior urethral valve (PUV) anomaly.

   a. In almost all cases, the fetus is male. Urogenital and cloacal abnormalities may present similarly in female fetuses.

   b. Retrograde pressure forms behind the obstruction and

causes progressive cystic dilatation of the urinary tract. Left unrelieved, this results in irreversible damage to and destruction of the kidneys.

   c. Bilateral uretropelvic junction obstruction presents with similar-appearing fetal kidneys, but the megacystis of PUV is absent.

4. Percutaneous and operative attempts to relieve obstruction may be of value in select cases where fetal renal function is preserved (by analysis of sampled fetal urine) and irreversible pulmonary hypoplasia is absent. Percutaneous vesicoamniotic catheters have been successfully placed, and open fetal cystostomy has been described. These techniques are available in a few centers but are still considered experimental.

5. Nonobstructive renal causes of severe oligohydramnios include fetal infantile polycystic kidney disease (IPKD) and multicystic dysplastic kidney disease. In IPKD, markedly enlarged, solid-appearing kidneys are noted, with nonvisualization of the fetal bladder and oligohydramnios. Multicystic, dysplastic kidneys are macrocystic and enlarged. Again, the critical factor is the absence of amniotic fluid. Termination before 24 weeks' gestation and nonaggressive management are appropriate for most cases treated after 24 weeks.

I. **Urinary tract disease not associated with oligohydramnios.** Partially obstructive, unilaterally obstructive, and nonobstructive cystic renal diseases that are not associated with oligohydramnios do not require in utero therapy and rarely, if ever, necessitate altering the timing or route of delivery. In general, as long as the amniotic fluid volume remains within normal limits, serial observation of amniotic fluid volume is appropriate. As with most antenatally diagnosed conditions, a careful search for coexisting anomalies is necessary, as these will often alter the prognosis. Delivery in a tertiary center equipped to evaluate and care for such infants is suggested.

J. **Nonimmune hydrops fetalis (NIHF).** *Nonimmune hydrops fetalis* is a general term describing a fetal condition of skin edema associated with effusions of the abdominal, pleural, and/or pericardial cavities. It is distinguished from immune causes (red cell antigen sensitizations) by a negative indirect Coombs' test.

1. **Incidence.** The overall occurrence of NIHF is 1/2500 pregnancies.

2. **Cause.** There are more than 100 reported causes of NIHF that can be grouped into cardiac, infectious, hematologic, chromosomal, anatomic (thoracic, gastrointestinal, renal), placental, metabolic, and other causes. A detailed discussion of the management of each of these causes is beyond the scope of this chapter.

3. **Diagnosis.** When NIHF presents, every attempt should be made to gather evidence of a cause.

    a. A detailed maternal and family history is important.

    b. A maternal complete blood count (CBC), Kleihauer-Betke screen (to exclude fetal-maternal hemorrhage), hemoglobin electrophoresis, TORCH (toxoplasmosis, rubella, cytomegalovirus, and herpes) titers, serologic tests for syphilis, glucose-6-phosphate dehydrogenase and erythrocyte pyruvate kinase studies, and glucose tolerance tests are appropriate. A Level II ultrasound examination and a fetal echocardiogram are essential.

    c. In most cases, a cause is not readily apparent. Percutaneous umbilical vein blood sampling is frequently helpful. Fetal blood should be sent for karyotype, blood type, hemoglobin electrophoresis, CBC, protein electrophoresis, TORCH, parvovirus B-19 (Fifth's disease) IgM, and total protein.

  4. **Prognosis** depends on the cause, but in general, the mortality rate is expected to range from 50 to 98 percent.

  5. **Management.** Therapy is directed at identified causes.

    a. Intrauterine blood transfusion has been reported for both spontaneous fetal-maternal hemorrhage and to treat the fetal aplastic anemia induced by parvovirus. Supraventricular fetal tachycardia has induced NIHF and has been reversed with several agents, including digoxin and quinidine. NIHF associated with chromosomal aneuploidy is almost always lethal. Spontaneous resolution of NIHF associated with cystic hygroma has been reported.

    b. Delivery at a tertiary center is of value for several reasons.

      (1) Antenatal care and postnatal evaluation are facilitated.

      (2) Ancillary services are available.

      (3) Perinatal autopsy can be performed in cases where perinatal death occurs.

    c. NIHF requires individualization of management. Proper care choices include the entire range from aggressive to nonaggressive management to termination of pregnancy. Postnatal survival may be enhanced by antenatal interventions and by aggressive neonatal support. Multispecialty involvement both before and after delivery is advised.

K. **Cardiac anomalies**

  1. **Incidence.** Congenital heart defects (CHDs), when grouped together, occur in 0.6 to 0.8 percent of births and are the most frequently occurring congenital anomalies.

  2. **Cause.** When diagnosed antenatally, 44 percent of fetuses are found to have additional extracardiac anomalies, and 19 percent are found to have chromosomal aneuploidy. This rate is higher than that reported for liveborns and is explained by an increased risk of second- and third-trimester spontaneous demise in this group.

3. **Diagnosis.** Most cases (90 percent) occur in families with no antecedent history. Frequently, they are discovered during ultrasound examinations for other purposes. The value of visualization of a normal four-chambered heart during Level I ultrasound examination has recently been emphasized.

   a. Ninety-six percent (71/74 cases) of CHD identified antenatally in a recent series of 1022 pregnancies were associated with an abnormal four-chambered heart. The positive predictive value was 95.8 percent and the negative predictive value was 99.4 percent.

   b. Failure to obtain a four-chambered view of the heart at Level I ultrasound examination (after 17 to 18 weeks' gestation) should prompt referral for evaluation.

   c. Certain historical and clinical factors are associated with an increased risk of CHD (Table 15.2), and their presence should prompt referral for Level II ultrasound and echocardiography.

4. **Prognosis.** In general, antenatally identified heart defects are amenable to postnatal medical therapy and/or surgical repair. The overall prognosis for survival of newborns with isolated CHD is good.

   a. However, the subgroups that are identified antenatally tend to exclude simple atrial and ventricular septal defects and patent ductus arteriosus, which account for the best survival rates.

Table 15.2. Risk Factors for Congenital Heart Disease

Prior affected child
Parental CHD
Parental autosomal recessive or dominant or sex-linked disease with risk of CHD Noonan's, Apert's, Marfan's syndromes, etc.
Maternal type I diabetes mellitus
Maternal autoimmune disease
Maternal teratogen exposure
 Phenytoin, trimethadione, isotretinoin, lithium, etc.
Maternal infection
 Toxoplasmosis, cytomegalovirus, mumps, rubella, etc.
Fetal aneuploidy
 Trisomies (particularly 13, 18, and 21), 45XO (Turner's syndrome), etc.
Symmetric intrauterine growth retardation
Oligohydramnios/polyhydramnios
Fetal cardiac arrhythmia
NIHF
Identified extracardiac fetal anomalies
 Hydrocephalus, microcephaly, holoprosencephaly, agenesis of the corpus callosum, esophageal or duodenal atresia, diaphragmatic hernia, omphalocele, renal dysplasia, NTD, etc.

b. When evidence of congestive heart failure (CHF) or extreme (NIHF) is present, the prognosis worsens. A recent study by Ferraszzi et al. (1989) reports an overall perinatal survival rate of 24 percent (7/29) for antenatally diagnosed CHD, and only 1/12 fetuses survived when CHF was noted. The reported management of CHD when CHF or NIHF is present has been aggressive, with cesarean section performed in most cases. However, neonatal death occurs commonly.

c. When CHF or NIHF is identified in association with tachyarrhythmia, reversal of the arrhythmia and resolution of the hydrops may improve postnatal survival.

d. Hypoplastic left ventricle has been diagnosed antenatally, and its discovery creates difficult management decisions. While the recently introduced Norwood procedure has created the potential for survival, lethality of the condition remains high. The potential for survival associated with the procedure precludes nonaggressive management in most cases.

5. **Management.** The management of antenatally diagnosed CHD depends on the anomaly identified and the presence or absence of chromosomal aneuploidy, NIHF or CHF, associated anomalies, associated syndrome identification, and fetal arrhythmia.

a. Chromosomal analysis via amniocentesis, placental biopsy, or fetal blood sampling is recommended.

b. Careful anatomic evaluation for coexisting anomalies may reveal syndromic causes for CHD. Even in the best centers, the limitations of fetal echocardiography are such that the full extent of cardiac disease is, at times, underestimated. The limitations of antenatal diagnosis should be explained so that the findings of postnatal evaluations that differ from antenatal findings are not unanticipated.

c. Whenever a CHD is suspected, delivery in a center capable of providing complete postnatal medical and surgical care of the newborn is recommended.

BIBLIOGRAPHY

Adzick NS, Harrison MR, Glick PL, et al. Diaphragmatic hernia in the fetus: Prenatal diagnosis and outcome in 94 cases. J Pediatr Surg 1985; 20:2357–2361.

Bastide A, Manning F, Harman C, et al. Ultrasound evaluation of amniotic fluid: Outcome of pregnancies with severe oligohydramnios. Am J Obstet Gynecol 1986; 154:895–900.

Bensen JT, Dillard RG, Burton BK. Open spina bifida: Does cesarean section delivery improve prognosis? Obstet Gynecol 1988; 71:532–534.

Berkowitz RL, Glickman MG, Smith GJW, et al. Fetal urinary tract obstruction: What is the role of surgical intervention in utero? Am J Obstet Gynecol 1982; 144:367–375.

Carpenter MW, Curci MR, Dibbins AW, et al. Perinatal management of ventral wall defects. Obstet Gynecol 1984; 64:646–651.

Chervenak FA, Berkowitz RL, Tortora M, et al. The management of fetal hydrocephalus. Am J Obstet Gynecol 1985; 151:933–942.

Chervenak FA, Duncan C, Ment LR, et al. Perinatal management of meningomyelocele. Obstet Gynecol 1984; 63:376–380.

Chervenak FA, Farley MA, Walters L, et al. When is termination of pregnancy during the third trimester morally justifiable? N Engl J Med 1984; 310:501–504.

Chervenak FA, McCullough LB. Ethical analysis of the intrapartum management of pregnancy complicated by fetal hydrocephalus with macrocephaly. Obstet Gynecol 1986; 68:720–725.

Copel JA, Pilu G, Green J, et al. Fetal echocardiographic screening for congenital disease: The importance of the four-chamber view. Am J Obstet Gynecol 1987; 175:648–655.

Crombleholme TM, Harrison MR, Golbus MS, et al. Fetal intervention in obstructive uropathy: Prognostic indicators and efficacy of intervention. Am J Obstet Gynecol 1990; 162:1239–1244.

Davis CL. Diagnosis and management of nonimmune hydrops fetalis. J Reprod Med 1982; 27:594–600.

Elias S, Annas GJ. Perspectives on fetal surgery. Am J Obstet Gynecol 1983; 145:807–812.

Ferrazzi E, Fesslova V, Bellotti M, et al. Prenatal diagnosis and management of congenital heart disease. J Reprod Med 1989; 34:207–214.

Fitzsimmons J, Nyberg DA, Cyr DR, et al. Perinatal management of gastroschisis. Obstet Gynecol 1988; 71:910–913.

Ghidini A, Sirtori M, Vergani P, et al. Ureteropelvic junction obstruction in utero and ex utero. Obstet Gynecol 1990; 75:805–808.

Graves GR, Baskett TF. Nonimmune hydrops fetalis: Antenatal diagnosis and management. Am J Obstet Gynecol 1984; 1248:563–565.

Hadi HA, Loy RA, Long EM, et al. Outcome of fetal meningomyelocele after vaginal delivery. J Reprod Med 1987; 32:597–600.

Harrison MR, Adzick NS, Longaker MT, et al. Successful repair in utero of a fetal diaphragmatic hernia after removal of herniated viscera from the left thorax. N Eng J Med 1990; 322:1582–1584.

Hobbins JC, Romero R, Grannum P, et al. Antenatal diagnosis of renal anomalies with ultrasound. I. Obstructive uropathy. Am J Obstet Gynecol 1984; 148:868–877.

Hsieh FJ, Chang FM, Ko TM, et al. Percutaneous ultrasound-guided fetal blood sampling in the management of nonimmune hydrops fetalis. Am J Obstet Gynecol 1987; 1547:44–49.

Hutchison AA, Drew JH, Yu VYH, et al. Nonimmunologic hydrops fetalis: A review of 61 cases. Obstet Gynecol 1982; 59:347–352.

Kirk EP, Wah RM. Obstetric management of the fetus with omphalocele or gastroschisis: A review and report of one hundred twelve cases. Am J Obstet Gynecol 1983; 146:512–518.

Machin GA. Hydrops revisited: Literature review of 1,414 cases published in the 1980s. Am J Med Genet 1989; 34:366–390.

Maidman JE, Yeager C, Anderson V, et al. Prenatal diagnosis and management of nonimmunologic hydrops fetalis. Obstet Gynecol 1980; 56:571–576.

Michejda M, Queenan JT, McCullough D. Present status of intrauterine treatment of hydrocephalus and its future. Am J Obstet Gynecol 1986; 155:873–882.

Nyberg DA, Mack LA, Hirsch J, et al. Fetal hydrocephalus: Sonographic detection and clinical significance of associated anomalies. Radiology 1987; 163:187–191.

Saltzman DH, Frigoletto FD, Harlow BL, et al. Sonographic evaluation of hydrops fetalis. Obstet Gynecol 1989; 74:106–111.

Sipes SL, Weiner CP, Sipes DR, et al. Gastroschisis and omphalocele: Does either antenatal diagnosis or route of delivery make a difference in perinatal outcome? Obstet Gynecol 1990; 76:195–199.

Spinnato JA, Shaver DC, Flinn GS, et al. Fetal supraventricular tachycardia: In utero therapy with digoxin and quinidine. Obstet Gynecol 1984; 64:730–735.

Van den Hof MC, Nicolaides KH, Campbell J, et al. Evaluation of the lemon and banana signs in one hundred thirty fetuses with open spina bifida. Am J Obstet Gynecol 1990; 162:322–327.

Vintzileos AM, Ingardia CJ, Nochimson DJ. Congenital hydrocephalus: A review and protocol for perinatal management. Obstet Gynecol 1983; 62:539–549.

CHAPTER 16

Antenatal Fetal Assessment

Susan Baker

I. **Indications for assessment.** Antenatal fetal assessment is usually reserved for those pregnancies deemed "high-risk." These pregnancies are at risk for the development of uteroplacental insufficiency which may result in restricted fetal growth, fetal hypoxemia, fetal acidosis, and fetal demise.

Indications for antenatal testing include maternal hypertensive disorders, maternal diabetes mellitus (insulin-requiring), post-term pregnancies, collagen vascular disease, homozygous hemoglobinopathies, fetal growth restriction, oligohydramnios, and isoimmunized pregnancies.

Fetal testing usually begins at 32–34 weeks of gestation, and the interval between tests is 7 days. Testing may begin earlier or be performed more frequently with severe disease or a deteriorating condition.

II. **Biochemical testing.** Initial efforts to assess fetal well-being involved measurement of placental hormonal products that were thought to reflect placental function and/or the status of the fetus. These tests may reflect chronic fetal compromise but contribute little to acute assessment of the fetus. They are generally expensive and difficult to reproduce, exhibit wide individual variation, and are often inaccurate due to maternal and fetal factors unrelated to immediate fetal jeopardy. A discussion of the most widely used biochemical tests follows.

A. **Estriol.** In late pregnancy, the primary circulating estrogen is estriol, 90 percent of which is produced by the fetoplacental unit. Estriol production is dependent on the availability of maternal precursors, an intact fetal hypothalamic-pituitary-adrenal axis, and placental enzymes such as sulfatase. The size and growth of the fetoplacental unit are reflected by estriol levels, and conditions related to uteroplacental insufficiency such as hypertension and fetal growth restriction are expected to produce low estriol values.

Estriol has been measured in 24-h urine collections (the

majority of conjugated estriol is excreted in urine), random urine samples for estriol: creatinine ratios, and in plasma using radioimmunoassay techniques. Since there is wide individual and diurnal variation in estriol synthesis, each patient must serve as her own control, and serial measurements are required to determine a trend. There are a number of factors that alter estriol levels, including maternal antibiotic ingestion, maternal hepatic or renal disease, fetal anencephaly, and placental sulfatase deficiency.

The complexity and variability of estriol synthesis and excretion, and the inability to identify acute fetal problems, have led to a decline in its use as a monitor of high-risk pregnancies. Biophysical techniques of fetal surveillance have virtually replaced estriol measurements as an indicator of fetal status.

B. **Human placental lactogen.** Human placental lactogen (hPL) is synthesized by syncytiotrophoblasts in the placenta and secreted into the maternal circulation. Maternal serum concentrations rise progressively until approximately 37 weeks' gestation, at which time they decline slightly until delivery. The major determinant of hPL concentration is the functional mass of the placenta, and hPL maternal serum levels have been used to monitor placental function as an indirect evaluation of fetal well-being. Abnormally low values may reflect decreased placental function and thus fetal compromise, but their accuracy and predictive value are variable. Biophysical fetal assessment has also replaced hPL determination as a test of fetal well-being.

III. **Biophysical testing**
   A. **Assessment of fetal movement**
      1. **Definition.** This test involves measuring the number of fetal movements in a prescribed period of time and is based on the premise that fetal compromise reduces the level of gross fetal body movements. There are no standard protocols and published criteria vary, but most protocols involve the recording of maternally perceived fetal movement rather than ultrasound detection of fetal movement. Some of the commonly used protocols are discussed in part 5 of this section.
      2. **Physiology.** The monitoring of gross fetal body movements is thought to be an indirect method of evaluating central nervous system (CNS) function and integrity. The control and coordination of fetal movements require complex neurologic interaction; such activity may begin as early as the seventh gestational week and become more complex with maturation of the CNS. Real-time ultrasonography studies have shown that the human fetus spends approximately 10 percent of its time making gross body movements, and 10 to 30 such movements may be observed in a 30- to 60-min period. Fetal activity appears to be greatest between 28 and 34

weeks' gestation, with a gradual decline in the number of movements as the pregnancy progresses to term. The use of fetal movement counting as a means of antepartum surveillance is based on animal studies showing a reduction or cessation of fetal forelimb movement in the presence of fetal hypoxemia and reports of maternal detection of a change in fetal activity (more infrequent and weaker movements) prior to cessation of fetal movement.

3. **Effectiveness.** Fetal movement counting appears to be a simple, inexpensive, and efficacious method of antepartum fetal surveillance for high- and low-risk pregnancies. The mother may perceive 80 to 85 percent of fetal movements, as well as a change in the type of activity. The false-positive rate is high (> 50 percent in some studies) but the false-negative rate is relatively low (< 10 percent in most studies). Sensitivity is > 50 percent and specificity is > 80 percent in a number of studies. There is only one reported prospective trial, and this indicated that fetal movement counting was a useful predictor of fetal well-being. Most studies indicate a decrease in the stillbirth rate in the monitored population. This method of surveillance is primarily effective in detecting chronic fetal compromise and may be normal in fetuses that die secondary to an acute event such as cord compression, placental abruption, or uterine rupture.

4. **Limitations.** Several factors may influence the maternal perception of fetal activity. These include hydramnios, placental location (anterior), maternal sedation, obesity, and maternal position (increased perception in the left lateral decubitus position). Fetuses with major malformations may have decreased activity compared to normal fetuses; this is particularly true with CNS involvement. This test may also be less useful in multiple gestations because independent assessment of each fetus is not possible.

5. **Clinical implementation.** Various protocols have been reported as effective. To improve patient compliance and reduce confusion, each institution should be consistent in the protocol it adopts. A few of the reported protocols are as follows:

   a. Cardiff Count-to-Ten Chart: 12-h daily recording periods; abnormal is defined as < 10 movements per 12-h study interval.

   b. Movement alarm signal: 30 to 60-min recording period two or three times daily. Fewer than three movements per hour or no movement in 12 h demands further evaluation.

   c. One-hour recording periods at least once per day; abnormal is defined as four or fewer movements per hour for 2 consecutive hours.

   If any of the above counts are abnormal, the patient is instructed to contact her physician or institution for further evaluation. The patient's record of fetal movement should be reviewed at every prenatal visit for reinforcement of the technique and its value in assessing fetal well-being.

6. **Intervention.** Each fetus develops its own pattern of activity. Therefore, the absolute number of movements in some fetuses may not be as important as the degree of change in those movements. If there is a significant change in the pattern of fetal movement or a significant decrease in fetal movement, then further evaluation with other biophysical tests is required prior to intervention. These tests usually include the nonstress test, the contraction stress test, and the biophysical profile.

B. Nonstress test

1. **Definition.** The term *nonstress test (NST)* refers to a group of tests that rely on determination of fetal heart rate (FHR) accelerations in response to fetal movement in a defined period of time as a measure of fetal well-being. There are no universally accepted criteria for classification of a reactive or nonreactive test. The most widely accepted criteria are:

   a. Reactive: two or more FHR accelerations of at least 15 beats per minute for at least 15 s duration in a 20-min period (Fig. 16.1).

   b. Nonreactive: no acceptable FHR accelerations over a 40-min period. Some institutions also use the category of "uncertain reactivity," which includes those FHR tracings that have accelerations < 15 beats per min or < 15 s

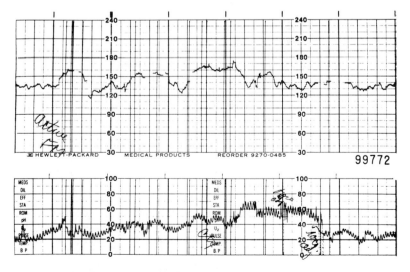

FIGURE 16.1. Reactive NST with a spontaneous contraction.

duration, fewer than two fetal movements in 20 min, or an abnormal baseline rate.

Overall, 85 percent of NSTs will be reactive on initial testing and 15 percent will be nonreactive.

2. **Physiology.** As gestation progresses, the healthy fetus will exhibit up to 30 accelerations above the baseline heart rate each hour. FHR accelerations require intact neurologic coupling between the fetal CNS and the fetal heart. Hypoxia or acidosis disrupts this pathway, and chronic hypoxia results in decreased FHR variability. In late gestation, accelerations are associated with fetal movement > 85 percent of the time and > 90 percent of gross movements are accompanied by an increase in heart rate. These accelerations may be absent during fetal sleep and may be diminished with maternal use of CNS depressant drugs such as narcotics or other sedatives. Beta blockers and smoking also reduce accelerations. A fetus may not exhibit FHR accelerations for up to 80 min and still be normal.

3. **Effectiveness.** The NST is used as the primary screening test at many institutions because it is easily and quickly performed in an outpatient setting. The classification criteria and technique for performing the test have not been standardized, making comparison of published reports difficult. In most studies, the sensitivity is reported as > 50 percent and the specificity as > 80 percent for perinatal morbidity and mortality. The false-positive rate is > 75 percent in most studies, and the false-negative rate ranges from < 2 percent for perinatal mortality to < 10 percent for perinatal morbidity. There have been four randomized controlled trials evaluating the NST, none of which suggested a clinical benefit. However, the numbers in these studies were insufficient to substantiate discarding the NST as a method of antepartum fetal surveillance.

4. **Limitations.** The NST was introduced primarily as a test of fetal condition, in contrast to the contraction stress test, which is a test of uteroplacental function. Several factors can affect the result and interpretation of an NST. Maternal obesity, hydramnios, maternal or fetal movement, and a very small fetus may interfere with accurate categorization of a test. In addition, a higher incidence of nonreactive tests may be seen with maternal ingestion of CNS depressant drugs, recent tobacco use, fetuses with a congenital anomaly, normal fetuses in a sleep state, and preterm fetuses (< 28 weeks).

Many centers extend the observation period when a nonreactive test is encountered. One study found that 24 percent had nonreactive tests in the first 20 min, 5 percent at 40 min, and only 2 percent by 80 min. A reactive NST may be predictive of continued fetal health for approximately 7 days, but it does not predict acute events that lead to fetal demise such as cord accidents or placental abruption.

5. **Clinical implementation.** The NST is used as the primary surveillance technique in many centers. It is generally reserved for those pregnancies deemed high risk, rather than used as a screening tool for the entire gravid population. The criteria for a reactive or nonreactive test must be established for each institution, as well as the gestational age at which surveillance begins. In general, FHR testing begins at 32 to 34 weeks' gestation, but may begin earlier in pregnancies with severe disease or a deteriorating condition.

The test is performed in the semi-Fowler or lateral tilt position, and FHR is monitored by an ultrasound transducer. The patient should be in a nonfasting, relaxed state and without a history of recent drug or tobacco ingestion. The FHR is then recorded for the prescribed period of time, and fetal movement is recorded on the tracing. If a test is nonreactive, it may be extended for 20 to 40 min. Some centers use fetal acoustic stimulation to lessen the testing time and to decrease the incidence of nonreactive tests. The test is generally repeated once per week, but recent studies have recommended more frequent evaluation in patients with specific conditions such as insulin-dependent diabetes mellitus, postterm pregnancies, intrauterine growth retardation, and hypertension.

6. **Intervention.** When a nonreactive test is encountered, further evaluation should be performed. This is particularly critical in a preterm gestation. The observation period can be extended, or another biophysical test such as the contraction stress test or biophysical profile can be performed. Subsequent management is based on the results of these further tests. The occurrence of fetal bradycardia or a sinusoidal heart rate pattern has been associated with poor perinatal outcome, and demands further evaluation and possibly delivery. Mild variable decelerations have not been associated with increased perinatal mortality, but they should lead to an assessment of the amniotic fluid volume.

C. **Contraction stress test**
1. **Definition.** The contraction stress test (CST) was the first biophysical test for antepartum surveillance to be widely used. It was developed to assess the status of fetuses at high risk for uteroplacental insufficiency and is based on the FHR response to uterine contractions.

An adequate test is defined as three completed contractions of at least 40 to 60 s duration in a 10-min interval. The results are interpreted as follows:

Negative: no late decelerations (Figs. 16.2 and 16.3)

Positive: late decelerations following ≥ 50 percent of the contractions (See Fig. 16.4)

Equivocal: (1) suspicious — intermittent late or variable decelerations with < 50 percent of the contractions; (2) hyperstimulation — FHR decelerations associated with excessive uterine activity (contraction frequency > every 2 min or duration > 90 s)

Unsatisfactory: fewer than three contractions in 10 min or a poor-quality FHR tracing

The FHR tracing is further categorized as **reactive** (at least two accelerations of 15 beats per minute and 15 s duration in a 20-min interval) (see Fig. 16.2) or **nonreactive** (less than these criteria) (see Fig. 16.3). The recommended intervention and follow-up for each of these test categories will be outlined in a following section (see Intervention). The testing interval is generally 7 days.

2. **Physiology.** Uterine contractions cause intrauterine pressure to rise, resulting in impedance or cessation of blood flow to the intervillous space and transiently decreasing fetal oxygenation. In a fetus with adequate oxygen reserve, these periodic falls in Po_2 do not drop below a critical level (17 to 18 mm Hg). However, in a fetus with diminished reserve, this transient fall in Po_2 may be sufficiently low to activate an

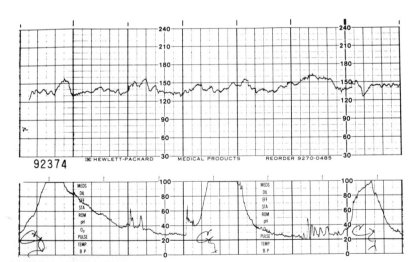

FIGURE 16.2. Negative CST. The baseline heart rate is 140 beats per min, with an acceleration noted.

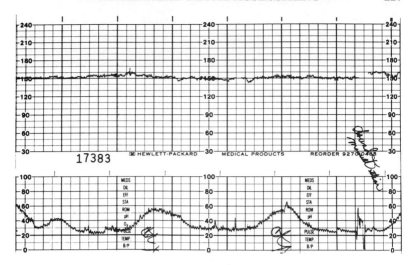

FIGURE 16.3. Negative CST. The tracing is also nonreactive, with a very flat baseline heart rate.

autonomic reflex mechanism that causes the FHR to decrease. When the fetal oxygen level rises above a threshold value the FHR will increase, and the resulting pattern is late decelerations. Another mechanism resulting in FHR decelerations is direct myocardial depression. This usually occurs when hypoxia is of sufficient duration and severity to lead to metabolic acidosis. Late decelerations associated with metabolic acidosis are shallow in depth and associated with decreased FHR reactivity.

The CST is based on the concept that fetuses with marginal basal oxygenation will exhibit FHR decelerations when

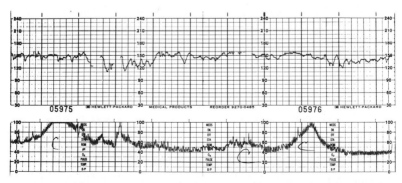

FIGURE 16.4 Positive CST with a baseline heart rate of 150 beats per min.

exposed to the hypoxic stress of uterine contractions. Once a fetus has been identified as being at risk for an adverse outcome related to uteroplacental insufficiency, management plans can be formulated based on gestational age and other maternal and fetal factors.

3. **Effectiveness.** The CST has been characterized as a test with good reliability in predicting a normal outcome but poor reliability in predicting an adverse outcome. The sensitivity for perinatal morbidity and mortality in published reports is low, exceeding 50 percent in only a few studies. The specificity is > 80 percent for perinatal morbidity and mortality in most studies. False-positive rates as high as 50 to 70 percent have been reported, but this may be affected by the technique, equipment employed, and experience in interpretation of results. The false-negative rate is low, generally < 1 percent, and has been reported to vary from 2 to 10/1000 high-risk patients tested.

When reviewing the efficacy of the CST, one must keep in mind that the purpose of this test is to detect **early** fetal compromise in order to prevent further morbidity or fetal death. Therefore, a positive test with a normal fetal outcome is deemed false positive when, in fact, it may have accomplished its goal. The other advantage of the CST is its low false-negative rate, allowing nonintervention in some high-risk pregnancies, particularly those that are premature in gestation.

4. **Limitations.** Many of the factors that affect the results and interpretation of the NST also affect the CST. These include maternal obesity, recent tobacco use, CNS depressant drugs, fetuses with congenital anomalies, and extremely preterm fetuses (< 28 weeks' gestation). The CST is an acute indicator of oxygen and acid-base status but is not effective in predicting the neurologic outcome. Previous damage to the fetal cerebral cortex may not be elucidated with the CST if the brainstem has not been damaged, providing a false sense of reassurance.

Like other biophysical tests, the CST reflects the intrauterine environment at the time of testing, but it will not predict acute events that may occur in the interval between tests such as placental abruption and cord accidents.

5. **Clinical implementation.** Testing begins at 32 to 34 weeks' gestation for most conditions associated with uteroplacental insufficiency, but severe disease or a deteriorating status may require earlier initiation of testing.

The CST may be performed in an inpatient or outpatient setting. The contractions are produced via intravenous administration of low-dose oxytocin (initial dose of 0.5 mU/min) — the oxytocin challenge test (OCT) — or with intermittent nipple stimulation — the nipple stimulation contraction stress test (NS-CST). The patient is placed in the semi-Fowler position with a tilt to the left to prevent maternal hypotension and decreased uterine blood flow from the supine position. The FHR is recorded using an ultrasound transducer, and uterine activity is monitored with a tocodynamometer. Maternal blood pressure and heart rate are determined every 5 to 10 min throughout the testing period. A baseline FHR and uterine activity tracing are obtained for 15 to 20 min. If adequate uterine activity (three contractions in 10 min) occurs spontaneously, additional uterine stimulation is not necessary. If uterine activity is absent or inadequate, uterine stimulation is performed via the OCT or NS-CST until an adequate test is achieved. Uterine stimulation should then cease, and the patient should be observed until uterine activity has returned to its baseline level.

Contraindications to the CST involve conditions associated with preterm delivery, uterine bleeding, or uterine rupture and include the following:

Premature labor

Premature rupture of membranes

Incompetent cervix

Vertical uterine scar

Placenta previa or abruptio placentae

6. **Intervention.** Eighty to 90 percent of CSTs will be interpreted as negative and reactive. A follow up test should be performed in 7 days unless the clinical situation mandates more frequent testing, such as with worsening hypertension.

A negative but nonreactive test is generally reassuring, but the FHR tracing should be inspected carefully for subtle late decelerations and evidence of long-term variability. The mother should also be questioned regarding ingestion of drugs, recent tobacco use, or other factors that might reduce FHR accelerations. If an ultrasound scan has not been obtained, a detailed scan for fetal anomalies should be performed. The timing of a repeat test with a negative, nonreactive result depends on the clinical situation and the degree of concern regarding fetal status. If no fetal abnormalities are found and there is evidence of long-term FHR variability, the test may be repeated in 7 days.

Equivocal tests should be repeated in 24 h, whether they are hyperstimulated or suspicious. Only 10 to 15 percent of suspicious tests will become positive when repeated, and studies have found no excess adverse outcome with a 24-h waiting period. In certain clinical situations such as postterm pregnancy, or when other indications for delivery exist, an equivocal test may initiate intervention. An unsatisfactory test should also be repeated in 24 h and will generally be satisfactory upon retesting.

A positive CST requires further evaluation and possibly delivery. The decision to intervene is usually determined by fetal maturity, the clinical condition, and the presence or absence of FHR reactivity. If a maternal condition such as diabetic ketoacidosis or severe sickle cell crisis exists, then continuous fetal monitoring may be employed until the condition is corrected; the fetus can then be reassessed.

A preterm fetus with a positive CST should initiate an evaluation of (1) correctable conditions such as the supine hypotensive syndrome, (2) adequacy of the amniotic fluid, and (3) possible fetal karyotypic abnormalities and major malformations. The test may be repeated after this evaluation, or a decision for delivery may be made based on these results and the clinical condition that prompted the CST. In these circumstances, some authors also recommend further testing with a biophysical profile.

A positive CST in a mature fetus demands evaluation for delivery, as well as investigation of the above-mentioned factors. If no obstetric contraindications exist, induction of labor may be attempted when delivery is indicated. Careful monitoring of the FHR pattern and intrauterine resuscitation techniques should be employed in these patients.

In summary, equivocal or unsatisfactory tests should be repeated within 24 h. The management of a positive test is individualized and is based upon the clinical condition and fetal maturity status.

D. Biophysical profile
   1. Definition. The fetal biophysical profile is a method of fetal risk surveillance based on the composite assessment of five discrete biophysical variables that encompass both acute and chronic markers of fetal compromise. These variables are FHR reactivity (or the NST), fetal breathing movements, fetal gross body movements, fetal tone, and adequacy of the amniotic fluid volume. Each of these variables is evaluated and a score assigned. The sum of these scores is then used in clinical decision making, as outlined below.
   2. Physiology. The presence of normal biophysical activity in a fetus is thought to be indirect evidence of an intact CNS, since this activity requires complex intregration of nervous system functions. Factors that cause CNS depression may reduce or abolish fetal biophysical activity. Hypoxemia has been demonstrated to decrease FHR reactivity, fetal breathing movements, and fetal movements and tone.

   FHR, gross body movements, and respiratory activity are considered to be acute markers of fetal condition, while amniotic fluid volume is thought to be a chronic marker. The presence or absence of adequate amniotic fluid enhances

the information gained from other biophysical variables and is critical in the continued management of a pregnancy.
3. **Effectiveness.** The biophysical profile was introduced as a more comprehensive method of evaluating fetal condition because several biophysical variables are assessed as part of the test. The underlying premise is the number of false-positive and false-negative tests can be reduced by including both chronic and acute markers of fetal compromise.

The detection of major fetal anomalies is also possible with the biophysical profile, since ultrasonography is required to perform the test. Greater than 90 percent of tests have been normal (score 8 to 10) in published reports, leaving only a small percentage that need further evaluation. The false-negative rate is low, approximately 1/1000 high-risk patients tested.
4. **Limitations.** Many limitations of the other biophysical antepartum fetal tests also apply to the biophysical profile. CNS depressants such as sedatives and analgesics, and CNS stimulants such as catecholamines, may affect fetal activity, leading to false-positive or false-negative tests. Maternal hyperglycemia increases fetal respiratory movement, and this component of the test may be falsely reassuring in a compromised fetus.

The biophysical profile was designed to reflect the fetal condition at the time of testing, with some indication of the chronic intrauterine environment (amniotic fluid level). This test cannot predict acute events that occur between testing periods, such as cord accidents and placental abruption.
5. **Clinical implementation.** The gestational age for initiation of testing varies among studies, but generally testing begins at 32 weeks for most high-risk conditions, and the interval between tests is 7 days. A deteriorating maternal or fetal condition or severe disease may require earlier and more frequent testing. Twice-weekly testing is recommended for postterm pregnancies, severe maternal hypertension, and patients with insulin-dependent diabetes mellitus. The FHR portion of the biophysical profile is performed similarly to the NST. An initial survey ultrasound scan is then done on each patient to determine the fetal position and placental location, as well as the presence of major structural fetal anomalies. The uterine cavity is scanned to identify the largest pocket of amniotic fluid, and the largest vertical axis of this fluid pocket is measured. The fetus is then scanned, and a proper plane for observing the fetal thorax, limbs, trunk, and back is identified. Once the desired plane is found, the time is noted and observation continued until normal fetal activity is seen or 30 consecutive min of scanning have elapsed. A score is then assigned based on the interpretation of the five biophysical variables. Table 16.1 gives the recommended technique, interpretation, and scor-

Table 16.1. Biophysical Profile Scoring: Technique and Interpretation

BIOPHYSICAL VARIABLE	NORMAL (SCORE = 2)	ABNORMAL (SCORE = 0)
Fetal breathing movements (FBM)	At least 1 episode of FBM of at least 30-sec duration in 30-min observation	Absent FBM or no episode of > 30 sec in 30 min
Gross body movement	At least 3 discrete body or limb movements in 30 min (episodes of active continuous movement considered as single movement)	2 of fewer episodes of body or limb movements in 30 min
Fetal tone	At least 1 episode of active extension with return to flexion of fetal limb(s) or trunk. Opening and closing of hand considered normal tone	Either slow extension with return to partial flexion or movement of limb in full extension, absent fetal movement.
Reactive FHR	At least 2 episodes of FHR acceleration of > 15 beats/min and of at least 15-sec duration associated with fetal movement in 30 min	Less than 2 episodes of acceleration of FHR or acceleration of > 15 beats/min in 30 min
Qualitative AFV	At least 1 pocket of AF that measures at least 1 cm in two perpendicular planes	Either no AF pockets or a pocket < 1 cm in two perpendicular planes

Abbreviations: FBM = fetal breathing movement; FHR = fetal heart rate; AFV = amniotic fluid volume; AF = amniotic fluid.
Source: Manning FA, Harman CR. The fetal biophysical profile. In: Eden RD, Boehm FH, Haire M, et al. Assessment and Care of the Fetus. East Norwalk, CT: Appleton & Lange; 1990:389.

ing for each component. A score of 2 is assigned for each normal component and a score of 0 for each abnormal portion of the test, giving a maximum test score of 10 and a minimum score of 0.

6. **Intervention.** Clinical management is based on the test score in conjunction with obstetric factors (e.g., a favorable cervix), the severity and progression of maternal disease, and fetal factors such as gestational age and the presence or absence of anomalies. Integration of all of these factors in decision making is important, since one of the primary purposes of fetal assessment is to allow the high-risk pregnancy to progress safely, without adding undue risk to the mother

Table 16.2. Interpretation of Fetal Biophysical Profile Score Results and Recommended Clinical Management Based on These Results

TEST SCORE RESULT	INTERPRETATION	PNM[a] WITHIN 1 WK WITHOUT INTERVENTION	MANAGEMENT
10 of 10 8 of 10 (norm fluid) 8 of 8 (NST not done)	Risk of fetal asphyxia extremely rare	<1 per 1000	Intervention only for obstetric and maternal factors. No indication for intervention for fetal disease
8 of 10 (abnorm fluid)	Probable chronic fetal compromise	89 per 1000[b]	Determine that there is functioning renal tissue and intact membranes; if so deliver for fetal indications
6 of 10 (norm fluid)	Equivocal test possible fetal asphyxia	Variable	If the fetus is mature—deliver. In the immature fetus repeat test within 24 hr; if <6/10 deliver
6 of 10 (abnorm fluid)	Probable fetal asphyxia	89 per 1000[b]	Deliver for fetal indications
4 of 10	High probability fetal asphyxia	91 of 1000[a]	Deliver for fetal indications
2 of 10	Fetal asphyxia almost certain	125 per 1000[a]	Deliver for fetal indication
0 of 10	Fetal asphyxia certain	600 per 1000[a]	Deliver for fetal indication

[a]From Johnson JM, Harman CR, Lange IR, Manning FA. Biophysical Profile Scoring in the management of the postterm pregnancy: An analysis of 307 patients. Am J Obstet Gynecol. 1986; 154(2):269–273.

[b]From Seeds AE. Am J Obstet Gynecol. 1980; 138:575.

Source: Manning FA, Harman CR. The fetal biophysical profile. In: Eden RD, Boehm FH, Haire M, et al. Assessment and Care of the Fetus. East Norwalk, CT: Appleton & Lange; 1990:390.

or fetus. Table 16.2 presents a recommended interpretation and clinical management scheme for each possible test score result.

   E. **Fetal acoustic stimulation.** Fetal acoustic stimulation tests attempt to elicit a FHR response and fetal body movement with an external source of sound and vibration. Vibroacoustic stimuli have been demonstrated to change the behavior state and induce heart rate reactivity in most fetuses. The stimulus source varies among investigators and includes the electronic artificial larynx, the electric toothbrush, and an oscillating amplifier, as well as others. The stimulus is usually applied near the fetal head, and the fetal response is observed and recorded (changes in heart rate, increase in body movements).

The neurologic pathways for reception of and response to vibroacoustic stimuli appear to develop early and mature as gestation advances. An intact cochlea and peripheral sensory end organs have been demonstrated as early as 24 weeks' gestation in human fetuses, and there is evidence that fetal auditory receptors are functional by 26 weeks' gestation. Thus, most fetuses ≥ 26 weeks' gestation will respond to a vibroacoustic stimulus with FHR changes (usually accelerations and/or an increase in basal FHR) and an increase in gross body movements.

The FHR response to vibroacoustic stimulation may be gestational age dependent, with fetuses < 30 weeks responding with a single long-duration FHR acceleration, and fetuses > 30 weeks responding with an increase in basal heart rate and/or in the number of accelerations. Fetal acoustic stimulation has been suggested as a test of fetal well-being and as a means to shorten other biophysical tests such as the NST by increasing the number of FHR accelerations.

Although fetal acoustic stimulation shows great promise as an antepartum surveillance test, no uniform criteria have been established for the intensity, frequency, or duration of the stimulus, and the effect of the stimulus on neonatal hearing is unknown. The test response nomenclature also varies among investigators, making comparison of published studies difficult. A positive, reactive, or normal test refers to the presence of FHR accelerations and/or an increase in body movement. The absence of these changes in activity is described as negative, nonreactive, nonresponsive, or impaired.

Fetal acoustic stimulation may be of great value as an adjunct to existing antepartum surveillance tests, but its efficacy and safety are still being determined, and it remains an experimental research tool at the present time.

BIBLIOGRAPHY

ACOG Technical Bulletin No. 107. Antepartum fetal surveillance. August 1987.

Freeman RK, Lagrew DC. The contraction stress test. In: Eden RD, Boch FH, Haire M, et al. Assessment and Care of the Fetus. East Norwalk, CT: Appleton & Lange; 1990; 351–364.

Gagno R. Stimulation of human fetuses with sound and vibration. Semin Perinatol 1989; 13:393–402.

Huddleston JF, Quinlan RW. Clinical utility of the contraction stress test. Clin Obstet Gynecol 1987; 30:912–919.

Lee CY, Drubber B: The nonstress test for the antepartum assessment of fetal reserve. Am J Obstet Gynecol 1929; 134:460.

Leveno KJ, Cunningham FG. Forecasting fetal health. Williams Obstet Suppl. 1988; 19:1–12.

Manning FA, Harman CR. The fetal biophysical profile. In: Eden RD, Boehm FH, Haire M, et al. Assessment and Care of the Fetus. East Norwalk, CT: Appleton & Lange; 1990:385–396.

Pearson JF, Weaver JB. Fetal activity and fetal wellbeing: An evaluation. Br Med J 1976; 1:1305.

Rayburn WF, Zuspan FP, Motley ME. An alternative to antepartum fetal heart rate testing. Am J Obstet Gynecol 1980; 138:223.

Romero R. A critical appraisal of fetal acoustic stimulation as an antenatal test for fetal well-being. Obstet Gynecol 1988; 71:781–786.

Sadovsky E, Polishuk WZ. Fetal movements in utero. Obstet Gynecol 1977; 50:49.

Thacker SB, Berkelman RL. Assessing the diagnostic accuracy and efficacy of selected antepartum fetal surveillance techniques. Obstet Gynecol Surv 1986; 41:121–141.

Vintzileos AM. The use and misuse of the fetal biophysical profile. Am J Obstet Gynecol 1987; 156:527–533.

Weingold AB, Yonekura ML, O'Kieffe J: Nonstress testing. Am J Obstet Gynecol 1980; 138:195.

CHAPTER 17

Intrapartum Fetal Assessment

J. Martin Tucker

Intrapartum fetal assessment is an attempt to identify those fetuses that become seriously compromised and thus require intervention to prevent fetal damage or death. Currently, this assessment is made most often by reviewing changes in fetal heart rate patterns and/or evaluating the fetal acid/base status. Ideally, these methods would be both sensitive and specific in identifying a fetus in jeopardy. Practically, the ideal technique or procedure has not been found.

I. **Relationship of intrapartum events to the subsequent neurological deficit**
   A. **Background.** Despite technologic advances, the occurrence of cerebral palsy remains 1–2/1000 term pregnancies. This rate has not changed over the last 20 years. The task of the obstetrician during labor is frequent assessment of both the maternal and fetal conditions. Although a great deal about intrapartum events has been learned, it is not possible to ensure or expect a perfect obstetric outcome in each case.
   B. **Intrapartum events.** Most cases of cerebral palsy are *not* caused during the labor and delivery process. Less than 15 percent can be linked to intrapartum events. One can assume the presence of substantial fetal cerebral hypoxia leading to cerebral palsy only if the following criteria are met:
      1. Apgar score less than or equal to 3 at 10 min, without another identifiable cause
      2. Neonatal seizures
      3. Several hours of hypotonia
      4. Confirmation of metabolic acidemia in umbilical artery cord blood
   C. **Other associations.** The vast majority of cases of cerebral palsy can be linked to a variety of factors. These factors include premature birth, genetic factors such as congenital anomalies and chromosomal abnormalities, congenital infections including cytomegalic virus and toxoplasmosis, environmental toxins, and other antenatal insults, the mechanisms of which are poorly understood.

II. Pathophysiology

   A. The fetus is dependent on placental exchange for oxygen, nutrients, and the transfer of waste products. Fetal life is normally maintained through oxidative metabolism. However, during periods of diminished oxygen supply, fetal metabolism converts to anaerobic glycolysis. Prolonged interruptions of the fetal oxygen supply will eventually result in metabolic acidosis in the fetus.

   B. Labor is stressful for the fetus. During labor, the supply of oxygen to the fetus is interrupted briefly during each contraction. A healthy fetus generally tolerates the stresses of labor quite well.

   C. Special receptors in the fetus are responsive to changes that can occur during labor. These receptors regulate the fetal circulation and can alter fetal heart rate patterns.

   1. Pressure on the fetal head is presumed to cause an alteration of fetal cerebral blood flow. This, in turn, causes central vagal stimulation and a reflex drop in the fetal heart rate (early deceleration).

   2. Fetal baroreceptors are responsive to pressure changes in the fetal circulation. The fetus can become transiently hypertensive due to umbilical cord compression, leading to baroreceptor stimulation. Baroreceptors trigger the vagal nerve, leading to a drop in the fetal heart rate (variable deceleration).

   3. Chemoreceptors are responsive to fetal hypoxemia with or without acidemia. Through a similar vagally mediated reflex, changes in fetal acid/base status can cause changes in the fetal heart rate pattern (variable and late decelerations). It is the evaluation of fetal acid/base status and subsequent changes in fetal heart rate patterns that form the basis of intrapartum fetal assessment.

III. Diagnostic techniques

   A. Fetal heart rate monitoring. Fetal heart rate monitoring is the mainstay in the assessment of intrapartum fetal status. The fetal heart rate can be monitored through auscultation with a fetal stethoscope or Doppler device or by the use of continuous electronic recording of the fetal heart rate.

   1. Intermittent auscultation. Auscultation should be performed during a contraction and for 30 s afterward. In high-risk patients, auscultation should be performed every 15 min in the first stage of labor and every 5 min in the second stage. In low-risk patients, auscultation should be performed every 30 min in the first stage and every 15 min in the second stage. If this method is chosen as the primary means of intrapartum assessment, a patient : nurse ratio of 1 : 1 should be used.

   When auscultation is used, three patterns are considered nonreassuring:

   a. A baseline fetal heart rate of less than 100 beats per min

   b. A fetal heart rate of less than 100 beats per min 30 s after a contraction

   c. Unexplained baseline tachycardia in excess of 160 beats per min

When a nonreassuring assessment is made, auscultation should be performed at more frequent intervals (every 3 to 5 min). If corrective measures are not successful in returning the fetal heart rate to a normal baseline, then other methods of assessment may be necessary. Preparations for emergency delivery should be made if the fetal heart rate remains below 100 beats per min after three successive contractions.

2. **Continuous electronic fetal monitoring (EFM).** This method of intrapartum assessment allows the obstetrician to focus on baseline variability and periodic fetal heart rate changes, as well as baseline fetal heart rate changes. Continuous EFM has great sensitivity but poor specificity and low positive predictive value in correlating abnormalities with subsequent adverse outcomes. Therefore, terms like *asphyxia* and *fetal distress* should be avoided when describing a nonreassuring fetal heart rate pattern.

When continuous EFM is used, the record should be evaluated at the frequency described for heart rate auscultation above.

   a. **Variability.** The fetal heart rate is driven by an intraatrial pacemaker. Normally, the fetal heart rate is alternately increased and decreased by impulses from the fetal brain via the autonomic nervous system. This generates variability in the fetal heart rate of up to 8 beats per min from baseline. Absence of variability may represent fetal hypoxia, acidemia, the fetal sleep state, or a drug effect.

   b. **Periodic changes.** Periodic changes in fetal heart rate include accelerations and early, variable, and late decelerations. Only certain late and variable decelerations are considered nonreassuring.

A variable deceleration (Fig. 17.1) is a reflex-mediated decrease in the fetal heart rate, usually due to umbilical cord compression. Variable decelerations vary in shape and do not bear a constant relationship to the contraction. They are usually clinically insignificant

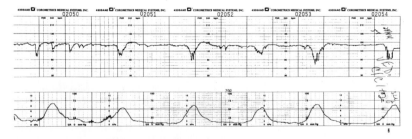

FIGURE 17.1. Variable decelerations with prompt return to the baseline.

but should be considered nonreassuring when there are repetitive decreases to less than 70 beats per min for at least 60 s and/or when there is a late recovery component (Fig. 17.2).

Early decelerations (Fig. 17.3) are usually seen during the latent phase of labor. Their shape and location mirror those of the associated contraction. They have no clinical importance.

A late deceleration (Fig. 17.4) is a decrease in the fetal heart rate that begins after the onset of a contraction and does not return to baseline until the contraction is over. Late decelerations may be mediated by the vagal nerve, and if associated with normal variability, they probably are clinically insignificant. However, repetitive late decelerations in the presence of diminished fetal heart rate baseline variability are associated with fetal acidemia in 50 percent of cases, and such decelerations should be considered nonreassuring.

c. **Baseline changes.** Persistent fetal bradycardia of less than 70 beats per min is worrisome even with good beat-to-beat variability. Mild tachycardia may be due to maternal medications, maternal fever, or fetal infection. Severe, persistent tachycardia (greater than 180 beats per min) should be considered nonreassuring.

d. **Sinusoidal pattern.** Another nonreassuring fetal heart rate pattern is the sinusoidal pattern. This is an undulating pattern of three to five cycles per min with an ampli-

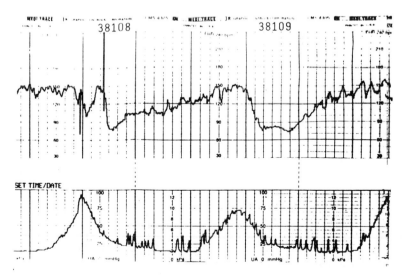

FIGURE 17.2. Variable deceleration with marked late recovery to the baseline.

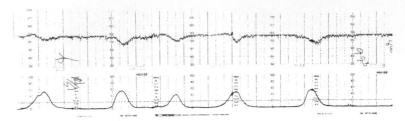

FIGURE 17.3. Early decelerations.

tude of 5 to 15 beats per min and markedly decreased beat-to-beat variability. This pattern has been associated with fetal anemia or with administration of certain maternal drugs like alphaprodine (Nisentil).

B. Fetal scalp pH assessment. Fetal scalp capillary blood sampling was introduced by Saling in 1962. This method of assessment can be used as an adjunct to fetal heart rate monitoring when the fetal heart rate pattern is nonreassuring. For example, if there are uncorrectable severe variable or late decelerations and vaginal delivery is anticipated within a reasonable amount of time, then fetal scalp pH assessment is useful in documenting fetal well-being. It can also be used as a primary means of assessment in cases of fetal bradycardia due to complete heart block. Fetal scalp capillary blood sampling is contraindicated in cases of maternal genital infection, human immunodeficiency virus (HIV), and bleeding disorders. Because of its limited availability and prerequisites for use, this method is used in less than 1 percent of all deliveries.

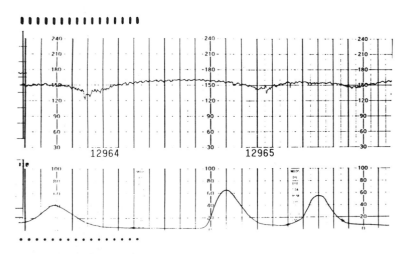

FIGURE 17.4. Repetitive late decelerations with poor beat-to-beat variability.

Fetal scalp blood sampling is performed via vaginoscopy. The cervix must be 2 to 3 cm dilated, the membranes must be ruptured, and the presenting part should be engaged. A fetal scalp pH of 7.25 or greater is considered normal, and the test should be repeated as necessary. Values between 7.20 and 7.25 are borderline and should be repeated every 15 to 30 min. Values below 7.20 are generally thought to be an indication for delivery.

C. **Alternatives to fetal scalp pH assessment.** Investigators have shown that fetuses that have accelerations in heart rate following scalp or sound stimulation are extremely unlikely to be acidotic. If the fetus does not respond to either of these stimuli, then there is a 50 percent chance of fetal acidemia. Given these data, fetal scalp or acoustic stimulation (with an artificial larynx) would seem to be a reasonable alternative to fetal scalp capillary blood sampling.

D. **Meconium staining.** Meconium passage by the fetus is often equated with fetal distress. Many theories exist as to the cause of this phenomenon. By itself, meconium is *not* indicative of fetal distress, but it should be considered as part of the total clinical picture along with other previously described means of intrapartum fetal assessment.

E. **Umbilical cord blood acid/base assessment.** Intrapartum events can be retrospectively assessed through the use of umbilical cord blood analysis. Immediately after delivery of the neonate, a segment of umbilical cord can be doubly clamped and divided. Umbilical arterial blood can be obtained for objective analysis of the acid/base status of the neonate. In the depressed newborn, documentation of normal acid/base measurements can exclude intrapartum hypoxemia as the cause of neonatal depression. In addition, this knowledge may aid providers in the assessment and care of the depressed infant.

Historically, neonatal acidemia has been defined as an umbilical artery pH below 7.20. More recently, investigators have shown that this value may be arbitrarily high. Clinically, pH values as low as 7.00 may be considered normal.

Finally, it is important to classify the type of neonatal acidemia (Table 17.1). Respiratory acidemia is usually indicative of acute

Table 17.1. Classification of Neonatal Acidemia*

TYPE OF ACIDEMIA	pCO_2 (mmHg)	HCO_3 (mEq/L)	BASE DEFICIT (mEq/L)
Respiratory	High ($\geq$ 65)	Normal ($>$ 17)	Normal ($<$ 9)
Metabolic	Normal ($<$ 65)	Low ($\leq$ 17)	High ($>$ 9)
Mixed	High ($\geq$ 65)	Low ($\leq$ 17)	High ($>$ 9)

*Umbilical artery pH $<$ 7.20.

changes, such as those seen in umbilical cord compression. Metabolic acidemia reflects more long-standing changes in fetal acid/base status.

IV. Management

A. **Preventive measures.** Although we cannot precisely define fetal distress, we are often faced with situations of suspected fetal compromise. Treatment of fetal compromise begins with preventive measures. Laboring patients should avoid the supine position and have adequate hydration. Oxytocin should be administered precisely with infusion pumps and be discontinued if a nonreassuring fetal heart rate pattern develops. Regional anesthetics are occasionally associated with profound maternal hypotension, which can result in fetal compromise. Finally, abrupt decompression of the uterus by rupture of membranes may result in sudden fetal decompensation in some instances. Careful attention to all of these matters may prevent fetal jeopardy.

B. **Intervention.** Despite preventive measures, nonreassuring fetal heart rate patterns may develop or persist. Intervention should proceed in a stepwise process. Moderate or severe fetal bradycardia is the most serious of the nonreassuring patterns. An immediate vaginal exam should be performed to rule out prolapsed umbilical cord and, if present, the presenting part should be elevated. Oxytocin, if being used, should be discontinued. If uterine hypertonia persists, one may consider the use of a tocolytic agent to stop or reduce contractions. Tocolytic agents such as terbutaline or magnesium sulfate that can be administered in a bolus fashion may be useful in reducing uterine hypertonus and restoring a reassuring fetal heart rate pattern. The mother should be placed in the right or left lateral tilt position or in a more exaggerated position such as the knee-chest position if fetal bradycardia persists. Supplemental oxygen should be administered, and maternal blood pressure should be assessed and aggressively treated with intravenous crystalloid, blood products, or ephedrinelike drugs as indicated. If fetal bradycardia persists despite these measures, immediate delivery is indicated.

C. **Evaluation.** Other nonreassuring fetal heart rate patterns are often less dramatic in their presentation. Decreased variability of the fetal heart rate, tachycardia, and severe variable or late decelerations fit this description. Evaluation of the maternal condition for such underlying problems such as fever or metabolic derangement (e.g., ketoacidosis, thyrotoxicosis) must be undertaken and corrected if possible. Intervention should proceed in a manner similar to that described for fetal bradycardia.

D. **Delivery.** Despite efforts to improve a nonreassuring fetal heart rate pattern, there is sometimes no improvement or even deterioration of the pattern. When a nonreassuring pattern persists, especially if supported by decreased pH on fetal scalp sampling, it is usually prudent to perform either vaginal or abdominal delivery, as appropriate.

BIBLIOGRAPHY

American Academy of Pediatrics and American College of Obstetricians and Gynecologists. Guidelines for Perinatal Care. 2nd ed. Washington, DC: AAP/ACOG; 1988.

American College of Obstetricians and Gynecologists Committee Opinion. Use and misuse of the APGAR score; 1986:49.

American College of Obstetricians and Gynecologists Technical Bulletin. Intrapartum Fetal Heart Rate Monitoring; 1989:132.

American College of Obstetricians and Gynecologists Committee Opinion. Utility of umbilical cord blood acid-base assessment; 1991:91.

Arias F. Intrauterine resuscitation with terbutaline: A method for the management of acute intrapartum fetal distress. Am J Obstet Gynecol 1978; 131:39.

Freeman RK, Garite TJ, Nageotte MP, eds. Fetal Heart Rate Monitoring. 2nd ed. Baltimore: Williams and Wilkins; 1991.

Gilstrap LC, Hauth JC, Hankins GDV, et al. Second stage fetal heart rate abnormalities and type of neonatal acidemia. Obstet Gynecol 1987; 70:191.

Nelson KB, Ellenberg JH. Antecedents of cerebral palsy. N Engl J Med. 1986; 315:81.

Paul RH, Huey JE Jr, Yaeger CF. Clinical fetal monitoring. Postgrad Med 1977; 61:160.

Sandmlre HF. Whither electronic fetal monitoring? Obstet Gynecol 1990; 76:1130.

Tucker JM, Hauth JC. Intrapartum assessment of fetal well-being. Clin Obstet Gynecol 1990; 33:515.

Winkler CL, Hauth JC, Tucker JM, et al. Neonatal complications at term related to the degree of umbilical artery acidemia. Am J Obstet Gynecol 1991; 164:637.

CHAPTER 18

Altered Fetal Growth

Ralph K. Tamura
Rudy E. Sabbagha

Altered fetal growth, either suboptimal or accelerated, may be caused by distinctly different fetal and maternal conditions. Diagnostic ultrasound in obstetrics makes it possible to observe fetal growth abnormalities. In this chapter, detection and management of the intrauterine growth-retarded fetus, and the small-for-gestational age fetus, as well as of the accelerated fetal growth or large-for-gestational age fetus, are outlined.

I. **Intrauterine growth retardation (IUGR) or small-for-gestational-age (SGA) fetuses**
   A. **Definitions of growth retardation**
      1. Birth weight ≤ 10th percentile for a given gestational age. This is determined by accurate menstrual dates, or fetal sonar examination using the crown-rump length (CRL) from 8 to 12 weeks or the biparietal diameter (BPD) and femur length (FL) from 14 to 26 weeks, and/or pediatric exam of the neonate.
      2. Presence of fetal malnutrition. This is evidenced by tissue wasting, including a decrease in muscle mass, subcutaneous tissue, or fat. Note: In fetal malnutrition, birth weight may fall above the 10th percentile for dates.
      3. IUGR is considered moderately severe if birth weight is ≤ 3rd percentile for dates, especially if it is accompanied by reduction in body length.
   B. **Morbidity, mortality, and perinatal risk**
      1. There is up to a seven- to eightfold increase in perinatal mortality in cases of IUGR.
      2. There is a tenfold increase in perinatal mortality if birth weight falls below two standard deviations of the mean for gestational age.
      3. Long-term physical and neurologic sequalae are described in approximately one-third of cases.
   C. **Cause, pathogenesis, and pathophysiology**
      1. Normally, early fetal growth occurs primarily by cell hyperplasia, or cell division. This is followed later in development by both cell hyperplasia and hypertrophy. Finally, in the latter stage of a pregnancy, the number of fetal cells is

latter usually constant, and growth occurs by cellular hypertrophy alone.

    a. Consequently, **early onset of growth retardation** is likely to affect cell division adversely, leading to irreversible diminution in organ size and possibly function. Factors associated with early IUGR include heritable causes (e.g., trisomies), immunologic abnormalities, fetal infections, chronic maternal disease (e.g., cardiovascular, metabolic), poor maternal nutrition, multiple pregnancy, and irradiation.

    b. By contrast, **delayed onset of growth retardation** (after organ cell number is completed) tends to result only in decreased cell size and is usually reversible. The most common cause of this condition is uteroplacental insufficiency.

  2. IUGR is usually classified as symmetric or asymmetric.

    a. Symmetric IUGR implies that the insult is of long duration, and measures of cephalic growth [BPD or head circumference (HC)] and abdominal growth [abdominal circumference (AC)] are both diminished.

    b. Asymmetric IUGR is of later onset, with a decrease in abdominal circumference but sparing the head (normal or nearly normal BPD or HC).

D. **Antenatal diagnosis of IUGR**

  1. Clinical methods (e.g., serial fundal height [FH] measures, weight gain) allow diagnosis in only one-third of the cases of IUGR. The reasons for this low yield are related to inaccurate assessment of gestational age and fetal weight by parameters such as menstrual dates and uterine FH. This inaccuracy is due to issues outside of the provider's control such as later care, maternal obesity, uterine leiomyoma, uncertain dates, or irregular menses.

  2. Serial cephalometry

    a. There are ranges of success in the antenatal diagnosis of IUGR by serial cephalometry (BPD), with variable rates of false-positive and false-negative results. Discrepancy in the ability to diagnose is due to a number of problems.

      (1) There is no uniformity in the method of obtaining sonar BPDs.

      (2) There are no early sonographic parameters for dating. In general, early pregnancy parameters are much more accurate than similar measurements made late in gestation.

      (3) A constitutionally small fetus will have decreased BPD growth in relation to a mean value derived from a heterogeneous population of fetuses. It is necessary to establish the growth potential of each fetus by at least two sonographic examinations, the first obtained prior to 26 weeks' gestation.

(4) There is similarity in the mean BPD growth rate for IUGR (especially asymmetric) and normal fetuses over short intervals (2 to 3 weeks).

b. These discrepancies suggest that cephalometry should not be used to diagnose IUGR definitively. Instead, serial BPDs should be used to identify fetuses at high risk for IUGR, with the undertanding that a certain proportion of these infants will be normal.

c. The sensitivity of cephalometry for diagnosing IUGR is about 50 percent.

3. Fetal AC measurements

a. The fetal AC is more likely to predit IUGR since the measurement reflects the size of the fetal liver and subcutaneous tissue. Both the liver and subcutaneous tissues are small in SGA fetuses, whether symmetric or asymmetric.

b. AC measurements correctly detect IUGR in approximately **70 to 80 percent** of cases in the third trimester of pregnancy.

4. Head to abdomen circumference (H/A) ratios

a. In normal pregnancies, the H/A circumference ratio is > 1.0 until 35 to 37 weeks' gestation. Following this interval, the AC enlarges at a faster rate and the H/A ratio is reversed to < 1.0. Nonetheless, in approximately 70 percent of cases with asymmetric IUGR, the H/A ratio remains not only > 1.0 but at least two standard deviations above the mean H/A value. Like most ultrasound evaluations, accuracy of H/A ratio depends on objective knowledge of dates.

5. Total intrauterine volume (TIUV)

a. The TIUV is obtained from multiple ultrasound measurements of the uterus (length × width × height × 0.5).

b The sensitivity of TIUV (proportion of undergrown fetuses with TIUV less than one standard deviation is about 50 percent.

c. It should be noted that placental hypertrophy or polyhydramnios invalidates TIUV for detection of IUGR. In addition, dates should be objectively defined by fetal CRL or early BPD measurement for proper interpretation of TIUV.

d. The TIUV method is currently utilized infrequently, as it offers no advantage relative to direct fetal measurements and requires a static scanner for measurement, which is not available in most ultrasound units.

6. Assessment of individual fetal growth potential using both BPD and AC

a. BPD measurements are obtained in the intervals of 18 to 26 and 30 to 33 weeks of pregnancy. Based on curves relating BPD to gestational age, the fetus is assigned a BPD growth percentile that (1) defines its gestational age in 90 percent of fetuses to within ±3–5 days by using the growth-adjusted sonar age (GASA) method and (2) establishes its potential cephalic growth for the rest of the pregnancy.

b. AC measurements are obtained between 30 and 33 or between 34 and 37 weeks' gestation, depending on the BPD percentile rank and/or the presence of adverse clinical conditions. Based on curves relating AC to gestational age, the fetus is assigned a growth percentile for the AC. The AC percentile measurement primarily serves to estimate fetal body size.

c. The above sonar measurements allow classification of each of the BPD and AC values into three possible growth patterns: large (≥ 90th percentile), small (≤ 10th percentile), or average, (10th to 90th percentiles). By relating the three BPD growth patterns to a specific AC percentile rank, nine fetal growth combinations are possible (Fig. 18.1). Preliminary data indicate the following:

(1) LGA (large-for-gestational-age) fetuses are likely to fall into growth patterns 1 and 4.

(2) Asymmetric IUGR fetuses are likely to fall into growth patterns 3 and 6.

(3) Symmetric IUGR fetuses are likely to fall into growth patterns 6 and 9.

(4) AGA (appropriate-for-gestational-age) fetuses are likely to fall into growth patterns 2, 5, 7, and 8.

Percentile Growth Patterns

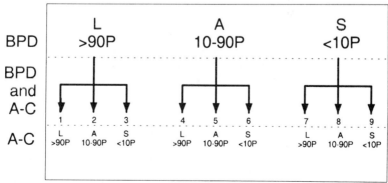

L=large A=average S=small

FIGURE 18.1. Nine fetal growth patterns noted by using BPD and AC percentile (p) (Modified from Tamura RK, Sabbagha RE. Percentile ranks of sonar fetal abdominal circumference measurements. Am J Obstet Gynecol 1980; 138(5):478. Reprinted with permission.)

    d. Preliminary results indicate that approximately 75 percent of IUGR fetuses would be detected by this method.

7. Diagnosis of IUGR based on estimated fetal weight (EFW) by ultrasound
    a. Numerous formulas for EFW determined by ultrasound are available, with predictive accuracy ranging from ±12 to ±20 percent (two standard deviations).
    b. The degree of accuracy is related to the size of the fetus, with larger infants having greater inaccuracy.
    c. The use of targeted formulas may improve accuracy (i.e., different formulas for SGA, AGA, and LGA; term vs. preterm fetuses). Overall, the sensitivity is about 70 to 75 percent.
    d. FL by itself is of limited use in EFW.

8. Oligohydramnios as a predictor of IUGR
    a. Oligohydramnios is a poor predictor, with sensitivity rates of 8 to 16 percent when only a single measurement of subjective assessment is used. However, the positive predictive value for IUGR is 40 percent when oligohydramnios is present [amniotic fluid index (AFI)].
    b. The four-quadrant amniotic fluid assessment by ultrasound may be a more sensitive indicator of IUGR.
    c. The quantification of fluid volume is more useful in assessment of fetal well-being in postdated pregnancies.

9. Doppler velocity studies
    a. EFW determined by ultrasound is more sensitive than Doppler studies for detecting IUGR.
    b. Doppler studies are better able to predict fetal compromise. This is particularly true if absent or reversed end-diastolic velocity is found.
    c. The role of fetal cerebral Doppler velocimetry is not fully established.

E. Antenatal management of IUGR
1. The determination of BPD and AC at intervals of approximately 3 weeks can be used to diagnose and prospectively evaluate the course of the individual fetus with suspected IUGR.
2. Bioelectric testing can be done weekly using nonstress tests (NST). A contraction stress tests (CST) can be done as indicated by the NST or the clinical course.
3. Dynamic ultrasound modalities to assess fetal breathing movements, fetal body movements, fetal tone, and quantitative amniotic fluid volume together with the NST constitute the biophysical profile of the fetus. The advantage of the biophysical profile relative to bioelectric testing in the diagnosis of fetal compromise is not established.
4. The assessment of pulmonary maturity will guide the deliberations for the most optimal time for delivery.

F. Neonatal complications: More common in IUGR infants
1. Intrauterine asphyxia, with the associated meconium aspira-

tion syndrome, pneumonia, and intracranial hemorrhage, are seen more frequently in infants with IUGR.
   2. Hypoglycemia (blood glucose values less than 30 to 40 mg/mL) has an incidence of 29 to 67 percent in IUGR infants. It is most frequently observed in preterm IUGR neonates and in the presence of hypoxia or hypothermia or both. The cause is related to deficient reserves, a high brain/liver ratio (resulting in a glucose demand that outstrips the rate of production), and delayed onset of gluconeogenesis.
   3. Other events that occur with increased frequency in IUGR neonates include polycythemia, electrolyte disturbances, and hypothermia.
G. **Prognosis for growth and development**
   1. The prognosis is difficult to assess because of the heterogeneity of IUGR fetuses, that is, symmetric versus asymmetric.
   2. With appropriate postnatal nutrition there is evidence of "catch-up" growth in the first year of life, especially in neonates with asymmetric IUGR due to placental insufficiency.
   3. In one prospective study, IUGR infants progressed to develop normal IQs. However, 25 percent of 96 full-term SGA infants had evidence of minimal cerebral dysfunction, such as poor school performance and dyslexia.

II. **Accelerated fetal growth (AFG) or large-for-gestational-age (LGA) fetuses**
A. **Definition**
   1. Large for gestational age implies a birth weight that meets one of the following criteria:
      a. > 4000 g, 10 percent incidence
      b. ≥ 4500 g, 1 percent incidence
      c. > 90th percentile for gestational age
   2. Recent pediatric studies using skinfold thickness measurements in the immediate neonatal period, should serve to delineate further these LGA infants.
B. **Morbidity, mortality, and perinatal risk**
   1. It is important to identify these fetuses antenatally, since they experience a threefold increase in perinatal mortality.
   2. As might be anticipated, fetuses weighing more than 4000 g are at increased risk for prolonged second-stage labor, midforceps delivery, shoulder dystocia, and immediate neonatal injury.
   3. There is an increase in severe neurologic disability as a result of great trauma.
C. **Cause, pathogenesis, and pathophysiology**
   1. Accelerated fetal growth is observed in a variety of conditions, including maternal obesity, excessive maternal weight gain, fetal insulinomas, nesidioblastosis, and Beckwith-Wiedeman syndrome. Among diabetic pregnancies,

particularly White's classes A to C, the frequency of AFG is 16 to 45 percent.
   2. Similar to retarded growth, there are two types of accelerated growth.
      a. Symmetric accelerated growth is proportionate accelerated growth (> 90th percentile) of all fetal parameters. This occurs in patients with prolonged pregnancies and in those of large physical stature.
      b. Asymmetric accelerated growth is disproportionate. Fetal head and limb growth is large but is usually at or below the 90th percentile; however, the fetal abdomen is above the 90th percentile. This occurs in White's class A to C diabetic mothers.
   D. **Antenatal diagnosis of AFG** depends on the definition used by the institution. For that reason, there are numerous screening tests.
      1. Recent studies utilizing ultrasound measurement of the BPD and AC (see Section I.D.6) appear promising for detection of AFG. For example, in 23 infants of diabetic mothers (White's classes A to C), the BPD values for all fetuses fell in the normal range, whereas the AC values of 10 of the 23 fetuses were more than two standard deviations above the mean. The birth weights and skinfold thicknesses of the latter infants were significantly greater than those of the others.
      2. A difference by ultrasound between the fetal trunk diameter and BPD of more than 1.4 cm may be predictive of an LGA fetus at term.
      3. Fetal sonar abdominal circumference and weight estimations are also useful in the prediction of AFG.
      4. Correct antenatal prediction of AFG is possible in about 88 to 90 percent of cases if both AC and ultrasonic predicted weight utilizing AC exceed the 90th percentile.
   E. **Antenatal management of suspected AFG**
      1. The antenatal management of suspected AFG is essentially directed to those women who are determined to be diabetic. Early active intervention may help to minimize the AFG. Prevention of excessive weight gain may also be beneficial.
      2. Ultrasound assessment of fetal weight and size may be of some assistance in determining the mode of delivery.
      3. If macrosomia is suspected, a thoughtful deliberation is indicated before doing a forceps delivery since this may cause iatrogenic shoulder dystocia.
   F. **Neonatal complications**
      1. Birth injury is increased in macrosomic infants, primarily as a result of shoulder dystocia.
      2. AFG secondary to maternal diabetes is associated with the additional complications of hypoglycemia, polycythemia, hypocalcemia, and renal vein thrombosis.

G. Prognosis for growth and development

1. When AFG is associated with infants of diabetic mothers, 40 percent of these infants are obese at 7 years of age compared to 5 percent of normally grown infants.
2. Infants of nondiabetic mothers with AFG may be at increased risk for developing diabetes mellitus.

BIBLIOGRAPHY

Sabbagha RE. Intrauterine growth retardation. In: Sabbagha RE, ed. Ultrasound Applied to Obstetrics and Gynecology. 2nd ed. Philadelphia: JB Lippincott; 1990:112–131.

Tamura RK, Dooley SL: Diabetes mellitus and fetal macrosomia. In: Sabbagha RE, ed. Ultrasound Applied to Obstetrics and Gynecology. 2nd ed. Philadelphia: JB Lippincott; 1990:165–173.

Tamura RK, Sabbagha, RE: Altered fetal growth. In: Sicarra JJ, ed and Droegemuller W, assoc ed. Gynecology and Obstetrics, Vol III: Maternal-Fetal Medicine. Rev. ed. Philadelphia: JB Lippincott; 1990; chap 74.

CHAPTER 19
Isoimmunization

David C. Shaver

Hemolytic disease of the fetus and newborn has been a known complication of pregnancy for hundreds of years. It was not until 1940, with identification of the Rh antigen, that the cause of most cases of hemolytic disease of the newborn began to be unraveled. Subsequent to its identification, the Rh antigen was described as the agent most commonly responsible for hemolytic disease; further work has led not only to management of the disease process, but also to its prevention. Due to the success in preventing Rh sensitization, it is no longer the leading cause of hemolytic diseases, and sensitization to other antigens, once relatively uncommon, has now become the major contributor to this disease process.

I. **Definition**
  A. **Isoimmunization** refers to development of antibodies as a result of antigenic stimulation with material on the red cells of another individual of the same species. Rh sensitization has historically been the most common cause of isoimmunization. The Rh system is actually made up of three groups of antigens in pairs: Dd, Cc, and Ee. It is the presence of D that determines Rh positivity. The presence of d has never been documented.
  B. There are numerous other blood groups on the red blood cells, and antibodies to any of these antigens can occur. Fortunately, most antibodies that develop to these other blood groups, the **irregular antibodies,** tend to be weak or are IgM and therefore usually do not produce the severe disease in the newborn. However, some, notably Kell, Duffy, and the other Rh blood group antigens, are associated with severe disease (Table 19.1).
  C. **Erythroblastosis fetalis** refers to the presence of erythroblasts, nucleated immature red blood cells, that are found in the circulation of infants with hemolytic disease of the newborn.

II. **Incidence**
  A. The incidence of patients who are candidates for Rh isoimmunization (i.e., Rh negative) is 15 percent in whites and 8 percent in blacks. It is rare in Asians.
  B. In Rh-negative women delivering their first Rh-positive baby, the risk of antibody formation following the pregnancy is 8 percent.

Table 19.1. Antibodies Causing Hemolytic Disease*

BLOOD GROUP SYSTEM	ANTIGENS RELATED TO HEMOLYTIC DISEASE	SEVERITY OF HEMOLYTIC DISEASE
ODE	D	Mild to severe
	C	Mild to moderate
	c	Mild to severe
	E	Mild to severe
	e	Mild to moderate
Lewis		Not a proved cause of hemolytic disease of the newborn
		Not a proved cause of hemolytic disease of the newborn
Kell	K	Mild to severe with hydrops fetalis
	k	Mild to severe
Duffy	Fy^a	Mild to severe with hydrops fetalis
	Fy^b	Not a cause of hemolytic disease of the newborn
Kidd	Jk^a	Mild to severe
	Jk^b	Mild to severe
MNSs	M	Mild to severe
	N	Mild
	S	Mild to severe
	s	Mild to severe
Lutheran	Lu^a	Mild
	Lu^b	Mild
Diego	Di^a	Mild to severe
	Di^b	Mild to severe
Xg	Xg^a	Mild
P	PP P* (Tj^a)	Mild to severe
Public	Yt^a	Moderate to severe
	Yt^b	Mild
	Lan	Mild
	En^a	Moderate
	Ge	Mild
	Jr^a	Mild
	Co^a	Severe
Private antigens	Co^{a-b}	Mild
	Batty	Mild
	Becker	Mild
	Berrens	Mild
	Evans	Mild
	Gonzales	Mild
	Good	Severe
	Heibel	Moderate
	Hunt	Mild
	Jobbins	Mild
	Radin	Moderate
	Rm	Mild

Table 19.1. *(Continued)*

BLOOD GROUP SYSTEM	ANTIGENS RELATED TO HEMOLYTIC DISEASE	SEVERITY OF HEMOLYTIC DISEASE
	Ven	Mild
	Wright[a]	Severe
	Wright[b]	Mild
	Zd	Moderate

*Note that conditions listed as being "mild" only can be treated like ABO incompatibility. Patients with all other conditions should be monitored as if they were sensitized to D.

Modified from Weinstein L. Irregular antibodies causing hemolytic disease of the newborn: A continuing problem. Clin Obstet Gynecol 1982:25(2):327–328.

However, the incidence of Rh antibodies demonstrated during the next pregnancy as a result of sensitization during the first pregnancy is 16 percent. This delayed appearance of the antibody in the subsequent pregnancy is referred to as **sensibilization,** and is presumably due to a secondary immune response resulting in an adequate level of antibody production for laboratory confirmation.

    C. In *ABO-incompatible* pregnancies (e.g., a mother of type O and a baby of type A, a mother of type A and a baby of type B), the incidence of isoimmunization falls to 2 percent, apparently due to destruction of the fetal red blood cells in the liver by reticuloendothelial cells, thereby avoiding sensitization to the Rh antigen.

    D. Approximately 1 percent of women become sensitized to Rh **during pregnancy,** primarily during the third trimester.

    E. Although it might be expected that repeated exposure of an Rh-negative woman to Rh-positive fetal cells would ultimately result in a 100 percent incidence of sensitization, this is not the case. Only about 50 percent of women become sensitized, regardless of the number of exposures to Rh-positive red blood cells.

III. **Morbidity and mortality.** The basic disease process in isoimmunization is transplacental passage of IgG, resulting in destruction of fetal red blood cells. In some cases of isoimmunization, the antibody is IgM (such as the Lewis antibodies, Le[a] and Le[b]). Other antibodies may not cause problems simply because they are found only on adult red blood cells and are not present during fetal life.

    A. The result of transplacental passage of the antibody is destruction of the red blood cells, usually within the spleen. This hemolytic process causes stimulation of fetal erythropoietin and may exceed the ability of the bone marrow to replace red blood cells. If this happens, extramedullary hematopoiesis will occur, primarily in the liver and spleen.

1. The result of this process is severe fetal anemia due to the inability of the fetus to replace the hemolyzed red blood cells. Severe anemia is associated with erythroblastosis.
2. The increase in erythropoiesis within the fetal liver results in a decrease in the production of albumin. In addition, portal hypertension develops due to replacement of the liver by areas of erythropoiesis. The result is development of hydrops fetalis.
3. Fetal death will ensue if the disease process is not arrested.

B. The severity of isoimmunization can be classified as mild, moderate, or severe.

1. Mild disease generally is associated with only mild anemia at the time of birth (i.e., > 12 g of hemoglobin per 100 mL). Most babies with mild disease do not have severe hyperbilirubinemia and will not require exchange transfusions.
2. In infants with moderate disease, the fetus will not develop such severe disease as to become hydropic in utero, but may be born anemic, and will develop hyperbilirubinemia and potentially kernicterus after birth if exchange transfusion is not done in the neonatal period.
3. Severe disease is associated with significant anemia and the development of hydrops fetalis. These infants will be either stillborn or severely affected at birth.

IV. **Cause**

A. The cause of virtually all cases of Rh isoimmunization occurring today is pregnancy with an Rh-positive fetus in an Rh-negative mother. Maternal exposure to fetal red blood cells, which is necessary for sensitization, occurs as a result of transplacental fetal-maternal hemorrhage. This transplacental hemorrhage occurs in the majority of pregnancies, primarily during the last trimester and around the time of delivery. The amount of hemorrhage is usually less than 1 mL of fetal blood but is great enough to stimulate an immune response in many cases.

B. Certain events may increase the risk of transplacental fetal-maternal hemorrhage during pregnancy. These include amniocentesis, external cephalic version, abruptio placenta, and cesarean section.

C. There is a possibility of sensitization following abortion. This incidence is probably negligible with very early abortions, since the number of fetal red blood cells may be too low to stimulate an immune response. However, abortion late in the first trimester or in the second trimester is associated with a risk of sensitization of up to 2 to 5 percent. A similar response can occur following ectopic pregnancy.

D. Since blood transfusions are usually compatible only for the ABO and Rh systems, the cause of most irregular antibodies is secondary to blood transfusion. However, in many cases, sensitization to irregular antigens develops by the same mechanism as Rh sensitization, namely, exposure to fetal blood during pregnancy.

V. **Diagnosis.** The diagnosis of isoimmunization requires detection of antibodies in maternal serum.
   A. The most commonly utilized method for screening for maternal antibodies is the indirect Coombs' test (indirect antiglobulin or antibody screening). Briefly, this test depends upon the ability of anti-immunoglobulin G (Coombs') serum to agglutinate red blood cells coated with immunoglobulin G. To perform the test, the patient's serum is mixed with red blood cells that are known to contain all significant red blood cell antigens and, following incubation, the cells are washed. A substance is then added to reduce the electrical potential of the red blood cell membranes, which is necessary to facilitate red blood cell agglutination. Coombs' serum is then added, and if maternal immunoglobulin is present on the red blood cells, then agglutination will occur. If the test is positive, further evaluation to determine the specific antigen is required. The result is then reported as the reciprocal of the highest dilution of maternal serum that will cause agglutination.
   B. Older methods for reporting antibody titers relied upon saline and albumin. Briefly, the saline method utilizes the patient's serum incubated with Rh-positive red blood cells suspended in saline. Due to the electrical potential of the cells, only large immunoglobulins such as IgM can bridge the gap between cells and precipitate agglutination. The albumin method utilizes albumin for incubating the specimen. Albumin reduces the electrical potential of the blood red cells and allows the red blood cells to lie closer together and thus be precipitated by both IgG and IgM antibodies. In general, these methods will produce an antibody titer severalfold lower than that achieved by the more sensitive indirect antiglobulin test.

VI. **Differential diagnosis.** Occasionally, a patient will present with hydrops fetalis of unknown cause. In these circumstances, immune and nonimmune hydrops fetalis must be differentiated. An antibody screening test at this time should determine whether immune hydrops fetalis exists; if not, then nonimmune causes should be explored (see Chapter 15).

VII. **Management.** The management described will be that for Rh isoimmunization. However, sensitization to other antigens known to cause severe fetal disease should be managed in a similar manner.
   A. **Predicting the severity of fetal disease.** The major goal in managing patients who are isoimmunized is to predict which babies will develop severe disease. In general, severity of disease is related to two factors: antibody titer and past obstetric history.
      1. A **critical level of antibody** must be present before severe

fetal anemia can occur. In the absence of a previous hydropic infant or a neonate who required exchange transfusion, it is safe to delay fetal investigation until a critical antibody titer has been reached. Unfortunately, due to differences in technique, the critical antibody titer varies from laboratory to laboratory. Although it is generally recommended that each laboratory determine its own cutoff for the critical titer, it is likely that many laboratories will not have enough experience with severely isoimmunized pregnancies to determine this critical level. If no critical level is available for a laboratory, then the following can generally be used as guidelines:

    a. An albumin titer of $< 1:16$ is rarely if ever associated with hydrops.

    b. Since the indirect antiglobulin titer is more sensitive than the albumin titer, a titer of $< 1:16$ to $< 1:32$ should not be associated with a severe fetal outcome. Once the critical titer of an antibody is reached, the patient is considered to be at risk for a severe outcome, and fetal investigation at the appropriate gestational age should be carried out.

  2. The **obstetric history** is very important in determining the fetal risk. As a general rule, the severity of fetal disease increases with each sensitized pregnancy.

B. Management of the first sensitized pregnancy. Obviously, in the patient with the first pregnancy complicated by Rh sensitization, the obstetric history is of no benefit in management. Therefore, the decision about the necessity for further evaluation is based primarily on the antibody titer (Fig. 19.1).

  1. Once the diagnosis of Rh sensitization is made, the **paternal antigen status** should be determined. If the father is Rh positive, then the fetus may be Rh positive and therefore may be affected. Conversely, if the father is Rh negative, then the fetus will by necessity be Rh negative and no further evaluation will be necessary. If the status of the father cannot be assured or obtained, then the father should be presumed to be Rh positive.

  2. If the father's antigen is positive, antibody titers should be obtained every 2 to 4 weeks for the remainder of the pregnancy. If the titer does not rise to a level $\geq 1:16$, then the fetus can be presumed to be at minimal risk and no further evaluation should be carried out. If the antibody titer rises to $\geq 1:16$, then some method for evaluating the fetus [amniocentesis or percutaneous umbilical blood sampling (PUBS)] should be instituted.

    a. Amniocentesis allows evaluation of the amniotic fluid for spectrophotometric examination for bilirubin. It has been known for some time that the severity of the fetal hemolytic process is reflected by the amount of bilirubin in the amniotic fluid, and the bilirubin can be measured

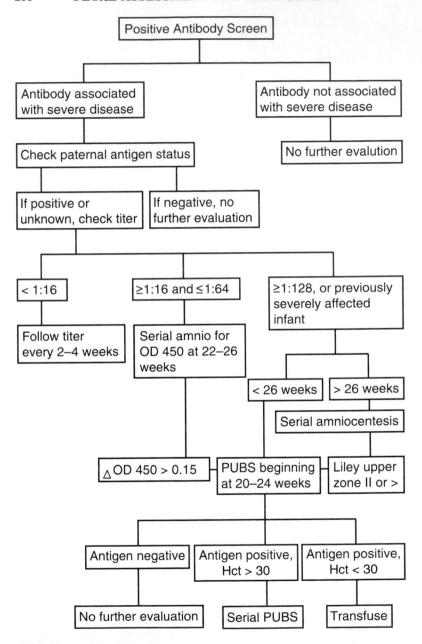

FIGURE 19.1. A proposed management scheme for isoimmunization during pregnancy.

by the change in the optical density at a wavelength of 450 nm (Δ OD 450). The amount of bilirubin in the amniotic fluid is also affected by gestational age. Therefore, Liley (Fig. 19.2) instituted the use of a semilogarithmic graph to plot the Δ OD 450 vs. gestational age for predicting the severity of fetal anemia.

Amniocentesis should be performed on all patients who develop a critical titer in the third trimester or who have a good obstetric history without an extreme elevation of the antibody titer. The value is then plotted on the Liley graph and a decision about subsequent amniocentesis is made, depending on the zone.

(1) Repeated values within zone 1 indicate an unaffected or mildly affected fetus and the pregnancy can continue to term, although it should not be allowed to go past 40 weeks' gestation.

(2) Values in the upper part of zone 2 or values that are increasing in zone 2 indicate moderate to severe disease and require early delivery, PUBS, or repeat amniocentesis within a week.

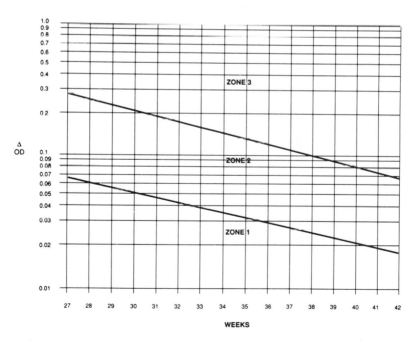

FIGURE 19.2. Liley graph used to depict degrees of sensitization. (Liley AW. Liquor amnii analysis in management of pregnancy complicated by rhesus sensitization. Am J Obstet Gynecol 1961;82(6):1362. Reprinted with permission.)

(3) Values within zone 3 indicate a high likelihood of the development of hydrops fetalis and should be managed by either PUBS or early delivery.

(4) The initial study by Liley reported on patients who were managed during the third trimester. The use of amniocentesis in the second trimester has been shown to be less reliable. If midtrimester amniocentesis is used, the following can be said to apply:

(a) A Δ OD 450 value of ≥ 0.4 is associated with a high risk of hydrops fetalis, regardless of the gestational age.

(b) The trend in Δ OD 450 may be helpful even if a single value does not correlate well with the fetal condition.

(c) Severe disease in the fetus is unlikely at a value < 0.15 to 0.2.

b. PUBS has been utilized more frequently over the last few years in the management of Rh isoimmunization. The advantage of this method is that the fetal hematocrit can be directly measured, the fetal antigen status can be ascertained, and the blood is available for additional tests such as direct Coombs' tests and reticulocyte counts. For these reasons, PUBS is generally felt to be indicated for the following circumstances:

(1) Early sampling (e.g., at 20 to 22 weeks) is indicated due to previous severe disease or extremely high maternal antibody titers.

(2) If the father is believed to be heterozygous, consideration may be given to PUBS since there is a chance that the fetus may be antigen negative. This can be determined directly by evaluation of the fetal blood, obviating the need for continued surveillance.

The disadvantage of PUBS is primarily related to potential complications, which are still poorly elucidated but may approach a fetal mortality rate as high as 1 to 2 percent. Additionally, the expertise necessary to perform PUBS is significantly greater than that needed for amniocentesis, and generally a referral to a maternal-fetal medicine subspecialist would be indicated for this procedure. Therefore, PUBS should be reserved for those cases in which the additional information is clearly felt to compensate for the increased risk over amniocentesis.

C. **Management of the patient with a previous immunized pregnancy.** For patients who have had a previous severely affected infant who required exchange transfusion or developed hydrops fetalis, fetal evaluation is indicated early in gestation, preferably by 20 to 24 weeks of gestation. If the previous infant developed hydrops, then evaluation should be carried out at least 4 weeks prior to the previous onset of hydrops fetalis (e.g., if the previous infant developed hydrops at 26 weeks of gestation, then evaluation should carried out by 20 to 22 weeks of gestation). A patient with a previously immunized pregnancy in which the neonate required no treatment can probably be managed the same as the patient with the first immunized pregnancy.

D. **Management of the severely affected fetus.** For patients who are determined to have probable severe fetal disease, as determined by serial Δ OD 450 determinations or PUBS, management depends upon the gestational age.

1. In patients of $\geq$ 34 weeks of gestation, especially if pulmonary maturity is present, delivery is indicated.

2. For patients of $\geq$ 34 weeks of gestation with immature lungs, consideration of steroid therapy prior to delivery vs. intrauterine transfusion can be debated.

3. For patients of $<$ 34 weeks of gestation with suspected severe disease, intrauterine transfusion is probably indicated. Intrauterine transfusion can be performed by one of two methods.

    a. Intraperitoneal transfusion was first described by Liley in 1963. Administration of red blood cells into the fetal abdomen is associated with absorption of the intact red cells via the lymphatics into the fetal vascular system. In general, the red blood cells are absorbed over the course of approximately 1 week unless hydrops fetalis is present, in which case absorption is delayed. Intraperitoneal transfusion is performed under ultrasound guidance with insertion of a needle into the fetal abdomen, preferably into the lower quadrants away from the enlarged liver and spleen. Type O-negative, maternal-compatible, packed red blood cells are injected. The volume to be infused is predicted by the gestational age:

$$\text{Volume} = (\text{weeks gestation} - 20) \times 10 \text{ mL}$$

    For example, a fetus at 27 weeks of gestation would be given 70 mL of packed red blood cells intraperitoneally. A second transfusion would be given in approximately 10 days, and then at intervals of 3 to 4 weeks until the fetus reaches near-term gestation.

    b. Direct intravascular transfusion under ultrasound guidance has recently gained favor and has been increasingly performed as expertise with PUBS has improved. With this procedure, the fetal hematocrit can be directly measured and blood given directly into the fetal circulation, and a posttransfusion hematocrit can be obtained. As is true for PUBS, the expertise of the operator is extremely important for direct intravascular transfusion. In addition, an expert sonographer is required for both procedures.

c. The choice of transfusion technique depends on the operator's preference, the location of the umbilical cord insertion site, and the fetal condition. Success rates appear to be similar for both procedures, with the exception of hydrops fetalis, for which direct intravascular transfusion is associated with an improved outcome.

VIII. Prevention of isoimmunization. Rh sensitization can be prevented in the vast majority of cases with passive immunization. High-titer Rh immunoglobulin (RhIG) has been developed for administration to prevent Rh sensitization. A standard dose of RhIG of 300 μg has been demonstrated to prevent sensitization after exposure to 30 mL of Rh-positive fetal blood. RhIG should be administered to the Rh-negative mother (unless the father is also known to be Rh negative) in the following circumstances:

A. Following elective or spontaneous abortion. If the abortion occurs in the first trimester, a smaller dose of 50 μg is probably adequate for protection.

B. A dose of 300 μg should be given following amniocentesis. If delivery occurs within 3 weeks after amniocentesis, then the RhIG need not be repeated.

C. At 28 to 30 weeks of gestation. Administration of 300 μg of RhIG to the mother early in the third trimester will prevent most cases of isoimmunization that occur during this period as a result of small transplacental fetal-maternal hemorrhages.

D. A dose of 300 μg is repeated following delivery if the neonate is demonstrated to be Rh positive.

The vast majority (> 99 percent) of Rh sensitization can be prevented by following these guidelines. A small number of patients may become sensitized due to various factors, including unrecognized early abortion or massive transplacental hemorrhage. Hemorrhage in excess of 30 mL of fetal blood is rare but may occur. If more significant hemorrhage does occur, it tends to take place around the time of delivery, especially in association with events such as abruptio placenta or manual extraction of the placenta. In these cases, a Kleihauer-Betke stain on the maternal blood may be indicated to determine if a larger hemorrhage has occurred. If so, the volume of hemorrhage can be calculated and an appropriate amount of RhIG administered to protect against sensitization.

IX. Prognosis. With current therapy, most cases of Rh immunization can be managed quite successfully. Although the risk of intraperitoneal transfusion historically approaches 3 percent per procedure and that for intravascular transfusion up to 1 percent per procedure, most large series reported today are generally quite good. In general, for fetuses who do not develop hydrops, even if transfusion is necessary, survival should approach 100 percent, whereas that of hydropic fetuses may approach 70 to 80 percent with intravascular transfusion. These good outcomes reflect not only emerging techniques, but also the expertise of high-risk maternal-fetal medicine subspecialists in various centers. Patients in whom a high likelihood of severe disease is possible should be referred to these centers for management.

BIBLIOGRAPHY

ACOG. Prevention of D Isoimmunization. ACOG Technical Bulletin, No. 147, October 1990.

ACOG. Management of Isoimmunization in Pregnancy. ACOG Technical Bulletin, No. 148, October 1990.

Ananth U, Queenan JT Does midtrimester ΔOD_{450} of amniotic fluid reflect severity of Rh disease? Am J Obstet Gynecol 1989; 161:47–49.

Bowman JM The management of Rh-isoimmunization. Obstet Gynecol 1978; 52:1–16.

Nicolaides KH, Fontanarosa M, Gabbe SG, et al. Failure of ultrasonographic parameters to predict the severity of fetal anemia in rhesus isoimmunization. Am J Gynecol 1988; 158:920–926.

Nicolaides KH, Rodeck CH, Mibashan RS, Kemp JR Have Liley charts outlived their usefulness? Am J Obstet Gynecol 1986; 155:90–94.

Parer JT Severe Rh isoimmunization—Current methods of in utero diagnosis and treatment. Am J Obstet Gynecol 1988; 158:1323–1329.

Watts DH, Luthy DA, Benedetti TJ, et al. Intraperitoneal fetal transfusion under direct ultrasound guidance. Obstet Gynecol 1988; 71:84.

Weiner CP, Williamson RA, Wenstrom KD, et al. Management of fetal hemolytic disease by cordocentesis. Am J Obstet Gynecol 1991; 165:546–553.

Weinstein L. Irregular antibodies causing hemolytic disease of the newborn. Obstet Gynecol Surv 1976; 31:581–591.

CHAPTER 20

Perinatal Infections

Jessica L. Thomason

Toxoplasmosis, rubella, cytomegalovirus, and herpes (TORCH) infections during pregnancy are difficult to diagnose and treat. Patients often ask pointed questions regarding statistical risks to their unborn children. Individual TORCH infections are discussed, with particular reference for the practicing physician. Other infections, such as **syphilis and hepatitis,** also carry significant obstetric maternal risks, requiring careful evaluation and treatment as well as explanation to parents.

TOXOPLASMOSIS

I. **Characteristics of the organism**
   A. **Microbiology of toxoplasmosis.** The causative organism of toxoplasmosis is an intracellular parasite, *Toxoplasma gondii.* There are three forms of the protozoan:
   1. **Trophozoites** are seen in the acute stage of the infection. They invade cells, dividing to produce either a **tissue cyst** or **destruction** of the **host cell** by lysis. Desiccation, freezing, thawing, and normal gastric secretions are lethal to trophozoites.
   2. **Tissue cysts** may contain up to 3000 organisms and are a major mode of transmission of the disease. Undercooked, infected meat (e.g., lamb) is eaten with the cyst wall disrupted by normal gastric juices, allowing viable organisms to invade the host's gastrointestinal tract. Freezing, thawing, heating, and desiccation destroy cysts.
   3. **Oocytes** are produced only in the intestines of the cat family. Oocytes undergo both an asexual and a sexual cycle. Noninfectious, unsporulated oocytes are defecated by cats. With sporulation, which takes 4 or 5 days, oocytes become infectious. Infectious oocytes can remain in moist soil for more than 1 year and are easily airborne. **Only** cats who hunt and kill their prey are capable of being reservoirs. Cats eating only canned, frozen, or dried food are **not** at risk for transmitting the disease.

II. Epidemiology and disease

A. Human infection in nonpregnant women. Thirty percent of reproductive-age women have antibodies to the disease. Most infections in children and adults are totally **asymptomatic.** Seroconversion in the United States occurs at a rate of 0.5–2/1000 pregnant women. With appropriate cellular and hormonal immunity, trophozoites disappear from tissue and blood and encyst especially in skeletal muscle. But in immunocompromised hosts, cysts may occur in the brain, heart, and other vital organs.

B. Human infection during pregnancy. Toxoplasmosis acquired during pregnancy **can cause fetal disease.** The **severity** of fetal disease is greater, although the rate of infection is less, if disease is acquired in the **first** trimester of pregnancy. Conversely, the **rate of fetal infection** is higher, although the severity is less when disease is acquired in the **third** trimester of pregnancy. Of women **acquiring disease during pregnancy,** up to 60 percent of infants show serologic evidence of congenital infection. The **majority** (75 percent) of congenitally infected infants show no gross signs of infection at birth. However, congenital disease can cause **severe mental retardation** with chorioretinitis, blindness, epilepsy, intracranial calcifications, and hydrocephalus.

C. Animal infection. In domestic animals, toxoplasmosis has a severe economic impact, producing repeated abortions in sheep and swine. However, it does **not produce** similar disease in **human gestations.**

III. Diagnosis.

Although isolation of *T. gondii* from blood or body secretions or demonstration of trophozoites in tissue establishes that the infection is acute, most acquired infections are **totally asymptomatic.** Therefore, the clinician must rely on **serologic evidence** of disease. The Centers for Disease Control does **not** currently **recommend routine screening** of all pregnant patients. Serologic testing should be performed only at reliable laboratories having excellent control standards. Incorrect test values are reported in over 65 percent of routine laboratories.

A. Serologic testing. Available tests include identification of IgG and IgM antibodies. The presence of **high IgG and positive IgM** levels may support the diagnosis of recently acquired infection. However, **IgM titers** can **remain elevated** for long periods of time after an acute infection — more than one year in some cases. In addition, IgM levels may rise spontaneously years after an acute infection, making interpretation of a positive IgM level very difficult. With **asymptomatic** patients it is often impossible to determine with accuracy the time of onset of disease. **IgG antibody levels** are detected by:

1. Sabin-Feldman dye test **(DT)** (most frequently used)
2. Indirect immunofluorescent test **(IFA)**
3. Indirect hemagglutination test **(IHA)**
4. Enzyme-linked immunosorbent assay **(ELISA).** Recommended.

IgM antibody levels are detected by:
   1. **IgM immunofluorescent test** and **IgM immunoabsorbent assay.** Both tests can have false-positive reactions secondary to rheumatoid factors and antinuclear antibodies.
   2. A double-sandwich IgM enzyme-linked immunosorbent assay **(DS-IgM-ELISA),** which is recommended.
   B. **Serologic interpretation. Paired** sera drawn 3 weeks apart, indicating **no** antibodies previously, or a fourfold rise in titer with an IgG test helps to confirm a diagnosis of acute infection. A **negative** DT or IFA virtually **excludes the diagnosis** of acute infection if only one serum is available for testing. A **single** high titer of DT, IFA, or IHA is **not** diagnostic of an acute infection. A **low** DS-IgM-ELISA titer makes recent infection unlikely. A **negative** IgM level rules out an acute infection.

IV. **Prevention.** Prevention of disease is most important in pregnant women since therapy for disease during pregnancy is inadequate to prevent congenital disease.
   A. All meats should be thoroughly cooked or frozen prior to cooking.
   B. The hands should be thoroughly washed after handling raw milk, eggs, and vegetables.
   C. Disposable gloves should be worn for garden or outdoor yard work.
   D. Cats should be kept indoors and fed only store-bought food. Other members of the family should change cat litter since the infective oocytes are easily airborne. Cat feces should be avoided altogether.

V. **Treatment**
   A. **First-trimester infection.** Women in whom disease is documented in the first trimester should be counseled about the risk of serious congenital infection and given information about therapeutic pregnancy termination.
   B. **Medical treatment.** In the United States, the only effective medication marketed is a combination of sulfadiazine (or triple sulfonamide) and pyrimethamine (Daraprin). Daraprin is a folic acid antagonist that depresses the bone marrow. Folinic acid or Baker's yeast helps to prevent this toxicity. Pyrimethamine is **teratogenic** in laboratory animals and **cannot** be used in the first trimester of pregnancy. Spiramycin (pyrimethamine + sulfonamide) is available only in Europe and decreases but does **not** eliminate congenital infection.

RUBELLA VIRUS

I. **Characteristics of the organism.** The rubella virus belongs to the Toga group, is composed of RNA, and is commonly known as *German* or *3-day measles.*

II. Epidemiology and disease characteristics

A. Susceptibility. From 10 to 15 percent of all reproductive-age women are susceptible to infection. A history of prior infection is unreliable in 50 percent of patients.

B. Transmission. Transmission from an infected individual occurs after contact with nasopharyngeal secretions by droplet spread or airborne transmission. **Communicability** is possible approximately 7 days prior to rash development and persists for 4 days after rash onset. The **incubation period** ranges from 14 to 21 days postexposure.

C. Clinical presentation. Clinical **signs of disease** range from an asymptomatic state (70 percent of all patients) to low-grade fever, headache, malaise, and rash. **Rash** may be the first sign of disease. Discrete, pink-red maculopapules appear first on the face and spread rapidly to the neck, arms, trunk, and extremities. Frequently, lesions coalesce to form a **blush.** Usually, the rash is gone by the third day after its appearance, leaving in the same sequence as its appearance. Postauricular or suboccipital lymphadenopathy suggests acute rubella infection, and conjunctivitis is frequent.

D. Antibody formation. Antibody formation begins at the same time as the rash (14 to 21 days postexposure). IgM antibodies generally do not persist longer than 4 to 5 days after onset of the illness.

E. Congenital rubella syndrome. Babies with congenital rubella syndrome can have a wide variety of significant organ defects. Although 50 to 70 percent of babies with congenital rubella may appear normal at birth, many subsequently develop signs of infection. Common defects include cataracts, patent ductus arteriosus, and deafness.

F. Risk of congenital rubella. The risk of congenital rubella (CR) after maternal infection is related to the gestational age at the time of infection. There is a

1. 90 percent CR risk if the disease occurs at ≤ 11 weeks.
2. 33 percent CR risk if disease occurs at 11 to 12 weeks.
3. 24 percent CR risk if disease occurs at 13 to 14 weeks.
4. 11 percent CR risk if disease occurs at 15 to 16 weeks.
5. 5 percent CR risk if disease occurs in the third trimester.

III. Diagnosis

A. Virology. Direct **virus isolation** from the pharynx is possible from 7 days prior to the rash up to 14 days after rash resolution. Clinical signs of disease should always be confirmed by laboratory tests.

B. Serology. Serology testing is accurate for both IgG and IgM. Demonstration of IgM is indicative of recent infection. Hemagglutination inhibition (HAI), IFA, and ELISA testing are available for IgG antibody. Paired sera drawn 2 to 4 weeks apart demonstrating a fourfold or greater rise (e.g., HAI) indicates recent infection. **ELISA testing** very accurately demonstrates antibody to the disease and is the **recommended** test for routine antenatal screening of all patients.

IV. Prevention
A. **Vaccination.** Vaccination of all rubella-susceptible women in the United States is advocated since there is **no cure** for the maternal or neonatal disease. The available **vaccine** (RA 27/3) is a **live, attenuated** rubella virus that induces antibodies in ≥ 95 percent of vaccinations. Patients should be **checked** for evidence of rubella antibodies 6 weeks after vaccination. Susceptible postpartum women should receive vaccine but should be cautioned to avoid pregnancy for at least 3 months after vaccination, although CR syndrome has never been documented to occur in women who received the vaccine while pregnant or who became pregnant within 3 months after vaccination. Breast-feeding is not contraindicated after vaccination.
B. **Rh immune globulin and rubella vaccination.** Rh immune globulin may be administered in patients receiving the vaccine.

V. Treatment.
Pregnant patients documented to have rubella should **not** receive human immune gamma globulin since it will **not** prevent or lessen infection or viremia to the fetus. No antiviral chemotherapy for rubella is available. Maternal treatment is supportive care. Fetal treatment depends on the gestational age of the fetus at the time of infection and the parents' desires about continuing the pregnancy, depending on the risk of CR.

CYTOMEGALOVIRAL DISEASE

I. Characteristics of the organism.
Cytomegalovirus (CMV) is a DNA virus and belongs to the **Herpes** group. Being composed of DNA, CMV can undergo **latency** and **reactivate** at later times, just as **herpes simplex** infections can. **Primary** infections have more clinical importance than recurrent infections.

II. Epidemiology and disease
A. **Perinatal infection.** CMV is the most frequent cause of perinatal infection, occurring in 1 percent of all births in the United States. Acquisition of the virus requires intimate contact with an infected person's body secretions. CMV can be transmitted in saliva, semen, cervical secretions, breast milk, blood, and urine.
1. **Breast milk.** One of the most efficient sources of perinatal transmission from mother to infant is through breast milk after delivery. More than 60 percent of uninfected neonates may acquire the infection by this route, although little morbidity is seen in such infants.
2. **Cervical shedding.** Cervical shedding of CMV, including primary and reactivated virus, occurs in 2 to 30 percent of women during pregnancy, generally increasing in prev-

alence as the pregnancy proceeds. Isolation of CMV from the cervix will not differentiate between primary and recurrent disease.

B. Demographics. In the United States, 10 to 65 percent of reproductive-age women are seronegative and thus susceptible to infection during pregnancy. The lower the socioeconomic status, the more likely a patient is to have a positive antibody status to CMV. In poor socioeconomic circumstances, 40 to 60 percent of individuals are seropositive by 5 years of age.

C. Infection risks. The **risk of maternal infection causing intrauterine infection is 0.5 to 1.5 percent** and occurs with either **primary** seroconversion or **recurrent** (reactivation) infection. However, the **highest risk** of delivering a severely infected infant is with primary seroconversion during pregnancy. Only 50 percent of mothers with primary disease (seroconversion) during pregnancy will transmit the infection to their infants. Fetal infection at birth that is clinically apparent occurs virtually **only** after primary seroconversion during pregnancy in 10 to 15 percent of such women. Despite incomplete protection against transmission in utero, mothers who are seropositive prior to their pregnancy bestow a beneficial immunologic effect on the fetus and developing infant by reducing the virulence of the transmitted CMV infection. Although the risk of delivering a baby shedding CMV is the same in primary or recurrent disease, most babies (> 99 percent) shedding CMV born to mothers having recurrent (or reactivated) virus during pregnancy are asymptomatic at birth.

D. Neonatal infection. Neonatal infection with CMV (severe disease) is clinically evident in only 5 percent of infected babies. Although another 5 percent at birth will have an atypical presentation, the majority (90 percent) of babies infected in utero are asymptomatic at birth, although shedding CMV. Severe infection is manifested as microcephaly with or without intracranial calcifications, intrauterine growth retardation, hepatosplenomegaly, or petechiae. **From 10 to 15 percent** of **asymptomatic** CMV-infected babies will eventually develop sensorineural hearing loss, chorioretinitis, mild neurologic defects, and dental defects. Currently, it is unknown if infection during different trimesters will predict the severity of neonatal infection. From 40 to 60 percent of infants acquire CMV infection at **delivery** from the infected birth canal when a mother is shedding virus from the cervix. Recovery of CMV from the urine or cervix of pregnant women around the time of delivery does not indicate the need for a cesarean section, since acquisition of the disease by this method is rarely associated with detectable clinical illness subsequently in the neonate. Infants infected with CMV may be delivered subsequently to mothers whose pregnancy was complicated by a previous CMV-infected infant. However, in all such reported cases, the first baby was severely infected or died, whereas the subsequent sibling simply shed the virus at birth (an asymptomatic CMV shedder at birth).

III. Diagnosis

    A. Clinical signs of CMV infection. Clinical signs of CMV infection are those of a mononucleosis-like syndrome. However, more than 95 percent of mothers acquiring the disease are asymptomatic. At the present time, there is no way to prevent or treat CMV infections.

    B. Virus isolation. Virus isolation from infected tissue (e.g., nasopharynx, urine, cervix) is the "gold standard" for microbiologic diagnosis. However, classic cytopathologic effects in tissue culture can take as long as 42 days to occur. Isolation cannot differentiate between primary and recurrent disease.

    C. Serologic testing. Serology is **not** recommended unless performed by the Centers for Disease Control or certain research laboratories elsewhere in the country.

        1. Complement fixation, IHA, IFA, and ELISA (recommended) are available for IgG testing. Paired sera drawn 3 weeks apart with a fourfold titer rise are needed for diagnosis, although high titers alone may be suggestive of recent infection.

        2. **IgM** testing in adults is **totally unreliable** and is not recommended, since IgM can persist for months and can reappear when recurrent shedding occurs. In adults, it cannot be used to document primary infection.

    D. Amniocentesis for viral isolation is not recommended due to the large number of false-negative reports.

IV. Prevention

    A. Contact. In job-related situations where pregnant women come in contact with secretions of patients at risk for CMV shedding (e.g., day care centers, nurseries, mental institutions), careful hand washing after exposure to potentially infected sources is probably sufficient protection against acquiring the disease.

    B. Vaccines are being developed but will probably **not** be effective since recurrent (or reactivation of) latent virus during pregnancy can result in neonatal CMV infection.

V. Treatment

    A. No chemotherapy or immunotherapy is currently effective.

    B. Vaccines: See Section IV.B.

HERPES SIMPLEX VIRUS

  I. Herpes simplex virus (HSV) during pregnancy. During pregnancy, acquiring HSV for the **first time** results more frequently in pregnancy loss. The effect on the fetus of **recurrent** disease is of no concern, except when the disease is acquired through vaginal birth. Recurrent episodes do not occur more frequently or with prolonged viral shedding during pregnancy.

 II. Risk to the fetus. Seventy percent of babies infected with HSV are delivered from mothers who are asymptomatically shedding virus (no clinical signs or symptoms of disease at delivery). The risk to the neonate of acquiring HSV through an infected birth canal can be as high as 50 percent with primary infections. The risk with secondary or asymptomatic shedding is significantly less (probably less than 1 to 2 percent). Of the infants infected with HSV, 50 percent die and 65 percent of the remaining living infants develop significant neurologic sequelae. The risk to the neonate, even if delivered by cesarean section from a mother with intact membranes known to be shedding HSV, is 6 percent.

III. **Management of the pregnant patient with HSV**
   A. **Antepartum monitoring. Cervical virologic monitoring** should be abandoned. HSV weekly cultures do not accurately predict if a patient will be shedding virus at delivery. Amniocentesis is **not** recommended since isolation of virus from fluid does not predict intrauterine infection.
   B. **Rules for labor and delivery.**
      1. Any evidence of active clinical disease at the time of delivery dictates **abdominal** delivery.
      2. Clinical evidence of HSV with:
         a. **Membranes intact:** abdominal delivery
         b. Membranes ruptured < 4 to 6 h: abdominal delivery
         c. Membranes ruptured > 6 h: no absolute proven advantage to cesarean section, but discussion of risks with the patient should dictate the delivery method.
      3. Do **not** use a scalp electrode when monitoring the fetus.

SYPHILIS

I. **Characteristics of the organism. Treponema pallidum (TP)** is a motile, tightly coiled spirochete that cannot be grown in vitro. TP causes syphilis, while yaws and pinta are diseases caused by other treponemal spirochetes not endemic to the United States. The spirochete can invade intact mucous membranes or areas of abraded skin.

II. **Epidemiology and disease**
   A. **Maternal.** Although believed to cross the placenta only after 16 weeks' gestation, TP has been documented to infect the fetus as early as 6 weeks. Women having primary or secondary disease are more likely to transmit the disease to their offspring than those with latent disease. Abortion, stillbirths, and neonatal deaths are more frequent in mothers having untreated disease during pregnancy.
   B. **Neonatal.** Infants born with congenital syphilis may range from totally asymptomatic to having classic stigmata, although **most** infants do not develop evidence of active disease for 10 to 14 days after delivery. The early signs and symptoms of congenital syphilis include a maculopapular rash, snuffles, mucous patches on the oropharynx, hepatosplenomegaly, jaundice, lymphade-

nopathy, and chorioretinitis. Later in life, signs of congenital syphilis that was undiagnosed and untreated include hutchinsonian teeth, mulberry molars, saddle nose, and saber shins.

III. **Diagnosis**
   A. **Serologic testing.** Serologic testing is the mainstay of diagnosis. It is divided into two types of tests.
      1. **Nontreponemal tests.** Nontreponemal tests identify antibodies (called *reagin* antibodies) developed by the body in response to nonspecific antigens from the immunologic inflammatory response to the spirochete. These tests are quantitated and reported in titers (e.g., 1:8, 1:64). The higher the titer, the higher the inflammatory reaction to infection. **False-positive tests** occur and are seen with chronic diseases (e.g., leprosy), with autoimmune diseases (e.g., lupus), and in drug addiction.
      2. **Treponemal-specific tests.** Treponemal-specific tests identify specific antibody directed against TP. A positive result indicates either **active disease** or **previous exposure** to syphilis. Microhemagglutination assay for TP (MHA-TP) is frequently used in testing neonates, while the fluorescent treponemal antibody absorption (FTA-ABS) test is the standard adult test.
   B. **Dark-field microscopy.** Dark-field microscopy is useful in lesions with active motile spirochetes (primary and secondary lesions). The skin lesion should be scraped and the exudate from the lesion touched to a glass slide, covered, and sealed at the edges (i.e., petroleum jelly). Spirochetes remain motile in an anaerobic environment for hours.

IV. **Treatment.** Treatment for syphilis is based on clinical and serologic staging of the disease.
   A. **Antibiotic therapy**
      1. **Early disease (primary or secondary stage) or latent disease less than 1 year's duration**
         a. Benzathine penicillin, 2.4 million U IM
         b. Penicillin-allergic patients: tetracycline HCl, 500 mg p.o. q.i.d. for 15 days in the non-pregnant patient
         c. The penicillin-allergic patient who is pregnant must undergo penicillin desensitization. Penicillin is the only antibiotic that will cross the placenta in adequate amounts to treat the fetus.
      2. **Latent disease greater than 1 year's duration or late disease**
         a. Benzathine penicillin, 2.4 million U IM weekly for 3 weeks, or
         b. Aqueous procain penicillin, 600, 000 U IM q.d. for 15 days, or
         c. Penicillin-allergic patients: tetracycline HCl 500 mg p.o. q.i.d. for 30 days if not pregnant. If pregnant, the patient must undergo penicillin desensitization.

B. **Follow-up evaluation after treatment.** Patients should be reevaluated with nontreponemal quantitative tests at 3, 6, 12, and 24 months posttherapy. A **fourfold rise in titer** indicates inadequate treatment or reinfection and requires retreatment.

C. **Neurosyphilis.** Consultation with an infectious disease expert is required for the treatment of these complicated patients

GROUP B BETA-HEMOLYTIC STREPTOCOCCI

I. **Characteristics of the organism.** *Streptococcus agalactiae* is a β-hemolytic streptococcus with Lancefield group B polysaccharide antigen that is associated with two types of perinatal infections.

II. **Epidemiology and disease characteristics.** Although up to 30 percent of pregnant women are colonized and up to 75 percent of the babies born to these women will be colonized with the organism, the overall infection rate is only 2–3/1000 live births. There are two manifestations of neonatal infection. **Early-onset syndrome** appears within the first week of birth, usually within the first 2 days. **Late-onset** syndrome appears after the first week.

Early-onset syndrome is devastating, with mortality rates exceeding 50 percent. Septic shock accompanied by respiratory distress can result in infant death within a few hours despite appropriate antibiotic therapy. Meningitis is present in 30 percent of cases. There is a strong association between early-onset infection and chorioamnionitis or early-onset endometritis. Late-onset syndrome is generally less severe, but the majority of these infants develop meningitis and over 50 percent of them show subsequent neurologic defects.

III. **Diagnosis.** Mothers can be tested by vaginal and rectal culture. Infants are identified by culture of blood and cerebrospinal fluid. Rapid antigen tests allow a presumptive diagnosis within hours, in contrast to culture, which requires 18 to 24 h.

IV. **Management.** Penicillins or cephalothin remain the drugs of choice for treatment. Penicillin resistance is extremely rare. Twenty million units of penicillin G given daily in individual doses is one accepted regimen. An alternative is a loading dose of 2 g IV ampicillin or cephalothin followed by 1 g IV every 4 to 6 h. In penicillin-sensitive individuals, erythromycin and clindamycin are alternatives.

V. **Prevention.** Routine antepartum cervical culturing or antigen testing is not predictive of disease in the baby. Even treatment of the mother and her partner in the antepartum period is not helpful. Recolonization can occur in such couples prior to delivery. Mothers at risk for beta-streptococci (e.g., previous fetal demise from such disease, urinary tract infection caused by the organism) should be encouraged to enter the labor and delivery area early in labor and IV antibiotic prophylaxis begun until cultures and/or rapid test detection results are known.

ACQUIRED IMMUNODEFICIENCY SYNDROME (AIDS)

I. Characteristics of the virus/microbiology

A. The causative virus is a human retrovirus, first isolated in 1983. The Human Retrovirus Subcommittee of the Committee on the Taxonomy of Viruses has proposed that all AIDS-related viruses be designated by a single name: **human immunodeficiency virus (HIV).** Previous virus names have included *human T-lymphotropic virus III (HTLV-III)* and *lymphadenopathy-associated virus (LAV).*

B. Retroviruses have the unique ability to convert their own viral RNA into DNA (classically, transcription occurs by DNA conversion to RNA) by a specific enzyme, **reverse transcriptase.** Viral DNA is incorporated into infected cell (T-cell lymphocyte) DNA and exists in a *provirus* form until the infected cell is signaled to reproduce itself by antigenic stimulation. New viral particles form by budding from the T-cell membrane, and the infected T cell itself dies. The new viral particles subsequently invade new T cells. HIV has a marked predilection for invasion of T4 (helper/inducer) lymphocytes, since the surface protein of the T4 cell distinguishes it from other lymphocytes acting as the receptor for the virus.

C. It is the continued destruction of the T4 cell population that causes:
   1. The gradual depletion of this lymphocyte population, causing
   2. A reversal of the T4 (helper)/T8 (suppressor) ratio of lymphocytes, leading to
   3. Defects in cell-mediated immunity, ultimately producing clinical opportunistic infections in patients with HIV infection.

D. T4 lymphocytes play a pivotal role in immune modulation of both cellular and humoral immunity.

E. HIV can infect monocytes, tissue macrophages, and neural tissue cells of the brain, spinal cord, and peripheral nerves, although its main target is the T4 lymphocyte. It may be that cells other than lymphocytes serve as a potential reservoir for the virus, since cell invasion does not produce cell destruction.

F. Live virus has been isolated from blood, semen, urine, breast milk, vaginal secretions, bone marrow, lymph nodes, spleen, cerebrospinal fluid, brain, and neural tissues. Although it has been isolated from tears and saliva, there is no evidence that transmission through saliva can occur.

G. **Antibody** to the virus **does not** indicate immunity to or protection from further infection. Antibody is a reliable clinical sign that can be accurately measured and indicates that a person has **live** virus capable of causing and transmitting disease.

H. Patients having antibody or from whom the virus has been isolated are at risk for opportunistic infections and certain common bacterial infections normally handled by B lymphocytes.

II. Incidence and epidemiology

A. HIV was probably introduced into the United States after 1978.

B. The majority of AIDS patients fall into three groups:
   1. Homosexual/bisexual males
   2. IV drug users
   3. Recipients of blood products (e.g., hemophiliacs).
   Women partners of AIDS patients are at risk (range, 7 to 70 percent; mean, 20 percent) for acquiring the virus. Perinatal cases currently account for a small but growing percentage (~4 percent) of AIDS patients.

C. Only three routes of transmission are important:
   1. Blood
   2. Sexual
   3. Perinatal

D. Acquisition of the virus (seroconversion) depends upon many factors: the amount of encountered virus (inoculum amount), the number of times inoculation was possible (e.g., the number of sexual episodes, sexual partners, units of infected blood), the immunologic status of the host (e.g., the pediatric immune status differs significantly from adult immune mechanisms), and other currently unknown factors. After the virus is acquired, cofactors are **not** needed for the development of AIDS. There is evidence that cofactors may help the virus to divide more rapidly. Seroconversion may occur as early as 1 week or as long as 3 months postexposure. **Rarely,** seroconversion has been documented to occur 3 months after exposure. Seroconversion is possible without any signs or symptoms of disease.

E. After seroconversion, subsequent clinical signs of AIDS-related complex (ARC) and AIDS depend on many of the same factors discussed in Section III.E. However, there may be unknown factors that contribute as well. Currently, it is **not** known if **all** individuals with HIV infection will progress to AIDS. However, the long-term outlook of patients who have the virus looks grim. More than 98 percent of patients first reported to have the virus have died. Because the disease has been studied only since the early 1980s, definitive statements about the natural history are difficult. Some estimates can be given.
   1. The incubation period of seroconversion after contacting the virus (e.g., sexual intercourse) is unknown but may range from 1 week to several years. The mean time of seroconversion after acquiring the virus is approximately 120 days. **Rarely,** individuals have seroconverted at a later time.
   2. The incubation period of perinatally acquired AIDS is 1 to 80 months (mean, 10 months). Signs of the disease appearing in the first year of life portend a very poor outcome with rapid demise.
   3. The mean incubation period of transfusion-acquired AIDS in adults is 30 months.
   4. The mean interval between seroconversion with HIV and the onset of AIDS exceeds 7 years.

F. The risk of transmission of HIV-positive mothers to babies is approximately 30 percent by prospective studies. The risk is not lowered by cesarean section delivery of the infant.

G. HIV has been transmitted through artificial insemination.

H. There is strong evidence that HIV infection is **not transmitted through**

1. Household contact
2. Close personal contact except sexual
3. Animal vectors (e.g., mosquitos)

I. The risk of transmission of HIV from a needle or mucous membrane exposure is < 1 percent (contrast the risk of acquiring hepatitis B through a needle stick: ~ 2.5 percent).

III. Clinical disease

A. Currently, over 90 percent of individuals infected with HIV are without signs or symptoms of disease. Although most patients have no signs when they acquire the infection, some patients have a mononucleosis-like syndrome. Rarely, acute neurologic syndromes have been associated with early disease. A staging system combining clinical signs of disease and serologic tests is useful.

B. As patients progress with the HIV infection, they develop the pre-AIDS syndrome. An HIV infection must be seen as an evolving, dynamic process. Patients with this stage of disease (previously called *AIDS-related complex*) should be examined regularly and cautioned about the development of opportunistic infections or developing malignancies. Laboratory evaluations are needed during this stage and may include a complete blood count (CBC), liver function tests, sedimentation rates, chest x-ray, cultures of the stool, and so on. Some investigators suggest following the p24 antigen, with reappearance signaling that the patient is about to develop full-blown AIDS.

C. AIDS is the end stage of the HIV infection.

D. The infectious and/or neoplastic complications of AIDS to which the patient ultimately succumbs is explained by the chronic, progressive depletion and malfunction of the T4 lymphocyte immune response of the host. Infections with relatively nonvirulent organisms result in opportunistic and life-threatening diseases in the immunocompromised hosts.

1. Protozoal infections include *Pneumocystis carinii* (the most common opportunistic infection; 70 percent of patients acquire it), *Toxoplasma*, *Cryptosporidium*, and *Isospora*.
2. Common fungal infections include *Candida* and *Cryptococcus*.
3. Viruses of importance include CMV, herpes, varicella-zoster, and Epstein-Barr virus.
4. Mycobacterial infections include *Mycobacterium avium, M. intracellulare,* and *M. tuberculosis,* among others.
5. Common neoplasms include Kaposi's sarcoma, non-Hodgkin's lymphoma, and carcinoma of the oropharynx.

  E. The diagnosis of an opportunistic infection should alert the clinician about the possibility of HIV, especially if it is *P. carinii.*

IV. Diagnosis
  A. Physical examination is important to identify skin lesions indicating opportunistic infections or neoplasms, to document the size and number of lymph nodes, and to stage a patient clinically.
  B. A standard CBC with differential and a platelet count are useful but may be normal in the early stages of the disease.
  C. Skin testing is useful to evaluate delayed hypersensitivity.
  D. Serologic testing of T cells is useful to:
   1. Indicate the need to perform ELISA testing for HIV
   2. Clinically stage the patient's disease. The total T4 cell count should be > 400 cells/mm^3. The T4/T8 ratio should be > 1 (recommended).
  E. Because no test is perfect and false-positive tests occur, all **positive** test results should be repeated. If the serum remains positive, a Western blot test (electrophoresis) will confirm the ELISA test. A positive ELISA test with a positive Western blot test confirms seroconversion to HIV. Due to the legal, social, and psychological impact of HIV testing, a patient should be informed of a positive test result only after the confirmatory Western blot test.
  F. Investigations of serologic tests for IgM antibody are not widely available.
  G. Virus isolation also indicates HIV infection.
  H. Diagnosis of opportunistic infections should be directed to the specific organism suspected.

V. Therapy/prevention
  A. Currently, **no** therapy is available to reverse the underlying immunodeficiency.
  B. Palliative therapy in an attempt to inhibit HIV replication has been most promising with AZT (3'-azido-3'-deoxythymidine, Retrovir). Other trials with reverse transcriptase inhibitors include suramin, ribivirin, phosphonoformate, HPV-23, and dideoxycytidine. Trials with immune modulating agents have involved alpha interferon, gamma interferon, isoprinosine, and interleukin 2.
  C. Vaccine research is in progress, but due to the inherent qualities of retroviruses, a vaccine will not be developed in the near future.
  D. Safe sex practices are the most logical method for prevention of disease. Epidemiologic data confirm the low risk of transmission in groups practicing safe-sex rules: use of condoms, limiting the number of sexual contacts (monogamy), avoiding intercourse with an HIV-infected individual, and so on.
  E. Female partners known to be HIV positive should **avoid** pregnancy, since transmission rates can be high and pregnancy itself may have an adverse effect on the latent infection.

F. The virus is easily destroyed outside the human host. Destruction is possible with common detergents, sodium hypochlorite (household bleach), hand soaps, H_2O_2, phenolics, alcohols, high and low pH, and exposure to high temperatures.

BIBLIOGRAPHY

Baker DA, ed. Viral diseases in pregnancy. Clin Obstet Gynecol 1990; 33:1–290.

Boyer KM, Gotoff SP. Prevention of early-onset neonatal group B streptococcal disease with selective intrapartum chemoprophylaxis. N Engl J Med 1986; 314:1665–1669.

Preblud SR, Williams NM. Fetal risk associated with rubella vaccine: Implications for vaccination of susceptible women. Obset Gynecol 1985; 66:121.

Prober CG, Hensleigh PA, et al. Use of routine viral cultures at delivery to identify neonates exposed to herpes simplex virus. N Engl J Med 1988; 318:887–891.

Sever JL, Larsen JW, Grossman JH. Handbook of Perinatal Infections. Boston, Little, Brown; 1989.

Sperling RS, Stratton P. Treatment options for human immunodeficiency virus–infected pregnant women. Obstet Gynecol 1992; 79:443–448.

Part IV

Obstetric Complications

CHAPTER 21

Premature Labor and Delivery

David C. Shaver

Premature labor and delivery is an important event in obstetrics because of its impact on neonatal mortality and morbidity. Currently, it is responsible for the majority of perinatal deaths in this country, and statistics reveal that the incidence of premature delivery has not changed significantly over the last 20 to 30 years. Approaches to management of the patient with premature labor are complicated by varying definitions of what actually constitutes premature labor and by controversies regarding therapy.

I. **Definition**

   A. **Premature labor** is defined as labor that occurs prior to 37 completed weeks of gestation. Since delivery prior to 20 weeks of gestation is generally considered an abortion, premature labor is labor that occurs between 20 and 37 weeks of gestation.

   B. Progressive dilatation and effacement coupled with regular uterine activity is generally required for the diagnosis of labor. Thus, one of the most common controversies in diagnosis of premature labor concerns the degree of dilatation and effacement that must have taken place and the frequency of uterine contractions. Regular uterine activity may occur in patients who are not in premature labor and may resolve spontaneously. Cervical effacement is very subjective and is difficult to quantitate. Cervical dilatation of up to 1 to 2 cm may occur during normal pregnancy. Therefore, true premature labor can best be defined as regular, painful uterine activity associated with progressive dilatation and/or effacement, or regular uterine activity associated with the cervix that is either $\geq$ 2 cm dilated or $\geq$ 80 percent effaced.

II. **Incidence.** The incidence of preterm delivery varies according to the population study. Overall in the United States, the incidence is between 8 and 9 percent of all deliveries. Within different population subgroups, the incidence varies from approximately 5 to 15 percent.

III. Morbidity and mortality

A. There does not appear to be any significant inherent risk of increased maternal morbidity and mortality secondary to preterm labor and delivery.

B. The primary concerns are the significant associated fetal and neonatal risks.

1. **Fetal distress** appears to be more common in premature labor and delivery, presumably as a result of decreased fetal reserve and the inability of the premature fetus to tolerate labor. Additionally, many of the factors that predispose to premature delivery, such as abruptio placentae, also contribute to fetal distress.

2. Although accounting for only 5 to 10 percent of deliveries in developed countries, premature infants are estimated to account for 50 to 75 percent of **perinatal deaths.** Perinatal mortality rates are gestational age dependent. In spite of improving survival rates at any gestational age beyond 24 weeks, the percentage of perinatal deaths attributable to prematurity has not changed.

3. **Perinatal morbidity** is also gestational age dependent. Morbidity can generally be classified as either short-term or long-term.

   a. **Short-term morbidity** includes complications such as respiratory distress syndrome and necrotizing enterocolitis. These complications are frequently life-threatening, and their incidence at various gestational ages is variable. Obstetric factors such as maternal medical complications, and other issues such as associated fetal growth retardation and peripartum steroid administration, may influence the incidence of these problems.

   b. **Long-term morbidity** includes problems such as neurologic handicaps and bronchopulmonary dysplasia. The incidence of these complications appears to be stable, with perhaps some decrease as neonatal care has improved.

IV. Cause

A. The specific factors that predispose to premature delivery are quite variable and frequently cannot be determined in each case. It must also be remembered that premature labor is not the most common cause of preterm delivery. In general, preterm delivery can be attributed to three broad causes:

1. Indicated preterm delivery such as might occur with hypertensive or other medical complications of pregnancy

2. Premature delivery secondary to premature rupture of the membranes

3. Premature labor

B. The causes of **premature labor** are varied, often poorly understood, and in many cases obscure. Due to the difficulty of describing specific causes of preterm delivery, various epidemiologic factors have been evaluated to demonstrate an association with preterm delivery. Unfortunately, most of these factors are associated with preterm delivery per se, and not necessarily with preterm labor.

1. **Socioeconomic** factors. It is known that women of lower socioeconomic status have a higher incidence of preterm delivery. This may be accounted for to some extent by low-birth-weight infants as well as preterm infants. In addition, blacks appear to have a higher incidence of both preterm labor and small-for-gestational-age infants.

2. **Maternal characteristics**
   a. Extremes of **maternal age** are also associated with an increase in the incidence of preterm delivery.
   b. Poor **maternal nutrition** may also play a role, although it is debatable whether this actually increases the risk of preterm labor.

3. **Infections**
   a. Serious **systemic** maternal illnesses such as pyelonephritis and pneumonia have long been known to be associated with premature labor.
   b. Asymptomatic **urinary tract infections** have also been associated with preterm delivery, although the relationship is debatable.
   c. **Cervical and vaginal infections** have recently been associated with many studies of preterm labor and delivery. In some studies, chlamydia trachomatis infection has been shown to be associated with preterm labor. Other studies have implicated beta-hemolytic streptococci, genital mycoplasmas, trichomonas vaginitis, and bacterial vaginosis.
   d. **Chorioamnionitis**, either overt or occult, may cause premature labor and may well account for many cases of premature labor of unknown origin. Current estimates are that positive amniotic fluid culture can be obtained in 5 to 10 percent of patients in premature labor with intact membranes.
   e. **Syphilis** is also frequently associated with premature delivery.

4. **Obstetric factors.** Many obstetric factors are known to be associated with an increased risk of premature delivery.
   a. **Maternal obstetric history** is an important indicator of the risk of premature labor. For women with a previous preterm infant, the recurrence risk is severalfold above that of the general population. This risk rises with the increasing number of previous infants born prematurely. Other factors, such as a history of previous abortions and first-trimester bleeding, have also been associated with preterm delivery.
   b. **Uterine abnormalities** are also associated with an increased risk of premature labor. Conditions such as a

subseptate uterus or duplication of the upper tract are linked with a high incidence of preterm labor. Diethylstilbestrol (DES) exposure in utero is also associated with a high incidence of uterine abnormality and with subsequent incompetent cervix and premature labor.

    c.   Any obstetric factor that is associated with **overdistention of the uterus** also predisposes to premature labor. Examples include multiple gestation and hydramnios. On average, each additional fetus in excess of one is associated with a shortening of the gestational age by 3 to 4 weeks.

V. Diagnosis

  A.   The diagnosis of premature labor requires excessive uterine activity associated with progressive dilatation and/or effacement of the cervix. Since each of these factors (uterine activity, cervical dilatation, and cervical effacement) can occur during normal gestation, the definition of when premature labor begins is arbitrary. In general, with intact membranes, premature labor can be diagnosed when the following criteria are met:

    1.   Regular, usually painful uterine contractions and progressive cervical dilatation and effacement or

    2.   Uterine activity associated with cervical finding of ≥ 2 cm dilatation and/or ≥ 80 percent effacement.

  B.   Since digital examinations of the cervix are contraindicated with premature rupture of the membranes, and since premature labor occurs frequently following membrane rupture, the presence of regular uterine activity in a patient with premature rupture of the membranes is adequate for a diagnosis of preterm labor.

  C.   In addition to the above findings, which are necessary for a diagnosis of premature labor, several events have frequently been demonstrated to precede the onset of preterm labor.

    1.   **Maternal symptoms.** Patients frequently complain of a change in cervical discharge and a feeling of low back and pelvic pressure in the days preceding the onset of premature labor.

    2.   **Cervical ripening.** Pelvic exam may reveal softening of the cervic associated with some cervical dilatation and shortening prior to the onset of labor. In addition, development of the lower uterine segment can be noted by feeling the bulging of the lower uterus through the vaginal fornices.

    3.   **Uterine activity.** Uterine activity is present throughout later gestation in all patients, although it is not always perceived by the patient.

        a.   Patients with twin pregnancies who deliver at term have more uterine activity than do those with singleton pregnancies.

        b.   Recent data indicate that patients who are destined to develop preterm labor often have excessive uterine activity throughout pregnancy and that this activity may increase markedly in the hours to days prior to the onset of premature labor.

c. Diurnal variation in uterine activity is frequently demonstrated, with increased activity noted more often during the evening hours.

VI. Differential diagnosis. Patients who present with increased uterine activity must be distinguished as being in premature labor, as opposed to threatened preterm labor or false labor.

A. **False labor** is generally recognized as irregular uterine activity unassociated with cervical changes. The uterine contractions are most consistent with Braxton Hicks contractions.

B. **Threatened premature labor** (preterm contractions) occurs when regular, usually painful uterine contractions occur without progressive changes.

VII. Management. Unfortunately, when most patients present in premature labor, they are not candidates for long-term tocolysis due to advanced cervical dilatation or associated rupture of membranes. Therefore, effective management is dependent upon early diagnosis and effective therapy.

A. **Early diagnosis**

1. All patients should be aware of the **symptoms** that may precede the onset of preterm labor. Patients should be encouraged to present for evaluation if these symptoms occur, especially if other risk factors are present.

2. **Preterm birth prevention programs** have been evaluated by many investigators. These programs consist of the following components:

   a. First, risk assessment is done to identify those patients who are at increased risk for preterm delivery. Using these epidemiologic factors, the majority of patients who are destined to deliver prematurely can be identified. However, the specificity of this method is quite low.

   b. Second, education of the patient and the health care personnel is carried out to increase awareness of premature labor and, hopefully, lead to earlier diagnosis.

   c. Finally, regular examinations of the cervix may detect changes that indicate a high likelihood of premature labor.

   The success of preterm labor prevention programs has been quite varied. In general, preterm delivery has been reduced primarily in middle class populations. In contrast, high-risk indigent populations have demonstrated less benefit from these programs.

3. **Ambulatory uterine contraction monitoring.** Several devices for home contraction monitoring have been developed. These devices have been demonstrated to be quite accurate in assessing uterine activity.

   a. Most protocols call for the patient to monitor uterine

activity for 1 h twice daily. This information is transmitted by telephone to a central office, where it is assessed by nursing personnel. In addition, these services provide daily nursing contact with the patient. Most services also allow the patient to monitor or discuss with the nursing personnel problems that may come up at any time during the day.

b. Some studies have demonstrated that ambulatory uterine contraction monitoring identifies patients earlier in premature labor and decreases the incidence of premature delivery. The improvement in outcome appears to be due both to early identification of increasing uterine contractions and to the daily nursing contact that is provided.

c. Widespread use of ambulatory monitoring is restricted by its cost. The service is expensive and thus should be restricted to patients at high risk of premature labor and delivery.

VIII. Treatment

A. When the patient is admitted to the hospital with the diagnosis of premature labor, a stepwise approach to management is undertaken.

1. Intravenous hydration is begun following admission. Although there is little evidence that hydration alone will arrest true premature labor, there is some suggestion that these patients may have decreased intravascular volume, and they will generally need to be kept NPO while initial therapy is being carried out.

2. Urinalysis is performed for evaluation for any asymptomatic infection that requires treatment.

3. A sterile speculum exam should be performed to obtain cervical culture for chlamydia, hemolytic streptococci, and gonorrhea and to rule out premature rupture of the membranes. While there is no evidence that these organisms are the cause of premature labor, if a culture is positive, therapy may need to be instituted to prevent exposure of the premature infant to the organisms if delivery ensues.

4. Amniocentesis may be indicated in a variety of situations.

a. Obtaining amniotic fluid for **fetal lung maturity** testing may be advisable at advanced gestational ages, such as after 34 weeks of gestation, or with larger fetuses ($\geq$ 2000 g). In these situations the benefits of tocolytic therapy in the face of fetal lung maturity may not outweigh the risks.

b. If **chorioamnionitis** is suspected due to maternal fever or other symptoms, amniocentesis may be necessary. The presence of bacteria on Gram stain or positive culture indicates chorioamnionitis. At present, there is no reason to perform amniocentesis routinely in all cases of idiopathic premature labor to rule out chorioamnionitis.

B. Once the diagnosis of premature labor is confirmed, tocolytic therapy may be initiated if no contraindications exist (Table 21.1).

    1. Narcotic agents are often given prior to initiation of tocolytic therapy, but there appears to be no evidence that they are of benefit in treating true preterm labor.

    2. The efficacy of tocolytic agents has been proven in delaying delivery for > 48 h, but long-term delay in delivery and the ability to prevent delivery prior to 37 weeks are less clearcut. In addition, there is little proof that the overall incidence of respiratory distress and neonatal mortality has been altered by tocolytic therapy.

    3. Although it has generally been recommended, long-term maintenance therapy for prevention of recurrent premature labor has also not been clearly proven.

C. Specific tocolytic agents

    1. Beta sympathomimetics. The beta-adrenergic agents that are commonly used for therapy of preterm labor include ritodrine (Yutopar), which is the only Food and Drug Administration (FDA)-approved drug for therapy of premature labor, and terbutaline (Brethine).

        a. Mechanism of action. Beta-adrenergic agents achieve their effect by stimulating the $beta_2$ receptors on the uterine smooth muscle wall. There are no pure $beta_2$ stimulants, however, with all these agents retaining some $beta_1$ activity.

        b. Dosage and administration. The initial administration should be intravenous.

            (1) Terbutaline or ritodrine is infused as outlined in Tables 21.2 and 21.3.

            (2) The infusion is decreased or discontinued if excessive maternal symptoms occur or if the maternal pulse rate exceeds 140 beats per min. Once uterine

Table 21.1. Contraindications to Tocolytic Therapy

Absolute Contraindications
  Fetal death or an anomaly incompatible with life
  Severe preeclampsia
  Significant abruptio placentae
  Chorioamnionitis

Relative Contraindications
  Mild preeclampsia
  Advanced cervical dilatation ($\geq$ 5 cm)
  Fetal growth retardation
  Suspected abruptio placentae

Table 21.2. Administration of Ritodrine for Preterm Labor

1. Mix 3 ampules of ritodrine (150 mg) in 500 mL of 5% dextrose in water, which provides 300 μg of ritodrine per milliliter of solution.
2. Using a pump, the infusion is started at a rate of 100 μg/min (20 mL/h).
3. The rate is increased every 10 to 15 min by 50 μg/min (10 mL/h) until contractions either stop or occur no more than once every 15 to 20 min.
4. The maximum rate of infusion is 350 μg/min (70 mL/h).

activity has been eliminated, the infusion is continued for another 8 to 12 h.

   (3) Thirty minutes prior to discontinuing the intravenous infusion, an oral tocolytic agent (ritodrine, 20 mg, or terbutaline, 2.5 to 5 mg) is given by mouth.

   (4) During intravenous administration, the total volume of intravenous fluids is kept to a minimum, and maintenance fluids are given as dextrose solution without saline to minimize the possibility of fluid overload and pulmonary edema.

   (5) Maintenance may be continued with an oral tocolytic agent (ritodrine, 10 to 20 mg every 2 to 4 h, or terbutaline, 2.5 to 5 mg every 4 to 6 h).

  c. **Adverse effects.** Adverse effects, both mild and severe, occur frequently with beta–adrenergic therapy.

   (1) The beta$_1$ effects of these agents have a stimulatory effect on the heart. This results in tachycardia and increased cardiac output.

   (2) Arrhythmias and myocardial ischemia have been shown to occur with increased frequency during beta-mimetic therapy, especially at higher heart rates.

   (3) Pulmonary edema is the most serious and most commonly reported serious adverse effect of beta-mimetic therapy, and appears to be related to the duration of therapy and an excessive sodium load. A predisposing factor is multiple gestation, which is

Table 21.3. Administration of Terbutaline for Preterm Labor

1. Mix 5 ampules of terbutaline (5 mg) in 250 mL of 5% dextrose in water, which provides 20 μg of terbutaline per milliliter of solution.
2. Using a pump, the infusion is started at a rate of 5 μg/min (15 mL/h).
3. The rate is increased every 10 to 15 min by 5 μg/min (15 mL/h) until contractions either stop or occur at no more than once every 15 to 20 min.
4. The maximum rate of infusion is 30 μg/min (90 mL/h).

associated with a higher plasma volume. Pulmonary edema appears to be decreased by limiting saline infusions.

(4) Increased glycogenolysis results in elevated glucose levels during therapy. In the average patient, this minimal degree of hyperglycemia appears to have no adverse effect; however, the effect on diabetics may be more profound.

(5) Hypokalemia is frequently seen in association with hyperglycemia. The total body potassium level appears to remain normal, however, and therapy does not appear to be indicated.

  d. **Contraindications.** Beta-adrenergic therapy is contraindicated in patients with cardiac disease or with hyperthyroidism. Due to the effect on glucose metabolism, it is relatively contraindicated in diabetics.

2. Magnesium sulfate

  a. **Mechanism of action.** It is presumed that magnesium sulfate works by competing with calcium for intracellular uptake into smooth muscle cells, a necessary part of smooth muscle contractions.

  b. **Dosage and administration**

(1) Magnesium sulfate infusion is begun as outlined in Table 21.4.

(2) Magnesium sulfate infusion can be increased or decreased, depending on the patient's response. Additionally, magnesium sulfate levels can be checked every 6 to 12 h, with the aim of maintaining levels between 6 and 8 mEq/L.

(3) Urine output and deep tendon reflexes should be assessed frequently. Magnesium sulfate is excreted solely by the kidneys; therefore renal function is a major determinant of the serum level.

(4) Once contractions have been controlled, the infusion should be continued for a minimum of 8 to 12 h and an oral tocolytic agent may be begun prior to discontinuation of the infusion. Unless a contraindication exists, the oral agent of choice is a beta-mimetic.

Table 21.4. Administration of Magnesium Sulfate (MgSO₄) for Preterm Labor

1. Mix 6 g of $MgSO_4$ in 100 to 150 mL of 5% dextrose in water and infuse over 15 to 20 min as a loading dose.
2. Mix 40 g of $MgSO_4$ in 1000 mL of 5% dextrose in water, which provides 1 g of $MgSO_4$ per 25 mL of solution.
3. Using a pump, the maintenance infusion is begun at a rate of 2 g/h (50 mL/h).

c. **Adverse effects.** Magnesium sulfate has been used extensively for therapy of preeclampsia, and serious adverse effects are unusual.

   (1) **Pulmonary edema** has been associated with prolonged therapy associated with large volume loads.

   (2) Many patients complain of significant **flushing** due to transient vasodilatation after the initial infusion of magnesium sulfate.

   (3) **Hypermagnesemia** may be associated with respiratory and cardiac decompensation if toxic levels are achieved. It can be treated acutely with 1 ampule (1 g) of calcium gluconate.

   (4) Magnesium sulfate freely crosses the placenta; therefore the **neonatal level** will reflect the maternal level. Depressed Apgar scores and neonatal flaccidity have been reported with magnesium sulfate therapy but are difficult to correlate with specific levels.

d. **Contraindications.** Contraindications to magnesium sulfate therapy are unusual. Since excretion is exclusively by the kidneys, care should be taken in administering it to patients with renal compromise. Magnesium sulfate should not be used in patients with myasthenia gravis or severe hypocalcemia.

3. **Prostaglandin synthetase inhibitors.** The most commonly used agent is indomethacin. The efficacy of indomethacin appears to be similar to that of beta-mimetics and magnesium sulfate.

   a. **Mechanism of action.** Prostaglandins are necessary for normal uterine contraction. Indomethacin is a potent but reversible prostaglandin synthetase inhibitor.

   b. **Dosage and administration.** The usual initial dose is 50 to 100 mg, usually given either orally or rectally. The maintenance dose is 25 mg by mouth every 6 h. The dose can be increased to 50 mg every 6 h if necessary. The drug is rapidly absorbed and freely crosses the placenta.

   c. **Adverse effects.** Indomethacin is a potent prostaglandin synthetase inhibitor, and since it crosses the placenta freely, it affects fetal as well as maternal prostaglandin synthesis. The major maternal side effect noted is gastrointestinal disturbance. Fetal effects are more frequent and potentially much more significant.

      (1) The fetal ductus requires prostaglandin E to remain patent, and ductal narrowing has been reported with indomethacin administration. Theoretically, ductal narrowing in utero may be associated with development of pulmonary hypertension. Although ductal narrowing has been demonstrated with short-term indomethacin therapy, significant pul-

monary hypertension in the neonate has not. However, pulmonary hypertension is a frequently reported complication of long-term indomethacin therapy. Ductal narrowing also seems to be more common with advancing gestation. Therefore, either indomethacin administration should be limited to a short term (48 h) or the ability to monitor the flow through the fetal ductus should be available.

(2) Fetal urine output also is significantly affected by indomethacin administration. Since fetal urine production is a major determinant of amniotic fluid volume, indomethacin administration is associated with oligohydramnios. Development of oligohydramnios is not consistent or predictable. Therefore patients talking indomethacin must be followed at regular intervals with amniotic fluid volume determination.

   d. **Contraindications.** An absolute contraindication to indomethacin therapy is ulcer disease in the mother. Indomethacin is also relatively contraindicated with oligohydramnios or fetal cardiac abnormalities.

D. Delivery

   1. In general, the route of delivery should not be affected by the gestational age; that is, there appears to be no benefit from abdominal delivery of the preterm infant in vertex presentation.

   2. Fetal reserve and the ability to tolerate stress appear to be decreased in the preterm fetus. This should be kept in mind when evaluating the fetus in preterm labor.

   3. The use of prophylactic outlet forceps to prevent intraventricular hemorrhage in the very small infant is controversial. However, every effort should be made to protect the head, regardless of the route of delivery.

BIBLIOGRAPHY

Besinger RE, Niebyl JR. The safety and efficacy of tocolytic agents for the treatment of preterm labor. Obstet Gynecol Survey 1990; 45:415–440.

Besinger RE, Niebyl JR, Keyes WG, Johnson TRB. Randomized comparative trial of indomethacin and ritodrine for the long-term treatment of preterm labor. Am J Obstet Gynecol 1991; 164:981–988.

Caritis SN, Toig G, Heddinger LA, Ashmead G. A double-blind study comparing ritodrine and terbutaline in the treatment of preterm labor. Am J Obstet Gynecol 1984; 150:7.

Goldenberg RL, Davis RO, Copper RL, et al. The Alabama preterm birth prevention project. Obstet Gynecol 1990; 75:933.

Grimes DA, Schulz KF. Randomized controlled trials of home uterine activity monitoring: A review and critique. Obstet Gynecol 1992; 79:137–142.

King JF, Grant A, Keirse MJNC, Chalmers I. Beta-mimetics in preterm labour: An overview of the randomized controlled trials. Br J Obstet Gynaecol 1988; 95:211–222.

Main DM, Main EK, Strong SE, Gabbe SG. The effect of oral ritodrine therapy on glucose tolerance in pregnancy. Am J Obstet Gynecol 1985; 152:1031–1033.

Moise KJ, Huhta JC, Sharif DS, et al. Indomethacin in the treatment of premature labor: Effects on the fetal ductus arteriosus. N Engl J Med 1988; 319:327–331.

Mou SM, Sunderji SG, Gall S, et al. Multicenter randomized clinical trial of home uterine activity monitoring for detection of preterm labor. Am J Obstet Gynecol 1991; 165:858–866.

Philipsen T, Eriksen PS, Lynggård F. Pulmonary edema following ritodrine-saline infusion in premature labor. Obstet Gynecol 1981; 58:304.

Wilkins IA, Lynch L, Mehalek KE, et al. Efficacy and side effects of magnesium sulfate and ritodrine as tocolytic agents. Am J Obstet Gynecol 1988; 159:685–689.

CHAPTER 22

Premature Rupture of the Membranes

Brian Mercer

Premature rupture of the membranes (PROM) indicates membrane rupture prior to the onset of active labor at any gestational age. Differentiation from preterm labor with membrane rupture may be difficult, as membrane rupture is usually associated with some uterine activity.

This chapter will deal with spontaneous membrane rupture. The clinical significance and management of preterm PROM and PROM after 37 weeks' gestation are different.

ACRONYMS

The following acronyms are related to membrane rupture:
AROM — artificial rupture of the membranes
PROM — premature rupture of the membranes
SPROM — spontaneous premature rupture of the membranes
SROM — spontaneous rupture of the membranes

PRETERM PROM

I. **Incidence.** Preterm PROM complicates only 2 to 6 percent of pregnancies, but it is responsible for one-third of perinatal loss.

II. **Morbidity and mortality**
   A. The primary risk of preterm PROM is **prematurity.** The latent period (time from membrane rupture to labor onset) increases with decreasing gestation at PROM. In the late second trimester, latencies of 1 week are commonly seen with conservative management (30 to 50 percent). In the mid-third trimester, 70 to 80 percent of women will deliver within 1 week of PROM.
      1. Preterm delivery carries the risks of respiratory distress syndrome (RDS), intraventricular hemorrhage (IVH), neonatal infection including pneumonia, necrotizing enterocolitis, and sepsis, as well as the costs of prolonged neonatal intensive care and increased perinatal mortality.
      2. The incidence of abnormal fetal presentation requiring cesarean delivery also increases with decreasing gestational age.

B. Maternal infection is the second most common complication of preterm PROM.

1. **Amnionitis** (diagnosed antenatally by maternal temperature > 100.4°F) with the presence of two or more of the following: uterine tenderness, contractions, foul-smelling amniotic fluid, increasing white blood cell (WBC) count, or positive amniotic fluid cultures occurs in up to 30 percent of patients.

2. An increasing incidence of amnionitis is seen with decreasing gestational age at PROM, severity of oligohydramnios, and positive cervical cultures for *Neisseria* gonorrhea and group B streptococcus (GBS).

3. Amnionitis carries increased risks of neonatal respiratory and infectious morbidity. Some authors suggest an increase in neonatal intraventricular hemorrhage (IVH) with amnionitis. This may be related to the earlier gestational age at delivery and/or to the increased incidence of pulmonary complications in these infants.

C. Premature placental separation (abruptio placentae) is an obstetric complication commonly associated with PROM, occurring in 7 to 10 percent of cases. Whether this results from the rapid decrease in uterine size with shearing of the placental bed or is the underlying cause of PROM in these cases is not clear.

D. Fetal distress may result from umbilical cord compression in the presence of oligohydramnios. Variable-type fetal heart rate decelerations are frequently seen in this situation. Intrauterine fetal death complicates 1 to 2 percent of cases. This may be related to severe cord compression, intrauterine infection, or placental abruption.

E. Pulmonary hypoplasia is a serious complication of PROM prior to 26 weeks' gestation. Between 17 and 26 weeks, the glandular lungs are very sensitive to the presence of oligohydramnios. Lack of fluid results in a failure of development of alveoli. At birth these infants cannot be adequately ventilated and soon succumb to hypoxia or other barotrauma from high-pressure ventilation (pneumothorax, pneunomediastinum).

F. Fetal skeletal deformities may occur subsequent to prolonged oligohydramnios with intrauterine crowding.

G. An increased incidence of congenital fetal anomalies is seen in patients with PROM. While the association is frequently unclear, polyhydramnios, which may be associated with decreased fetal swallowing due to central nervous system or gastrointestinal abnormalities, may predispose to PROM.

III. Cause. PROM is multifactorial, with membrane weakness and increased intrauterine pressure being common denominators.

A. **Membrane weakness** may result from various causes, including structural abnormalities (such as type III collagen, copper, and vitamin C deficiencies) or microbial and antimicrobial enzyme activity (granulocyte elastase, peroxide antimicrobial factors).

  B. **Increased distention pressure** on the membranes over the internal cervical os is seen with cervical dilatation (cervical incompetence) or with increased intrauterine pressure (e.g., multifetal pregnancy and polyhydramnios, and abruptio or trauma with increased myometrial tone).

IV. Differential diagnosis
  A. Urinary incontinence
  B. Increased vaginal secretions in pregnancy (physiologic)
  C. Increased cervical discharge (pathologic infection)
  D. Exogenous fluids (semen, douches)
  E. Vesicovaginal fistula

V. Diagnosis
  A. An adequate clinical **history** will usually provide a high level of suspicion. A sudden gush of fluid followed by continued leakage is characteristic of uncontrollable membrane rupture. However, some patients will notice only intermittent slight leakage.
  1. A history of urinary tract infection, urgency prior to fluid loss, or an isolated episode related to increased intraabdominal pressure (coughing, straining) is more suggestive of urinary incontinence.
  2. If the history is not characteristic, the patient should be questioned with regard to recent cervical infections, sexual activity, douching practices, and a history of previous pelvic surgery (particularly fourth-degree lacerations with previous delivery) or inflammatory bowel disease.
  B. **Physical examination** should begin with inspection of the perineum for the presence of fluid with a characteristic odor. Then, using **sterile technique,** a speculum should be inserted into the vagina.
  1. Visualization of fluid passing from the cervical os is diagnostic of membrane rupture. If this is not seen, it can be stimulated with gentle uterine fundal pressure or by asking the patient to cough or bear down.
  2. Frequently, a pool of fluid will be identified in the posterior fornix, or the vaginal sidewalls will appear to be moist. Useful ancillary tests in this situation are the nitrazine and ferning tests.
  C. **Diagnostic procedures**
  1. **Nitrazine test.** Sterile pH paper is applied to the vaginal sidewall or pool of fluid. Amniotic fluid characteristically has a neutral pH and will turn the paper blue. Urine is usually acidic, and the paper will remain yellow. This test is 95 percent sensitive in the detection of membrane rupture (Table 22.1).
  2. **Ferning test.** A sterile swab is placed in the vaginal pool or wiped along the vaginal sidewalls and then streaked on a microscope slide. After drying, sodium chloride crystals will form on protein in amniotic fluid. The resultant arborized pattern in confirmatory of membrane rupture (Table 22.2).

Table 22.1. Nitrazine Test

FALSE POSITIVE	FALSE NEGATIVE
Basic urine	Remote PROM with little residual fluid
Semen	Minimal leakage
Cervical mucus	
Blood contamination	
Some antiseptic solutions	
Vaginitis (trichomonas)	

3. Other methods, including Nile blue staining for fetal cells (with orange fat globules), amniocentesis with injection of indigo carmine or saline (with inspection for passage of vaginal fluid), and vaginal fluid alpha fetoprotein, have been suggested. Ultrasonic demonstration of oligohydramnios may confirm the clinical suspicion; however, close examination to rule out urinary tract obstruction should be performed.

VI. Management
A. The patient with preterm PROM who presents with overt amnionitis, fetal distress, or advanced labor does not pose a significant management problem, with delivery being achieved using the standard obstetric protocol. The management decision for the patient without these complications is controversial. The approach will depend on the clinical experience and patient population where the physician practices, as well as the gestational age of the patient and specific physical findings.
1. Populations of low socioeconomic status are at increased risk not only for PROM, but also for amnionitis. Other factors increasing the risk of intrauterine and neonatal infection, such as positive amniotic fluid Gram stain, positive cervical cultures, or poor fetal biophysical activity, lead to more aggressive management and delivery of the fetus near term with a lower risk of neonatal morbidity and mortality (e.g.,

Table 22.2. Ferning Test

FALSE POSITIVE	FALSE NEGATIVE
Cervical mucus	Blood contamination
	Urine contamination
	Antiseptic solutions

34 to 36 weeks). Pulmonary function tests demonstrating fetal lung maturity further encourage this approach.

2. Alternatively, at gestation remote from term, in a middle- or upper-class population with reassuring fetal test results, conservative (expectant) management may be of significant benefit.

3. PROM prior to fetal viability (16 to 26 weeks) is a particularly difficult situation. Patients who choose conservative management are faced with the potential for prolonged hospitalization, with a high risk of delivery before viability and a high risk of perinatal morbidity and mortality. These patients require extensive counseling and support.

B. **General guidelines for active management (delivery)**
 1. Suspected amnionitis
 2. Cervical dilatation ≥ 4 cm
 3. Persistent abnormal fetal heart rate test results
 4. Estimated fetal weight > 2500 g with demonstrable fetal lung maturity
 5. Vaginal bleeding suggestive of placental abruption
 6. Estimated fetal weight 2000 to 2500 g, with mature lung test results and a positive Gram stain
 7. Positive amniotic fluid cultures for GBS, Neisseria gonorrhea, Listeria monocytogenes at any gestation
 8. Transverse fetal lie or footling breech presentation, with demonstrable fetal lung maturity after 32 weeks' gestation

C. **General guidelines for conservative (expectant) management**
 1. Estimated fetal weight < 2500 g
 2. Gestational age < 35 weeks
 3. Cephalic/frank breech lie
 4. Gestation < 30 weeks, with positive cervical cultures for GBS, Neisseria gonorrhea
    a. Initial evaluation for conservative management. The patient should be examined for signs of infection (fever, tachycardia, uterine tenderness, palpable contractions; digital pelvic examination and repeated speculum examination should be avoided where possible).
       (1) Vaginal culture for GBS should be performed. GBS is associated with amnionitis and neonatal pneumonia that is frequently severe or fatal. Rapid diagnostic tests for GBS have been promoted in this circumstance; however, they are insensitive and should be accompanied by a routine culture, if possible.
       (2) Cervical cultures should be obtained for Neisseria gonorrhea and chlamydia trachomatis. Gonorrhea is associated with amnionitis and neonatal infection. The role of chlamydia in amnionitis is controversial; however, this organism is seen more frequently in the setting of PROM and is associated with neonatal conjunctivitis, late-onset endometritis, and neonatal pneumonia.

(3) Vaginal fluid should be collected for the assessment of pulmonary maturity, if possible.
  b. Once the diagnosis of PROM is confirmed, fetal heart rate and uterine activity monitoring should be initiated. Fetal tachycardia may be the earliest sign of amnionitis. Fetal heart rate deceleration, usually variable, may be seen in the presence of oligohydramnios and uterine contractions.
  c. The WBC count is normally elevated in pregnancy; therefore, an isolated value of 18 000/mm^3 or less is not helpful in the diagnosis of infection. The presence of segmented neutrophils *(left shift)* may be suggestive of infection. C-reactive protein is a nonspecific reactant to inflammation and infection. Levels above 2 mg/dL may be predictive of subsequent infection. Preliminary study has not demonstrated maternal serum alpha fetoprotein (MSAFP) to be a sensitive predictor of subsequent amnionitis, though levels appear to rise in the presence of clinical infection.
  d. Amniocentesis for Gram stain, as well as aerobic and anaerobic cultures, is a good predictor of subsequent clinical amnionitis. The demonstration of bacteria on Gram stain is a rapid test with a positive predictive value for infection of 75 to 80 percent. The presence of WBCs on Gram stain does not predict infection in the setting of PROM. While amniotic fluid culture results may take 48 h to return, an early test may demonstrate specific organisms or sensitivities should amnionitis or neonatal infection occur. This allows early specific therapy for the infection.
  e. Urine culture should be performed via a catheterized specimen in order to rule out this treatable cause of increased uterine activity. Because of the abundant bacterial flora and large numbers of WBCs in pregnancy, a clean-catch specimen is not suitable for urine culture.
  f. Once the initial evaluation has been completed, most physicians admit the patient to a hospital for prolonged bed rest. This allows aggressive monitoring for signs of infection or labor and early intervention or monitoring as required. Some physicians keep the patient in the hospital until delivery if facilities permit. Others allow the patient to be discharged following prolonged bed rest if leakage stops and fluid reaccumulation occurs.
  g. **Serial maternal evaluation** to assess for signs of early infection is essential. The patient should be assessed frequently for tachycardia or fever. She should be examined for uterine tenderness and monitored for uterine activity. Serial laboratory testing, including a WBC count, differential count, and C-reactive protein testing

may be helpful in the early diagnosis of amnionitis. However, they are insensitive and nonspecific predictors of subsequent infection. As such, their role is primarily adjunctive to clinical assessment.

   h. **Serial fetal evaluation** should include fetal heart rate monitoring (non-stress test) daily. Oligohydramnios is associated with an increased risk of subsequent infection, as well as with abnormal fetal heart rate tracings. Fetal heart rate evaluation, either daily or twice daily, is suggested in this setting. Decreased fetal biophysical activity is related to increased perinatal infectious morbidity. As such, aggressive serial testing may help to identify patients early in the disease process so that treatment can be initiated.

D. Delivery location. Preterm rupture of the membranes carries a significant risk of maternal-fetal and neonatal morbidity and mortality. The major risks are related to prematurity, maternal and neonatal infection, and fetal distress. As such, the patient with preterm PROM should be cared for by an experienced team of medical and support personnel, with facilities available for fetal evaluation, immediate delivery (including cesarean section), and aggressive neonatal respiratory and infectious disease support. Centers that do not have adequate facilities should arrange for maternal transfer prior to the onset of labor and, if possible, immediately after initial assessment and stabilization.

E. Tocolysis of preterm labor. Again controversial, this subject has been discussed widely (without a consensus). Some authors believe that labor in the setting of PROM is a sign of intrauterine infection. They fear that tocolysis will delay delivery and increase the risk of maternal and neonatal sepsis. Further, tocolysis has not consistently been demonstrated to delay delivery significantly in the setting of intact or ruptured membranes. Finally, use of beta-mimetic tocolytics in the setting of infection may predispose the patient to tocolysis-induced pulmonary edema. Our practice is to use tocolysis in the absence of clinical or laboratory evidence of infection if pulmonary function studies demonstrate fetal immaturity.

F. Steroids for the induction of pulmonary maturity. Some authors suggest the administration of steroids (e.g., betamethasone) for the patient with preterm PROM. There is controversy in the literature. Meta-analysis of these studies suggests similar efficacy of steroids with either intact or ruptured membranes. A decrease in the incidence of IVH has also been suggested. Several researchers have demonstrated an increased risk of maternal and neonatal infection with the use of steroids. This has not been confirmed in a review of similar studies. As such, it is our practice to administer steroids when studies demonstrate fetal lung immaturity.

G. Antibiotics

   1. Prophylactic. Prophylactic antibiotics are used from the time of admission to delivery for the prevention of amnionitis and neonatal infection. Early results are promising, but this form of treatment is still investigational.

2. **GBS.** The treatment of conservatively managed patients with vaginal GBS is again controversial. Some authors suggest ampicillin therapy from admission to delivery; others suggest intrapartum parenteral ampicillin to prevent vertical transmission during passage through the birth canal.

3. **Chorioamnionitis.** Antibiotics have traditionally been withheld in the setting of chorioamnionitis until after clamping of the umbilical cord at delivery. There has been concern that subtherapeutic fetal antibiotic levels might confuse the neonatal picture and suppress bacterial growth on culture. Some neonatologists treat prophylactically all infants being delivered of mothers with prolonged preterm PROM. Aggressive intrapartum antibiotics in this situation may reduce the risk of maternal sepsis and lead to earlier attainment of therapeutic levels. The decision on when to administer antibiotics should be made jointly with the attending pediatrician.

VII. Term PROM

A. **Incidence.** While membrane rupture usually occurs subsequent to the onset of labor, up to 10 percent of women present with PROM at term.

B. **Morbidity and mortality**
   1. **Maternal.** In this circumstance, maternal and neonatal infectious outcomes are of prime importance. As with preterm PROM, membrane rupture allows a route for ascent of bacterial pathogens. Again, the loss of intrinsic defense mechanisms, including the physical membrane barrier, endocervical mucus plug (mechanical barrier, lysozyme, immunoglobulins), and amniotic fluid factors (lysozyme, betalysin, IgG, IgA), predispose these patients to infection. In addition, patients presenting with membrane rupture remote from delivery may undergo repeated pelvic examinations prior to delivery, again placing them at increased risk for intrauterine infection.
   2. **Fetal.** In the setting of oligohydramnios, the fetus is at increased risk of abnormal umbilical cord compression, which may lead to fetal distress and death. Alternatively, there is no significant fetal/neonatal benefit to prolonged delay in delivery subsequent to PROM at term.

C. The **cause** is presumed to be similar to that of preterm PROM.

D. The **differential diagnosis** is presumed to be similar to that of preterm PROM.

E. **Management.** Given the risks of infection and fetal distress, early delivery is generally preferable. Most women (80 percent) will progress to spontaneous labor within 24 h of membrane rupture at term. Unfortunately, with a mean labor duration of 12 to 14 h, a significant number of expectantly managed women will not deliver within 24 h of membrane rupture. Alternatively, induction of labor may be prolonged or unsuccessful if the cervix is not ripe. A significant risk of premature rupture of the membranes at any gestational age is cesarean section for failed induction of labor.

The need for active intervention with labor induction will vary from center to center. Physicians serving a population with primarily a low risk of infection will be more conservative, observing for spontaneous labor. In a high-risk population, active intervention with early delivery is generally preferred. In either population, expectant management (including a baseline WBC count, cervical cultures for GBS and *Neisseria* gonorrhea, and fetal heart rate monitoring for signs of fetal compromise) may be indicated in the presence of an unfavorable cervix. **Under all circumstances, digital pelvic examinations should be avoided prior to the onset of active labor.**

BIBLIOGRAPHY

Amon E, Lewis SV, Sibai BM, et al. Ampicillin prophylaxis in preterm rupture of the membranes. A prospective randomized study. Am J Obstet Gynecol 1988; 159:539–543.

Baker CJ. Summary of the workshop on perinatal infections due to group B streptococcus. J Infect Dis 1977; 136:137.

Beydoun SN, Yasin SY. Premature rupture of the membranes before 28 weeks: Conservative management. Am J Obstet Gynecol 1986; 155:471–479.

Christensen KK, Ingemarsson I, Leideman T, et al. Effect of ritodrine on labor after premature rupture of the membranes. Obstet Gynecol 1980; 55:187–190.

Collaborative Group on Antenatal Steroid Therapy. Effect of antenatal dexamethasone administration on the prevention of respiratory distress syndrome. Am J Obstet Gynecol 1981; 141:276–287.

D'Alton M, Mercer B, Riddick E, et al. Serial thoracic versus abdominal circumference ratios for the prediction of pulmonary hypoplasia in premature rupture of the membranes remote from term. Am J Obstet Gynecol 1992; 166:658–663.

Garite TJ, Freeman RK. Chorioamnionitis in the preterm gestation. Obstet Gynecol 1982; 59:539–545.

Garite TJ, Freeman RK, Linzey EM, et al. Prospective randomized study of corticosteroids in the management of premature rupture of the membranes and the preterm gestation. Am J Obstet Gynecol 1981; 141:508–515.

Garite TJ, Keegan KA, Freeman RK, et al. A randomized trial of ritodrine tocolysis versus expectant management in patients with premature rupture of membranes at 25 to 30 weeks of gestation. Am J Obstet Gynecol 1987; 157:388–393.

Gibbs RS, Blanco JD. Premature rupture of the membranes. Obstet Gynecol 1982; 60:671–679.

Gonik B, Cotton DB. The use of amniocentesis in preterm premature rupture of membranes. Am J Perinatol 1985; 2:21–24.

Gravett MG, Nelson HP, DeRouen T, et al. Independent associations of bacterial vaginosis and *Chlamydia* trachomatis infection with adverse pregnancy outcome. JAMA 1986; 256:1751–1752.

Guzick DS, Winn K. The association of chorioamnionitis with preterm delivery. Obstet Gynecol 1985; 65:11–16.

Johnston M, Sanchez-Ramos L, Benrubi GI. Premature rupture of membranes prior to 34 weeks gestational age. One year experience at a tertiary center. J Fla Med Assoc 1989; 76:767–771.

Levy DL, Warsof SL. Oral ritodrine and preterm premature rupture of membranes. Obstet Gynecol 1985; 66:621–623.

Mead PB. Management of the patient with premature rupture of the membranes. Clin Perinatol 1980; 7:243–255.

Mercer B, Moretti M, Rogers R, et al. Erythromycin therapy in preterm premature rupture of the membranes: A prospective, randomized trial of 220 patients. Am J Obstet Gynecol 1992; 166:794–802.

Minkoff H, Grunebaum AN, Schwarz RH, et al. Risk factors for prematurity and premature rupture of membranes: A prospective study of the vaginal flora in pregnancy. Am J Obstet Gynecol 1984; 150:965–972.

Moberg LJ, Garite TJ, Freeman RK. Fetal heart rate patterns and fetal distress in patients with preterm premature rupture of membranes. Obstet Gynecol 1984; 64(1):60–64.

Morales WJ, Angel JL, O'Brien WF, et al. Use of ampicillin and corticosteroids in premature rupture of membranes: A randomized study. Obstet Gynecol 1989; 73(5 pt 1):721–726.

Morales WJ, Diebel ND, Lazar AJ, et al. The effect of antenatal dexamethasone administration on the prevention of respiratory distress syndrome in preterm gestations with premature rupture of membranes. Am J Obstet Gynecol 1986; 154:591–595.

Morales WJ, Washington SR III, Lazar AJ. The effect of chorioamnionitis on perinatal outcome in preterm gestation. J Perinatol 1987; 7:105–110.

Naeye RL, Dellinger WS, Blanc WA. Fetal and maternal features of antenatal bacterial infections. J Pediatr 1971; 79:733.

Ohlsson A. Treatments of preterm premature rupture of the membranes: A meta-analysis. Am J Obstet Gynecol 1989; 160:890–906.

Pankuch GA, Appelbaum PC, Lorenz RP, et al. Placental microbiology and histology and the pathogenesis of chorioamnionitis. Obstet Gynecol 1984; 64:802–806.

Savitz DA, Blackmore CA, Thorp JM. Epidemiologic characteristics of preterm delivery: Etiologic heterogeneity. Am J Obstet Gynecol 1991; 164:467–471.

Simpson JL, Elias S, Morgan C, et al. Does unexplained second trimester (15–20 weeks' gestation) maternal serum alpha fetoprotein elevation presage adverse perinatal outcome? Am J Obstet Gynecol 1991; 164:829–836.

Skoll A, Mercer B, Baselski V, et al. Evaluation of rapid diagnostic tests in the detection of group B streptococcus colonization of women in labor. Obstet Gynecol 1991; 77:322–326.

Taylor J, Garite TJ. Premature rupture of membranes before fetal viability. Obstet Gynecol 1984; 64:615–620.

Vintzileos AM, Campbell WA, Nochimson DJ, et al. Degree of oligohydramnios and pregnancy outcome in patients with premature rupture of the membranes. Obstet Gynecol 1985; 66:162–167.

Vintzileos AM, Campbell WA, Nochimson DJ, et al. The fetal biophysical profile in patients with premature rupture of the membranes—an early predictor of fetal infection. An J Obstet Gynecol 1985; 152:510–516.

Vintzileos AM, Campbell WA, Nochimson DJ, et al. Preterm premature rupture of the membranes: A risk factor for the development of abruptio placentae. Am J Obstet Gynecol 1987; 156:1235–1238.

Weiner CP, Renk K, Klugman M. The therapeutic efficacy and cost-effectiveness of aggressive tocolysis for premature labor associated with premature rupture of the membranes. Am J Obstet Gynecol 1988; 159:216–222.

Zeevi D, Sadovsky E, Younis J, et al. Antepartum fetal heart rate characteristics in cases of premature rupture of membranes. Am J Perinatol 1988; 5:260–263.

CHAPTER 23

Multifetal Pregnancy

John Dacus

Multifetal pregnancy has fascinated medical and lay communities for centuries. Occurring in about 1 percent of all pregnancies, multiple pregnancy results in an inordinately high proportion of perinatal morbidity and mortality. Most of the common obstetric complications are increased in multifetal gestations. Therefore, early diagnosis, with careful antepartum, intrapartum, and postpartum management, is necessary to ensure an optimal outcome for the mother and her fetuses.

I. **Incidence.** Twin gestation occurs at a frequency of approximately 1/100 births, with triplets and quadruplets occurring much less frequently. Hellin's law proposes the following incidences: twins, 1/89 births; triplets, 1/7921 births (89^2); quadruplets, 1/704 969 births (89^3); and quintuplets, 1/62 742 241 births (89^4).

   A. **Monozygotic twins** (i.e., arising from a single fertilized ovum) appear to be relatively constant in incidence throughout the world, occurring in 1/250 births. This rate is not influenced by maternal age, parity, heredity, or ovulation induction agents.

   B. **Dizygotic twins** (i.e., arising from two separate fertilized ova) account for approximately two-thirds of all twin gestations (Fig. 23.1).

II. **Predisposing factors.** Advancing maternal age up to 40 and parity up to 7 increase the likelihood of twinning. Race greatly influences the rate of multiple gestations. According to the Collaborative Cerebral Palsy Study, twin births among whites occurs in 1/100 pregnancies. In Nigeria, twinning occurs in 1/22 births.

In orientals the rate is much lower, occurring in 1/155 births. Additional factors increasing the frequency of dizygotic twins are heredity and ovulation induction agents. Women who themselves are twins are more likely to carry multiple gestations. Men who are dizygotic twins do not appear to have an increased frequency of multiple gestations in their offspring. The use of clomiphene citrate and gonadotropins markedly increases the rate of multifetal gestation to as high as 20 to 40 percent.

III. **Morbidity and mortality.** The perinatal mortality (PNM) for twin gestation is reported to be three to four times greater than that for

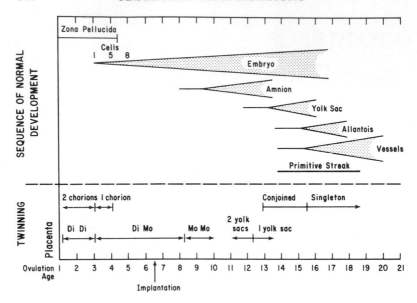

FIGURE 23.1. Diagram correlating the timing of embryolic events in the first part of zygote development (top) with types of placenta developing (bottom) when monozygotic twinning occurs. (From Benirschke K, Kim CK. Multiple pregnancy. N Engl J Med 1973; 288:1278. Reprinted by permission.)

singleton gestation. This is due to myriad factors, the most significant of which is an increase in premature delivery. The frequency of certain pathologic conditions of the fetus and placenta are increased with multiple gestations. These include velamentous cord insertion, placenta previa and vasa previa, fetus papyraceus, acardiac twin, and partial mole.

A. **Premature delivery.** The average length of gestation for twins is 37 weeks (260 days) and, for triplets, 35 weeks (247 days). The cause of premature labor in multiple gestation is not entirely known, but it may be related to an increase in protaglandin production resulting from an overstretched uterus.

B. **Spontaneous abortion.** Spontaneous abortion appears to occur more frequently in multiple gestation than in singleton gestation. Two or more gestational sacs may be visualized by ultrasonography at 5 to 7 weeks of gestation, with subsequent ultrasound examination demonstrating loss of one or more sacs. Thus, the true incidence of conceived multifetal pregnancies probably is far greater than that reported clinically.

C. **Intrauterine growth retardation.** Intrauterine growth retardation occurs more frequently in multiple gestation. This may affect one or more of the fetuses and is seen more often in the third trimester. This may be due to competition among the multiple fetuses for the supply of nutrients or premature placental dysfunction. Ultrasound studies have shown that fetal growth in twin gestation begins to lag behind that of singleton gestation beginning at 28 to 30 weeks. In pregnancies with more than two fetuses, this phenomenon may occur at an earlier gestational period (24 to 26 weeks). Biparietal diameter tables developed specifically for twin gestations show a slowing of the increase in biparietal diameter in twins compared to singletons (Table 23.1).

D. Preeclampsia. Pregnancies associated with an overabundance of

Table 23.1. Observed BPDs* of Twin and Singleton Fetuses between 16 and 40 Weeks' Gestation

WEEKS' GESTA-TION	TWIN FETUSES			SINGLETON FETUS (Mean mm)
	N	MEAN (mm)	2 SD (mm)	
16	6	37.2	5	37.5
17	6	34.0	5	41.9
18	4	42.5	4	42.8
19	12	43.6	7	47.7
20	21	48.2	6	51.8
21	18	48.2	9	54.9
22	17	55.9	8	57.2
23	11	56.9	5	58.5
24	9	59.3	5	65.1
25	10	64.8	7	66.6
26	30	65.6	6	70.1
27	26	68.0	7	71.3
28	25	71.2	6	74.5
29	37	74.2	8	76.8
30	38	75.8	7	80.1
31	27	79.0	7	81.6
32	44	80.0	6	84.4
33	43	81.7	8	85.5
34	38	85.2	7	87.0
35	63	85.4	8	89.9
36	37	87.6	8	90.8
37	38	89.2	6	93.4
38	15	90.4	7	92.6
39	6	89.7	3	94.0
40	8	89.8	8	96.3

*Measurements on bistable scope using outer-to-outer edge.

Source: Leveno KJ, Santos-Ramos R, Duenhoelter JH, et al. Sonar cephalometry in twins: A table of biparietal diameters for normal twin fetuses and a comparison with singletons. Am J Obstet Gynecol 1979; 135:727.

trophoblastic tissue show an increase in the preeclampsia/eclampsia syndrome. In multiple gestation, preeclampsia has a twofold increased incidence over single gestation (30 percent in primigravidas with multiple gestation).

E. **Placenta and cord problems.** Placenta previa and abruptio placenta are seen more frequently in multiple gestation.

F. **Congenital anomalies.** Especially in monozygotic twin gestation, an increased incidence of anomalies has been reported.

G. **Polyhydramnios.** Multifetal gestation increases the development of polyhydramnios.

H. **Twin-to-twin transfusion.** Arteriovenous shunting results in twin-to-twin transfusion, in which the donor shows growth retardation, anemia, and hypotension and the recipient becomes hydropic, polycythemic, and hypertensive. The amniotic sac of the recipient often demonstrates polyhydramnios, and the amniotic sac of the donor may show severe oligohydramnios with amnion nodosum. If ultrasonography reveals more than an 8-mm difference in the biparietal diameters of the twins, discordance is likely. In addition, a difference of more than 20 percent in ultrasonographically determined fetal weights is highly suggestive of this phenomenon. Twin-to-twin transfusion occurs almost exclusively in monozygotic twins with monochorionic placentation. Tocolysis and/or serial amniocentesis may be beneficial with delivery after fetal pulmonary maturity is assessed. A possible therapeutic entity may utilize fetoscopy with laser obliteration or clipping of the arteriovenous shunt in certain circumstances.

I. **Intrauterine death of one twin.** If one twin dies in utero, disseminated intravascular coagulation (DIC) may develop. If the pregnancy is premature, weekly clotting studies (plasma fibrinogen, prothrombin time, partial thromboplastin time, platelets, and fibrin split products) should be obtained. Heparin may be employed in the treatment of DIC if there is no evidence of abruptio placentae. DIC has also been reported in the surviving twin.

J. **Zygosity.** Monozygotic twins have a higher perinatal mortality than dizygotic twins. This increase is related to an increased incidence of congenital anomalies, twin-to-twin transfusions, conjoining, and cord accidents. The highest perinatal mortality is seen in monoamniotic, monochorionic twins.

K. **Birth trauma.** Due to the increase in abnormal presentations, vaginal delivery increases the likelihood of birth trauma, especially for the twin delivered second.

L. **Undiagnosed twins.** Before the widespread use of ultrasonography, approximately 50 percent of twins were undiagnosed until delivery. Presently, less than 10 percent of all twin gestations fall in this category. Undiagnosed twins may markedly increase the morbidity and mortality of the second twin, especially if there is an attempt to deliver the placenta before recognition of the second twin.

IV. Cause

A. **Monozygotic twins** account for approximately one-third of all twin gestations. The number of fetal membranes varies, depending upon the time of pregnancy at which twinning occurs.

1. If division occurs within the first 72 h following fertilization, two amnions and two chorions will develop.
2. Division between 3 and 8 days results in two amnions and one chorion.
3. If division occurs between 8 and 14 days, a monoamniotic, monochorionic twin pregnancy is formed.
4. After 14 days, a division produces conjoined twins (1 in 50 000 pregnancies), the most common location of fusion being at the thorax (thoracopagus).

B. **Dizygotic twins.** This occurrence is presumed to be secondary to two ovulatory events. It may happen spontaneously and is increased in certain ethnic groups. Nigerian women, with higher levels of gonadotropins, are at increased risk of twinning. Polyovulation may occur with ovulation induction agents. Superfetation occurs in lower animals and possibly also in humans. This is the development of a twin gestation resulting from two fertilizations by two separate acts of intercourse within one ovulatory cycle. Superfetation may occur in which a twin gestation results from two acts of intercourse further apart than one ovulatory cycle (not documented in humans).

V. Differential diagnosis

A. **Common problems**

1. Uterine size greater than the gestational age calculated from the last menstrual period often is the result of **wrong dates.**
2. Leiomyomata uteri will increase the uterine size, possibly causing the clinician to suspect multiple gestation.

B. **Less common problems**

1. The occurrence of a **hydatidiform mole** will increase the uterine size in relation to the menstrual dates 50 to 60 percent of the time.
2. The accumulation of **excessive amounts of amniotic fluid (polyhydramnios)** may cause a suspicion of multifetal pregnancy.

VI. Diagnosis

A. **Signs and symptoms.** Statistically, there is an increase in **nausea and vomiting** during multiple gestation compared to singleton gestation, presumably due to an increased amount of human chorionic gonadotropin (hCG). Many women with multifetal pregnancies report greater **fetal activity** compared to previous singleton pregnancies.

B. **Physical examination**

1. Uterine size may be larger than menstrual dates would suggest.

    2. Multiple fetal parts may be palpable.

    3. Occasionally more than one set of fetal heart tones will be auscultated.

C. Laboratory examination

    1. **Hematocrit levels** may be lower in multiple gestation due to an increase in the dilutional effect of pregnancy and the fetal demands.

    2. **Plasma volume** increases exceed those of singleton pregnancy, approaching a 100 percent increase in pregnancies with triplets over nonpregnant values.

    3. **Maternal serum alpha fetoprotein** is more commonly elevated in multifetal pregnancy.

    4. **Serum hCG and human placental lactogen (HPL) levels** may also be elevated.

D. Diagnostic procedures

    1. **Abdominal radiography** will visualize more than one fetal skeleton after 16 weeks of gestation.

    2. **Ultrasonography** is capable of identifying two gestational sacs by 5 to 6 weeks after the last menstrual period. This technique has virtually replaced the use of radiography.

    3. A single anterior-posterior radiograph of the abdomen during the third trimester is recommended by some to verify the correct number of fetuses, since there have been cases of triplets misdiagnosed by ultrasonography.

VII. Management

A. Antepartum

    1. The **caloric intake** of the average woman carrying twins should result in a total weight gain of 30 to 35 pounds, or 15 to 17 kg. It may be desirable to increase this gain slightly in the cases of triplets or quadruplets.

    2. **Iron and folate supplements** are extremely important to ensure that maternal and fetal needs are met (see Chapter 3).

    3. **Liberal use of bed rest,** especially in the left lateral recumbent position, maximizes uterine blood flow and may reduce the incidence of premature births and intrauterine growth-retarded infants. Routine hospitalization at 26 to 28 weeks is advocated by some in an attempt to decrease prematurity and growth retardation.

    4. In addition, the prompt administration of a tocolytic drug is indicated in the event of cervical effacement and/or dilatation (see Section V.B.1.a.).

    5. **Serial ultrasonography** is recommended in the management of all multiple gestations. Ultrasonography should be performed every 3 to 4 weeks to accomplish the following:

        a. Accurate determination of gestational age

        b. Evaluation of fetal growth

        c. Diagnosis of congenital anomalies

        d. Detection of conjoined twins

        e. Assessment of amniotic fluid volume

    f. Comparison of fetal weights

    g. Early detection of twin-to-twin transfusion

  6. Antepartum fetal surveillance testing, routinely beginning at 32 to 34 weeks of gestation, is advocated by many. If there are complications (e.g., preeclampsia, discordance of growth), antepartum fetal monitoring is mandatory. **Nonstress testing with either a contraction stress test or a biophysical profile** as a backup in cases of a nonreactive nonstress test is the preferred technique (see Chapter 16).

B. Premature labor

  1. Tocolytic drug therapy. If premature labor ensues and there are no contraindications to tocolysis, several options are available (see Chapter 21).

    a. **Ritodrine hydrochloride** (Yutopar), a betamimetic drug, is currently the only Food and Drug Administration (FDA)-approved tocolytic agent in the United States. Its use in multiple gestation may cause maternal pulmonary edema due to the already overexpanded plasma volume. Restriction of intravenous (IV) fluids, accurate fluid intake and output records, and limiting exposure of the patient to IV ritodrine to 24 h will minimize this risk.

    b. IV magnesium sulfate, 4 to 6 g as an initial dose followed by a maintenance dose of 2 to 3 g/h, is a reasonable alternative to ritodrine and other tocolytic agents, but it also has been reported to cause maternal pulmonary edema. Thus, the same precautions as those described for ritodrine (see Section VII.B.1) should be followed.

    c. Prostaglandin synthetase inhibitors (e.g., Indocin, Motrin) are currently being investigated as potential tocolytic agents. Due to their possible harmful fetal effects, at present these drugs should be administered only under research protocols.

    d. Calcium channel blockers (e.g., Nifedipine) are also being investigated as tocolytic agents.

  2. Steroid therapy. The enhancement of pulmonary maturity in multiple gestation by antepartum maternal administration of corticosteroids has not been established in the medical literature but is widely used (see Chapter 21). Thus their use in multifetal pregnancy remains controversial.

  3. Amniotic fluid analysis. In cases of premature labor, amniotic fluid analysis is essential in order to identify those patients who are candidates for the use of tocolytic agents. In the absence of discordance and premature rupture of membranes, fetal pulmonary maturation of multiple fetuses proceeds consistently. Therefore, pulmonary assessment of amniotic fluid from one sac should be sufficient; however, when chromosome analysis is indicated or in patients with isoimmunization, amniotic fluid must be obtained separately from both sacs.

C. **Intrapartum.** All deliveries of multiple gestation should be performed in an operative suite, regardless of the route of delivery. Blood should be typed and crossmatched, and an anesthesiologist, two experienced obstetricians, and two experienced pediatricians should be in attendance.

1. **Term twins**
   a. **Vertex/vertex presentation.** For twin births in which both fetuses are vertex in presentation (approximately 40 percent of all term twins), delivery by the vaginal route can be successfully performed, barring other obstetric difficulties (e.g., fetal distress, placental abruption). The **continuous use of electronic fetal monitoring** of both twins is preferred, and **judicious use of oxytocin (Pitocin)** for induction or augmentation of labor is permissible. Following delivery of the first twin, ultrasonic reevaluation of the presenting part of the second twin should be done if the presenting part of the second twin is not known. If regular uterine contractions have not been reestablished within 10 to 15 min after the birth of the first twin, a diluted Pitocin solution (1 mL in 1000 mL 5% dextrose in Ringer's lactate) may be administered IV while carefully monitoring the second fetus. The second twin need not be delivered within a specific time interval after the first twin, provided that continuous monitoring of the fetus and uterine contractions is utilized and descent of the presenting part occurs as in a normal labor pattern.
   b. **Vertex/nonvertex presentation.** There are several acceptable approaches to the delivery of a twin birth in which the first fetus is in the vertex presentation and the second is in a nonvertex presentation.
      (1) One approach is universal use of cesarean section.
      (2) A second approach is routine vaginal delivery of the first twin followed by breech delivery of the second twin. In this case, an x-ray, or ultrasound examination, is used to rule out a hyperextended fetal head, and simply awaiting descent of the fetus utilizing continuous fetal monitoring is permissible. Delivery is then accomplished with standard breech maneuvers.
      (3) A third approach is routine vaginal delivery of the first twin and total breech extraction or internal podalic version of the second twin. This technique should be attempted only in the absence of a hyperextended fetal head and requires the greatest degree of skill, especially in distinguishing the fetal feet from the hands. Ideally, the second amniotic sad is left intact, and the feet are grasped by the operator's hand, with gentle traction applied to

bring the fetal buttocks into the pelvis. Then an amniotomy is performed and the fetus is delivered by standard breech maneuvers.

(4) A fourth approach that has recently been used is external version of the second twin following routine vaginal delivery of the first. This technique requires a portable, real-time ultrasound unit to assess accurately the lie of the second twin. With gentle pressure and simultaneous fetal heart rate monitoring, the fetus may be maneuvered from a breech or transverse lie to a vertex presentation, and subsequent vaginal delivery may be accomplished.

c. **Nonvertex/vertex or nonvertex/nonvertex presentation.** In this situation, cesarean section is the preferred route of delivery.

2. **Term triplets and other multiple births.** With more than two fetuses, cesarean section is the preferred method of delivery.

3. **Preterm twins**

a. **Vertex/vertex presentation.** In births with both twins presenting vertex, vaginal delivery may be accomplished with careful monitoring of the second fetus, as described for the term twins (see Section VIII.C.1.a.).

b. **Vertex/nonvertex presentation.** In this situation, the deliveries may be managed as outlined for term twins (see Section VII.C.1.b.), but routine cesarean section is preferred by most obstetricians.

c. **Nonvertex/vertex or nonvertex/nonvertex.** As for term twins, cesarean section is indicated.

4. **Preterm triplets and other multiple births.** With more than two fetuses, cesarean delivery should be undertaken.

D. **Locking of twins.** Locking of twins occurs when one twin prevents the descent and delivery of the other. The management should be immediate cesarean delivery to avoid compromise of either fetus. There are **three types** of locking of twins.

1. **Collision.** Contact between fetal parts of both twins, preventing engagement of either.

2. **Compaction.** Engagement of the presenting part of both twins simultaneously, preventing further descent.

3. **Interlocking.** Contact of the fetal chins so as to prevent further descent. Interlocking occurs when the first fetus presents as a breech and the second as a vertex, and the fetuses are facing each other.

E. **Postpartum.** Due to the likelihood of a distended uterus, the frequency of postpartum hemorrhage secondary to uterine atony is increased in multiple births. The mother should be routinely given a dilute intravenous Pitocin solution (2 mL in 1000 mL 5% dextrose in Ringer's lactate) postpartum and should be closely observed in the recovery room for signs of excessive vaginal bleeding.

BIBLIOGRAPHY

Acker D, Liberman M, Holbrook H, et al. Delivery of the second twin. Obstet Gynecol 1982; 59:710.

Barrett JM, Staggs SM, Van Hooydonk JE, et al. The effect of type of delivery upon neonatal outcome in premature twins. Am J Obstet Gynecol 1982; 143:360.

Chervenak FA, Johnson RE, Youcha S, et al. Intrapartum management of twin gestation. Obstet Gynecol 1985; 65:119.

Jeffrey RL, Bowes WA, Delaney JJ. Role of bedrest in twin gestation. Obstet Gynecol 1974; 43:822.

Leveno KJ, Santos-Ramos R, Duenoelter JH, et al. Sonar cephalometry in twins: A table of biparietal diameters for normal twin fetuses and a comparison with singletons. Am Obstet Gynecol 1979; 135:727.

Marshall CL. Coping with an unsuspected second twin. Contemp Ob/Gyn 1984; 24:165.

Pritchard JA, MacDonald PC, Gant NF. Multifetal pregnancy. In: Williams Obstetrics. 17th ed. New York: Appleton-Century-Crofts; 1984:503.

Saunders MC, Dick JS, Brown IM, et al. The effects of hospital admission for bedrest on the duration of twin pregnancy: A randomized trial. Lancet. 1985; 1:793.

Weekes ARL, Menzies DN, de Boer CH. The relative efficacy of bedrest, cervical suture, and no treatment in the management of twin pregnancy. Br J Obstet Gynaecol 1977; 84:161.

CHAPTER 24

Prolonged Pregnancy

John R. Barton

The postterm pregnancy represents a significant area of concern for both the physician and the patient. This obstetric problem is associated with an increase in perinatal morbidity and mortality compared to the term gestation. Increased antenatal fetal surveillance (including ultrasound assessment) with selective induction or delivery has improved the outcome in recent years. This chapter outlines the evaluation and management of this high-risk complication of pregnancy.

I. **Definitions.** By convention, a term gestation is considered to be between 38 and 42 weeks from the first day of the last menstrual period (LMP). The terms *prolonged pregnancy, postdates, postterm,* and *postmaturity* have been used to describe pregnancies that exceed 42 weeks (294 days) of amenorrhea. A review of the literature by Lagrew and Freeman (1986) noted the appropriate definitions as follows:

Prolonged pregnancy: Should be used to describe pregnancies that are well documented to be > 294 days.

Postterm or **postdate pregnancy:** Should be used to describe pregnancies that are probably > 294 days, but the dating criteria are less strict.

Postmaturity: Prolonged pregnancy with the syndrome of dysmaturity.

II. **Incidence.** The incidence varies between 3.5 and 14 percent, depending on the diagnostic criteria used. However, the more accurate the estimate of gestational age, the lower the frequency of prolonged gestation.

III. **Cause.** The physiologic mechanism responsible for the failure of labor initiation prior to 42 weeks is not understood. Several causes are associated with postterm pregnancy.
   A. **Inaccurate or unknown date of the last menstrual period.** This is the most common cause and is frequently associated with late or no prenatal care.
   B. **Irregular ovulation or variation in the length of the follicular**

313

phase. Since ovulation and fertilization are presumed to have occurred 2 weeks following the LMP, an abnormally long follicular phase will result in overestimation of the actual length of gestation.

C. **Normal estrogen/progesterone ratio** is necessary for the onset of labor. Several factors are associated with decreased fetal production of estrogen and, therefore, delay in onset of labor. These include:

1. Anencephaly, which is associated with decreased production of 16α-hydroxydehydroepiandrosterone sulfate, the precursor for production of estriol.

2. Fetal adrenal hypoplasia, which also results in decreased fetal production of precursors for estriol synthesis.

3. Placental sulfatase deficiency, an X-linked inherited disease, which prevents conversion of sulfated estrogen precursors to estrogens by the placenta and is characterized by low estriol levels.

D. **Extrauterine pregnancy**

E. **Previous prolonged pregnancy,** in which the recurrence risk may be as high as 50 percent.

IV. **Morbidity and mortality.** Postterm pregnancies are associated with a significant increase in maternal and fetal complications. This risk is compounded in patients with other high-risk factors.

A. **Maternal problems**

1. Unripe cervix in 70 percent of cases

2. Maternal anxiety

3. Traumatic delivery due to fetal macrosomia (20 percent)

4. Increased cesarean section rates for fetal distress, failure to progress in labor, or cephalopelvic disproportion due to macrosomia

5. Increased postpartum hemorrhage, possibly due to fetal size or the frequent use of oxytocin for labor augmentation or induction

B. **Fetal problems.** These can be divided into two main categories: those related to intrauterine fetal growth and those of diminished amniotic fluid volume.

1. **Fetal growth abnormalities**

a. **Macrosomia.** This occurs three to seven times more frequently in the postterm than the term pregnancy. Fetal macrosomia predisposes the fetus to dysfunctional labor and is associated with birth trauma, including:

(1) Shoulder dystocia

(2) Clavicle fracture

(3) Erb-Duchenne palsy

All of these conditions are more common with a prolonged second stage of labor and midpelvic delivery.

b. **Placental dysfunction syndrome.** Although the majority of postterm fetuses continue to have normal intrauterine

growth, a definite subset with growth failure due to placenta dysfunction exists. Due to failure of the placenta to provide adequate nutrients and gas exchange, these infants have a higher incidence of neonatal complications including seizures, hypoglycemia, respiratory distress, persistent fetal circulation, and meconium aspiration. Physically, they are characterized by:
  (1) Loss of vernix caseosa
  (2) Dry, cracked, wrinkled skin
  (3) Decreased subcutaneous fat deposits
  (4) Long nails and abundant hair
  (5) Growth retardation or growth failure

2. **Oligohydramnios.** Decreased amniotic fluid is associated with an increased risk of:
  a. Fetal distress
  b. Meconium passage. This may be present in 25 to 50 percent of postterm pregnancies. Prognostically, thick meconium is more closely related to a compromised fetus than thin meconium.
  c. Cord accidents with sudden fetal death

V. **Patient assessment.** Before intervention or management decisions are made concerning the postterm pregnancy, it is important to review the prenatal history in order to confirm the assigned gestational age. An ultrasound examination of the fetus is also beneficial in the management of postterm pregnancy. Fetal anomalies can be detected, and fetal weight, placental condition, fetal presentation, and amniotic fluid volume (AFV) can be assessed. However, ultrasound will not be able to establish the gestational age accurately this late in pregnancy (± 3 weeks).

A. **Determination of the estimated date of confinement (EDC).** This determination is one of the most important parts of prenatal care because it provides the basis for many management decisions later in pregnancy. It is most accurate and reliable if performed early in pregnancy and can be predicted based on several parameters.

  1. If the LMP is known with certainty, then a term gestation is defined as 280 days ± 14 days from the LMP or 266 days ± 14 days from ovulation. The estimated delivery date can be calculated from Nagele's rule by subtracting 3 months from the first day of the LMP and adding 7 days. These calculations assume that the menstrual cycle is regular, occurs at 28-day intervals, and does not occur following cessation of oral contraceptive use.

  2. Early pelvic exams (less than 14 weeks) are reasonably accurate in predicting the gestational age when performed by an experienced examiner.

  3. The fundal height can also be used to estimate the gestational age; for example, the gestational age is approximately 20 weeks when the fundus is at the level of the umbilicus, and

the gestational age in weeks is roughly equivalent to the fundal height in centimeters after 20 weeks. However, the accuracy is only ± 4 weeks and decreases with advancing gestation.

4. Quickening is usually felt at 20 weeks by primiparas and may occur as early as 17 weeks in multiparas. Again, however, this prediction is not very accurate, is subjective, and is often not well documented.

5. Fetal heart tones can be heard by a Doppler stethoscope at an average of 10 to 12 weeks (but as early as 8) or by a DeLee fetoscope, usually by 19 to 20 weeks (but as early as 17).

6. Ultrasound is a very accurate predictor of gestational age. Several parameters can be measured. The ones most commonly utilized are the gestational sac as early as 5 to 6 weeks; the crown-rump length at < 12 weeks; and the biparietal diameter, preferably between 14 and 26 weeks. Numerous other parameters that can be measured, such as long bones and abdominal size, also have been found to correlate with gestational age. In general, the earlier in pregnancy a measurement is made, the more accurate the prediction of gestational age.

7. A positive serum pregnancy test (quantitative beta-human chorionic gonadotropin [b-HCG] values) may be correlated with gestational age < 10 weeks.

8. Assisted reproduction, such as in vitro fertilization or gamete-intrafallopian transfer, provide the most accurate dating criteria.

B. **Antenatal assessment of the fetus.** Before a postterm pregnancy can be allowed to remain undelivered, there must be assurance that the fetus is tolerating the intrauterine environment. Placental function tends to diminish after 38 weeks' gestation, and fetal oxygenation and nutrient delivery may be compromised. Further, amniotic fluid volume tends to decrease after 37 weeks' gestation, and cord compression is frequently associated with oligohydramnios.

1. **Ultrasonographic evaluation.** Biometry for estimated fetal weight (EFW) should be obtained. Placental grade and fluid status should be documented. Absence of a 2 × 2 cm pocket of amniotic fluid or an amniotic fluid index (AFI) < 5 cm is an indication for delivery in a postterm pregnancy. Evaluation for intrauterine growth retardation and macrosomia is also important.

2. Some form of fetal heart rate testing should be done on a regular basis. The options are:

a. **Nonstress test (NST).** This test evaluates the functional integrity of the fetal central nervous system and myocardium. It should be performed biweekly. Spontaneous late-appearing decelerations or recurrent variable decelerations are an indication for delivery. A nonreactive

NST is an indication for further tests such as a biophysical profile or a contraction stress test.

    b. **Contraction stress test (CST).** This test evaluates uteroplacental reserve in response to spontaneous or oxytocin-induced contractions. It should be performed weekly. A positive test is an indication for delivery. An equivocal test is divided into suspicious, hyperstimulation, and unsatisfactory categories. In any of these cases, the test should be repeated within 24 h.

    3. **Biophysical profile** is the dynamic ultrasonographic evaluation of fetal breathing movements, gross fetal body movements, fetal tone, and AFV, combined with results of the NST. Normal tests are repeated biweekly (Table 24.1).

C. **Assessment of cervical ripening.** The degree of cervical ripening is usually assessed with the use of a modified cervical Bishop scoring test that considers cervical dilatation, effacement (length), consistency, position, and the station of the presenting part (Table 24.2). An unripe cervix is defined by a Bishop score of < 6. A study of the Bishop score in postterm gestation indicated that only dilatation, effacement, and station correlated with the interval from examination to spontaneous onset of labor.

The success rate and outcome of induction of labor are related to the state of cervical ripening. If the Bishop score is ≥ 7, the cesarean section rate is < 10 percent; by contrast, the cesarean section rate is about 30 percent if the score is < 6.

VI. **Management.** Numerous articles have been published regarding the best approach in the management of prolonged pregnancy. The two most popular methods remain induction of labor and antepartum fetal testing until the onset of spontaneous labor or the development of parameters requiring delivery.

Some investigators now suggest that postterm protocols be initiated at 41 weeks. This trend is prompted by the increase in adverse perinatal outcome noted after 40 weeks' gestation in addition to the increased incidence of fetal macrosomia.

A. **Delivery algorithm**

    1. For patients with a definite gestational age of 41 weeks, management depends on an evaluation of the degree of cervical ripening.

        a. A ripe cervix (Bishop score ≥ 7) is seen in 8 to 36 percent of cases.

            (1) These patients are best managed by induction or augmentation of labor, assuming that no evidence of macrosomia exists.

            (2) Cesarean section should be seriously considered if the estimated fetal weight is ≥ 4500 g in nondiabetic patients or ≥ 4000 to 4200 g in diabetic patients.

            (3) Intrapartum fetal heart rate monitoring is employed, and a pediatrician should be in attendance

Table 24.1. Biophysical Profile Scoring: Techniques and Interpretation

BIOPHYSICAL VARIABLE	NORMAL (SCORE = 2)	ABNORMAL (SCORE = 0)
Fetal breathing movements	At least one episode of FBM of at least 30-s duration in a 30-min observation	Absent FBM or no episode of ≥ 30 s in 30 min
Gross body movement	At least three discrete body or limb movements in 30 min (episodes of active, continuous movement considered single movement)	Two or fewer episodes of body or limb movements in 30 min
Fetal tone	At least one episode of active extension with return to flexion of fetal limb(s) or trunk; opening and closing of hand considered normal tone	Either slow extension with return to partial flexion or movement of limb in full extension, absent fetal movement
Qualitative AFV	At least one pocket of amniotic fluid that measures at least 2 cm in two perpendicular planes or amniotic fluid index ≥ 5 cm	Amniotic fluid pocket < 2 cm in two perpendicular planes or amniotic fluid index < 5 cm
NST	At least two episodes of FHR acceleration of ≥ 15 beats/min and of at least 15-s duration in 20 min	Fewer than two episodes of acceleration of FHR or acceleration of < 15 beats/min in 20 min

Source: Adapted from Manning FA, Platt LD, Sipos L. Antepartum fetal evaluation: Development of a fetal biophysical profile. Am J Obstet Gynecol 1980; 136(6):788.

Abbreviations: FBM = fetal breathing movement; FHR = fetal heart rate; AFV = amniotic fluid volume.

       for the delivery if meconium is present. DeLee suction and tracheal intubation should be performed as needed.

   b. An unripe cervix (Bishop score ≤ 6) is frequently encountered in these patients, and requires that further evaluation of fetal well-being be done if delivery is not carried out.

      (1) NST and evaluation of AFV by ultrasound are performed. If both are normal, the pregnancy can be

Table 24.2. Modified Bishop Score

CATEGORY	SCORE 0	1	2	3
Dilatation (cm)	0	1–2	3–4	> 5
Effacement (%)	0–30	40–50	60–70	≥ 80
Station	≥ −3	−2	−1 or 0	≥ + 1
Position	Posterior	Mid	Anterior	
Consistency	Firm	Medium	Soft	

Source: Adapted from Bishop EH. Pelvic scoring for elective induction. Obstet Gynecol 1964; 24(2):267. Reprinted with permission from The American College of Obstetricians and Gynecologists.

allowed to continue and reassessment performed twice weekly.

(2)   If oligohydramnios (< 2 cm vertical pocket or amniotic fluid index < 5 cm) is present or variable decelerations are noted on NST, then induction of labor and delivery are considered.

(3)   If the AFV is normal and the NST is nonreactive, a CST or biophysical profile should be performed. A positive CST would dictate delivery, whereas a negative CST would allow the pregnancy to continue and be reevaluated in 3 days.

(4)   The cervical status (Bishop score) should be reevaluated at each visit, and delivery should be considered once cervical ripening occurs.

(5)   Consider delivery in all patients beyond 301 days (44 weeks).

2.   For patients with an uncertain gestational age > 287 days, management is the same, except that certainty must exist that the pregnancy is not premature. Amniocentesis for fetal lung maturity or another method of confirming maturity may be indicated.

3.   Postterm patients with serious maternal or fetal complications (such as diabetes, preeclampsia, Rh isoimmunization, or intrauterine growth retardation) should be delivered regardless of the cervical condition. Indeed, these high-risk pregnancies should not be allowed to enter the postterm period even with reassuring antenatal test results.

B.   **Role of cervical priming.** Numerous mechnical and pharmacologic methods have been employed to improve the degree of cervical ripening.

1.   Laminaria tents (from the seaweed *Laminaria digitata* or *L. japonicum*). Hydrophilic sticks, when placed in the cervical os, absorb moisture and expand to dilate the cervix.

2.   Foley catheter. Placement in the cervix and inflation may be

effective by causing physical dilation and local release of tissue prostaglandins.

3. Oxytocin is an octapeptide hormone produced in the hypothalamus and transported to and released into the blood by the posterior pituitary. This hormone produces a dose-dependent increase in uterine smooth muscle activity. Synthetic preparations are available that may be used to initiate cervical softening and effacement and to induce coordinated myometrial responsiveness.

4. Prostaglandin E_2 (PGE_2) has gained wide popularity for cervical priming. In vitro data indicate that PGE_2 may alter the membrane excitability of myometrial cells. There is significant experience with this drug in the induction of labor for pregnancy termination prior to 24 weeks' gestation, but currently there are no randomized placebo-controlled trials that prove that PGE_2 is efficacious in the induction of labor at term. Although it has been successful in promoting cervical priming, the cesarean section rate has not been shown to be reduced. Further, PGE_2 use may be associated with a significant risk of uterine hyperstimulation and fetal distress. If PGE_2 is used for labor induction, it is administered as a cream either intracervically (0.5 mg) or intravaginally (3 mg). Currently, clinical trials of a PGE_2 pessary are being conducted. Preliminary results are favorable, but the efficacy and safety are yet to be established.

5. Relaxin is a polypeptide hormone that produces inhibition of uterine contractions but may promote softening of the cervix. Clinical trials with relaxin are underway, but currently neither PGE_2 nor relaxin has been approved by the Food and Drug Administration for use in preinduction cervical priming.

C. **Intrapartum management**
1. Left lateral positioning of the patient is utilized to afford uterine displacement off the inferior vena cava.
2. Continuous electronic fetal monitoring is employed.
3. Supplemental oxygen is used liberally if abnormalities in the fetal heart rate pattern are detected.
4. Amniotomy is performed when deemed safe and feasible. Membrane rupture is associated with increased prostaglandin formation, and therefore may increase uterine activity and decrease the induction-to-delivery interval. Further, it allows examination of the amniotic fluid for blood or meconium staining.
5. Intravenous oxytocin is administered with a volume-controlled infusion pump. Recent American College of Obstetrics and Gynecology guidelines emphasize a low-dose protocol whereby oxytocin is increased by no more than 2 mU/min or at intervals of less than 30 minutes, resulting in a decreased incidence of hyperstimulation and fetal distress.
6. Amnioinfusion should be considered for oligohydramnios or

the presence of fluid meconium. Instillation of warmed normal saline in the uterine cavity may dilute meconium-stained amniotic fluid or produce abatement of variable fetal heart rate decelerations. A typical protocol is for an initial infusion of 300 to 500 mL over 15 to 30 minutes followed by a continuous infusion of 3 mL/min.

7. Fetal scalp blood sampling or another method of confirming fetal well-being is used as indicated by fetal monitoring.

8. Close attention is paid to the progress of labor (Friedman curve). Intrauterine pressure catheter use may allow a more timely diagnosis of dysfunctional labor.

9. Once delivered, the infant should be carefully assessed for hypoglycemia, hypovolemia, hypothermia, and polycythemia.

VII. Prevention of meconium aspiration. If meconium-stained fluid is noted, a person skilled at neonatal resuscitation should be present at the delivery. Management should include the following:

A. Aggressive suctioning of the nasopharynx and posterior oropharynx is done prior to delivery of the fetal chest.

B. If meconium is seen at the level of the vocal cords, positive-pressure ventilation is delayed until the trachea is intubated and adequately suctioned.

C. Routine tracheal intubation should be performed in the presence of thick meconium and a depressed neonate.

D. Saline amnioinfusion for dilution of meconium-stained fluid has been reported to reduce the risk of meconium aspiration and the need for positive-pressure ventilation in the neonate.

BIBLIOGRAPHY

American College of Obstetrics and Gynecologists. Diagnosis and management of postterm pregnancy. Technical Bulletin No. 130. Washington, DC; ACOG; July 1989.

American College of Obstetrics and Gynecologists. Induction and augmentation of labor. Technical Bulletin No. 110. Washington, DC: ACOG; November 1987.

Arias F. Predictability of complications associated with prolongation of pregnancy. Obstet Gynecol 1987; 70:101.

Bishop EH. Pelvic scoring for elective induction. Obstet Gynecol 1964; 24:266.

Lagrew DC, Freeman RK. Management of postdate pregnancy. Am J Obstet Gynecol 1986; 154:8.

Leveno KJ, Quirk JG, Cunningham FG, et al. Prolonged pregnancy I. Observations concerning the causes of fetal distress. Am J Obstet Gynecol 1984; 150:465.

Manning FA, Platt LD, Sipos L. Antepartum fetal evaluation: Development of a fetal biophysical profile. Am J Obstet Gynecol 1980; 136:787.

Phelan JP, Platt LD, Yeh S, et al. The role of ultrasound assessment of AFV in the management of the postdate pregnancy. Am J Obstet Gynecol 1985; 151:304.

CHAPTER 25

Peripartum Infections

Jessica L. Thomason

ENDOMETRITIS

I. **Epidemiology.** Endometritis, infection of the uterine cavity, is a common complication of the postpartum period. Other names for endometritis include *endomyometritis, endoparametritis,* and *metritis.* Endometritis follows approximately 3 percent of vaginal deliveries and 12 to 25 percent of abdominal deliveries. Maternal sepsis, which may follow untreated or especially severe endometritis, is the second most common cause of maternal death.

   A. **Peurperal morbidity.** Endometritis is commonly associated with puerperal morbidity, which is clinically defined as a temperature $\geq$ 100.4°F (38°C) on any 2 of the first 10 days postpartum, exclusive of the first 24 h. Other definitions define morbidity as occurring with any temperature > 99.4°F on any occasion or if a temperature > 101°F occurs at any point during labor, delivery, or the puerperium.

   B. **Low-grade fever postpartum.** Endometritis is often confused clinically with a low-grade fever ($\geq$ 100.4°F) or isolated spiking temperatures that occur and resolve spontaneously in 6 to 10 percent of deliveries. The cause of such temperature spikes is unknown.

II. **Risk factors.** Accurate prediction of which patients will develop endometritis is difficult. Causative factors associated with endometritis may help in this determination.

   A. **Factors associated with endometritis.** Four factors are repeatedly associated with endometritis.

   1. **Length of labor.** Patients experiencing no labor (e.g., elective cesarean section [C-section]) have lower infection rates than those who require surgery after labor, especially if lasting for more than 6 to 12 h. Although the amniotic fluid is usually sterile, bacteria can be found in the intact amniotic sac of women in labor. Length of labor prior to cesarean section is the most significant factor for predicting the development of infection after C-section.

2. **Rupture of membranes (ROM).** The longer the time of ruptured membranes, the more likely the finding of microorganisms contaminating the amniotic cavity. Compared with labor, membrane status plays less of a role in the development of infection after C-section. Many bacteria produce phospholipase A_2, the rate-limiting enzyme of the prostaglandin cascade involved in the initiation of labor. Patients with known abnormal vaginal flora **(bacterial vaginosis)** have a higher rate of rupture of membranes and premature labor.

3. **Number of vaginal examinations.** As the number of vaginal examinations increases, the rate of infection (especially after C-section) also increases. The critical number of examinations at which the rate of infection increases sharply is three or more. There is no difference in infection rates between patients examined vaginally or rectally. The length of labor has a higher correlation with infection than does the number of examinations.

4. **Intraoperative factors. Operative delivery (C-section) is the most important predisposing factor** associated with both the frequency and severity of endometritis, with the highest infection rate noted after emergency or nonprimary C-sections. Elective C-sections with intact membranes, whether primary or repeat, carry lower infection rates than nonelective C-sections. Rates of endometritis after intraperitoneal versus extraperitoneal approaches do not differ.

B. **Other factors associated with endometritis**
1. **Socioeconomic status.** The socioeconomic status of the patient independent of race is critical to predicting increased infectious morbidity. Nutritional status contributes to this factor. Anemia is difficult to separate from the social status, and low hematocrit is frequently seen in women with endometritis after C-section.

2. **Adolescents.** Adolescents are at increased risk for endometritis. They frequently have increased rates of sexually transmitted diseases (STDs) and lack the protective immunologic status seen in older women.

3. **Obesity.** Obesity is a factor more closely related to an increased risk for **wound** infections than endometritis.

4. **Amniotic fluid factors.** The **antibacterial component** inherent in amniotic fluid plays an important role in halting infection and is seen even with bacteria isolated from the intact amnion. A **phosphorus-sensitive peptide bound to zinc** is a major antibacterial factor for gram-negative aerobes. There is a progressive increase in the antibacterial activity of amniotic fluid from 20 weeks until term.

5. **Immunosuppressed patients.** Although patients being treated with immunosuppressive drugs are relatively uncommon, their flora and immune responses to infection are altered, placing them at higher risk for endometritis.

6. **Steroids.** Steroids are frequently given to women who are anticipated to deliver premature infants to induce fetal lung maturity. Most studies confirm a higher rate of maternal infection after steroid administration.
7. **Serious maternal systemic disease.** Serious systemic medical disease (e.g., diabetes) alters host responses to infectious challenges, usually increasing susceptibility.
8. **Adjuvants in amniotic fluid affect infection rates. Meconium** detrimentally alters the antibacterial activity of amniotic fluid. Leaving adjuvants at the operative site (i.e., fetal vernix, blood clots, meconium) increases the postoperative infection rate.

III. **Diagnosis.** The diagnosis of endometritis is suspected in any patient with fever (defined in Section I) unexplained by infection at other sites (i.e., urine, lungs, wound). From 10 to 20 percent of patients have concomitant bacteremia. **Pelvic examination** is necessary to rule out hematoma or abscess as a source of infection and obtaining endometrial cultures. *Endometrial cultures* for aerobes, anaerobes, and STDs must be obtained by double- or triple-lumen catheter technique to avoid contamination of cervical and vaginal flora. The average number of isolates from such cultures may vary from three to eight organisms (Table 25.1 and 25.2 for a description of common organisms in obstetric-gynecologic infections and their relative virulence).

IV. **Treatment.** Because endometritis is polymicrobial, a broad-spectrum antibiotic is required. Initial antibiotic coverage is empiric based on the expected organisms (especially gram-negative aerobes and gram-positive and -negative anaerobes). Antibiotics are changed if necessary at 72 h based on culture data and clinical response. It is important **not** to change the antibiotic regimen after only 24 h of therapy except when the clinical situation is worsening rapidly enough that the empiric addition of antibiotics is warranted.

A. **Representative antibiotic regimens.** There are several representative antibiotic regimens that provide such initial broad-spectrum coverage. As the regimens are essentially equivalent for initial therapy, the choice among them depends primarily on the clinical experience and preferences of the physician.
   1. Cefoxitan, 2 g IV q6 h
   2. Piperacillin, 4 g IV q6 h
   3. Clindamycin (900 mg IV q8 h) plus aminoglycoside (such as gentamycin, 80 mg IV q8 h).
   4. Claforan, 2 g IV q8 h
   5. Unasyn
B. **Chlamydia trachomatis.** When chlamydial infection is suspected, coverage with tetracycline or clindamycin is required.
C. **Neisseria gonorrhea.** When a gonorrheal infection is suspected, cefoxitin or piperacillin provides better coverage than clindamycin and an aminoglycoside.

Table 25.1. Important Organisms in Obstetric/Gynecologic Infections

AEROBIC/FACULTATIVE ORGANISMS	OBLIGATE ANAEROBIC ORGANISMS

GRAM-POSITIVE

Cocci	Cocci
Streptococcus spp.	*Peptococcus* spp.
Group B	*Peptostreptococcus* spp.
Group D	*Streptococcus* spp.
Staphylococcus* spp.	*Gaffkya* spp.
Rods	Rods
Lactobacillus spp.	*Lactobacillus* spp.
	Bifidobacterium spp.
	(Clostridium, Proprionibacterium, Eubacterium spp.)

GRAM-NEGATIVE

Cocci	Rods
Neisseria gonorrhoea	*Bacteroides fragilis* group
	B. distasonis
Rods	*B. fragilis*
Enterobacteriacae	*B. ovatus*
Escherichia coli	*B. thetaiotaomicron*
Klebsiella spp.	*B. vulgatus*
Proteus spp.	
	Prevotii group
	P. asaccharolyticus
	P. bivus
	P. capillosus
	P. disiens
	P. ruminicola
	P. uniformis
	Porphomonas / melaninogenicus
	Fusobacterium spp.
	Mobiluncus spp.
Other	
Chlamydia trachomatis	
Mycoplasmas	
Mycoplasma hominis	
Ureaplasma urealyticum	

*Only toxic shock.

Table 25.2. Organisms in Obstetric/Gynecologic Infections Ranked According to Virulence

	AEROBES	ANAEROBES
	LOW VIRULENCE	
Gram-positive	*Lactobacillus* spp. *Corynebacterium* spp. *Staph. epidermidis*	*Eubacterium* spp. *Propionibacterium* spp. *Gaffkya* spp.
Gram-negative		*Veillonella* spp. *Bifidobacterium* spp.
Other	*Candida* spp.	
	HIGH VIRULENCE	

Gram-positive	*Streptococcus* spp.
	Beta-hemolytic
	  Group B
	  Entercoccus (Gr.D)
		Peptococcus spp.
		Peptostreptococcus spp.
		Clostridium spp.

Gram-negative	*Enterobacteriacae* spp. *Escherichia coli* *Proteus* spp. *Klebsiella* spp.	*Bacteroides* spp. *B. fragilis* group *Prevotii* group *Fusobacterium* spp.

D. **Antibiotic dosages for patients with renal dysfunction.** Dosages of antibiotics that involve kidney excretion must be increased because glomerular filtration rates are one and one-half to two times normal in pregnant and immediately postpartum patients.

CHORIOAMNIONTIS
(INTRAAMNIOTIC INFECTIONS [IAI])

I. **Epidemiology.** One percent of all pregnancies are complicated by IAI, resulting in both maternal and neonatal infectious complications. Other names for this condition include *chorioamnionitis, amnionitis,* and *intrapartum infection*. Risk factors include poor socioeconomic status, anemia, adolescent pregnancy, altered vaginal flora (bacterial vaginosis), and premature labor or premature rupture of membranes. The organisms commonly involved are the same as those for endometritis (see Tables 25.1 and 25.2). IAI virtually always results in **premature labor** and/or **premature rupture of membranes. Neonatal outcome** includes sepsis, pneumonia, meningitis, and intracranial hemorrhage in 30 to 50 percent of patients.

II. Diagnosis

A. Clinical suspicion of IAI should be entertained in a pregnant patient with:
   1. **Fever** (> 100.4°F or 38°C) with no other site infection
   2. **Maternal** or **fetal tachycardia**
   3. **Uterine tenderness**
   4. **Foul odor** of the amniotic fluid
   5. **Leukocytosis** (usually > 20,000/mL³ in labor, > 15,000 mL³ when not in labor)

B. **Sepsis.** Maternal sepsis may accompany IAI and requires antibiotic management after blood cultures.

C. **Evaluation of amniotic fluid.** If amniotic fluid can be obtained, the unspun specimen should be examined for the following:
   1. The presence of one or more polymorphonuclear leukocytes (PMNs) per high-powered microscopic field
   2. The presence of any bacteria on Gram stain. **Note:** Although the identification of bacteria and PMNs is very specific (90 percent) for the identification of patients with IAI, sensitivity is low (≤ 50 percent)
   3. Culture for anaerobes, aerobes, chlamydia trachomatis, and mycoplasmas.

D. **Cultures.** Cultures of blood found to have high-virulence organisms predict IAI quite accurately while isolation of low-virulence organisms does not correlate with IAI.

E. **Tissue evaluation.** Histologic evaluation of maternal tissues has proven to be of little benefit. Histologic evaluation of endometrial tissue biopsied at the time of C-section has not been found to be clinically useful. Examination of amniotic membranes by Gram stain or culture is very specific but repeatedly has < 50 percent sensitivity.

III. Treatment

A. **Delivery.** Evacuation of the infected uterus is the treatment of choice. No definite data suggest that delivery must be effected within a certain time period to avoid excess maternal and neonatal morbidity. There is no evidence that abdominal versus vaginal delivery provides a better outcome. Likewise, there is no difference in outcome between a transperitoneal vs. an extraperitoneal approach to C-section. Cesarean delivery is increased with IAI, however, due to an increase in dysfunctional labor. It is appropriate to begin antibiotics at the time of diagnosis to decrease maternal morbidity from sepsis and initiate therapy to the fetus.

B. **Antibiotic choice** is based on the expected organisms. As IAI infections are **polymicrobial** involving the same organisms as endometritis, therapy should be directed especially against gram-negative aerobes and gram-positive and -negative anearobes, as in the treatment of endometritis (see the previous section).

BIBLIOGRAPHY

Duff P. Pathophysiology and management of postcesarean endomyometritis. Obstet Gynecol 1986; 67:269–276.

Lee GL, Thomason JL. Diagnosis of chorioamnionitis. Contemp Obstet Gynecol 1988; 32:47–54.

Soper DE, Kemmer CT, Conover WB. Abbreviated antibiotic therapy for the treatment of postpartum endometritis. Obstet Gynecol 1987; 69:127–130.

CHAPTER 26

Antepartum Bleeding in Advanced Pregnancy

Jeffrey C. King

Vaginal bleeding in the second or third trimester is always unexpected and usually results in immediate contact between the patient and her obstetrician. The physician must decide if the cause is benign or life-threatening to the mother, the fetus, or both.

The differential diagnosis of antepartum bleeding in advanced pregnancy is extensive, and includes as its two primary diagnoses placenta previa and abruptio placentae. Other elements of the differential diagnosis include the bloody show of early labor, severe vulvovaginitis and/or cervicitis, bleeding from endocervical polyps, cervical cancer, vasa previa and other placental anomalies, and trauma.

Even though the rate of maternal mortality has been significantly reduced by the ready availability of crossmatched blood and blood products, deaths resulting from antepartum obstetric hemorrhage continue to be listed in the majority of maternal mortality reports. Approximately 3 percent of all pregnancies are complicated by significant bleeding from the birth canal. The term *significant* is used to differentiate abnormal antepartum bleeding in advanced pregnancy from *show* or *bloody show,* which occurs near the onset of labor in most pregnant women. Of the antepartum causes of bleeding, placenta previa is discovered in 22 percent of cases and strong clinical evidence of abruptio placentae is found in 31 percent. The causes of the remaining 47 percent of cases of antepartum bleeding are classified as unknown.

General approach to antepartum bleeding. Whenever a patient informs her care providers of vaginal bleeding during late pregnancy, they must obtain historical information regarding the amount of blood loss, associated pain or trauma, and previous episodes of bleeding during pregnancy. The patient should usually be referred to the hospital if there is any question about the significance of the blood loss so that the fetus and gravida can be fully evaluated and laboratory studies, including ultrasonography, obtained. Vital signs should be monitored frequently, and fetal health should be evaluated by external electronic fetal monitoring. A complete physical examination should be performed; however, digital and speculum examinations of the birth canal and cervix are initially contraindicated. If a complete ultrasound examination to determine the cause of the bleeding is not diagnostic, a careful speculum examination may be helpful.

Baseline laboratory studies should include a complete blood count with platelet count, fibrinogen level, and a Kleihauer-Betke test for evidence of fetomaternal bleeding. The determination of fibrin splint products has been suggested, but since they are present in about 15 percent of normal pregnancies, a positive result may be misleading. In the face of suspected significant bleeding, a large-bore intravenous line should be inserted, and a blood type and screen should be obtained to speed blood crossmatching should it be required. If the blood bank is unable to provide blood products promptly upon request (e.g., in a small hospital or in the presence of maternal antibody), O-negative blood may be used in an extreme emergency. However, in general, blood bank facilities should be available in obstetric units and 2 U of packed red blood cells should be crossmatched and available at all times when significant loss has occurred.

PLACENTA PREVIA

I. **Definition.** Placenta previa is implantation of the placenta in the lower uterine segment in a position in advance of the fetal presenting part. Different degrees of placenta previa are described based upon the relationship of the placental margin to the internal cervical os prior to the onset of labor. This definition may apply to the placenta's relationship to the internal os at any time in pregnancy, but its clinical significance is greatest after the time of fetal viability. This condition is often detected early in pregnancy (before fetal viability and even in the first trimester), but fortunately, it persists into advanced pregnancy in only a small proportion of cases. The types of placenta previa are as follows:

   A. **Total or complete placenta previa** covers the internal os entirely.
   B. **Partial placenta previa** covers part of the internal os.
   C. **Marginal placenta previa** just reaches the internal os but does not cover any part of it.
   D. **Low-lying placenta** describes the placenta when it is implanted in the lower segment but does not reach the internal os.

II. **Incidence.** The reported incidence of placenta previa varies widely in published reports but averages approximately 1/250 births. The variability in incidence may be due to the varying definitions of placenta previa that have been employed.

III. **Morbidity and mortality**
   A. **Maternal morbidity and mortality.** The maternal mortality from placenta previa is less than 1 percent of maternal deaths. The morbidity of placenta previa is high, and is dependent on the extent of hemorrhage and the adequacy of volume replacement upon hemorrhage. **Placenta accreta** may occur in combination with placenta previa (placenta previa accreta) in up to 15 percent of cases. Placenta accreta is the invasion of trophoblastic tissue

into the myometrium in such a manner that placental separation cannot occur. If this abnormal adherence of the placenta to the uterus occurs, total abdominal hysterectomy may prove lifesaving if separation of the placenta from the uterus is impossible and uncontrollable hemorrhage ensues. **Intrauterine growth retardation** is associated with placenta previa in 16 percent of cases, and there is an approximate doubling of the rate of serious **congenital malformations** in cases of placenta previa. **Fetomaternal bleeding** is also a common complication of placenta previa, which may cause the additional complication of **Rh isoimmunization** unless RhoGAM is given in appropriate doses.

B. **Perinatal morbidity and mortality.** The total perinatal (fetal and neonatal) mortality is between 10 and 12 percent. The principal causes of perinatal death are hypoxia from placental insufficiency and prematurity. Neonatal morbidity depends upon the amount of blood loss, growth disturbances, presence of fetal malformations, and gestational age at the time of necessary delivery.

IV. Pathogenesis and pathophysiology

A. **Pathogenesis of placenta previa.** It has been suggested that previous placental implantation results in defective vascularization of the decidua, making those areas unsuitable for placentation in subsequent gestations. Multiparity, advancing maternal age, and previous cesarean delivery increase the risk of placenta previa. Pregnancies involving large placentas, such as erythroblastosis or multifetal gestations, are often complicated by spread of the placenta into the region of the internal os.

B. **Pathogenesis of the bleeding of placenta previa.** The bleeding of placenta previa is associated with the normal progressive development of the lower uterine segment and, presumably, dislocation of the placenta from its inappropriate implantation site on the lower uterine segment.

V. Differential diagnosis

A. **Abruptio placentae.** Abruption must always be considered with third-trimester bleeding until ultrasound examination has revealed the placental location.

B. **"Bloody show."** The most common cause of bleeding in late pregnancy is bloody show, characterized by the discharge of dark blood mixed with copious mucus as the mucous plug is expelled in early labor.

C. **Severe vulvovaginitis/cervicitis.** Trichomonas vaginitis may cause bleeding, but it is usually only a slight pink staining (see Chapter 31).

D. **Endocervical polyps.** Coitus may result in bleeding from an endocervical polyp, but the bleeding is usually limited. Removal of the polyp is indicated only if bleeding persists or neoplasia is suspected.

E. **Cervical cancer.** Inspection of the cervix for gross cancerous lesions and a Pap smear during pregnancy should always be performed to rule out this rare cause of antepartum bleeding.

F. **Vulvar varicose veins.** Due to elevated venous pressure below the level of the uterus, the vulvar vessels may dilate. This common condition may result in spontaneous rupture of the dilated vessels, causing bleeding.

G. **Trauma.** Abdominal or pelvic trauma, coital or otherwise, is an uncommon cause of antepartum bleeding.

H. **Vasa previa.** Vasa previa is a rare condition in which the fetal vessels of the umbilical cord pass over the internal os preceding the presenting fetal part, thus putting the fetus in jeopardy for hemorrhage if the vessels are torn. These vessels usually cannot be visualized by ultrasonography. Thus the greatest risk to the mother and fetus is that during spontaneous or artificial rupture of membranes, the vessels may be torn and the bleeding misinterpreted as maternal rather than fetal. Continuous electronic fetal monitoring may be lifesaving for the detection of acute fetal decompensation from fetal hemorrhage/hypovolemia.

VI. Diagnosis

A. **Signs and symptoms.** The classic symptom of placenta previa is **painless hemorrhage.** Fortunately, the initial episode of bleeding is rarely fatal to the fetus or mother. Bleeding usually ceases spontaneously, only to recur when least expected. The peak incidence for the first episode of bleeding is about the 34th week, although one-third of patients with placenta previa manifest antepartum bleeding before the 30th week and one-third after the 36th week.

B. **Physical examination.** Vital signs are usually within normal limits unless hemorrhage has been massive. The uterus will usually be soft upon palpation, and palpable uterine contractions are absent in the majority of cases of placenta previa. If contractions are felt upon palpation, abruptio placentae is a more likely diagnosis. In 35 percent of cases of placenta previa, the fetus is either in breech or in transverse lie. If the fetus is in the cephalic presentation, it is often high above the pelvic brim. However, malpresentations are no more frequent when the gestational age is adjusted. Speculum or digital pelvic examination is deferred until ultrasound examination has demonstrated that placenta previa does not exist or that another cause of bleeding is ascertained. Generally the patient is extremely anxious about this unexpected event, so attention to the patient's emotional status and reassurance is an important part of the physical examination procedure.

C. **Laboratory examination and diagnostic procedures**

1. **Ultrasonography.** Ultrasonography is highly accurate but not infallible in the diagnosis of placenta previa. Because there are no anatomic markers to locate the internal os precisely, the relationship between the placenta and the

internal os is often very hard to ascertain. The false-negative rate of ultrasound examination for placenta previa is about 7 percent due to the fetal head's obscuring the region of the cervix and to failure of complete scanning of the lateral uterine walls as they approach the cervix. Fortunately, a 90 percent rate of spontaneous resolution can be anticipated in asymptomatic women with ultrasonographically detected placenta previa in the second trimester; thus conservative care will suffice in these cases. This concept of *placental migration* explains the relative unimportance of placenta previa until 28 to 30 weeks. Careful transvaginal ultrasonography may be very helpful, particularly when the placenta is posteriorly implanted.

2. **Hematology and coagulation studies.** A complete blood count should be obtained to ascertain if maternal anemia exists and to provide information for the decision as to whether to proceed with maternal transfusion. While coagulation defects are uncommon in placenta previa, coagulation studies (prothrombin time, partial thromboplastin time, platelet count) are appropriate precautions.

3. **Blood bank.** The patient's ABO and Rh antibody status should be ascertained and 2 U of crossmatched blood made available at all times. RhoGAM should be administered as indicated.

4. **Tests for fetal hemoglobin and hence fetal bleeding.** The Apt and Kleihauer-Betke tests identify fetal hemoglobin and thereby the fetus as the source of antepartum bleeding. These tests have limited clinical utility in the face of massive fetal hemorrhage, as electronic fetal monitoring will identify the fetus affected by hemorrhage. If there is continuous vaginal bleeding without fetal distress, an Apt test may be helpful to determine if the bleeding is from vasa previa and hence is of fetal origin. The test involves mixing blood from the vaginal vault with an equal quantity of 0.25% NaOH. Fetal blood containing fetal hemoglobin will remain pink on examination, whereas maternal blood with adult hemoglobin will become light brown.

VII. Management. The goal of management of placenta previa is to obtain the maximum fetal maturation possible while minimizing the risk to both the fetus and mother. This conservative approach, even late in pregnancy, may allow sufficient time to reduce perinatal morbidity and mortality, especially in association with prematurity.

A. **Expectant management**
   1. **Initial management: Hospitalization.** Since placenta previa is characterized by recurrent episodes of vaginal bleeding, an expectant plan of management is encouraged. Patients with symptomatic placenta previa should be hospitalized for a minimum of 72 h, since almost one-third of patients will fail expectant management and require delivery within this

time. Initially, the patient should be placed on bed rest, with frequent monitoring for bleeding, fetal heart rate, and changes in maternal vital signs. If no bleeding occurs, a progressive increase in ambulation is permissible. Despite an aggressively expectant management plan, 20 percent of these patients are delivered prior to 32 weeks; this group represents approximately 75 percent of the perinatal deaths.

2. **Management at home after initial hospitalization.** While continued hospitalization is the ideal, the current costs of hospitalization and diagnostic related groups make outpatient management an option that may have to be considered. Approximately 50 percent of patients can be managed as outpatients, with careful selection based on severity of bleeding, gestational age, maternal status, and the home environment to which the patient will return. The patient must be highly motivated, educated about the serious nature of her condition, attended by a responsible adult, and must have readily available transportation for transport to the hospital within approximately 15 min.

3. **Tocolysis.** The use of tocolytics remains controversial, but some studies suggest that aggressive blood replacement and tocolytics can result in significant advancement of the gestational age without adversely affecting the perinatal outcome. If blood loss continues and is in excess of replacement, tocolysis should be discontinued.

4. **Blood transfusion.** Blood should be transfused as necessary to maintain a hematocrit at 30 percent or greater.

B. **Aggressive management: Delivery**
   1. **Cesarean section.** In the presence of a living, viable fetus, cesarean section is the delivery mode of choice. The uterine incision should be decided at the time of delivery. If the fetal lie is longitudinal and the placenta is not implanted above the bladder reflection, a low transverse incision may be performed if the lower uterine segment is well developed. In other circumstances, a vertical incision, either in the lower segment or in the upper contractile segment (classic incision), is suggested. Delivery by cesarean section is appropriate:
      a. If the pregnancy has completed 35 weeks or more, the diagnosis is confirmed, and the patient is actively bleeding.
      b. If there is persistence at 36 to 37 weeks of a previously diagnosed placenta previa (fetal lung maturity should be determined prior to delivery).
      c. If there is evidence of coexistent abruption or nonreassuring fetal status, unless the fetus is severely immature and the mother's condition is stable.
      d. If blood loss is continuing in excess of replacement.
   2. **Vaginal delivery.** The only circumstances that allow consideration of vaginal delivery are a clearly previable fetus and advanced labor.

C. **Management of Rh status.** If a large **fetomaternal bleed** is documented in an Rh-negative, unsensitized woman, the appropriate dose of Rh immune globulin is immediately administered and sufficiency is documented by a positive indirect Coombs' test 48 h later.

VIII. **Prognosis.** While expectant management may allow significant advancement of gestational age, prematurity still poses a formidable obstacle and accounts for a majority of perinatal morbidity and mortality. Irrespective of fetal age and weight, perinatal mortality is somewhat greater for pregnancies not complicated by placenta previa than for the general population.

ABRUPTIO PLACENTAE

I. **Definition and classification**
   A. **Definition.** Abruptio placentae is premature separation of a normally implanted placenta prior to the third stage of labor. While this definition is cumbersome, it differentiates the placenta that separates prematurely but is implanted normally in the fundus from one that separates from an abnormal implantation site over the internal os (placenta previa). Abruptio placentae is also called simply *placental abruption* or *abruption.*
   B. **Clinical classification.** The bleeding of placental abruption is most commonly through the cervix, causing **external hemorrhage.** Occasionally, it is retained within the uterus, resulting in a **concealed hemorrhage.** Abruptio placentae with concealed hemorrhage has a greater likelihood of causing maternal and fetal hazard from coagulopathy and unappreciated extent of blood loss than from abruptio placentae with external hemorrhage. The clinical classification of abruptio placentae involves mild, moderate, and severe abruptions according to the amount of blood loss, the uterine tone, the fetal heart rate, and the maternal status. This classification is presented in Table 26.1.

II. **Incidence.** The reported incidence varies widely due to the population studied and the diagnostic criteria that are applied but has been estimated at 1/120 deliveries. Abruption severe enough to result in fetal death occurs in 1/420 deliveries. The risk of **recurrence** has been reported as 5 to 15 percent, 20 times the risk of abruptio placentae in the general population.

III. **Morbidity and mortality**
   A. **Maternal.** Maternal mortality depends on when in the pathologic sequence of events the diagnosis is made and the skill with which the condition is then managed. Generally, the risk of maternal mortality is less than 5 percent even in severe cases. Maternal morbidity has a similar relationship to diagnosis and treatment, although severe cases involving coagulopathy and renal failure are associated with higher mortality.

Table 26.1. Clinical Classification of Abruptio Placentae

CLASS OF ABRUPTIO PLACENTAE	MILD (~ 65% OF CASES)	MODERATE (~ 23% OF CASES)	SEVERE (~ 12% OF CASES)
Amount of vaginal bleeding	< 100 mL	100–500 mL	> 500 mL
Uterine tone	Slightly irritable, soft, nontender	Increased activity and some tenderness	Tense, tetanic, tender uterus
Fetal heart rate pattern	Normal	Possible evidence of fetal compromise or intrauterine fetal demise	Usually evidence of fetal compromise or intrauterine fetal demise
Maternal status	Normal	Mild shock, infrequent coagulopathy	Moderate to severe shock, frequent coagulopathy

      B. Perinatal. Fetal mortality depends not only on the extent of placental separation but also on the gestational age. The quoted mortality rate is between 30 and 40 percent for all cases and 25 percent for infants weighing 1000 g or more. The significance of the problem is better appreciated when it is noted that mortality associated with abruptio placentae accounts for almost 15 percent of all perinatal deaths. The three major causes of perinatal death in abruptio placentae are anoxia, prematurity, and exsanguination.

IV. Pathogenesis and pathophysiology. Many factors have been suggested as causes of abruptio placentae, but a single causative concept has not been identified. The wide range of associated conditions seems to be best explained by an underlying disorder of the decidua and uterine vessels. Associated conditions include trauma, short umbilical cord, uterine anomaly, hypertensive disease, cigarette smoking, folic acid deficiency, hydramnios with sudden uterine decompression, inferior vena cava compression, antiphospholipid antibody syndrome, and maternal age.

V. Differential diagnosis. With severe abruptio placentae the clinical diagnosis is rarely in doubt. However, with milder cases the diagnosis is sometimes difficult and is often made by exclusion (see Section V in the discussion of placenta previa).

VI. Diagnosis
    A. Signs and symptoms. The signs and symptoms of abruptio placentae vary widely, depending on the extent of placental

separation. The classic presentation is vaginal bleeding, abdominal pain, uterine contractions, and uterine tenderness. However, the complete set of signs and symptoms is rarely present, and the absence of one or more does not exclude the diagnosis or imply a milder form. In fact, approximately 10 percent of patients present with only concealed hemorrhage, making assessment of total blood loss from the maternal circulation difficult. **Abdominal pain** is observed in 50 percent of patients and usually indicates extravasation of blood into the myometrium. While often difficult to feel, **uterine contractions** are present in the majority of cases. **Uterine tenderness** may be found only at the site of placental attachment or may be generalized.

B. **Physical examination.** Cardiovascular compromise (associated with maternal hypovolemia) out of proportion to observed external blood loss is highly suggestive of placental abruption. Serial fundal height and abdominal girth measurements that may detect the uterus enlarging with blood as the placental abruption progresses may be extremely helpful in the diagnosis of both concealed and external hemorrhage from abruption. The baseline uterine tone is elevated, making the documentation of contractions difficult, either by palpation or on external electronic fetal monitoring. When the fetal membranes are ruptured, the amniotic fluid is often bloody and is referred to as *port wine*–stained amniotic fluid.

C. **Laboratory examination and diagnostic procedures**
   1. **Laboratory evaluation.** A baseline complete blood count and platelet count, and electrolytes levels should be obtained.
   2. **Coagulation evaluation.** Because the most common cause of consumptive coagulopathy during pregnancy is abruptio placentae, a serum fibrinogen level should be obtained on admission and followed serially. Other coagulation parameters should be obtained if the fribrinogen level is low or falling. Quantitative platelet counts are also useful in assessing the maternal status. Obviously pathologic levels of fibrin split products are found in all cases of severe placental abruption. The coagulopathy that results from abruptio placentae occurs intravascularly and, to a much lesser degree, retroplacentally.
   3. **Fetomaternal bleeding and Rh isoimmunization.** Severe fetomaternal bleeding may occur as a result of premature placental separation, although it is uncommon. A Kleihauer-Betke stain is helpful to quantify the extent of exchange. Appropriate doses of Rh immune globulin (RhoGAM) should be given as indicated.
   4. **Blood bank.** Blood products, including packed red blood cells and fresh frozen plasma, should be crossmatched when the diagnosis is strongly suspected.
   5. **Ultrasound.** Ultrasound examination is not usually diagnostic of abruptio placentae; in fact, a retroplacental hematoma

is seen rarely. A negative ultrasound examination does not exclude a life-threatening abruptio placentae, but it should be performed when the mother and fetus are stable to rule out placenta previa.

VII. Management

A. **Initial management.** In cases of suspected abruptio placenta, immediate hospitalization is mandatory because of the life-threatening risks to the mother and fetus. The following immediate therapy to safeguard the mother and fetus is required:

1. **Immediate and continued evaluation of fetal status.** If the fetus is alive on admission, any delay in fetal evaluation may have disastrous consequences. Perinatal death occurs after hospitalization but before delivery in over 20 percent of these deaths, with 30 percent of these deaths occurring within the first 2 h after admission. If there is a question about the presence of fetal heart activity on external electronic fetal monitoring, one of two procedures to determine if the fetus is alive should be performed immediately. Ultrasound can be used to determine the presence or absence of fetal heart activity, and the rate may be determined by an experienced ultrasonographer. If the cervix is dilated sufficiently and the obstetric situation warrants, artificial rupture of membranes may be performed and a scalp electrode placed for direct fetal heart monitoring. The latter maneuver, however, commits the patient to delivery and therefore should be performed only after a rapid consideration of the total clinical situation.

2. **Oxygen.** Oxygen by face mask at a 6- to 8-L flow rate should be started immediately, as there is presumed impairment of the fetoplacental unit.

3. **Fluid management.** A large-bore (14- or 16-gauge needle) intravenous line should be placed immediately and normal saline, lactated Ringer's solution (LR), or lactated Ringer's solution with dextrose (D5LR) infused, depending on the clinical situation and the patient's hemodynamic status. The patient should be aggressively treated for shock, if present, or for impending shock.

B. **Obstetric management**

1. **Method and timing of delivery.** The method and timing of delivery depend on the extent of placental separation, the condition of the mother and fetus, and the status of the cervix (see Table 26.1). In the face of fetal immaturity and mild separation, an expectant approach may be elected. However, if the clinical condition suggests moderate to severe abruption, prompt delivery is indicated. Generally, amniotomy and direct fetal monitoring is the first step. Oxytocin may be necessary to augment uterine activity, but it must be used cautiously since the uterine response is often unpredictable. Cesarean section should be performed as

necessitated by fetal compromise unless contraindicated by the maternal condition. If fetal death has already occurred, vaginal delivery is indicated to reduce potential maternal morbidity.

2. **General management considerations.** The major complications of abruptio placentae are related to blood loss, shock, and coagulopathy. Therefore, aggressive replacement of blood, blood products, and crystalloids is mandatory. In severe abruption, blood may be forced into the myometrium. The uterus appears bruised and edematous and has been described as a *couvelaire uterus*. Hysterectomy is occasionally necessary in these cases due to poor uterine contractile force. Placement of a Foley catheter and hourly assessment of urinary output are helpful to determine the adequacy of blood replacement and/or renal perfusion.

VIII. Prognosis. The likelihood of maternal survival is high, but morbidity depends on the extent of blood loss and the aggressiveness of replacement. Fetal survival obviously depends on gestational age, blood loss, and hypoxia resulting from the loss of placental exchange surface.

BIBLIOGRAPHY

Abdella TN, Sibai BM, Hays JM, et al. Perinatal outcome in abruptio placentae. Obstet Gynecol 1984; 63:365.

Comeau J, Shaw L, Marcell CC, et al. Early placenta previa and delivery outcome. Obstet Gynecol 1983; 61:577.

Cotton DB, Read JA, Paul RH, et al. The conservative aggressive management of placenta previa. Am J Obstet Gynecol 1980; 137:687.

Hurd WW, Miodovnik M, Hertzberg V, et al. Selective management of abruptio placentae: A prospective study. Obstet Gynecol 1983; 61:467.

Naeye RL, Harkness WL, Utts J. Abruptio placentae and perinatal death: A prospective study. Am J Obstet Gynecol 1977; 128:740.

Varma TR. Fetal growth and placental function in patients with placenta previa. J Obstet Gynaecol Br Commonw 1973; 80:311.

Wexler P, Gottesfeld KR. Second trimester placenta previa: An apparently normal placentation. Obstet Gynecol 1977; 50:706.

CHAPTER 27

Postpartum Hemorrhage

Peter A. Grannum

Postpartum hemorrhage is one of the major causes of morbidity and mortality in obstetrics. It is defined as blood loss in excess of 500 mL at the time of delivery. Blood loss exceeding 1500 mL at the time of delivery is considered massive postpartum hemorrhage. Postpartum hemorrhage can be further defined as (1) **early,** occurring in the first 24 h, or (2) **delayed,** occurring after 24 h. Delayed postpartum hemorrhage occurs most often between the 6th and 10th day after delivery. It should be noted that even though a blood loss of 500 mL or more technically constitutes a postpartum hemorrhage, almost half of all women delivered vaginally lose more than this amount. Since the blood volume of the pregnant woman increases by almost 50 percent, blood losses in excess of 500 mL are usually well tolerated at delivery, although the definition persists.

I. **Incidence.** Postpartum hemorrhage is the most common cause of serious blood loss associated with pregnancy. Based on an estimated blood loss significantly greater than 500 mL, it is thought to occur in approximately 5 percent of deliveries. In a recent series, postpartum hemorrhage accounted for 24 percent of all obstetric deaths.

II. **Cause**
   A. **Early postpartum hemorrhage.** The most frequent causes of early postpartum hemorrhage are (1) uterine atony or hypotonic myometrium, (2) lacerations of the cervix and vagina, and (3) retained placental fragments. Other causes include uterine rupture; uterine inversion; placenta accreta, increta, or percreta; and a poorly performed or repaired episiotomy.
   B. **Late or delayed postpartum hemorrhage.** Late or delayed postpartum hemorrhage is most often a result of retained products of conception, reinjury of a recognized or unrecognized obstetric injury (e.g., rupture of a vulvar or vaginal hematoma at the time of resumption of sexual intercourse postpartum), or cervical lacerations. Abnormal penetration into the myometrium by the placenta, as in placenta accreta, increta, or percreta, can lead to retained products. The removal of such retained products may

be quite difficult compared to removal of simple retained products left by failure to examine the placenta and uterus after delivery.

C. Factors associated with early and late postpartum hemorrhage

1. Genital tract trauma
   a. Lacerations of the perineum, vagina, or cervix
   b. Large episiotomy
   c. Ruptured uterus
   d. Isochiorectal hematoma
2. Hemostatic failure at the placenta site
   a. Hypotonic myometrium (atony)
      (1) General anesthesia
      (2) Poorly perfused myometrium (hypotension from hemorrhage or conduction or general anesthesia)
      (3) Multiple pregnancy
      (4) Polyhydramnios
      (5) Prolonged labor
      (6) Rapid, precipitous labor
      (7) Labor following vigorous oxytocin stimulation
      (8) High parity
      (9) Previous hemorrhage from uterine atony
      (10) Uterine infection
   b. Retained placental fragments
      (1) Placenta acreta, increta, and percreta
      (2) Succenturiate lobe
   c. Coagulation defects
3. Uterine inversion

III. Pathogenesis

A. Problems with uterine contraction. Normally after delivery of the infant, the uterus contracts, effecting placental separation by the development of a cleavage plane along the decidua basalis. The placenta is usually completely separated within the first few uterine contractions, although several contractions, along with expulsive bearing-down efforts by the mother, may be necessary to expel the placenta from the uterus. Following the separation of the placenta, large venous sinuses become patent. The bleeding from these sinuses is controlled by contractions of the uterine musculature about the sinuses, which closes them, and by thrombosis formation within the lumen of the sinuses. Conditions that lead to poor uterine contractility, such as an overdistended uterus, prolonged labor, or prolonged oxytocin stimulation, significantly increase the chances for postpartum hemorrhage.

B. Problems with uterine integrity. Laceration of the cervix or vagina and laceration or rupture of the uterine corpus, as a result of either a uterine scar or an operative obstetric procedure, are causes of postpartum hemorrhage. Operative vaginal deliveries are a frequent cause. Careful inspection of the cervix and vagina is essential in these situations. Vulvar trauma with development of a hematoma must also be recognized and treated.

IV. **Morbidity and mortality.** The complications of postpartum hemorrhage include hypovolemic shock, anemia, transfusion reactions, Sheehan's syndrome, and Asherman's syndrome.
  A. **Hypovolemic shock and anemia (and transfusion reactions).** Failure to recognize postpartum hemorrhage, and institute methods for the treatment of hypovolemic shock and reduction of blood loss may lead to maternal death. While transfusion of properly crossmatched blood is relatively safe, the possibility of transfusion complications such as transfusion reaction, contamination with hepatitis virus or other agents, and sensitization makes avoidance of transfusion the best choice.
  B. **Sheehan's syndrome.** Sheehan's syndrome is the development of hypopituitarism due to pituitary necrosis. It results from the spasticity or thrombosis of the portal vasculature secondary to rapid postpartum hemorrhage. Failure to lactate is a consistent finding and the earliest to appear.
  C. **Asherman's syndrome.** Asherman's syndrome may develop after vigorous and aggressive curettage of the uterus in an attempt to control bleeding. It is characterized by the development of extensive adhesions of the uterine cavity. Failure to menstruate after a postpartum hemorrhage should alert the physician to consider this syndrome, which is associated with chronic pelvic pain and infertility.

V. **Diagnosis**
  A. **Signs and symptoms.** Postpartum hemorrhage is usually diagnosed by the **onset of heavy bleeding following delivery of the infant.** The effect of the blood loss on the patient is dependent on the predelivery hematocrit and blood volume and on the degree of anemia that ensues from the postpartum hemorrhage. **The patient may appear pale and sweaty and may have cold, clammy skin, or she may initially appear relatively normal. If blood loss is massive, loss of consciousness may occur.** Assessment of blood loss by visual inspection is usually inaccurate. Several reports indicate that the assessment of blood loss by inspection is about half of the actual measured amount. Sometimes the blood loss in postpartum hemorrhage may not be rapid. Slow, steady blood loss may not be considered serious until the patient goes into hypovolemic shock. Careful examination of blood loss by experienced medical staff following delivery should be carried out, especially in a woman at high risk.
  B. **Physical diagnosis.** When the onset of postpartum hemorrhage is suspected on the basis of signs and symptoms, **blood pressure and pulse should** be taken immediately. A fall in blood pressure and a rising pulse may indicate the onset of severe hypovolemia. It is important to remember that a young woman's cardiovascular system may be able to compensate for a considerable loss of blood volume before her vital signs show a significant change. When such changes are manifest, she may have lost much more blood volume than a corresponding older patient who has suf-

fered a hemorrhage. In a patient with hypertension, a fall in blood pressure to the normotensive range may give a false sense of security in a situation in which a pressure that would be considered normal in other circumstances is markedly subnormal. It should also be noted that a rapid pulse rate may occur with an insignificant blood loss, or may remain normal or slow despite a brisk, steady blood loss. In these situations, severe hypovolemia may not be recognized until very late, a clinical situation to be avoided.

VI. **Management.** Once the fetus has been delivered, the uterine fundus should be palpated to determine its height and consistency. The fundus is easily palpable at about the level of the umbilicus or just below it by the abdominal hand. If the uterus is firm and no vaginal bleeding is noticed, uterine fundal massage is not necessary. The fundus should be examined frequently until the placenta is delivered. If the fundus is or becomes boggy or soft, gentle abdominal massage may be necessary to help the uterus become firm. After the placenta has been delivered and is thought to be complete, the fundus should be examined frequently for the first hour before the patient is transferred to the postpartum floor. The placenta and membranes should be carefully inspected after every delivery. If part of the placenta or membranes is unaccounted for, exploration of the uterine cavity is indicated.

If brisk bleeding occurs either before or after delivery of the placenta, the diagnosis of postpartum hemorrhage must be entertained and managed accordingly. Management of postpartum hemorrhage is divided into three categories: conservative (medical) management, surgical management, and intervention radiography. Conservative management should be attempted before resorting to either radiography or surgical modalities.

A. **Conservative management**
   1. **Management before delivery of the placenta**
      a. **If the fundus is boggy, the uterus should be massaged** until firm, using the abdominal hand.
      b. If the **signs of placental separation** are evident (globular uterus, sudden gush of blood, uterus "rising" into the abdomen, umbilical cord becoming slack), attempts should be made to delivery the placenta by **manual pressure on the fundus.**
      c. **If this is not successful and the bleeding continues, manual removal of the placenta** is mandatory. For this procedure, the fundus of the uterus is grasped by the abdominal hand. The vaginal hand is passed into the uterus along the umbilical cord. As soon as the placental margin is reached, the operator's fingers should attempt to develop a plane between the placenta and the decidua basalis. This process is continued until the entire placenta has been separated (Fig. 27.1). The placenta is then grasped by the uterine hand and slowly removed.

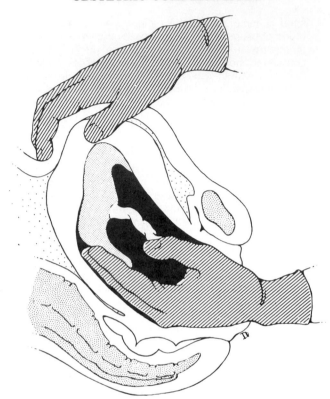

FIGURE 27.1. Manual removal of the placenta. The fingers are alternatively abducted, adducted, and advanced until the placenta is completely detached. (Reprinted with permission from Oxorn H. Human Labor and Birth. 5th ed. Norwalk, CT: Appleton-Century-Crofts; 1986:440.)

The membranes should be carefully teased off the uterine wall, using a sponge forceps if necessary to grasp the slippery membranes. A sponge held in or spread over the examining hand may then be used to wipe the uterine cavity free of remaining membranes. If bleeding persists, it is necessry to proceed to the next steps in conservative management.

2. **Initial management after delivery of the placenta.** After delivery of the placenta, the fundus should be palpated frequently. If the fundus is boggy and does not respond to vigorous abdominal massage, pharmacologic treatment and/ or bimanual palpation should be instituted. Precautionary measures such as the cross-matching of blood and a call for anesthesia support should be made early in the evaluation

and care of a patient with postpartum hemorrhage, as the sequence of events may be rapid and delays often cause serious problems.

a. **Initial pharmacologic treatment.** Initial treatment with oxytocic drugs, causing the uterus to contract, is common therapy. Some institutions have protocols that call for the routine administration of **methylergonovine (Methergine), 0.2 mg IM.** In other institutions, 20 U of **oxytocin** in 1000 mL of Ringer's lactate solution is administered IV at an infusion rate of 100 to 200 mL/h, depending on the clinical situation. If heavy bleeding continues after these measures, bimanual compression and other precautions should be begun.

b. **Bimanual uterine compression.** The abdominal hand is used to grasp the posterior aspect of the uterus, and the fist of the vaginal hand compresses the anterior wall of the uterus. This maneuver should initiate uterine contractions and usually controls most bleeding. (see Fig. 27.2).

c. **Precautionary measures early in the evaluation/treatment sequence for postpartum hemorrhage.** If bleeding continues despite oxytocin administration and bimanual uterine compression, the first step is to **obtain help,** which should include an anesthesiologist in case anesthesia is needed for uterine exploration or surgery. **IV access** if not already in place, should be obtained, preferably using a large-bore (16-gauge) needle. A small-bore needle or catheter may not be able to support the infusion rates of fluid and/or blood needed to manage a brisk postpartum hemorrhage. If a small-bore needle or catheter is in place, consideration should be given to starting a second IV line with a large-bore needle or catheter. A **complete blood count** and blood sample for **type and crossmatch** of at least 2 U of blood should be sent to the blood bank.

3. **Continued management after delivery of the placenta**

a. **Blood transfusion.** Blood transfusions may be begun in the presence of a falling blood pressure, thready rapid pulse, and/or heavy vaginal bleeding. The blood type of all pregnant patients should be known from the time of the first prenatal visit. In patients at risk for postpartum hemorrhage, such as overdistended uterus or prolonged oxytocin stimulation, or a previous history of postpartum hemorrhage, blood for typing and screening and a hematocrit should be requested on admission to the labor floor. If blood is not already crossmatched, non-crossmatched, type-specific blood may be given in an emergency situation when the risks of such transfusion are felt to be less than those caused by a delay in transfusion.

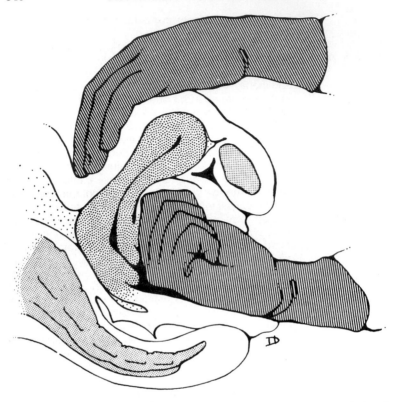

FIGURE 27.2 Bimanual compression of the uterus and massage with the abdominal hand usually will effectively control hemorrhage from uterine atony. (Reprinted with permission from Oxorn H. Human Labor and Birth. 5th ed. Norwalk, CT: Appleton-Century-Crofts; 1986:402.)

   b.   **Examination of the vulva, vagina, and cervix.** If vaginal bleeding persists despite a firm and contracted uterus, lacerations of the cervix and vagina should be suspected. They are more likely to occur following difficult operative vaginal deliveries or a precipitous, uncontrolled delivery, although it is certainly possible to sustain lacerations in a normal, spontaneous vaginal delivery. The vulva can be examined by inspection. The vagina and cervix can be easily inspected using a sponge on a ring forceps to elevate the cervix and allow a complete inspection of the vaginal mucosa, including the **fornices.** Lacerations of the vagina and cervix should be repaired after administration of proper anesthesia, usually a local or pudendal block, although general anesthesia may be required when the patient cannot remain still or is too uncomfortable with local anesthesia to allow surgical repair.

c. **Uterine exploration.** Uterine exploration is required if postpartum hemorrhage continues to ascertain if there are retained placental fragments or if there is trauma to the uterus itself. Uterine exploration requires manual skills that are developed with experience and a patient who is able to remain still during the examination. Anesthesia may be required to help the patient with the latter task, although the risk of anesthesia must be quickly weighed against the severity of the clinical situation. Although **retained placental fragments** are more usually a cause of late hemorrhage, they can cause immediate hemorrhage. If inspection of the placenta demonstrates a missing fragment, manual uterine exploration, or occasionally curettage with a blunt currette, or both should be performed to ensure complete evacuation. A succenturate lobe or placental polyp is part of the differential diagnosis and may be discovered as the cause of the postpartum hemorrhage in some cases. **Uterine perforation or rupture** is a rare cause of hemorrhage but may be discovered on careful examination of the intrauterine cavity. If a perforated or ruptured uterus is discovered in association with a postpartum hemorrhage, a laparotomy is mandatory to effect uterine repair and control bleeding. Occasionally a hysterectomy may be the only choice of treatment for a ruptured uterus.

d. **Oxytocic drug administration.** Oxytocics are administered in this clinical situation immediately upon suspicion of postpartum hemorrhage. Continued use of oxytocics may be required if hemorrhage continues. Ocytocics are drugs that cause the uterus to contract. **Oxytocin** (or syntocinon or pitocin, synthetic forms of the octapeptide oxytocin) is administered IV. It is usually given by adding 20 U of oxytocin to 1 L of Ringer's lactate solution or normal saline and administered at a rate of 10 mL/min. If bleeding persists or becomes heavier, this may be increased to 40 U in 1 L. After the uterus has become firm and the bleeding reduced significantly, the rate may be reduced to 1 to 2 mL/min until the patient is transferred to the postpartum floor. Oxytocin should not be given as a bolus IV since a fall in blood pressure or cardiac arrhythmias may result. In a patient who is already hypovolemic or has cardiac compromise, this may precipitate further deterioration in her condition. If bleeding persists despite oxytocin administration, Methylergonavine (Methergine), 0.2 mg IM or IV, should be administered. (**Note:** Women with hypertension should receive oxytocin first, since the ergot alkaloids [Methergine] may cause hypertension or exacerbation of preexisting hypertension.) If no effect is obtained and the uterus remains boggy with continued hemorrhage, prostaglandins may be given.

e. **Prostaglandins.** If uterine bleeding persists despite mechanical manipulation of the uterus and oxytocic drug administration, prostaglandins should be administered before proceeding to a surgical approach. Prostaglandins may be administered by IM or intramyometrial routes. 15 Methyl F2a (carbaprost, Hemabate), 0.25 mg, injected intramyometrially or IM, has been reported to be successful. (**Note:** The side effects of prostaglandins are significant and include nausea, vomiting, diarrhea, headache, fever, and chills. Perhaps the most significant side effect is transient diastolic hypertension, which would be contraindicated in the hypertensive and toxemic patient.)

B. **Surgical management.** The indication for surgical control of postpartum hemorrhage is primarily based on the failure of conservative measures and the failure or nonapplicability of intervention radiography methods.

1. **Uterine, ovarian, and hypogastric artery ligations** (Figs. 27.3 and 27.4). Uterine, ovarian, and hypogastric artery ligations are surgical methods used to control postpartum hemorrhage. Some surgeons suggest going directly to a bi-

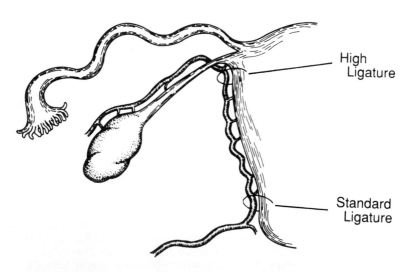

High Ligature

Standard Ligature

FIGURE 27.3 Technique of uterine artery ligation. (From Gleicher N. Principles and Practice of Medical Therapy in Pregnancy. 2nd ed. Norwalk, CT: Appleton & Lange; 1992:1266. Reprinted with permission.)

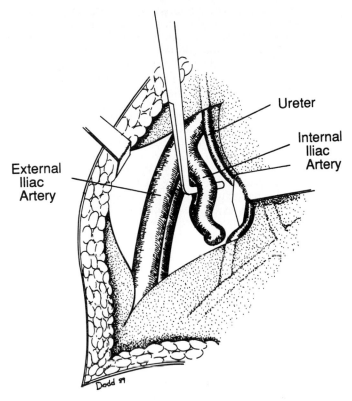

FIGURE 27.4 Technique of internal iliac (hypogastric) artery ligation. (From Gleicher N. Principles and Practice of Medical Therapy in Pregnancy. 2nd ed. Norwalk, CT: Appleton & Lange; 1992:1266. Reprinted with permission.)

lateral hypogastric ligation in an effort to reduce pulse pressure in the pelvic arteries, thereby accelerating coagulation and reduce bleeding. Uterine artery ligation has been reported to control bleeding in some patients with uterine atony. With the addition of bilateral ovarian artery ligation, persistent bleeding may be controlled without sacrificing the adnexa or uterus. In women who have had uterine, ovarian, and hypogastric artery ligations, successful pregnancies have been reported. One series (O'Leary) reported 12 patients out of a group of 110 who had previously undergone bilateral uterine artery ligation, who successfully carried a pregnancy. Before performing arterial ligation, patients should be counseled about the possibility of hysterectomy. The decisions about what specific procedure or procedures to perform should be made on an individual case basis by an experienced gynecologist.

2. **Hysterectomy.** If bleeding persists despite arterial ligation, a hysterectomy may be necessary to save the mother's life. With the changes in anatomy brought about by pregnancy (stretched cervix and lower uterine segment, enlarged blood vessels, a ureter that may be deviated from its normal position), special care must be taken in performing the surgical procedure to avoid damage to adjacent structures. Because the procedure is done under emergency circumstances, there is pressure to proceed rapidly, which compounds the surgical problem described. Considerable surgical skill and judgment are required in this emergency situation. A **supracervical hysterectomy** will usually suffice to control the bleeding, although a total hysterectomy is thought by many authorities to be the procedure of choice if time and the patient's clinical status permit.

C. **Selective pelvic artery embolization.** If conservative measures fail to control postpartum hemorrhage, invasive or surgical methods may become necessary. While surgery remains the treatment of choice in situations in which rapid clinical deterioration is occurring, if the patient's condition can be stabilized, selective pelvic artery embolization can be extremely helpful in controlling bleeding. However, it should be performed only by skilled arteriographers. With the development of arteriography as a subspecialty of radiography, catheterization of arteries such as the uterine branches of the internal iliac arteries can be safely achieved. Under fluoroscopy and with the use of contrast medium, the catheter can be directed to selected arteries and the site of extravasation visualized. The artery is then embolized using a surgical gelatin sponge (Gelfoam). Gelfoam injected into arteries causes thrombosis and forms a mechanical obstruction. This substance has been used for many years as a hemostatic material during surgery. The procedure may need to be repeated bilaterally if necessary to control bleeding.

1. **Advantages of the technique.** The advantages of using selective arterial embolization include the following: (a) it may be much easier to identify vessels under fluoroscopy prior to surgical intervention; (b) the bleeding sites may be difficult to identify at surgery; (c) a hysterectomy may be avoided; and (d) the risk of injury to the uterus, bladder, or bowel will be avoided.

2. **Complications of the technique.** Complications include (a) necrosis in the tissue supplied by that artery; (b) contrast medium toxicity to the kidneys; and (c) reflex of emboli back along a nontargeted artery, causing necrosis in a critical organ. The risks and benefits must be carefully examined with each patient.

BIBLIOGRAPHY

Burchell RC. Physiology of internal iliac artery ligation. J Obstet Gynaecol Br Commonw 1968; 75:642.

Clark SL, Phelan JP, Yeh SY, et al. Hypogastric artery ligation for obstetric hemorrhage. Obstet Gynecol 1985; 66:353.

Hayashi RH, Castillo MS, Noah ML. Management of severe postpartum hemorrhage due to uterine study using an analogue of prostaglandin $F_2\alpha$. Obstet Gynecol 1981; 58:426.

O'Leary JL, O'Leary JA. Uterine artery ligation in the control of intractable postpartum hemorrhage. Am J Obstet Gynecol 1966; 94:7.

Pritchard JA, Baldwin RM, Dickey JC, et al. Blood volume changes in pregnancy and the puerperium. Am J Obstet Gynecol 1962; 84:1271.

Part V

Medical and Surgical Complications in Pregnancy

CHAPTER 28

Cardiovascular and Thromboembolic Diseases

Jeffrey C. King

The successful outcome of pregnancy depends upon significant adaptation and alteration in the cardiovascular system. The presence of maternal cardiac disease may substantially interfere with the adaptive process, resulting in a detrimental effect on the mother, fetus, or both. The physiologic alterations of pregnancy may present a burden to women with known cardiac disease or exacerbate underlying cardiac disorders, causing them to progress to a clinically symptomatic or even lethal condition. Although the incidence of heart disease has declined dramatically in recent years, it is estimated to occur in approximately 1 percent of pregnant women. It is one of the four major causes of maternal mortality. Rheumatic fever previously accounted for the great majority of cases, but congenital heart disease is now seen more frequently. Because of advances in diagnostic and therapeutic procedures, survival for patients with congenital heart disease to reproductive age has become the rule rather than the exception.

Thromboembolic disease (especially pulmonary embolism) remains a major cause of morbidity and mortality during the childbearing period. An understanding of venous thromboembolic disorders is particularly important to the obstetrician because many thromboembolic events can be prevented. Between 5 and 30 percent of obstetric patients manifest some peripheral or central venous disorder during pregnancy. Pregnancy predisposes the patient to thromboembolic disease because of venous stasis and alterations in the coagulation system.

CARDIOVASCULAR DISEASE

I. **Classification of patients with cardiovascular disease.** It is impossible to determine the functional capacity and reserve of the heart accurately by noninvasive means. The use of invasive means in pregnancy, however, is fraught with dangers for the mother and fetus, and unless absolutely necessary, such maneuvers should be avoided. A useful clinical classification that avoids invasive diagnostic maneuvers has been provided by the New York Heart Association based on the patient's past and present disability and is not influenced by the presences or absence of physical signs.

Class I — Uncompromised: patients with cardiac disease but with no limitation of physical activity.

Class II — Slightly compromised: patients with cardiac disease and slight limitation of physical activity. They are comfortable at rest, but if ordinary physical activity is undertaken, discomfort results in the form of fatigue, palpitations, dyspnea, or anginal pain.

Class III — Markedly compromised: patients with cardiac disease and marked limitation of physical activity. They are comfortable at rest, but less than normal activity results in discomfort.

Class IV — Severely compromised: patients with cardiac disease who are unable to perform any physical activity without discomfort.

II. **Physiologic changes of the cardiovascular system in pregnancy**

A. **Blood volume.** There is a rapid expansion of total circulating blood volume during normal gestation to an increase of ~ 45 percent over the nonpregnant volume. Blood volume is made up of both plasma and red blood cell volume. The plasma begins to increase at 6 to 8 weeks of gestation and is 1200 to 1300 mL higher than the nonpregnant volume by 30 to 34 weeks. This increase then plateaus or decreases slightly until term. The red blood cell mass begins to expand after the increase in plasma volume and reaches 250 to 450 mL over the nonpregnant level, an increase of 20 to 30 percent. Since the percentage increase in plasma volume is greater than that of the red blood cell volume, a mild dilutional decrease in hemoglobin and hematocrit values is often found.

B. **Heart rate.** A gradual rise in the heart rate of 10 to 15 beats per min occurs during pregnancy. However, at term, heart rates greater than 90 beats per min in the supine or sitting position require an explanation other than pregnancy. In twin gestations, there is a greater increase in maternal heart rate than in singleton pregnancy: 40 vs. 21 percent.

C. **Stroke volume.** During the first half of pregnancy, an increase in the stroke volume to ~ 95 mL per beat occurs. Subsequently, there is a gradual decline to 70 mL per beat at term, which approximates the nonpregnant stroke volume.

D. **Cardiac output.** During pregnancy, there is a 30 to 50 percent increase in cardiac output, with an appreciable portion of the increase occurring prior to 20 weeks of gestation. The latter portion of pregnancy is characterized by variable cardiac output, with some women exhibiting a slight decrease. Measurements of cardiac output should be made with the patient in the left lateral recumbent position to avoid aortic/vena cava compression. Alterations of cardiac output caused by the supine position affect stroke volume rather than heart rate.

E. **Arterial blood pressure.** The **systolic pressure** is decreased in both the supine and left lateral recumbent positions during the entire pregnancy. At 32 weeks, the decrease is greater in the lateral recumbent position, reaching a nadir of 101 mm Hg, or 10 mm Hg below nonpregnant values. Similarly, the **diastolic pressure** is noted to decrease in both the supine and lateral recumbent positions. In the lateral recumbent position, the diastolic pressure decreases from 58 mm Hg in the nonpregnant state to about 45 mm Hg at 32 weeks. During the last 4 weeks of pregnancy, there is a sharp increase in the diastolic pressure taken in the left lateral position recumbent to within 4 mm Hg of the nonpregnant values.

F. **Systemic vascular resistance.** The slight decrease in arterial pressure and the marked increase in cardiac output result from a significant decrease in systemic vascular resistance. The uteroplacental circulation, with its low resistance, plays a major role in affecting systemic vascular resistance.

III. **Alterations in the cardiovascular system during labor and delivery.** Uterine contractions lead to a rise in central venous pressure caused by an increase in venous return to the heart. A rise in cardiac output is noted during the first stage of labor, the exact extent depending on the method of analgesia used. During the second stage, maternal bearing-down efforts can result in marked alteration of hemodynamic status. While the normal parturient easily tolerates these changes, the patient with moderate to severe heart disease should avoid bearing down because of its effect on venous return.

IV. **General management guidelines for cardiovascular disease in pregnancy.** The treatment of heart disease during pregnancy is dictated by the estimated functional capacity of the heart. A **multidisciplinary team approach to the management of pregnancy complicated by heart disease is essential.** An **obstetrician** and a **cardiologist** familiar with the hemodynamic changes of pregnancy are the basic members of the team. An obstetric anesthesiologist should be consulted during the antepartum period in order to contribute to the intrapartum management plan.

A. **Prenatal care**
   1. **Diet.** Adequate but not excessive nutritional intake is extremely important in the management of pregnant patients with cardiovascular disease. In order to avoid excessive weight gain, which places undue stress on the cardiovascular system, patients should be encouraged to limit their weight gain while maintaining a diet that is well balanced. A diet that eliminates table salt and food containing large amounts of salt (i.e., limiting salt intake to approximately 2 to 4 g/d) is appropriate for most cardiac patients.
   2. **Activity.** Patients with cardiac disease are known to be less tolerant of exercise during pregnancy. Therefore physical exertion should be restricted or eliminated if symptoms de-

velop. However, if the patient can tolerate mild forms of activity such as walking without the development of symptoms, such activity should be encouraged.

3. **Counseling.** Patients with congenital heart disease, either corrected or uncorrected, should be informed of the 3 to 5 percent risk that the fetus will develop a congenital heart defect. For some women with especially dangerous cardiac diseases such as cardiomyopathy, primary pulmonary hypertension, Marfan's syndrome, or Eisenmenger's syndrome, therapeutic abortion should be offered as a safer option than continuing pregnancy. Termination of pregnancy by suction curettage prior to 14 weeks of gestation places the patient at minimal risk. Beyond this stage, the new abortifacients, prostaglandins E_2 and F_2, are very successful for second-trimester evacuation of the uterus. However, these agents have significant cardiovascular side effects and should be used with extreme caution in women with cardiac disease.

4. **Drugs**
   a. **Quinidine and cardiac glycosides.** These drugs are not known to have any apparent teratogenic effects or to cause any problems with the developing fetus. They can usually be continued under proper medical supervision.
   b. **Anticoagulants.** Oral anticoagulants (e.g., warfarin) are potential teratogens when given during the first trimester of pregnancy. The *fetal warfarin syndrome* consists of nasal hypoplasia, optic atrophy, stippled epiphyses, and mental retardation and may occur in 15 to 25 percent of cases. Although pregnancy can be undertaken by a patient who is using oral anticoagulants, heparin is a safer alternative for both the mother and fetus. **Heparin** does not cross the placenta and has a short half-life, making it the anticoagulant of choice; however, the economic disadvantages of long-term parental heparin therapy are not trivial. In addition, long-term heparin therapy is associated with osteopenia, which is dose dependent.
   c. **Beta-adrenergic blockers.** The use of propranolol or other beta blockers during pregnancy needs further study because of their reported association with growth retardation, preterm labor and neonatal respiratory depression, bradycardia, and hypoglycemia. However, these drugs can be used if necessary with appropriate monitoring.
   d. **Thiazide diuretics.** These may produce harmful fetal effects especially if therapy is initiated in the third trimester, including severe electrolyte imbalance, jaundice, thrombocytopenia, liver damage, and even neonatal death. However, they are a mainstay in the treatment of congestive heart failure.

B. Intrapartum care

1. **Management of labor.** Spontaneous labor at term should be allowed for all cardiac patients, with the exception of those who are unstable. General anesthesia or segmental epidural analgesia is usually well tolerated to prevent prolonged Valsalva maneuvers and their associated hemodynamic changes. Patients should have the hemodynamically stressful second stage shortened by the use of outlet forceps or vacuum extraction. The parturient should be monitored by a continuous electrocardiogram (ECG) during labor and the early postpartum period. The use of an invasive Swan-Ganz catheter has been suggested to monitor cardiac output and chamber pressures and may be indicated in some patients, depending on the individual clinical situation. The decision to use such invasive measures is made by the multidisciplinary team.

2. **Antibiotic prophylaxis for bacterial endocarditis.** To prevent bacterial endocarditis, antibiotics should be used in patients with valvular abnormalities, congenital defects, or a prosthetic valve. Protection against gram-negative organisms is essential (Table 28.1).

V. Congenital heart disease in pregnancy

A. **Left-to-right shunts**

1. **Atrial septal defects (ASDs).** An ostium secundum defect is more common in women than in men. The defect is usually asymptomatic, and pregnancy is usually well tolerated. Prophylactic antibiotics are probably not necessary since bacterial endocarditis is rare. If either parent or a sibling has an

Table 28.1. American Heart Association Recommendations for Prevention of Bacterial Endocarditis in Patients Undergoing Genitourinary Procedures

DRUG	DOSAGE REGIMEN
	STANDARD REGIMEN
Ampicillin, gentamycin, and amoxicillin	IV or IM administration of ampicillin, 2.0 g, plus gentamycin, 1.5 mg/h (not to exceed 80 mg), 30 min before procedure; followed by amoxicillin, 1.5 g orally 6 h later, or repeat parental regimen 8 h after initial dose
	PENICILLIN ALTERNATE REGIMEN
Vancomycin and gentamycin	IV administration of vancomycin, 1.0 g over 1 h, plus IV or IM administration of gentamycin, 1.5 mg/h (not to exceed 80 mg), 1 h before procedure; repeat 8 h after initial dose.

Source: Dajani AS, Bisno AL, Chung KJ, et al. Prevention of bacterial endocarditis. JAMA 1990; 264(22): 2921. Copyright 1990, American Medical Association.

ASD, the risk for the child developing the same lesion is 2.5 percent.

2. **Ventricular septal defects (VSDs).** These defects are more common than ASDs, but more than half of them close spontaneously during childhood. If the defect persists, surgical correction is usually performed before the child reaches the reproductive age. While most patients with a VSD tolerate pregnancy well, if pulmonary hypertension exists the risk of pregnancy may be substantial. Prophylactic antibiotics are necessary because these patients are predisposed to bacterial endocarditis. There is a 3 to 4 percent risk of developing a VSD if a parent or sibling has the anomaly.

3. **Patent ductus arteriosus (PDA).** PDA is usually recognized and corrected in childhood; however, pregnancy is well tolerated when the condition is uncomplicated. However, if pulmonary hypertension develops, the risk of pregnancy is significant. Prophylactic antibiotics are indicated. The child of a parent with this lesion has a 4 percent chance of having the same defect and a 3 percent risk if a sibling had the anomaly.

B. **Right-to-left shunts**
   1. **Tetralogy of Fallot.** Affected patients have been cyanotic since childhood and suffer from dyspnea, tachypnea, or loss of consciousness. If the lesion has been totally corrected surgically, pregnancy does not represent an increased risk. If it has not been corrected, there is an increased risk of maternal as well as fetal mortality and morbidity. During labor and delivery and in the immediate postpartum period, antibiotic prophylaxis should be used and careful attention to maintaining venous return is essential. The fetal risk is 4 percent if a parent has the lesion and 2.5 percent if a sibling is affected.

   2. **Eisenmenger's syndrome** This condition is not surgically correctable and is characterized by right to left or bidirectional shunting plus high pulmonary vascular resistance. The maternal mortality ranges from 30 to 70 percent, depending on the degree of pulmonary hypertension. Maintenance of venous return is extremely important. Maternal death may occur at any time during pregnancy and usually results from an arrhythmia. Fetal survival is usually < 50 percent. Because these patients are at increased risk of pulmonary thrombosis, postpartum anticoagulation is recommended, along with prophylactic antibiotics. Because of the high maternal and fetal mortality associated with Eisenmenger's syndrome, therapeutic termination of pregnancy should be recommended.

   3. **Coarctation of the aorta.** The major risks for the pregnant patient with coarctation of the aorta are aortic dissection, bacterial endocarditis, cerebral hemorrhage, and complications of a long-standing hypertension. Maternal mortality ranges from 3 to 8 percent, with the highest value in

women with a bicuspid aortic value. Coarctation of the aorta in association with pregnancy is fortunately rare. If it occurs, control of hypertension and prophylactic antibiotics constitute the treatment plan. Surgical correction of a coarctation prior to pregnancy is indicated, since pregnancies following successful correction are generally unremarkable. The risk that a fetus will develop this defect is 2 percent if either a parent or a sibling is affected.

VI. Acquired cardiac lesions and pregnancy

A. Mitral stenosis

1. **Pathophysiology and mortality.** The hemodynamic defect of mitral stenosis is obstruction to blood flow between the left atrium and ventricle. This results in a decrease in cardiac output, elevated left atrial pressure, and pulmonary vascular congestion. Generally, the valve area must be < 2 cm^2 for pulmonary edema to occur. The maternal death rate in patients with mitral stenosis is approximately 1 percent, but it is increased to 4 to 5 percent if there is significant functional impairment. In patients who develop atrial fibrillation, the maternal death rate reaches 14 to 17 percent.

2. **Management**
   a. Symptoms should be controlled by **limitation of activity and sodium restriction.** If pulmonary congestion develops, further limitation of activity and sodium intake along with **diuretic therapy** is indicated. **Digitalis** should be started if atrial fibrillation develops and should be continued to ensure a relatively slow ventricular rate in case atrial fibrillation recurs.
   b. **Antibiotic prophylaxis** for bacterial endocarditis is indicated.
   c. **Surgical intervention** should be reserved for those patients unresponsive to medical management. Mitral commissurotomy is associated with a 1 percent maternal mortality. If necessary, open heart surgery with valve replacement can be considered, but fetal loss is high.

B. Aortic stenosis.
Experience with this cardiac disease in pregnancy is limited. The maternal mortality associated with aortic stenosis is described as 17 percent. Generally, patients do well as long as the gradient between the aorta and left ventricle is < 100 mm Hg. Hypovolemia must be avoided to prevent circulatory collapse and cerebral/myocardial ischemia. If severe stenosis is discovered prior to conception, valve replacement or commissurotomy should be suggested. Antibiotic prophylaxis is recommended.

C. Cardiomyopathy.
The cause of cardiomyopathy is unknown. It occurs most commonly in older, black, multiparous women; in women with multiple gestation; and in women whose pregnancy has been complicated by hypertension. The main findings is myocardial failure with pulmonary edema. It is associated with a

15 to 50 percent maternal mortality and usually becomes evident in the postpartum period. Therapy includes sodium restriction, diuretics, digoxin, and limitation of activity. Swan-Ganz catheter placement at the time of labor may be beneficial. Heart size usually returns to normal during the puerperium, but if persistent cardiomegaly occurs, the long-term prognosis is poor and future pregnancy is contraindicated because of the high likelihood of recurrence. Some type of residual damage is found in 50 percent of survivors, which has been shown to shorten the life expectancy.

VII. Miscellaneous heart disease in pregnancy

A. Marfan's syndrome. Marfan's syndrome is an autosomal dominant abnormality of the connective tissue characterized by aneurysm of the aorta, ectopia lentis, and long extremities. Pregnancy is particularly dangerous for patients with this condition because of the high risk of aortic rupture and dissection. Echocardiac evaluation of aortic root size may be helpful in predicting which patients are at risk for aortic dissection. If the diagnosis is proven, pregnancy is contraindicated and interruption of the pregnancy should be recommended if the aortic root diameter is >40 mm. There is a 25 to 50 percent maternal mortality, an overall reduced maternal life span, and a 50 percent chance that the offspring will inherit the disease. If the pregnancy continues, therapy should be directed at reducing cardiac work by limiting physical activity, treating hypertension, and decreasing systolic forces on the aortic wall with beta blockers.

B. Mitral valve prolapse. Mitral valve prolapse is a commonly encountered condition, found in 5 to 10 percent of young adults, particularly pregnant women. A late systolic murmur, along with a middle to late systolic click, is very suggestive and can be confirmed by echocardiography. While arrhythmias, chest pain, syncope, and peripheral arterial emboli may develop, there is no evidence that pregnancy increases the likelihood of these complications. In most cases, the pregnancy is unremarkable. No specific treatment is necessary. The necessity for antibiotic prophylaxis is unclear; hence treatment is recommended. However, in cases with mitral regurgitation, it is definitely indicated.

C. Idiopathic hypertrophic subaortic stenosis (IHSS). This autosomal dominant trait with variable penetrance can result in significant aortic outflow tract obstruction. Pregnancy is generally not well tolerated because the normal fall in peripheral resistance in pregnancy results in increased outflow tract obstruction. This condition may result in syncope, congestive failure, chest or epigastric pain, or sudden death. Treatment is aimed at avoiding hypovolemia, maintaining venous return, and diminishing the force of myocardial contractility. Excessive blood loss must be treated promptly. Epidural anesthesia is often not tolerated because of the possible development of sympathetic blockade and relative hypovolemia. Antibiotic prophylaxis is recommended at delivery to reduce the risk of endocarditis.

D. **Myocardial infarction.** This rare condition in pregnant women is encountered in 1/10 000 deliveries. The increased usage of beta mimetics to treat preterm labor has resulted in many complaints of cardiac "trouble" or chest pain, but these are usually not infarctions. The overall mortality of true infarction is 29 percent, but the outcome is dependent on the duration of pregnancy and the extent of the damage. Management of an acute myocardial infarcton is the same as for nonpregnant patients (see Chapter 43). Pregnancy occurring more than 6 months after a myocardial infarction is generally well tolerated.

E. **Pregnancy subsequent to cardiac surgery.** Totally corrected cardiac lesions allow pregnancy to be undertaken with no increased risk to the mother or fetus (except the intrinsic risk of recurrence). However, partial correction by mitral commissurotomy or prosthetic valve placement remains problematic.

1. **Mitral commissurotomy.** The maternal mortality in pregnancy following commissurotomy is 2 to 3 percent, with 95 percent of these deaths occurring in the third trimester or early puerperium. Close medical supervision and antibiotic prophylaxis are essential. Digoxin and/or diuretics may be necessary to treat impending congestive heart failure.

2. **Prosthetic valves.** All patients with mechanical prosthetic valves require complete anticoagulation. Coumadin has been associated with the development of morphologic abnormalities of the fetus, so long-term heparin anticoagulation is suggested. Prophylactic antibiotics are required since the development of endocarditis is associated with a 40 percent mortality in these patients. Porcine heterograft valves have the same risk for endocarditis but do not require anticoagulation. Young women contemplating pregnancy should consider this type of valve prosthesis even though reoperation replacement may be necessary.

THROMBOEMBOLIC DISEASE

I. **Superficial thrombophlebitis.** Superficial thrombophlebitis is the most common thromboembolic disorder in pregnant patients, occurring in 1/622 antepartum patients and 1/95 patients following delivery. There is an increased frequency of superficial thrombophlebitis in patients with preexisting varicose veins but not in those undergoing cesarean delivery. The coexistence of a deep vein thrombosis with a superficial one must be considered.

A. **Diagnosis.** The diagnosis of superficial thrombophlebitis is usually clinically obvious, with an erythematous superficial vein accompanied by pain and tenderness along its course. Eighty-seven percent of superficial cases of thrombophlebitis occur in the first 72 h following delivery.

    B. Management. Since superficial thrombi rarely embolize, patients should be treated with bed rest, elevation of the limb, local heat, and mild analgesics (e.g., acetaminophen with codeine).
    C. Prognosis. Recovery is usually seen in 1 to 2 weeks.

II. Deep vein thrombosis (DVT). The incidence of DVT during pregnancy is unknown but is generally felt to be equal to or moderately greater than that in the nonpregnant state. However, the incidence rises dramatically following delivery, ranging from 0.15 to 3 percent. Postpartum DVT occurs more frequently in patients who have undergone a traumatic or complicated vaginal delivery or have been delivered by cesarean section. The differential diagnosis includes rupture of a Baker cyst, muscle strain or hematoma, arterial insufficiency, arthritis, lymphangitis, myositis, bone disease, varicose veins, and superficial thrombophlebitis.

    A. Diagnosis
      1. Signs and symptoms. Pain, tenderness, and swelling are classically described but have poor sensitivity and specificity.
      2. Physical examination. The clinical diagnosis is both insensitive and nonspecific.
        a. **Homan's sign** is present in 33 percent of symptomatic patients with documented DVT but in 50 percent of normal patients.
        b. An **asymmetric limb,** usually more than 2 cm greater than the other limb in circumference, may be noted.
        c. **Localized warmth** and **dependent cyanosis** are variably present.
      3. Laboratory examination and diagnostic procedures
        a. Venography remains the standard for the diagnosis of DVT.
        b. Noninvasive tests such as impedance plethysmography and pulsed Doppler ultrasound are usually reliable, but their accuracy is reduced by the physiologic changes of pregnancy.
        c. Compressibility of veins under real-time ultrasound visualization is emerging as a very accurate diagnostic procedure.
        d. When the diagnosis remains in question, normal **fibrinopeptide A or antithrombin III activity** rules out active thrombotic disease.
        e. The **platelet count** should be checked before and intermittently following institution of heparin therapy.
    B. Anticoagulation therapy. Heparin is the anticoagulant of choice during pregnancy. Two treatment regimens are available: continuous infusion or subcutaneous injection.
      1. By the **intravenous** route, a loading dose of 100 to 110 U/kg of heparin is given, followed by a continuous infusion of 1000 U/h. The partial thromboplastin time (PTT) should be monitored frequently to achieve a one and one-half- to

twofold prolongation over baseline for 7 to 10 days. Once stable prolongation is attained, the PTT need not be repeated more frequently than every 24 to 48 h. Heparin resistance suggests extensive thrombosis, while a dropping requirement suggests cessation of thrombin production. Following the acute therapy, treatment with subcutaneous heparin (10 000 to 20 000 U) every 12 h is suggested for the remainder of the pregnancy and until 6 weeks postpartum, with a minimum duration of 3 months. The goal of this therapy is to maintain the mid-interval PTT (6 hours) at one and one-half times normal.

2. By the **subcutaneous** route, a loading dose of 150 U/kg of heparin is given intravenously followed by 15 000 to 20 000 U of heparin every 12 h. The PTT should be checked at the mid-interval and maintained at one and one-half times normal. Subcutaneous heparin should be continued as noted above. Patients treated with subcutaneous heparin should be instructed not to inject the heparin dose once uterine contractions have developed.

C. **Prognosis.** Eighty percent of venous thrombi lyse spontaneously, but only twenty percent lyse completely.

D. **History of DVT.** Patients with a previous demonstrated DVT or pulmonary embolus, especially if it occurred during a pregnancy or while taking oral contraceptives, are candidates for prophylactic low-dose heparin (5000 U bid) during pregnancy and the pueperium.

III. **Pulmonary emboli (PE).** The incidence of clinically diagnosed nonfatal PE during pregnancy and the puerperium ranges from 0.5 to 12 per 1000 deliveries. While only 50 percent of patients with documented DVT are symptomatic, most clinically symptomatic emboli arise from a thrombus in the deep venous system of the thigh. The differential diagnosis includes muscle strain, acute anxiety, and atelectasis.

A. **Diagnosis**

1. **Signs and symptoms.** The clinical diagnosis of pulmonary embolism lacks sensitivity and specificity.

a. **Dyspnea** and **tachypnea** are the most common findings. When a pleuritic component is noted > 70 percent of patients with documented PE have both dyspnea and tachypnea.

b. **Chest pain,** particularly in the lower chest, may occur secondary to pulmonary infarction or atelectasis.

c. **Hemoptysis** is uncommon. The reported classic triad of dyspnea, pleuritic pain, and hemoptysis is found in only 25 percent of patients with PE.

2. **Physical examination.** The cardiac manifestations and chest findings of PE include pleural effusions, localized rales, elevated jugular venous pressure with a prominent A wave, right ventricular heave, accentuated pulmonary second sound, and gallop rhythm.

   3. **Laboratory examination and diagnostic studies**
      a. **Chest radiography and (ECG)** usually show nonspecific abnormalities.
      b. A **perfusion (Q) scan** is performed by intravascular injection of labeled microspheres to detect areas of decreased flow. Almost all emboli occluding vessels > 2 mm are detectable by this technique. A **ventilation (V) scan** is performed with an inhaled gas immediately before or after the perfusion study. Perfusion/ventilation mismatches are consistent with PE. Only 10 to 15 percent of patients who are evaluated with a V/Q scan for suspected PE will require a pulmonary arteriogram which remains the ultimate "gold standard."
      c. **Arterial blood gases** While a decreased arterial oxygen level is common, 16 percent of patients with a documented PE have normal blood gases.
B. **Anticoagulation therapy.** Sixty-six percent of patients who die from PE do so within 30 min of the acute event.
   1. **Heparin.** A loading dose of heparin (110 to 120 U/kg) is given intavenously followed by continuous heparin infusion to maintain the PTT at twice normal. Anticoagulation in some form is indicated for 3 months or until 6 weeks postpartum.
   2. **Coumadin for postpartum therapy.** If the PE occurred following delivery, coumadin may be started after 7 to 10 days of heparin. (Sufficient coumadin is given orally to maintain a therapeutic prothrombinopenia of one and one-half to two and one-half times the normal prothrombin time [e.g., 21 to 35 s, with a control period of 14 s]).
C. **Thrombolytic therapy.** There is little experience with thrombolytic therapy during pregnancy, but it may be considered whenever massive PE are documented.
D. **Surgical therapy.** If the patient develops recurrent emboli, vena cava ligation or insertion of a balloon/filter distal to the renal veins should be considered.
E. **Prognosis.** PE is the most common nonobstetric cause of maternal deaths (3/100 000). If PE complicating pregnancy are untreated, there is a 13 percent mortality. This can be reduced to 1 percent with anticoagulation.

BIBLIOGRAPHY

Cardiac Disease

Barra Perey C, Arvalo-Toledo N, Cadena AO, et al. The course of pregnancy in patients with artificial heart valves. Am J Med 1976; 61:504.

Brinkman CR, Woods JR. Effects of cardiovascular drugs during pregnancy. Cardiovasc Med 1976; 1:231.

Chesley LC. Severe rheumatic cardiac disease and pregnancy: The ultimate prognosis. Am J Obstet Gynecol 1979; 136:552.

Elkayam U, Gleicher N. Cardiovascular Physiology of Pregnancy. New York: Alan R. Liss; 1982.

Hall JG, Pauli RM, Wilson KM. Maternal and fetal sequelae of anticoagulation during pregnancy. Am J Med 1980; 68:122.

Julian DG, Syekely P. Peripartum cardiomyopathy. Prog Cardiovasc Dis 1985; 27:223.

Lang RM, Borow KM. Pregnancy and heart disease. Clin Perinatol 1985; 12:551.

Lotgering FK, Gilbert RD, Longo LD. Maternal and fetal responses to exercise during pregnancy. Physiol Rev 1985; 65:1.

Naden RP, Redman CWG. Antihypertensive drugs in pregnancy. Clin Perinatol 1985; 12:521.

Selyer A. Risks of pregnancy in women with cardiac disease. JAMA 1977; 238:982.

Thromboembolic Disease

Anderson G, Fagrell B, Holmgren K, et al. Subcutaneous administration of heparin: A randomized comparison of intravenous administration of heparin to patients with deep vein thrombosis. Thromb Res 1982; 27:631.

Friend JR, Kakkar VV. The diagnosis of deep vein thrombosis in the puerperium. J Obstet Gynaecol Br Commonw 1970; 77:820.

Hall JG, Pauli RM, Wilson KM. Maternal and fetal sequelae of anticoagulation during pregnancy. Am J Med 1980; 68:122.

Hull R, Van Aken WG, Hirsh J, et al. Impedance plethysmography using the occlusive cuff technique in the diagnosis of venous thrombosis. Circulation 1976; 53:696.

Salyen EW, Deykin D, Shapiro RM, et al. Management of heparin therapy: Controlled prospective trial. N Engl J Med 1975; 292:1046.

White TM, Bernene JL, Marino AM. Continuous heparin infusion requirements: Diagnostic and therapeutic implications. JAMA 1979; 241:2717.

CHAPTER 29

Hypertensive Disease and Preeclampsia/ Eclampsia

Jeffrey C. King

BASIC CONSIDERATIONS

Hypertensive disorders are common complications of pregnancy and remain one of the most frequent causes of maternal death. Unfortunately, in spite of intensive research activity, how pregnancy unmasks or aggravates hypertension remains unknown. Hypertension can cause a wide spectrum of pathologic changes in multiple organ systems in pregnancy, including the fetoplacental unit. Long-term effects of hypertension have also been identified. Hypertension during pregnancy may have devastating consequences for both mother and fetus.

I. **Classification.** A major problem has hampered the interpretation of the literature: inconsistency of terminology. To solve this problem, the Committee on Terminology of the American College of Obstetricians and Gynecologists in 1972 developed a classification system for hypertension during pregnancy or the puerperium. In an attempt to separate the vasospasm that may induce hypertension during pregnancy from hypertension that merely coexists with pregnancy, the following classification is suggested:
   A. **Pregnancy-induced hypertension (PIH)**
      1. Preeclampsia
         a. Mild
         b. Severe
      2. Eclampsia
   B. **Chronic hypertension**
   C. **Pregnancy-aggravated hypertension**
      1. Superimposed preeclampsia
      2. Superimposed eclampsia
   D. **Gestational/transient hypertension**

II. **Definitions**
   A. **PIH.** An increase in blood pressure of 30 mm Hg systolic or 15 mm Hg diastolic over baseline is diagnostic of PIH. If early

pregnancy readings are not available, a pressure of $\geq$ 140/90 after 20 weeks' gestation is considered significant. This blood pressure elevation should be documented on two measurements taken at least 6 h apart with the patient at rest. Elevation of the mean arterial pressure (MAP = diastolic pressure + one-third pulse pressure) may also be used as a criterion for PIH. An increase of MAP of 20 mm Hg or an absolute value of 105 mm Hg indicates hypertension.

1. **Preeclampsia**
   a. **Mild preeclampsia.** Mild preeclampsia is defined as hypertension plus proteinuria (> 300 mg/24h) and/or nondependent edema after the 20th week of pregnancy.
   b. **Severe preeclampsia.** PIH may rapidly progress from mild to severe preeclampsia and even to eclampsia. The finding of one or more of the following allows classification of PIH as severe preeclampsia:
      (1) Blood pressure of $\geq$ 160 mm Hg systolic or $\geq$ 110 mm Hg diastolic on two occasions taken at least 6 h apart with the patient at rest
      (2) Proteinuria of $\geq$ 5 g/24 h or 3 to 4+ on Dipstick analysis of a random urine sample
      (3) Oliguria (< 500 mL/24 h)
      (4) Cerebral/visual disturbances (i.e., altered consciousness, blurred vision, scotomata, headache)
      (5) Pulmonary edema or peripheral cyanosis
      (6) Epigastric or right upper quadrant pain (probably due to subcapsular hepatic hemorrhage and stretching of Glisson's capsule)
2. **Eclampsia.** The development of seizures in a preeclamptic patient that cannot be attributed to another cause (e.g., epilepsy) is diagnostic of eclampsia.
B. **Chronic hypertension.** Hypertension (blood pressure $\geq$ 140/90) that is present and documented prior to pregnancy or develops prior to the 20th week of pregnancy is considered chronic. Hypertension that is first diagnosed during pregnancy but persists beyond the 42d week postpartum day is also considered chronic.
C. **Pregnancy-aggravated hypertension.** Chronic hypertension may become complicated by the development of superimposed preeclampsia/eclampsia, a condition called *pregnancy-aggravated hypertension.* The prognosis for mother and baby in this situation is worse than with either chronic hypertension or preeclampsia/eclampsia.
   1. **Superimposed preeclampsia.** The criteria are the same as those described in Section II.A.1.
   2. **Superimposed eclampsia.** The criteria are the same as those described in Section II.A.2.
D. **Gestational/transient hypertension.** Hypertension that develops during pregnancy or the first 24 h postpartum without other signs of preeclampsia or chronic hypertension is called *gestational/transient hypertension.*

PREECLAMPSIA

I. **Incidence.** PIH develops in 5 to 7 percent of pregnancies not terminating in first-trimester abortion. There is a bimodal frequency distribution, with teenage primigravidas and older multiparas at higher risk. There is a 30 percent incidence of PIH in twin pregnancies regardless of parity.

II. **Morbidity and mortality**
  A. **Maternal.** Maternal death is rare but may occur due to complications such as abruptio placentae, hepatic rupture, or progression of PIH/preeclampsia to eclampsia.
  B. **Perinatal.** The perinatal mortality in PIH increases progressively with each 5 mm Hg rise in MAP. In addition, perinatal mortality is significantly increased when proteinuria is > 3.5 g/24 h. The causes of the increase in perinatal mortality are placental insufficiency and abruptio placentae. For surviving infants, the incidence of intrauterine growth retardation is increased.

III. **Cause.** In spite of active research in this area, the cause of PIH remains unknown. Multiple theories have been suggested that include immunologic, endocrine, and genetic causes. In addition, social class and dietary deficiency have been proposed as causes. Unfortunately, no theory has been completely accepted. However, two theories do have substantial investigative support: women with PIH do have accentuated vascular sensitivity to vasoactive agents, and reduced prostacycline generation has been observed in PIH.

IV. **Differential diagnosis.** When the criteria for the diagnosis of preeclampsia have been fulfilled, the differential diagnosis is limited to chronic hypertension unmasked by pregnancy, superimposed preeclampsia, nephrotic syndrome, glomerulonephritis, and lupus nephritis.

V. **Diagnosis**
  A. **Signs and symptoms.** The majority of patients with early preeclampsia are asymptomatic. In general, **hypertension, edema,** and **proteinuria** develop prior to obvious symptoms and while the disease process is still mild. This fact reinforces the reason for frequent prenatal visits in late pregnancy, allowing early detection. Since PIH-associated vasospasm is found in all organ systems, it is not surprising to find symptoms in many systems. Excessive fluid retention may result in joint tightness or paresthesia due to ulnar/median nerve compression. Some symptoms also suggest the severity of the disease. Alterations in cerebral perfusion may result in headache or mental confusion. In addition, prior to developing convulsions, patients often complain of epigastric pain or pain penetrating to the back.
  B. **Physical examination.** The usual progression for the appearance of physical/laboratory findings is edema followed by hypertension and proteinuria. It is useful to keep this pathophysiologic

sequence in mind when evaluating a patient suspected of having preeclampsia.

1. **Blood pressure.** See Section II.A.
2. **Fluid status.** Fluid retention will result in rapid **weight gain** prior to the development of **edema.** A gain of 2.25 kg in 1 week is a warning sign.
3. **Reflexes.** While **hyperreflexia** is given significant attention, it is not consistently associated with preeclampsia. While often brisker than normal, deep tendon reflex changes are not part of the diagnostic criteria. In fact, patients may develop convulsions in the face of normal reflexes.
4. **Retina.** In over 50 percent of women with preeclampsia, local or generalized changes are seen in the retinal arterioles. These retinal changes have been shown to correlate with changes in the renal biopsy, and include localized narrowing of arterioles seen as narrowing during fundoscopic examination. Retinal sheen is of no clinical importance.
5. **Heart and lungs.** Examination of the heart and lungs is generally unremarkable unless congestive heart failure is present.
6. **Abdomen.** Abdominal examination is usually normal unless hepatic tenderness is found. Ascites is relatively rare, and other conditions causing ascites should be considered if it is present.
7. **Skin.** Ecchymoses and/or purpura may indicate ongoing thrombocytopenia of disseminated intravascular coagulation.

C. **Laboratory examination and diagnostic procedures**
   1. **Urinalysis.** See Section II.A for the defined limits of **proteinuria.** While the extent of **proteinuria** is related to perinatal mortality, eclampsia is often seen in the absence of proteinuria. Thus, the amount of proteinuria is not a good indicator of the potential for seizures. Microscopic evaluation of the urinary sediment is not a useful aid to the differential diagnosis except in patients with preexisting renal disease.
   2. **Complete blood count (CBC).** A CBC is extremely important in the evaluation of a patient for preeclampsia, as the discovery of a rising hematocrit compared to values found earlier in pregnancy may indicate the reduction in plasma volume seen in preeclampsia.
   3. **Renal functions. Creatinine clearance** is decreased in severe preeclampsia but is often normal in milder forms. Mild changes of **serum creatinine** and **blood urea nitrogen (BUN)** are usually not helpful in the diagnosis.
   4. **Liver function tests. (LFTs).** LFTs are generally not helpful in evaluating the severity of preeclampsia; however, when elevated serum glutamic-oxaloacetic transaminase (SGOT) and serum glutamic-pyruvic (SGPT) are found in conjunction with microangiopathic anemia (hemolysis) and thrombocy-

topenia, the HELLP syndrome (hemolysis, elevated liver enzymes, low platelets), a severe variant of preeclampsia, is diagnosed. Maternal and perinatal mortality are both significantly raised in this condition.

5. **Coagulation studies.** Active disseminated intravascular coagulation is uncommon in mild preeclampsia, but in severe preeclampsia a **platelet count** and measurement of **fibrinogen levels** will often show thrombocytopenia and depressed fibrinogen levels. Usually these studies become abnormal before alterations of the prothrombin time or partial thromboplastin time or before fibrin split products are seen. One must remember that elevated fibrin split products are seen in approximately 15 percent of normal pregnancies. Therefore, the finding of elevated fibrin split products alone does not indicate a coagulopathy.

6. **Fetal evaluations.** Ultrasonographic study of the fetus should be performed to evaluate fetal size and growth, amniotic fluid volume, fetal breathing/movement, and placental grading. Some form of fetal surveillance, in the form of biophysical profile, nipple stimulation test/contraction stress test, and fetal activity monitoring is required.

VI. Management. The clinical management of a patient with PIH depends on the severity of the disease and fetal maturity. There is no doubt that delivery will result in resolution of the disease for the mother; however, this course of action may not always be in the best interest of the fetus. In general, ambulatory treatment has no place in the management of PIH or pregnancy-aggravated hypertension.

A. **Mild preeclampsia**

1. **Initial care.** Patients with mild preeclampsia should be hospitalized for rest and evaluation.

   a. **If the fetus is at term and the condition of the cervix is favorable,** induction of labor is indicated, as delivery will resolve the maternal disease process and remove the fetus from further jeopardy.

   b. **If the patient is not at term or the condition of the cervix is unfavorable,** continued appraisal of the clinical status of the mother and fetus is required.

      (1) Patients should be maintained on **bed rest,** with bathroom privileges only. The **lateral recumbent position** is encouraged to increase uterine blood flow and to assist in mobilization of peripheral edema.

      (2) To determine fluid status, **weight is obtained on admission and every 2 days thereafter.**

      (3) An appropriate-size cuff should be used to obtain **blood pressure readings every 4 h.** Because of hydrostatic effects that may artificially lower blood pressure if determined in the upper arm, all blood

pressures should be determined in the lower arm when in the lateral recumbent position.

(4) **Serial evaluations** of blood count, platelets, proteinuria, creatinine clearance, and liver functions may be helpful.

(5) **Antepartum studies of fetal well-being** should be performed. If fetal well-being is established, further antepartum care is appropriate if the maternal status does not worsen. Indications of intrauterine fetal compromise should engender further fetal evaluation and/or delivery, depending on the severity of the findings.

2. **Continued care.** If 72 to 96 h of conservative therapy do not result in significant patient improvement (decreased edema, resolving hypertension, and onset of diuresis), induction of labor should be considered. In addition, if during the 72 to 96 h there is continued deterioration of the patient, delivery is indicated. Outpatient care may be considered in selected patients if diuresis and resolution of hypertension occurs during the initial 72 to 96 h of hospitalization.

3. **Intrapartum care**

   a. **Delivery.** The mode of delivery—vaginal delivery versus cesarean section—is dependent on the gestational age, the Bishop score of the cervix and fetal presentation, and the fetal and maternal status. Attempts at vaginal delivery by pitocin induction of labor with direct fetal/uterine monitoring should be made in cephalic presentations since the success rate has been shown not to be dependent on cervical status or parity.

   b. **Magnesium sulfate therapy.** Magnesium sulfate therapy should be initiated during the intrapartum period in all patients with PIH to prevent seizures and progression to eclampsia. While the mechanism whereby magnesium sulfate prevents convulsions is not completely understood, the principal effect is the result of peripheral neuromuscular blockade. Hypermagnesemia impairs acetylcholine release by the motor nerve impulses and decreases the sensitivity of the motor end plate to acetylcholine. It is generally held that the intravenous route of administration for magnesium sulfate is superior.

      (1) An initial **loading dose** of 4 to 6 g is given intravenously over 20 min followed by a continuous infusion of 1 to 2 g/h to prevent the development of eclamptic convulsion.

      (2) The magnesium sulfate should be **continued for approximately 24 h following delivery.** A Foley catheter should be inserted to ensure an accurate intake/output measurement.

      (3) Since magnesium is excreted almost exclusively by the kidneys and the half-time for excretion is de-

pendent on renal function, urine output < 30 mL/h places the patient at risk for magnesium toxicity. **Therapeutic levels** of magnesium are 4 to 6 mEq/L (4.8 to 9.6 mg/dl) and are generally found when deep tendon reflexes are present but slightly depressed. If the deep tendon reflexes are lost, a magnesium level of 10 mEq/L can be expected. When higher levels are found, respiratory depression progressing to general anesthesia and cardiac arrest may be anticipated.

(4)   Calcium gluconate, 10 mL of a 10% solution (1 g), may be given via slow intravenous push to reverse the overdosage effects of magnesium sulfate.

c.   **Anesthesia and analgesia and maternal monitoring for labor.** During labor, pain relief may be achieved by intravenous narcotics or segmental epidural anesthetic administration following adequate intravenous preloading with at least 500 mL of lactated Ringer's solution. In mild PIH, the use of central pressure monitoring (central venous pressure line or Swan-Ganz catheter) is encouraged but not mandatory. Paracervical blockade is contraindicated. Pudendal blockade supplemented by local perineal infiltration is sufficient for most vaginal deliveries. Cesarean section should be performed under balanced general or segmental epidural anesthesia. The use of segmental epidural anesthesia has been advocated to modulate maternal blood pressure and avoid the hypertensive response to endotracheal intubation. Careful attention to maternal blood pressure, adequate preload, and fetal heart rate is essential if segmental epidural anesthesia is used since hypotension from sympathetic blockade and subsequent utero-placental insufficiency may result.

B.   **Severe preeclampsia**
1.   **Antepartum management: preparation for labor and delivery.** When the criteria for severe PIH are met, conservative measures to prolong pregnancy are discouraged and delivery is generally indicated. Patients should be hospitalized immediately for evaluation. When severe PIH is being managed, the use of a Swan-Ganz catheter may be extremely helpful. The use of this monitoring technique is encouraged when regional anesthesia is employed for pain relief during labor or for cesarean section. Vaginal delivery can be performed safely under pudendal blockade supplemented by local perineal infiltration. The optimal route for delivery is not known, but close surveillance of fetal status by continuous electronic fetal monitoring is essential. Delivery should be accomplished promptly when the maternal and fetal status have been stabilized.
2.   **Magnesium sulfate therapy.** Magnesium sulfate therapy

should be initiated and maintained according to the previous guidelines. It should be maintained for at least 24 h following delivery. The criteria for discontinuing magnesium sulfate include onset of diuresis and modulation of hypertension.

3. **Hydralazine.** Hydralazine causes a reduction in arteriolar resistance, as seen by a greater decrease in diastolic than systolic pressure.
   a. **Administration.** The drug is given in a dosage of 5 to 10 mg intravenously every 2 to 4 h in emergency situations. When the drug is given intravenously, the maternal blood pressure must be monitored closely to avoid transient hypotension, which could be dangerous to both the mother and fetus.
   b. **Side effects.** Maternal side effects include headache, palpitations, nausea, and diarrhea. A false-positive lupus erythematosus cell preparation may be seen with the long-term use of hydralazine.

ECLAMPSIA

I. **Incidence.** Eclampsia may develop in fulminant cases of preeclampsia but is more commonly found in neglected cases. Therefore, its incidence is dependent on the quality of care provided to the parturient. Fortunately, the overall incident is low, occurring in 0.5–4.1/1000 deliveries. It should be remembered that in 26 percent of eclamptic patients, the previous diagnosis was mild preeclampsia. Approximately one-third of eclamptic episodes occur in each of the antepartum, intrapartum, and postpartum periods. Eclampsia occurs most often in the last trimester and becomes most frequent as term approaches. Nearly all cases of postpartum eclampsia appear within 24 h of delivery. Delayed cases, beyond 7 days, are usually due to some cause other than hypertensive complications of pregnancy.

II. **Morbidity and mortality**
   A. **Maternal.** Maternal mortality is reported as being between 2.2 and 17 percent. Morbidity is dependent on the extent of injury and may range from tongue injury to acute pulmonary edema to hemiplegia from a sublethal cerebral hemorrhage. Blindness may result from retinal edema, which usually resolves, but retinal detachment may have permanent sequelae. The usual cause of maternal death for eclamptic patients is cerebral hemorrhage.
   B. **Perinatal.** Perinatal morbidity and mortality depend on when the seizure occurs during the antepartum or intrapartum course. The reported mortality ranges from 13 to 30 percent.

III. **Causes.** Since eclampsia is a progression from preeclampsia, the cause of this condition is likewise unknown.

IV. Differential diagnosis. The development of seizures during pregnancy or the early puerperium is most commonly due to eclampsia, although other conditions such as epilepsy, encephalitis, meningitis, cerebral tumor, acute porphyria, ruptured cerebral aneurysm, and even hysteria must be considered. These conditions must be kept in mind and excluded before a definite diagnosis of eclampsia is made. Until eclampsia can be excluded, however, all pregnant women with convulsions should be considered and treated as eclamptic.

V. Diagnosis
  A. Signs and symptoms
   1. The definitive symptom is **tonic-clonic seizures** in a patient with PIH.
   2. The signs and symptoms described for PIH and preeclampsia are found in most patients with eclampsia (see **Section II.A.1**). Headache, visual disturbance, and epigastric or right upper quadrant pain in a preeclamptic patient should warn the physician of impending seizures and thus eclampsia.
  B. Physical examination
   1. The convulsion usually begins about the mouth in the form of **facial twitching.** After a few seconds, the entire body becomes rigid in a **generalized muscular contraction** that may last for 15 to 20 s. This is followed by **tonic-clonic movements** beginning at the jaw/mouth and progressing to the face and extremities. This phase may last for 1 min. During the tonic-clonic phase, the diaphragm is fixed and respiration ceases. Following the eclamptic convulsion(s), the respiratory rate is increased and breathing may be stertorous. Cyanosis may be seen in severe cases.
   2. The first convulsion is generally a forerunner of additional seizures, ranging from 1 or 2 in mild cases to 10 or 20, or even continuous seizure activity in untreated severe cases. The duration of coma following a convulsion is variable.
   3. When maternal temperatures of $\geq$ 39.5°C are found, the prognosis is grave.
  C. Laboratory findings
   1. **Proteinuria** is almost always present and frequently is marked ($>$ 3.5 g).
   2. **Hypercarbia** from lactic acidemia is thought to explain the tachypnea.

VI. Management. The general principles are to stop seizures, avoid maternal injury, and maintain the airway/oxygenation.
  A. Airway management. While placement of a **padded tongue blade** to prevent injury is ideal, if the patient's teeth and jaw are already closed, dental injury to the patient or finger injury to the personnel may result from such attempts. The **mouth and oropharynx should be suctioned** frequently to prevent aspiration. As the seizure resolves, an oral airway should be inserted until the patient regains complete consciousness. After acute

stabilization, an upright portable chest x-ray should be obtained to evaluate for aspiration.

B. **Treatment of the convulsive episode**
   1. Initiation of **magnesium sulfate** administration remains the mainstay of therapy. The dosage has already been outlined (see **Section VI.A.3.b**).
   2. The addition of **diazepam** (Valium) (5 to 10 mg) or **sodium amytal** (up to 250 mg) intravenously may be necessary to control repeated convulsions, but this therapy may result in severe fetal depression.
C. **Delivery.** Delivery should not be accomplished immediately following a maternal seizure, since both maternal and fetal physiology have been significantly altered.
   1. **Stabilization of maternal blood pressure** by intravenous hydralazine and of **maternal neuromuscular status** by magnesium sulfate must be achieved over the next 2 to 4 h. Only at this time can delivery be considered.
   2. If the obstetric criteria for induction of labor are met, **induction of labor** should be attempted with direct fetal monitoring.
   3. If the obstetric criteria for induction of labor are not met, or if direct monitoring is not feasible, delivery by **cesarean section** under balanced general anesthesia should be considered.
D. **Postpartum care**
   1. **Magnesium sulfate** therapy should be continued for 24 to 36 h postpartum.
   2. **Central pressure monitoring** is indicated to protect maternal cardiovascular function and assist in decision making with regard to fluid, blood, or blood replacement therapy.
E. **Prognosis.** Twenty-five percent of subsequent pregnancies are complicated by hypertension. Only 5 percent become severe and 2 percent of patients will develop eclampsia again. If the hypertension associated with eclampsia resolves in 6 to 12 weeks postpartum, the risk of developing essential hypertension is not increased. However, if hypertension develops in a subsequent pregnancy, the risk of chronic hypertension is high.

CHRONIC HYPERTENSION

I. **Incidence.** Approximately 50 percent of all cases of hypertension in pregnancy involve patients with underlying chronic hypertensive disease. The overall incidence of chronic hypertension complicating pregnancy is 3 to 4 percent.

II. **Morbidity and mortality**
   A. **Maternal.** Maternal mortality is uncommon with mild (< 100 mm Hg) diastolic hypertension, but there is an increased likelihood of a maternal morbid event when diastolic blood pressure

> 105 mm Hg. The major maternal risk is the development of intracranial bleeding. The finding of chronic hypertension increases the risk of placental abruption.

   B. **Perinatal.** There is no question that perinatal mortality is higher for infants of hypertensive compared to normotensive women. Perinatal mortality for patients with uncomplicated chronic hypertension ranges from 8 to 15 percent. The fetus is at significant risk for the development of intrauterine growth retardation. The risk to both mother and fetus is increased if superimposed preeclampsia develops.

III. Cause. Hypertensive disease during pregnancy is seen most frequently in older women. In addition, obesity is a prime risk factor, with 25 percent of women weighing > 90 kg having elevated blood pressure. Heredity has also been implicated, since many members of the family of an index case may also have hypertension.

IV. Differential diagnosis. Other causes of hypertension should be considered, such as chronic renal disease, pheochromocytoma, renal artery stenosis, and coarctation of the aorta. Patients who develop recurrent bouts of hypertension late in repeated pregnancies, with normal blood pressure between pregnancy, most likely have latent hypertensive vascular disease.

V. Diagnosis
   A. **Signs and symptoms.** As with hypertension in the nonpregnant patient, there are usually no definitive signs or symptoms of its presence.
   B. **Physical examination**
      1. The **retinas** should be examined closely for evidence of long-standing hypertension such as arteriolar narrowing and arteriovenous nicking. The presence of retinal hemorrhages or exudates indicates accelerated hypertension.
      2. A careful **cardiac examination** is indicated to evaluate for the presence of end organ damage, particularly cardiomegaly.
      3. **Auscultation over the renal arteries** for a bruit may diagnose renal vascular hypertension.
      4. Blood pressure measurements should be taken in all extremities. These measurements, together with simultaneous palpation of the femoral and radial pulses, may suggest coarctation of the aorta. Patients should be instructed about the importance of home blood pressure monitoring. Blood pressure readings should be made at least three times per week. Acute changes should be immediately reported.
   C. **Laboratory examinations and diagnostic procedures**
      1. **Urine tests.** The following tests of maternal urine are indicated for all patients with known or suspect hypertension:
         a. Urinalysis and culture and sensitivity performed on a clean-catch urine sample

b. A 24-h urine collection for creatinine clearance and total protein excretion to evaluate renal function
c. Tests for catecholamines and vanillylmandelic acid (VMA) to evaluate for pheochromocytoma.
2. **Blood tests.** Tests for BUN, serum creatinine, and serum electrolytes should be performed.
3. **Electrocardiography and chest x-ray.** A baseline electrocardiogram (ECG) is suggested for all patients, but if hypertension is severe, an ECG and a chest X-ray with an abdominal shield may be helpful.

VI. Management. Because women with chronic hypertension and their fetuses are at increased risk, they should be seen frequently. After 24 weeks of gestation, they should have prenatal visits at least every 2 weeks, with weekly evaluation after 32 weeks. These patients should be encouraged to increase their daily rest periods and to report any unusual symptoms promptly. If the chronic hypertension appears to worsen or if proteinuria develops, hospitalization is indicated.
A. Maternal management
1. **Rest.** The single most important aspect of management of these pregnant patients with chronic hypertension is **2 h of bed rest per day.** If the patient works outside of the home, coordination with the patient's employer will usually result in compliance with a 1-h period of lateral recumbent rest while the patient is having lunch. Patients should be encouraged to limit extra salt intake; their salt intake should be restricted only if excessive edema occurs.
2. **Antihypertensive therapy.** The value of antihypertensive therapy to prevent maternal complications and whether there is a distinct benefit for the fetus are unknown. The decision to use antihypertensive medications must be made on a case-by-case basis. In general, treatment of mild to moderate hypertension is discouraged since a clear benefit for the pregnancy is unlikely.
a. **Methyldopa** is a centrally acting agent that reduces sympathetic tone and decreases peripheral resistance. There is very little change in cardiac output or pulse. Methyldopa is the only drug whose long-term safety for the fetus has been adequately addressed. No significant adverse effects of this therapy on fetal or neonatal outcome have been noted, with the exception of a small reduction in neonatal blood pressure. Since this drug has undergone two randomized studies, it should be the **drug of first choice.**
(1) Therapy is begun at an initial dosage of 250 mg three or four times per day. The dosage is increased gradually until the desired antihypertensive effect is achieved or a maximum dosage of 2 g/d is obtained. The dosage should be altered no more than

every 72 h, as it takes this long for a new regimen's effect on blood pressure to be evaluable. If the maternal blood pressure cannot be controlled by methyldopa therapy alone, additional medications must be added to the patient's regimen.

(2) **Side effects.** Lethargy and drowsiness are common: Hemolytic anemia and hepatitis are rarely seen.

b. **Hydralazine** is a potent vasodilator whose primary indication for usage is acute elevation of blood pressure. The initial dosage is 10 mg four times daily, increasing to 200 mg/d.

c. **Labetalol** is a combined alpha- and beta-blocking drug. At low to moderate doses, its predominant action is beta-adrenergic inhibition. Labetalol also induces vasodilatation because of its apha-blocking properties. While studies indicate that labetalol can provide adequate blood pressure control with reasonable maternal safety, the fetal and neonatal effects have not been fully evaluated. There does not appear to be any major advantage of labetalol over methyldopa therapy.

(1) **Dosage.** If labetalol is used, the initial dosage is 100 mg orally three or four times a day. The dosage may be increased every 2 to 3 days until the desired antihypertensive effect is achieved or until the maximum dosage of 1200 mg/d is reached.

(2) **Side effects.** Side effects of therapy with labetalol include tremulousness and headache.

d. **Betablockers (inderal, atenolol, metoprolol, oxprenolol)** have been used most extensively in women with mild to moderate chronic hypertension. While previous reports of adverse fetal effects of therapy have been refuted, the reported maternal or fetal benefits have not been consistent. While beta blockers appear to be safe, their use during pregnancy may attenuate the usual signs of fetal distress.

(1) **Dosage.** The dosage is variable, depending on the drug being used, and should be evaluated on an individual basis with the maternal-fetal medicine consultant.

(2) **Side-effects.** Side effects of beta-blocker therapy are rare as long as contraindications to their use (asthma, Raynaud's phenomenon) are kept in mind.

e. **Diuretics** should, in general, be discontinued during pregnancy since their usage may alter the normal plasma volume expansion of pregnancy and is not justified. However, acute pulmonary or laryngeal edema, which occasionally complicates severe preeclampsia or eclampsia, requires aggressive therapy, which may include diuretic therapy.

    f. **Calcium channel blockers,** such as nifedipine, have recently garnered increased attention. The dosage is 10 to 20 mg four to six times daily.

    g. **Angiotensin-converting enzyme (ACE) inhibitors,** such as captopril, enalapril, or lisinopril, are contraindicated in pregnancy.

B. Fetal management

    1. Ultrasound. An early ultrasound examination is required to confirm the gestational age. Serial sonography at 4- to 6-week intervals is necessary to evaluate fetal growth and to diagnose growth retardation.

    2. Evaluation of fetal well-being. Testing should be initiated on at least a weekly basis after 32 weeks. The use of kick counts (a kick count is obtained by asking the mother to count the number of fetal movements she feels during a specified amount of time each day) provides additional information about fetal well-being and allows the patient to participate actively in her own management and in fetal assessment. A secondary gain is that during the kick count observation period, the patient is instructed to rest in the lateral position, which is always beneficial to the function of the fetoplacental unit. If electronic fetal monitoring, NST or CST, suggests fetal compromise, a biophysical profile is indicated.

C. Management of delivery. Pregnancy should be terminated by induction of labor if fetal growth ceases or if progressive organ failure occurs. Amniocentesis may help determine the optimal time for delivery, but in no case should pregnancy be allowed to progress beyond term. During labor, direct fetal/uterine monitoring is essential to evaluate fetal health and well-being. The use of steroids to enhance pulmonary maturation in the immature fetus has not been associated with worsening of maternal hypertension.

VII. Prognosis. Blood pressure can usually be well controlled during pregnancy, and there is no apparent worsening of maternal blood pressure following delivery.

PREGNANCY-AGGRAVATED HYPERTENSION

I. Incidence. The true incidence of pregnancy-aggravated hypertension is difficult to determine because of the use of variable criteria for diagnosis. However, the reported and projected incidence of preeclampsia complicating chronic hypertension ranges from 5.7 to almost 50 percent.

II. Morbidity and mortality. The outlook for both the fetus and the mother is grave when superimposed preeclampsia develops. Delivery should be strongly considered, particularly if the gestational age is >

32 weeks. The reported perinatal loss is 21 percent, and maternal mortality is < 1 percent. If the fetus is liveborn and survives the perinatal period, the long-term prognosis is good.

III. Cause. As with preeclampsia and chronic hypertension, the cause of pregnancy-aggravated hypertension is unknown.

IV. Differential diagnosis. Accelerated hypertension, acute glomerulonephritis, lupus nephritis, pheochromocytoma, nephrotic syndrome, and scleroderma should be considered. However, if the various diagnostic criteria for both preeclampsia and chronic hypertension are met (see **Sections II.A.1 and II.2**), the rare causes mentioned above can be easily ruled out.

V. Diagnosis. The same diagnostic criteria stated for preeclampsia and eclampsia should be used (see **Sections II.A.1 and II.2**). Typically, pregnancy-aggravated hypertension becomes manifest by a sudden rise in blood pressure, which may become complicated by oliguria and impaired creatinine clearance. The retina may develop extensive hemorrhages and cottonwool exudates. The syndrome of superimposed preeclampsia may progress rapidly to convulsions and become very similar to hypertensive encephalopathy.

VI. Management. The definitive therapy of pregnancy-aggravated hypertension is delivery. The timing of delivery, however, is a complex decision based on the severity of maternal and fetal disease. Maternal indications include organ failure such as renal failure, development of a coagulopathy, seizures associated with the development of eclampsia, and uncontrollable hypertension; fetal indications include intrauterine growth retardation and non-reassuring fetal parameters, such as oligohydramnios or nonreactive NST. The decision is best made by consultation among the obstetrician, maternal fetal medicine specialist, and neonatologist.

   A. Maternal management. Initiation of magnesium sulfate therapy to prevent convulsions, using the doses previously outlined, is essential. Blood pressure should be aggressively controlled with hydralazine. Many of these patients benefit from Swan-Ganz catheter monitoring for identification of workload of the heart and cardiac output measurements.

   B. Fetal management. Continuous electronic fetal monitoring is mandatory to make sure that lowering the maternal blood pressure does not result in utero-placental insufficiency.

   C. Delivery. Delivery probably is most easily accomplished by cesarean section. If possible, vaginal delivery is worth considering if the cervical status is favorable. Direct fetal heart and uterine pressure monitoring should be used if vaginal delivery is attempted. The risk/benefit ratio of conduction anesthesia must be weighed carefully.

VII. Prognosis. The risks for the future are apparently the same as for patients with preeclampsia or chronic hypertension alone. However, since the risk of recurrent superimposed preeclampsia in a subsequent pregnancy is 70 percent, these patients should be advised to avoid future pregnancy.

GESTATIONAL/TRANSIENT HYPERTENSION

This hypertensive disorder of pregnancy is poorly characterized. However, in most patients, the blood pressure returns to normotensive levels within 10 days postpartum. If blood pressure elevation persists beyond this period, the patient is more likely to have chronic hypertension unmasked by pregnancy. While many patients in this category are labeled as mild preeclamptics, it has been suggested that they really have latent essential hypertension that has become evident during gestation. Irrespective of the underlying cause, these patients should be watched closely for progression to actual preeclampsia, and many suggest that they be managed as if they do have preeclampsia.

BIBLIOGRAPHY

Benedetti TJ, Cotton DB, Read JC, et al. Hemodynamic observations in severe preeclampsia with a flow-directed pulmonary artery catheter. Am J Obstet Gynecol 1980; 136:65.

Chesley LC. Hypertensive Disorders in Pregnancy. New York: Appleton-Century-Crofts; 1978.

Cunningham FG, Lindheimer MD. Hypertension in pregnancy. N Engl J Med 1992; 326:927.

Lindheimer MD, Katz AI. Pathophysiology of preeclampsia. Annu Rev Med 1981; 32:273.

Naden RP, Redman CWG. Antihypertensive drugs in pregnancy. Clin Perinatol 1985; 12:521.

Pritchard JA. Management of preeclampsia and eclampsia. Kidney Int 1980; 18:259.

Rayburn WF, Zuspan FP, Piehl EJ. Self blood pressure monitoring during pregnancy. Am J Obstet Gynecol 1984; 148:159.

Rubin PC. Beta blockers in pregnancy. N Engl J Med 1981; 305:1323.

Sibai BM. The HELLP syndrome (hemolysis, elevated liver enzymes, and low platelet): Much ado about nothing? Am J Obstet Gynecol 1990; 162:311.

Sibai BM. Eclampsia: VI. Maternal-perinatal outcome in 254 consecutive cases. Am J Obstet Gynecol 1990; 163:1049.

Sibai BM, Abdella TN, Anderson GD. Pregnancy outcome in 211 patients with mild chronic hypertension. Obstet Gynecol 1983; 61:571.

Weiner CP, Brandt J. Plasma antithrombin III activity: An aid in the diagnosis of preeclampsia-eclampsia. Am J Obstet Gynecol 1982; 142:275.

CHAPTER 30

Renal Disease

Ana Tomasi

Due to anatomic and physiologic changes, the renal system is particularly susceptible to compromise during pregnancy. The major source of problems is infection, but the kidney may also be affected by diabetes, preeclampsia, and exacerbation of autoimmune diseases.

I. **Physiology.** During pregnancy, the renal plasma flow increases, with up to a 50 percent increase in the glomerular filtration rate (GFR). This, in turn, causes decreases in the normal laboratory values of blood urea nitrogen (BUN) and creatinine. The increased GFR also exceeds the tubular reabsorption capacity, resulting in glycosuria and loss of water-soluble vitamins and amino acids.

II. **Infections of the urinary tract.** Urinary tract infections are the most common medical complications of pregnancy, ranging from asymptomatic bacteriuria to symptomatic problems such as cystitis and acute pyelonephritis.

A. **Asymptomatic bacteriuria**

1. **Definition.** Asymptomatic bacteriuria is the presence of 100 000 organisms of the same species per milliliter of urine in the urine of a patient without the symptoms of a urinary tract infection.

2. **Incidence.** Asymptomatic bacteriuria is discovered in 2 to 12 percent of pregnant women, the incidence varying depending on race, parity, and socioeconomic status.

3. **Morbidity.** Although the majority of women with untreated, asymptomatic bacteriuria remain symptom free, 30 percent develop an acute symptomatic urinary tract infection during pregnancy such as cystitis or acute pyelonephritis. In addition, some studies have demonstrated an association between asymptomatic bacteriuria and preterm labor.

4. **Pathophysiology.** Factors that predispose to asymptomatic bacteriuria include the fact that the female urethra is fairly short, so that bacterial contamination from the vagina and rectum is more likely to occur. Because asymptomatic bacteriuria is more frequently seen in pregnant than nonpregnant women, it is probable that some factors present during

gestation may increase the ability of bacteria to replicate in the urine. The effect of progesterone on muscle tone and activity, and the mechanical obstruction produced by the enlarging uterus, predispose to increased capacity and incomplete emptying of the bladder. The pH is also an increased due to increased bicarbonate excretion, which enhances bacterial growth. Glycosuria is not uncommon during pregnancy and may predispose to an increased rate of bacterial multiplication in the urine.

5. **Differential diagnosis.** The differential diagnosis of asymptomatic bacteriuria is essentially whether the urine culture is contaminated with bacteria from the vagina and/or the rectum.

6. **History and physical examination.** Since the infection is totally asymptomatic, there are no signs or symptoms.

7. **Management**
   a. **Evaluation.** Because asymptomatic bacteriuria is ultimately associated with a very high incidence of symptomatic complications if it remains untreated, every pregnant patient should be screened at the first prenatal visit with a urine culture. If the culture is positive, she should be treated and urine cultures should be repeated periodically during the pregnancy. After an initial negative urine culture, < 1.5 percent of patients will acquire urinary tract infection during the subsequent months before delivery.
   b. **Treatment.** Because *Escherichia coli* has been the most common organism found in asymptomatic bacteriuria, oral treatment with an antibiotic to which *E. coli* is usually sensitive should be started. These antibiotics include a quick-acting sulfonamide such as sulfisoxazole (Gantrisin, 1 g q.i.d), or nitrofurantoin (Macrodantin, 50 mg p.o. q.i.d), or ampicillin (500 mg p.o. q6 h). Whichever regimen is chosen should be continued for 7 to 10 days. Single-dose treatment has been demonstrated to be effective in 75 to 80 percent of the cases. A single dose of sulfisoxazole (Gantrisin) 2g, nitrofurantoin (Macrodanazole) 200 mg, or ampicillin 2g plus probenecid 1g eradicated the bacteria. In the last trimester of pregnancy, ampicillin is the drug of choice, because sulfa compounds compete with bilirubin for albumin-binding sites in the fetus and theoretically may produce hyperbilirubinemia in the newborn. If infection recurs, the patient should be treated again, and then suppressive antimicrobial therapy with Macrodantin (50 to 100 mg p.o. q.d.) should be used for the remainder of the pregnancy. Women who do not respond to treatment, or who subsequently demonstrate reinfection, should be evaluated radiologically with an intravenous pyelogram after the puerperium to assess for renal parenchymal

abnormalities, as well as for abnormalities of the urinary collecting system.

8. **Prognosis.** Eradication of bacteriuria with antimicrobial agents has been shown to be effective in the prevention of nearly all clinically evident infections.

B. **Acute pyelonephritis.** The most frequent symptomatic urinary tract infection during pregnancy is acute pyelonephritis.

1. **Incidence.** The overall incidence of pyelonephritis in pregnancy is 1 to 2.5 percent, with an estimated 10 to 20 percent recurrence rate during the same pregnancy.

2. **Morbidity and mortality.** Twenty percent of affected women may have transient renal dysfunction, as measured by decreased creatinine clearance. Approximately 10 percent of all patients with acute pyelonephritis will be found to have bacteremia if blood cultures are taken. Acute pyelonephritis is associated with increased uterine activity and preterm labor in ~ 20 percent of the cases. With appropriate antimicrobial therapy, maternal mortality is almost negligible.

3. **Pathophysiology**
   a. **Microbiology.** Pyelonephritis generally results from an ascending infection from the lower urinary tract. Many different microorganisms can infect the urinary tract, but the most common agents by far are the gram-negative bacilli. *E. coli* causes approximately 90 percent of the cases of pyelonephritis, and other gram-negative rods, including *Proteus, Klebsiella, Enterobacter, Serratia,* and *Pseudomonas,* account for a smaller proportion of the other uncomplicated infections. *Proteus* species, by virtue of urease production, and *Klebsiella* species, through production of extracellular slime and polysaccharide, predispose to stone formation and are isolated more frequently from patients with urinary calculi.
   b. **Maternal factors.** The maternal factors leading to increased pyelonephritis in pregnancy are the same as those outlined for asymptomatic bacteremia.

4. **Differential diagnosis.** Pyelonephritis may be mistaken for labor, appendicitis, placental abruption, or infarction of a myoma, and in the puerperium for infection of the uterus and adjacent structures.

5. **Diagnosis.** The signs and symptoms of pyelonephritis are shaking chills, fever, flank pain, nausea and vomiting, urinary frequency and urgency, dysuria, and costovertebral angle tenderness. Physical examination reveals fever and marked tenderness in one or both lumbar regions and costovertebral angles. The abdominal examination is normal.

6. **Laboratory evaluation.** Urine analysis shows bacteriuria and pyuria. A quantitative urine culture with > 100 000 organisms per milliliter of urine is necessary to document the presence of infection. In the absence of a positive quantitative urine culture, the presence of bacteriuria on microscop-

ic examination in a drop of unspun urine usually indicates significant bacteriuria (more than 100 000 organisms per milliliter).

7. **Management.** Pyelonephritis poses a serious threat to maternal-fetal well-being; consequently, the patient should be hospitalized for vigorous treatment with intravenous fluids and antimicrobial agents. Urine culture and sensitivity should be done before starting any antimicrobial therapy in the patient with acute pyelonephritis.

   a. **Antibiotics.** Broad-spectrum antibiotics should be administered parenterally as soon as the diagnosis of acute pyelonephritis is made and urine cultures are taken. In most cases, therapy with **ampicillin** (2 g intravenously q6 h) will be sufficient. The antibiotic regimen should be changed if necessary according to subsequent urine culture and sensitivity reports. Forty-eight hours after the patient with acute pyelonephritis becomes afebrile, an oral route of antibiotic administration may be started to complete a 10-day course of therapy. In the patient allergic to penicillin, or in the patient who has a very high fever or who is very ill at the time of presentation, gentamicin (60 to 80 mg IV q8 h, with serial evaluation of serum gentamicin levels and urinary function) is a good alternative therapy. **Urinary tract obstruction** should be considered if improvement does not occur within 48 to 72 h, in which case an intravenous pyelogram should be done. Following therapy, urine cultures should be obtained monthly.

8. **Prognosis.** The prognosis for the mother and fetus for the patient with acute pyelonephritis is good with appropriate antimicrobial therapy; however, the recurrence rate during the same pregnancy is 10 to 20 percent. If pyelonephritis recurs after therapy has been completed, antimicrobial suppression with nitrofurantoin (Macrodantin, 50 mg p.o. q.d.) for the duration of the pregnancy should be performed.

III. Acute and chronic renal failure

A. **Acute renal failure.** Acute renal failure is defined as a rapid decline in GFR toward a value that approaches zero, a nearly linear increase in serum creatinine concentration at a rate of 0.5 to 1.5 mg/dL/d, a progressive, rapid rise in serum urea nitrogen, and usually a fall in the urine flow rate to < 400 to 500 mL/d. Sustained renal failure beyond a few days results in marked azotemia, metabolic acidosis, hyperkalemia, anemia, and eventually neurologic manifestations of uremia. In the absence of the appropriate treatment, death will occur within 1 to 2 weeks.

   1. **Incidence.** Acute renal failure is relatively infrequent in pregnancy, the estimated incidence being only 1/2000 to 1/5000 pregnancies. The frequency distribution of acute renal failure in pregnancy shows two peaks. The first occurs early in

gestation (12 to 18 weeks) and comprises most cases associated with abortion; the second is seen during the third trimester and represents mainly the acute renal failure caused by preeclampsia and its hemorrhagic complications.

2. **Morbidity and mortality.** The maternal mortality rate of acute renal failure is very high, between 35 and 65 percent, despite the introduction of dialysis and modern management of fluid and electrolyte abnormalities. The mortality rate tends to be higher in patients with preexistent renal disease or medical conditions not related to pregnancy. The leading causes of death are the primary illness that precipitated the renal failure, septicemia, and intractable shock. The prognosis for the fetus is even worse than that for the mother, and many pregnancies complicated by acute renal failure end in abortion or stillbirth, the perinatal mortality rate being nearly 40 percent.

3. **Cause.** Acute loss of renal function during pregnancy or post partum is usually due to pregnancy-related disorders (especially preeclampsia/eclampsia) or deterioration of preexistent renal disease.

4. **Pathophysiology.** Acute renal failure should be divided into three types: prerenal, renal, and postrenal.

   a. **Prerenal acute failure.** Prerenal acute failure implies that the GFR is markedly reduced owing to renal hypoperfusion without renal histopathologic changes or impaired tubular function. Acute renal blood flow falls, fractional sodium excretion is reduced to less than 1 percent, and urinary sodium excretion is low. Renal hypoperfusion can result from hypotension, volume contraction, and heart failure. Common causes of renal hypoperfusion during pregnancy include hyperemesis gravidarum, septic shock, and preeclampsia. These conditions result in volume contraction and abruptio placentae, which causes hypotension. Correction of renal hypoperfusion in these conditions promptly restores the GFR and reverses the metabolic consequences of renal failure.

   b. **Renal acute failure.** Renal parenchyma disorders that produce renal failure are acute tubular necrosis, which is reversible, and cortical renal necrosis, which is irreversible. These two situations can be caused by renal hypoperfusion due to hypotension, decreased circulating plasma volume, decreased cardiac output, and disseminated intravascular coagulation (DIC), as well as by nephrotoxins. **Acute tubular necrosis** occurs when the renal insult from severe ischemia or the action of nephrotoxin causes severe but reversible damage to renal tubular cells. The histopathologic lesion is characterized by interstitial edema and necrotic, sloughed tubular cells. Glomeruli appear normal by light microscopy, and DIC fragments of red blood cells and fibrin deposits are commonly seen in glomerular capillaries. In contrast to prerenal acute failure, tubular transport function is markedly impaired and results in increased fraction excretion of sodium $>$ 1 to 2 percent, a urinary sodium level $>$ 40 mEq/L, and impaired concentrating ability, demonstrated by a urine osmolarity $<$ 400 mOsm/kg H_2O. Restoration of renal function usually becomes clinically evident within 10 to 21 days and is dependent, at least in part, on regeneration of tubular epithelial cells and increased renal blood flow. Since the rise in GFR precedes full recovery of tubular function, the early phase of improved renal function is usually marked by a progressive rise in the urine flow rate with a urine sodium concentration of 70 to 90 mEq/L and a potassium concentration of 20 to 30 mEq/L. **Renal cortical necrosis** is a pathologic entity characterized by tissue death throughout the cortex in a diffused or patchy pattern, with sparing of the medullary portions of the kidney, and is a form of irreversible acute tubular necrosis. Although cortical necrosis is uncommon in nonpregnant women, it is a frequent complication of obstetric conditions. Cortical necrosis is more likely to occur in multigravidas who are beyond 30 years of age and is most commonly associated with abruptio placentae. The causes and clinical characteristics of cortical necrosis are the same as those of acute tubular necrosis, except for the lack of recovery of renal function.

    c. **Postrenal acute failure.** Postrenal causes of renal failure are obstruction of the ureters or bladder outlet and extravasation of urine for all urinary collecting system components. Factors that prevent the external elimination of final urine can result in uremia, with clinical features that are indistinguishable from those of the prerenal and renal types of acute renal failure.

5. **Diagnosis.** The clinical approach to acute renal failure begins with determining the category that most likely explains the cause for the sudden decline in renal function. Bladder outlet obstruction is evaluated by simple catheterization of the urinary bladder. Examination of the urine for fractional excretion of sodium and concentrating ability is useful in distinguishing prerenal from renal causes of acute renal failure. The presence of hypotension, or of clinically evident cardiac failure or dehydration, demands prompt corrective measures to maximize renal perfusion. A careful bedside examination to evaluate skin turgor and jugular venous pressure, and attention to changes in body weight and a history of vomiting or bleeding, will provide important clues regarding the maternal volume status. In cases of abruptio placentae, sufficient occult bleeding may have occurred by

the time the patient presents to warrant immediate volume replacement. Since effective plasma volume is often difficult to ascertain by physical examination (particularly in edematous patients), Swan-Ganz catheterization to determine the pulmonary wedge pressure is the most reliable means for evaluating volume status.

6. **Management.** If the diagnosis of acute tubular necrosis or cortical necrosis seems likely after exclusion of pre- and postrenal factors, therapy is begun to minimize the consequences of severe renal failure. Fluid administration is restricted to replacing the volume of external losses plus insensible loss of water (~ 400 to 500 mL/d). Intake of substances containing potassium, metabolic acid, and sodium should be eliminated. A caloric intake of at least 2000 kcal/d should be achieved through the administration of carbohydrate and lipids. Hypertension should be treated with vasodilator agents, hydralazine being the drug of choice in the undelivered patient. The serum magnesium level tends to rise in acute renal failure and may reach toxic levels. It should be evaluated (a toxic level is generally > 8 mg/dL) and magnesium sulfate therapy should be avoided in the clinical setting of renal insufficiency. Elevated plasma levels of potassium > 5.5 mEq/L should be reduced by the administration of a cation-exchange resin such as **sodium polystyrene sulfonate** (Kayexelate enema) by retention enema of 40 g of resin and 50 g of sorbitol mixed in 200 mL of water every 4 to 6 h. If sorbitol is unavailable, the resin may be mixed in 200 mL of $D_{10}W$ or $D_{20}W$. These resins remove approximately 1 mEq K^+ per gram of resin administered. In the patient whose serum K^+ is so high as to cause cardiac arrhythmias or similar immediate life-threatening problems, a glucose-insulin infusion may be given, which causes a rapid shift of potassium into the cells. The glucose and insulin are given intravenously, usually in a ratio of 1 U of regular insulin for every 2 g of glucose. Thus, for a 300-mL bolus of $D_{20}W$, 30 U of regular insulin should be administered over a 20- to 30-min interval. When the serum bicarbonate level falls to 12 to 14 mEq/L, acidosis is corrected by the administration of sodium bicarbonate to raise the level to a range of 18 to 20 mEq/L. Blood should be administered to maintain the hematocrit value above at least 25 percent in order to enhance fetal viability. Dialysis treatment should be established if renal failure persists for more than 3 to 4 days without signs of improvement or if the serum creatinine level rises above 5 mg/dL. Early dialysis has the advantage of preventing many of the severe manifestations of uremia and permits the administration of protein and calories in the large amounts that are often required in severely catabolic patients. The administration of a potent diuretic should not be used as a diagnostic test for prerenal acute renal failure or

in an attempt to hasten the rate of recovery in acute tubular necrosis. Although large, sustained doses of furosemide, a very popular potent loop diuretic, may result in increased urine volume, this treatment does not stimulate renal cellular recovery and is associated with a high incidence of ototoxicity.

B. **Chronic renal disease.** Chronic renal disease is characterized by a decline in GFR that occurs over days, weeks, or months, in contrast to the sudden fall in GFR that takes place in acute renal failure.

1. **Incidence.** The incidence of chronic renal failure in pregnancy is 1/5000 to 1/10 000 pregnancies. The incidence will depend on the underlying cause, maternal age, and prepregnancy serum creatinine level, since it is unusual for a woman to become pregnant or to complete a normal pregnancy if her prepregnancy creatinine level exceeds 3 mg/dL.

2. **Cause.** The cause of chronic renal disease is associated with glomerular lesions such as chronic glomerulonephritis; proliferative glomerulonephritis; membranous nephropathy; some diseases, such as diabetic glomerulosclerosis, systemic lupus erythematous, systemic vasculitis, amyloidosis, and toxemia of pregnancy; interstitial causes such as acute interstitial nephritis, chronic interstitial nephritis, and chronic pyelonephritis; and vascular lesions such as arterial nephrosclerosis, renal arteriosclerosis, and renal thrombosis.

3. **Pathophysiology.** Chronic renal failure is manifested by a progressive decrease in the GFR over a period of time. The decreased GFR will produce electrolyte, metabolic, and hematologic derangements that include hyperpotassemia, hyperphosphaturia, hypocalcemia, hypoproteinemia, metabolic acidosis, and anemia. These homeostatic alterations, known as **uremia,** are responsible for clinical neurologic manifestations that include nausea, vomiting, hypotension, somnolence, coma, and death.

4. **Diagnosis.** In most patients, the specific cause of renal failure will have been established before conception or in early pregnancy or will be evident from the clinical manifestations of a systemic disorder. The discovery of progressive renal insufficiency after the 20th week of gestation may present a difficult diagnostic problem because of the lack of specific criteria by which to distinguish preeclampsia from primary renal disease. Renal biopsy, which can usually provide a specific histologic finding of preeclampsia, is not a safe procedure in most centers; the clinician usually assumes that preeclampsia is present and will deliver the fetus, if the clinical features are highly suggestive of the disorder. Electrolyte alterations include a rise in the serum potassium level $>$ to 5 mEq/L, a serum phosphorus level of 5 to 8 mg/dL, and a calcium level that is usually normal or slightly reduced, and metabolic acidosis may be present. The latter condi-

tion is due to a decreased rate of excretion of metabolic acid. The metabolic and hemodynamic complications of severe renal failure include worsening anemia with a hematocrit values commonly < 25 percent, hypertension, impaired cardiac function, weakness, and anorexia. Manifestations of central nervous system dysfunction include somnolence, impaired intellectual function, hiccups, and depression. The final stage in renal failure is reached when the GFR is < 5 mL/min and is characterized by the severe toxic symptoms of nausea, vomiting, pruritus, hypothermia, and, if dialysis is not initiated, by the terminal events of myoclonus, convulsions, and coma.

5. **Management.** Disturbances in acid-base balance and electrolytes can be managed by conservative means before dialysis is instituted. Elevated levels of potassium can be reduced < 5 mEq/L by restricting the daily dietary intake of potassium to ~ 20 mEq. The complication of hyperphosphatemia can be managed by dietary reduction of phosphorus to 600 to 800 mg/d and by the administration of oral phosphate-binding agents such as Basogel to reduce serum phosphorus below 5 mg/dL. As in the treatment of acute renal failure, sodium bicarbonate should be administered to patients with a serum bicarbonate level < 12 to 14 mEq/L. An oral dose of 1 to 4 g/d is usually sufficient to titrate the daily production of metabolic acid. If there is demonstrated hypocalcemia, it seems reasonable to administer a dose of 1,25-dihydroxycalciferol in a dose of 0.25 μg/d. Dialysis should be instituted if the GFR is < 5 to 10 mL/min to prevent uremic complications.

C. **Dialysis in pregnancy.** Even though the use of dialysis in pregnancy is not as extensive as that in nonpregnant human beings, most authorities advocate initiating early treatment before uremic symptoms are manifest and using daily rather than intermittent dialysis. This can be done by either peritoneal dialysis or hemodialysis. Hypotension, vaginal bleeding, and premature contractions are known complications of dialysis; they can be minimized by reducing the hypotension and by using sequential ultrafiltration.

IV. **Renal stone disease in pregnancy.** Nephrolithiasis has been reported to occur with an incidence of 1/1500 pregnancies. This condition creates diagnostic problems because of the difficulty of distinguishing ureteral colic from obstetric causes of abdominal pain. Most patients manifest the typical symptoms of flank pain, urgency, and dysuria and are found to have microhematuria. Atypical clinical presentations, however, have been reported, and nephrolithiasis should be considered in patients with urinary tract infection that is refractory to antibiotics and in patients with recurring pyelonephritis. The principal causes of nephrolithiasis in this population are similar to those observed in the general population. Patients who pass stones during pregnancy for the first time should be evaluated, therefore, for hyperparathyroidism with at least three determinations of plasma calcium and for cystinuria by examination of the urine with a nitroprusside test. Although stones are passed spontaneously in most cases, operative intervention may be required to eradicate the infection or to correct complete ureteral obstruction. The incidence of induction of labor by operative procedures is estimated to be about 5 to 10 percent. To reduce the exposure to radiation of the fetus, it has been suggested that a modified intravenous pyelogram should include only a single plain film prior to the administration of dye and a repeat film after 20 min. Renal ultrasound may also prove useful.

V. Renal transplantation in pregnancy. Pregnancy after renal transplantation has become a more common challenge for the obstetrician in the last few years. In the past, these patients were counseled to avoid pregnancy, whereas now they are not so advised. Patients with a kidney transplant have a higher than normal incidence of kidney rejection (about 9 percent during pregnancy), a slightly higher incidence of increased abortions, and a questionable possibility of congenital abnormalities associated with the medications presently used to treat kidney transplant patients, such as immunosuppressive agents. These patients usually do very well during pregnancy. It is advised, however, that they employ contraception for at least 18 months after the transplant, because there is a higher incidence of renal transplant rejection in the first few months after transplantation. During pregnancy, these patients do have a slightly higher incidence of preeclampsia, especially those who have hypertension.

BIBLIOGRAPHY

Berkowitz R. Critical Care of the Obstetric Patient. New York: Churchill-Livingston; 1983.

Davison J, Lindheimer JD. Pregnancy in renal transplant recipients. J Reprod Med 1982; 27:613.

Gilstrap L, Cunningham F, Whalley P. Acute pyelonephritis in pregnancy. Obstet Gynecol 1981; 57:409.

Grunfeld J, Ganeval D, Bourncrias F. Acute renal failure in pregnancy. Kidney Int 1980; 18:179.

Harris R, Dunnihoo D. The incidence and significance of urinary calculi in pregnancy. Ann J Obstet Gynecol 1967; 99:237.

Kass E. Pyleonephritis and bacteriuria. Ann Intern Med 1962; 56:46.

Ober W, Reid D, Romney S, et al. Renal lesions and acute renal failure in pregnancy. Am J Med 1956; 21:781.

Strauch B, Hayslett Y. Kidney disease and pregnancy. Br Med J 1974; 2:578.

Whalley P. Bacteriuria of pregnancy. Am J Obstet Gynecol 1967; 97:123.

CHAPTER 31

Pulmonary Disease

Michael T. Parsons

I. **Respiratory physiology in pregnancy.** The mechanical and hormonal changes that naturally occur during pregnancy significantly alter the respiratory state of the patient and influence the results of physical and laboratory examinations of the pregnant patient when she is well and when she is ill. Changes in respiratory parameters that are seen in the pregnant patient include:
   A. Hyperemia, edema, and increased secretions that may cause nasal obstruction or epistaxis
   B. Elevation of the diaphragm
   C. Alterations in physiologic measurements (Fig. 31.1)
      1. Increased respiratory parameters: tidal volume, inspiratory capacity, minute ventilation, and alveolar ventilation
      2. Decreased respiratory parameters: functional residual capacity, residual volume, expiratory reserve volume, and total lung capacity
      3. No or minimal change in respiratory parameters: respiratory rate (may be slightly increased), forced vital capacity (FVC), forced expiratory volume (FEV), or forced expiratory volume in 1 second (FEV_1).
   D. The majority of pregnant women experience a sensation of increased breathing effort, which is often referred to as **dyspnea of pregnancy.**

II. **Acute respiratory disease**
   A. **Upper respiratory tract infection (URI)**
      1. **Incidence.** The incidence of URIs (colds) is unchanged from that encountered in the nonpregnant state. Overall, colds are most common in fall and winter.
      2. **Morbidity and mortality.** Because of the physiologic changes in the respiratory system during pregnancy, the respiratory compromise associated with URIs during pregnancy may be slightly increased over that in the nonpregnant state. The common, mild viral respiratory illnesses do not have a viremic phase, so that fetal involvement is not expected.

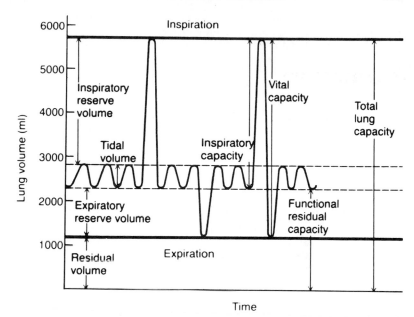

FIGURE 31.1. Pulmonary volumes and capacities during pregnancy. (From Guyton AC. Textbook of Medical Physiology. 8th ed. Philadelphia: WB Saunders; 1991:407. Reprinted with permission.)

3. **Cause.** The most common viruses causing URIs include rhinovirus, adenovirus, coronavirus, parainfluenza virus, and respiratory syncytical viruses.
4. **Pathogenesis and pathophysiology.** After the patient inhales exhaled respiratory tree droplets from affected individuals, the virus enters the patient's cells, replicates, and spreads locally from the infected nasopharyngeal mucosa.
5. **Differential diagnosis.** Major alternatives in the differential diagnosis of URI include influenza, mycoplasma pneumonia, and streptococcal pharyngitis.
6. **Diagnosis.** The patient with a URI has symptoms of the common cold, including congestion of the upper respiratory tract, sneezing, malaise, possible headache, and pharyngitis. A minimal fever may be present. The specific virus may be identified by isolation in tissue culture, identification of antigens in nasal secretions, or rising serum antibody titers against the specified virus.
7. **Management.** Supportive care is indicated for patients with URIs, including adequate hydration and treatment of excessive fever with antipyretics.
   a. Encourage oral hydration with liquids (water, juice), the

amount required varying with the patient's temperature elevation and degree of tachypnea.
   b. If the patient's temperature is > 102° and other causes are ruled out, acetaminophen (Tylenol, 1000 mg p.o. q4–6 h) may be used as an effective antipyretic.
   c. Admission to the hospital is not necessary for an uncomplicated URI.
   d. Decongestants (e.g., pseudoephedrine) should be avoided during pregnancy unless considered absolutely necessary because of severe respiratory compromise.
   e. If the throat is inflamed, a culture for Group A beta-hemolytic streptococcus should be obtained and appropriately treated.

B. Asthma
   1. **Incidence.** Asthma affects approximately 1 percent of pregnant patients.
   2. **Morbidity and mortality.** Severe asthma, requiring multiple trips to the emergency room, admission to a hospital, or high doses of prednisone, is associated with an increased incidence of prematurity, intrauterine growth retardation, and perinatal death. Mild asthma controlled by minimal or no medication is less likely to affect the pregnancy outcome adversely.
   3. **Cause.** Asthma may have either an allergic (extrinsic) or an idiosyncratic (intrinsic) cause, or may have features of both that irritate the tracheobronchial tree. Factors that may provoke asthma include airborne allergens such as pollens, aspirin, environmental factors (pollution), work-related irritants, exercise, emotional stress, and infections.
   4. **Pathogenesis and pathophysiology.** Edema of the bronchial walls, thick secretions, and smooth muscle contraction produce a reduced airway diameter. This leads to increased resistance, a decrease in expiratory flow rate, and an increased effort in breathing, with altered blood gases.
      a. Possible influences of pregnancy that improve the asthmatic states include:
         (1) Increased corticosteroid levels
         (2) Increased progesterone levels
         (3) Increased serum cyclic adenosine monophosphate (cAMP)
         (4) Decreased cell-mediated immunity
      b. Possible influences of pregnancy that adversely affect the asthmatic status include:
         (1) Antigenicity of the fetus
         (2) Nasal congestion
         (3) Decreased functional residual volume
         (4) Decreased cell-mediated immunity, leading to viral infections
         (5) Dyspnea of pregnancy, increasing the patient's anxiety

5. **Differential diagnosis.** The diagnosis of asthma is usually not difficult. Other diseases that may be confused with asthma are upper airway obstruction by tumor, localized endobronchial disease, chronic bronchitis, carcinoid tumors, pneumonias, and congestive heart failure.

6. **Diagnosis**
   a. A history of asthma attacks and symptoms of dyspnea, chest tightness, coughing, and wheezing are usually present. A history of recent exposure to allergens, infections, or irritants, or increased activity or unusual emotional stress, may precipitate an attack.
   b. Physical examination may not indicate the severity of the asthmatic disease state. The patient's wheezing may become less obvious as increased plugging of the respiratory tree occurs. The patient's use of accessory muscles of respiration and the presence of pulsus paradoxus may help to differentiate the severity of the disease but are not sensitive.
   c. Laboratory studies are of value. Arterial blood gases are very important to evaluate the ventilatory status. Hyperventilation is indicated by a low P_{CO_2}. Elevation of P_{CO_2} indicates CO_2 retention. A respiratory rate > 30 per min, a pulse of 120 beats per min, FEV < 1000 mL, or $P_{O_2} < 80$ mm Hg requires aggressive management. Sputum Gram stains containing eosinophils suggest an allergic cause of the asthma attack; such stains containing neutrophils suggest an infectious cause.

7. **Management.** The clinical management of an asthmatic attack in pregnancy requires a series of steps:
   a. Eliminate any identifiable causative agent (if applicable) or treat any recognized infection with an appropriate antibiotic.
   b. Give oxygen by nasal cannula (at a rate of 3 L/min for the initial rate) if $P_{O_2} < 70$ mm Hg.
   c. Provide hydration (100 to 200 mL/h of 0.5 normal saline or other suitable fluids).
   d. Administer a sympathomimetic, either epinephrine or terbutaline; 0.3 mL of a 1 : 1000 dilution subcutaneous is an initial therapy for acute respiratory distress. This can be repeated every 15 to 20 min.
   e. While the parenteral sympathomimetic agent may reverse the acute episode, the addition of **theophylline** will improve its effectiveness and provide long-term treatment. Theophylline inhibits phosphodiesterase, which increases the cyclic AMP level and controls bronchospasm. This is administered as a loading dose of 6 mg/kg in 100 mL D5/W given intravenously over 20 min, followed by a maintenance dose of 0.9 mg/kg/h. An oral dose of a long-acting theophylline should follow the intravenous infusion when the attack has subsided

sufficiently to discontinue intravenous therapy. For both intravenous and oral therapy, a therapeutic level of theophylline should be maintained. The therapeutic serum level is 10 to 20 μg/mL.

f. **Beta-adrenergic agents** elevate the level of cyclic AMP by activating adenyl cyclase. These agents are useful in the acute attack and especially in the long-term maintenance of the patient. Metaproterenol by oral spray, two puffs four times a day, and/or oral terbutaline, 2.5 to 5 mg three times a day, provide additional bronchodilation.

g. **Corticosteroids** are indicated if the patient does not respond to the initial therapy within several hours of its initiation, or if the attack is severe and the patient has a history of such attacks that required steroid therapy for successful treatment. Hydrocortisone is administered intravenously with a loading dose of 7 mg/kg, followed by a maintenance infusion of 100 to 300 mg q4–6 h. This should be decreased to 50 to 100 mg q6 h over the following 24 h, then changed to oral prednisone, 1 mg/kg/24 h in divided doses three or four times a day. Inhaled corticosteroids (beclomethasone) may be used to replace or reduce oral steroids.

h. Recently there is more emphasis on the use of inhalational agents in treatment of acute asthma.

i. **Antibiotics** should be administered if a fever, purulent sputum, or a pulmonary infiltrate on chest x-ray is present.

j. If the patient remains refractory to therapy with increasing P_{CO_2}, respiratory acidosis will develop and the patient requires transfer to an intensive care unit with intubation and mechanical ventilation. At delivery, regional anesthesia is preferable to general anesthesia.

k. **Determination of fetal well-being.** Evaluation of fetal status is important, and appropriate electronic fetal monitoring should be performed. If fetal distress is discovered, appropriate actions should be taken, but these must be tempered by consideration of the mother's status. As a general rule, the mother needs to be stable prior to extreme interventions such as cesarean section. Premature labor should be anticipated and treated if present.

C. **Pneumonia.** Pneumonia is an acute infection involving inflammation of the lung parenchyma.

1. **Incidence.** Pneumonia occurs in less than 0.8 percent of pregnancies.

2. **Morbidity and mortality.** An increased incidence of spontaneous abortions and premature labor has been reported in some studies of pregnant women with pneumonia. Pneumonia is a major cause of nonobstetric maternal deaths, with a reported mortality of 3.5 to 8.6 percent.

3. **Cause.** The two most common causative organisms are *Streptococcus pneumonia* and *Mycoplasma pneumoniae,* but all of the following causes have been reported:
   a. **Bacterial**
      (1) *Streptococcus* pneumonia
      (2) *Staphylococcus*
      (3) *Hemophilus* influenza
      (4) Gram-negative organisms are uncommon
   b. **Mycoplasma pneumonia**
   c. **Legionella pneumophila**
   d. **Viral**
      (1) Influenza
      (2) Varicella (rare, but may be life-threatening if a cause of pneumonia in pregnancy)
   e. **Fungal** (uncommon as a cause of pneumonia in pregnancy compared to other causes)
      (1) Coccidiomycosis
      (2) Histoplasmosis
      (3) Cryptococcosis
4. **Pathogenesis/pathophysiology.** The disease process may start by inhalation of organisms from the air or aspiration of organisms from the nasopharynx or oropharynx. Less common mechanisms are hematogenous spread or direct contiguous spread. The defense mechanisms of the lung, including ciliated lining epithelium, the cough reflex to expel material, and the immunologic system, are not always successful in preventing infection. Other conditions, such as alteration of consciousness, surgery, or other physical impairments, may predispose to increased infection. Pneumonia can lead to inadequate oxygenation. The viral infections may progress to respiratory failure and acute respiratory distress syndrome.
5. **Differential diagnosis.** The diagnosis of pneumonia is usually evident from the signs, symptoms, physical examination, and laboratory studies. Other causes that should be considered in the differential diagnosis include tumor, tuberculosis, bronchitis, and asthma.
6. **Diagnosis**
   a. **History.** Symptoms of pneumonia include cough, fever, dyspnea, sputum production, and chest pain; shaking chills may occur.
   b. **Physical examination.** Physical examination reveals fever, tachypnea, and tachycardia. There may be decreased respiratory excursion, and dullness on percussion. If consolidation is present, bronchial breath sounds may be present.
   c. **Laboratory examination.** The **white blood cell count** is often elevated, with increased immature cells. **Arterial blood gases** may reveal hypoxemia, hypocarbia, and respiratory allkalosis. **Roentgenographic examination**

may provide a clue to the causative factor. Homogeneous, nonsegmental consolidation in a lobe with air bronchograms suggests pneumococcal pneumonia. Interstitial pneumonia, in which a reticular pattern is present, suggests mycoplasma pneumonia. Identification of the specific organism is important and is best determined by **Gram stain and culture of the sputum.** Cough-produced sputum is usually sufficient. Other methods besides voluntary coughing to produce sputum include saline aerosolization, nasotracheal suction, and, if necessary, transtracheal aspiration. Blood cultures should be performed.

7. **Management.** General treatment guidelines include hydration, oxygen at a starting rate of 3 L/min, nasal cannula if hypoxia is present, and observation of fetal well-being and premature labor. Antibiotics should be selected on the basis of Gram stain of sputum and changed as indicated by culture and sensitivity results. Uncomplicated pneumococcal pneumonia is treated with penicillin G, 600 000 units q12 h. Mycoplasma and Legionella pneumonia are treated with erythromycin (not estolate), 500 mg q.i.d. for 14 days, and most gram-negative organisms are treated with aminoglycosides. Varicella pneumonia may require acyclovir. Fungal infections may require anti-fungal agents, such as amphotericin B.

D. Tuberculosis

1. **Incidence.** The incidence of tuberculosis is < 15/100 000 patients, and < 200 cases of congenital tuberculosis have been reported.

2. **Morbidity and mortality.** The death rate from tuberculosis is < 2/100 000. If a new tuberculosis infection is not treated, 5 to 15 percent of such patients will progress to a serious disease in the following 5 years. If tuberculosis is adequately treated, the pregnancy is unaffected. If, however, congenital tuberculosis occurs, the perinatal/infant mortality rate approaches 40 percent.

3. **Cause.** The organism causing tuberculosis is *Mycobacterium tuberculosis,* a 3 × 0.3-μm acid-fast aerobic bacillus.

4. **Pathogenesis/pathophysiology.** *M. tuberculosis* is spread by inhalation of droplets that are produced by infected individuals. The organism proliferates in the alveoli and causes an inflammatory response; spread may then occur through the lymphatic or hematologic system. The immunologic system fights the infection, and a cell-mediated response is established.

5. **Differential diagnosis**
   a. Pneumonia
      (1) Bacterial
      (2) Mycoplasma
      (3) Aspiration

   b. Fungal infection
   c. Sarcoidosis
   d. Carcinoma of the lung
6. **Diagnosis.** A tuberculin skin test is used to diagnose a tuberculosis infection, either clinically apparent or dormant. If it is negative, no further evaluation is necessary. If it is positive, a complete history and physical exam and a shielded chest x-ray are performed. The chest x-ray may reveal multiple bilateral infiltrates that are suggestive of tuberculosis. The upper lobes are most commonly involved. The only proof of active infection is **culture identification** of M. tuberculosis, most commonly from sputum, although on occasion positive blood cultures may be obtained. Microscopic examination of the smear from the sputum sample may give preliminary information if it is positive for tubercle bacilli.

   The initial infection by tuberculosis often does not produce a clinical illness. The diagnosis is usually made by examining the contacts of an infected person, when the disease progresses to a serious form, or by routine screening programs. If symptoms are present, they may include fever, malaise, night sweats, and cough. On exam, crepitant rales may be present.

7. **Management**
   a. **Inactive infection.** If the patient has a **positive skin test conversion and a negative chest x-ray,** treatment with **isoniazid,** 300 mg p.o. daily for 1 year, is required. Some feel that treatment may be delayed until after delivery if active infection is not present.
   b. **Active infection.** If a diagnosis of active infection is made, a common treatment modality is the following:
      (1) **Isoniazid,** 5 mg/kg/d p.o. for 9 months, plus **rifampin,** 10 mg/kg/d p.o. for 9 months. Isoniazid's toxicities include peripheral neuropathy by competition with pyridoxine, allergic reaction, and pathocellular toxicity. Pyridoxine may be given to combat the neuropathy. Rifampin's toxicities include jaundice, gastrointestinal symptoms, and thrombocytopenia. Both of these medications have been used during pregnancy without evidence of teratogenicity.
      (2) Other medications that are less commonly used are ethambutol and streptomycin.
      (3) Monitoring must be performed to be sure that:
         (a) The medications chosen are effective. Bacteriology should reveal negative cultures by 4 months.
         (b) Toxic side effects are not present.
   c. If congenital tuberculosis is present in the infant, antituberculosis medications are necessary. If the infant of a mother with tuberculosis does not have the disease,

isoniazid prophylaxis, purified protein derivative (PPD) skin tests, or bacille Calmette-Guérin (BCG) may be administered.

III. Chronic respiratory disease
A. Tobacco smoking
1. **Incidence.** It is estimated that 30 percent of women are smoking when they become pregnant. Many will either stop smoking or smoke less frequently during pregnancy, but others will continue to smoke as usual.
2. **Morbidity and mortality.** The general effects of smoking on the individual, including increased risk of lung cancer, emphysema, chronic bronchitis, and cardiovascular disease, are well known.

   Obstetric problems that have been reported from smoking cigarettes include mean decreased birth weight of 200 grams, increased incidence of placenta previa and abruptio placentae, and possible long-term neurologic abnormalities in the infant.
3. **Pathogenesis/pathophysiology.** The effects on the fetus in smokers have been attributed to:
   a. Poor nutrition
   b. Structural abnormalities of blood vessels
   c. Vasospasm of vessels
   d. Increased carbon monoxide in the bloodstream that competes with oxygen
   e. Increased cyanide in the bloodstream
4. **Management.** Management consists of encouraging the pregnant woman to stop or decrease her cigarette smoking. The importance of her infant's health as well as her own should be stressed. If growth retardation is evident, appropriate monitoring should be performed.
B. Kyphoscoliosis.
Kyphoscoliosis is a congenital lateral and backward curvature of the spine. It is seen in approximately 0.8 to 6/10 000 pregnancies and has been reported to be associated with increased rates of prematurity and stillbirth. Causes of kyphoscoliosis include idiopathic factors, poliomyelitis, trauma, tuberculosis, and rickets. Physiologically, the maternal effect of this problem is an alteration of the rib cage configuration, which may lead to compression of the lungs with emphysema and/or atelectasis. This can cause decreased vital capacity and cardiopulmonary complications including cor pulmonale.
1. **Diagnosis.** Careful physical examination should reveal the spinal deformity.
2. **Management**
   a. Monitor the maternal status for cardipulmonary compromise, and the fetal status for adequate growth and well-being, and for preterm labor.
   b. Give oxygen if indicated for hypoxia.
   c. Give antibiotics if indicated for pulmonary infection.

    d. Give digitalis if indicated.
  3. Prognosis. Successful pregnancies can usually be achieved.
C. Sarcoidosis
  1. Incidence. The incidence is 0.02 to 0.05 percent of pregnancies.
  2. Morbidity and mortality
    a. **Maternal.** Sarcoidosis itself does not damage the pregnancy, but any disease that has compromised pulmonary or cardiac function may lead to deleterious effects in pregnancy. Pregnancy does not worsen the clinical course of sarcoidosis, but an increased number of exacerbations have been reported several months postpartum.
    b. **Fetal.** No effects have been noted on the fetus or newborn. There may be a familial tendency.
  3. Cause. Sarcoidosis is a systemic granulomatosis disease. The cause is unknown.
  4. Pathogenesis/pathophysiology. The most common organs affected are the lungs. They may be affected by pulmonary granuloas and alveolitis. Progressive fibrosis with loss of volume may result. Other affected organs include lymph nodes, eyes, skin, bone, nerves, heart, kidneys, and liver.
  5. Diagnosis. The diagnosis is made by clinical exam and pulmonary function test, revealing restrictive lung disease, and noncaseating granulomas are demonstrated by biopsy from the lung, skin, conjunctiva, or other organs.
  6. Management
    a. Patients with mild, asymptomatic disease do not require treatment because the disease may resolve spontaneously.
    b. Corticosteroids suppress the granulomatous aspect of the disease in more severe cases. Give prednisone, 40 mg p.o. q.i.d. for 1 to 2 months, then taper the dose to 10 to 15 mg p.o. q.i.d. and continue it for 6 to 12 months.
    c. Oxygen may be needed during labor and delivery if hypoxia occurs.
  7. Prognosis. Pregnancy is well tolerated if the following conditions are not present:
    a. Vital capacity < 1 L
    b. Pulmonary hypertension
    c. $PaO_2 < 55$ mm Hg
    d. Dyspnea
    e. High doses of steroids required

BIBLIOGRAPHY

Benedetti TJ, Valle R, Ledger WJ. Antepartum pneumonia in pregnancy. Am J Obstet Gynecol 1982; 144:413.
Burrow GN, Ferris TF, eds. Medical Complications During Pregnancy. 3rd ed. Philadelphia: WB Saunders; 1988

Creasy RK, Resnik R, eds. Maternal-Fetal Medicine Principles and Practice. 2nd ed. Philadelphia: WB Saunders; 1989.

Cunningham FC, McDonald PC, Gant NF. Williams Obstetrics. 18th ed. New York: Appleton-Century-Crofts; 1989.

de Swiet M. Medical disorders in pregnancy. Clin Obstet Gynecol 1977; 4:287.

Dunagan WC, Ridner ML, eds. Manual of Medical Therapeutics. 26th ed. Boston: Little, Brown; 1989.

Fishburne JI. Physiology and diseases of the respiratory system in pregnancy. Reprod Med 1979; 22:4.

Gleicher N, ed. Principals of Medical Therapy in Pregnancy. 2nd ed. Norwalk, CT: Appleton and Lange; 1992.

Gluck JC. The effect of pregnancy on asthma: A prospective study. Ann Allergy 1976; 37:164.

Grossman JH II. Perinatal viral infections. Clin Perinatol 1980; 7:257.

Hageman J. Congenital tuberculosis: Critical reappraisal of clinical findings and diagnostic procedures. Pediatrics 1980; 66:1980.

Hernandez E. Asthma in pregnancy. Curr Concepts Obstet Gynecol 1980; 55:790.

Schatz M. Asthma during pregnancy: Interrelationships and management. Annals of Allergy 1992; 68:123.

Sever JL, Larsen JW, Grossman JH. Handbook of Perinatal Infections. 2nd ed. Boston: Little, Brown; 1989.

Snider DE. Treatment of tuberculosis during pregnancy. Am Rev Respir Dis 1980; 122:65.

Warkany J. Antituberculosis drugs. Teratology 1979; 20:133.

Weinstein AM. Asthma and pregnancy. JAMA 1979; 241:1161.

CHAPTER 32

Gastrointestinal Diseases

Michael T. Parsons
Shirley K. Sawai

I. **Anatomic and physiologic alterations in pregnancy.** During pregnancy there are several anatomic and physiologic alterations in the gastrointestinal and hepatobiliary tracts. These include increased appetite, abnormal taste sensations, pica (compulsive ingestion of various material such as starch, clay, or ice), ptyalism (excessive salivation), decrease esophageal sphincter tone, decreased gastric and gallbladder emptying, possible suppressed gastric acid secretion, and increased efficiency of intestinal absorption possibly due to slower intestinal transit time. Uterine enlargement leads to displacement of abdominal organs, altering their function.

II. **Nausea and vomiting**
   A. **Incidence.** Approximately 50 percent of pregnant patients experience **mild nausea and vomiting,** which is, indeed, a symptom in the presumptive diagnosis of pregnancy. In contrast, the more severe condition of hyperemesis gravidarum (intractable vomiting during pregnancy) occurs in < 0.5 to 2 percent of pregnancies.
   B. **Morbidity and mortality.** Maternal complications from nausea and emesis may include electrolyte disturbance, dehydration, ketosis, weight loss, dental caries, gastroesophageal mucosal (Mallory-Weiss) tears, and, rarely, aspiration pneumonia, as well as neurologic, hepatic, and renal damage. There is no clear evidence that nausea and vomiting increases perinatal mortality. On the contrary, nausea and vomiting in early pregnancy is considered a favorable prognostic sign of a lower risk of spontaneous abortion before 20 weeks. There is no significant difference in birth weight or maternal weight gain in patients who experience nausea and vomiting.
   C. **Cause.** The cause of nausea in pregnancy is poorly understood. Suggested causes include psychogenic factors; elevated human chorionic gonadotropin (hCG) and/or estrogen levels; allergic

reactions to the fetoplacental unit; altered carbohydrate metabolism; vitamin deficiencies; position and size of the corpus luteum, other less clearly specified endocrine disturbances; and possibly socioeconomic, dietary, and hereditary factors. Hormonal causes of hyperemesis gravidarum have been investigated, with progesterone, adrenocorticotropic hormone, cortisol, growth hormone, and prolactin shown to be no different between hyperemesis patients and controls. hCG has been variably reported to be elevated, depressed, or unchanged with severe nausea and vomiting; estrogen levels have been reported to be elevated or unchanged; and free T_4 has been shown to be elevated or unchanged, depending on the study.

D. Differential diagnosis. Many diseases must be considered in the differential diagnosis of nausea in pregnancy, including diabetes mellitus; Addison's disease; thyrotoxicosis and other endocrine disorders; molar pregnancy; multiple gestation; partial intestinal obstruction; gastrointestinal tract, gallbladder, liver, and pancreas disorders; infections; and preeclampsia; as well as psychogenic causes.

E. Diagnosis. The diagnosis is made on the basis of the history and physical examination and by the exclusion of other diseases. Laboratory studies should include serum electrolytes, ketones, and indices of hepatic, hematologic, and renal function in cases of severe nausea and vomiting. Should jaundice occur, the bilirubin level is generally < 3.5 mg/dL and serum transaminase activity is mildly elevated (less than threefold). Starvation may lead to metabolic acidosis, obscuring the alkalosis of hyperemesis. Increase urine concentration of bicarbonate, sodium, and potassium may occur. Urine that is isotonic with serum, Wernicke's encephalopathy, and hepatocellular jaundice may occur with chronic hyperemesis.

F. Management

1. Diet. Most patients with mild nausea and vomiting in pregnancy respond to avoidance of irritating foods, separation of solid and liquid meals, eating dry crackers upon waking, and the assurance that the condition is temporary, self-limiting, and not harmful.

2. Antiemetics. Antiemetics may be used if absolutely necessary (e.g., dehydration or ketosis), but avoidance of medications during pregnancy, especially in the first trimester, is desirable. Compazine, 10 mg p.o. or p.r. as a suppository, every 6 to 8 h as needed, may be used for this purpose.

3. Hospitalization for hyperemesis. Hospitalization with **intravenous fluid and electrolyte support** may be necessary in hyperemesis gravidarum and persistent cases of less severe nausea.

a. **Dextrose containing intravenous solution** should be started at a rate of 125 to 165 mL/h (e.g., $D_5 l/2NS$). If the serum potassium level is less than 3.5 mEq/L, **potassium supplementation** is indicated, either by the oral route if the patient can retain the preparation or by intravenous administration. The recommended regimen of potassium replacement is 40 mEq added to each liter of intravenous fluid. The patient's serum potassium level should be reevaluated every 4 to 6 h and the dosage modified if necessary to maintain a normal level.

   b. **Parenteral hyperalimentation** may be necessary in severe cases in which ketosis and weight loss continue, thus avoiding metabolic deterioration with hepatic and renal dysfunction.

4. **Psychogenic evaluation and treatment.** Patients suspected of having nausea and vomiting due to a psychogenic disorder should be referred for psychiatric evaluation. Organic causes should be eliminated before such referral.

III. Gastroesophageal reflux

A. **Incidence.** Gastroesophageal reflux, usually occurring in the third trimester, is a complaint in 30 to 50 percent of pregnancies.

B. **Morbidity and mortality.** Gastroesophageal reflux does not alter the course of pregnancy and is not detrimental to the fetus. Rare complications are esophagitis with bleeding, perforation, and stricture; Barrett's esophagus (replacement of the squamous mucosa of the esophagus by columnar epithelium); chronic pulmonary symptoms; and reflux aspiration syndrome.

C. **Cause.**
1. **Increased progesterone level.** An elevated maternal progesterone level may cause decreased lower esophageal sphincter (LES) tone and lead to reflux. Several studies have shown the basal LES tone to be decreased throughout the gravid state, reaching its nadir at 36 weeks. There is no difference in gastric pH or fasting plasma gastrin level during pregnancy. Reflux is exacerbated by delayed gastric emptying, which may also be caused by progesterone and the decreased mobility of the distal esophagus, preventing appropriate drainage of refluxed acid back into the stomach. Within 24 h of delivery, plasma progesterone decreases to levels similar to those seen in the luteal phase of the menstrual cycle.
2. **Hiatal hernia.** Hiatal hernia from decreased gastric tone, upward displacement of abdominal organs, and gastric atony may be responsible in 10 to 20 percent of cases.

D. **Diagnosis.** A burning sensation in the epigastric or substernal region that worsens with recumbency, regurgitation, nausea, and belching with an acid taste are suggestive of the diagnosis of gastroesophageal reflux. It can present with pulmonary symptoms or masquerade as atypical chest pain.

E. **Management**
1. **Position.** Using the maternal position to take advantage of gravity, including elevating the head of the bed 15 to 25 cm

and avoiding recumbent positions after meals, will help to reduce the reflux.

2. **Diet.** Small, frequent meals are helpful to reduce reflux, with the evening meal being light and ingested at least 4 to 5 h before retiring. Spicy foods, alcohol, and smoking should be avoided, as they increase acid secretion.

3. **Antacids.** Magnesium and aluminum hydroxide preparations ($Mg(OH)_2$ and $Al(OH)_3$ combinations), 15 to 30 mL p.o. at bedtime or after meals, are helpful.

   Note: H_2 receptor blockers such as cimetidine are not approved for use in pregnancy.

4. **Metoclopromide.** Metoclopromide increases LES tone, increases esophageal peristalsis, and increases gastric emptying by three postulated mechanisms: dopamine antagonism, cholinergic activity, and direct action on smooth muscle. Metoclopromide is excreted in breast milk; however, there have been no reported serious adverse effects in breast-feeding infants. It also crosses the placenta and appears in fetal blood in concentrations similar to those in maternal blood. Although no dysmorphogenic effects have been reported in animals, its effects on the human fetus have not been established. Therefore it should not be used in the first trimester of pregnancy.

IV. **Constipation.** Constipation is defined as excessively dry stool, less than 50 g/d of stool, or infrequent bowel movements (fewer than one every day). Pregnant women suffer from an increased incidence of constipation. Factors that may aggravate constipation in pregnancy include elevated maternal **progesterone** levels, which may decrease colon function, and the **mechanical pressure** of the uterus on the colon. Constipation in pregnancy is **treated by increased fiber in the maternal diet,** especially bran and roughage, and **increased fluid intake.** Other supplements, such as stool-softening agents (e.g., docusate sodium) or mild laxatives (e.g., milk of magnesia), may be necessary if diet manipulation is unsuccessful.

V. **Peptic ulcer.** The incidence of peptic ulcer in pregnancy is decreased from the nonpregnant state in women (0.8/1000 per year). There is overall improvement in peptic ulcers in up to 88 percent of women who become pregnant, and complications of peptic ulcer disease such as perforation and hemorrhage are rare. Proposed mechanisms for the improvement of peptic ulcer disease during pregnancy include (1) a reduction in peptic acid secretion secondary to histaminase produced by the placenta, which reduces the parietal cell response to endogenous histamine, and (2) decreased peptic acid secretion and increased mucus production secondary to the hormonal changes of pregnancy (elevated maternal estrogen and progesterone levels). Some investigators do not find altered secretion.

A. Diagnosis. A history of dyspepsia, which includes epigastric pain that is relieved by food or the ingestion of antacids, especially pain that awakens the patient 1 or 2 h after resting, is so highly suggestive of peptic ulcer that therapy may be considered in the pregnant patient on this basis alone. If simple therapy does not improve symptoms, tests such as **upper gastrointestinal radiographs or endoscopy** may be considered.

B. Management.

1. **Antacids.** The goal of treatment is to neutralize gastric hydrochloric acid. Antacids (magnesium and aluminum hydroxide) several hours after meals and at bedtime should be used for 6 weeks, regardless of symptoms, which correlate poorly with ulcer healing.

2. **Diet.** Avoidance of irritating foods, cigarettes, and alcohol may be helpful.

3. If **hemorrhage occurs,** management includes:
   a. **Nasogastric suction** and **ice water lavage**
   b. **Blood replacement** therapy
   c. **Surgery** if the bleeding is unresponsive to medical management.

   Note: Neither histamine (H₂) blockers nor mucosal surface protective agents such as sucralfate have been proven to be safe in pregnancy.

   Note: Misoprostol, a synthetic analogue of prostaglandin F₁, which inhibits gastric acid secretion, is contraindicated in pregnancy. Limited experience in the first trimester of pregnancy in women seeking abortion reveals an increased frequency and intensity of uterine contractions and increase uterine bleeding over placebo-treated women.

C. Prognosis. In women with improvement of peptic ulcer disease during pregnancy, 50 percent have recurrences within several months of delivery.

VI. Pancreatitis.

A. Incidence. The incidence of pancreatitis in pregnancy, most often occurring in the third trimester during the peak rise in plasma triglycerides or postpartum, is 0.1 to 0.01 percent of pregnancies. Primigravid patients have been reported to be more prone to pancreatitis; however, this has been contested by large reviews that note no difference in parity. Gallstones, a common cause of pancreatitis, occur more frequently in multigravidas.

B. Morbidity and mortality

1. **Maternal.** Maternal morbidity and mortality (studies estimate 5 to 15 percent) associated with pancreatitis are substantial and include congestive heart failure, pulmonary complications (pneumonia, emboli, pleural effusion), hypotension, hyperglycemia, acidosis, hypocalcemia, hypokalemia,

hypochloremia, jaundice, fatty liver encephalopathy, pre-eclampsia, disseminated intravascular coagulation, sepsis, and paralytic ileus.

2. **Perinatal.** There is a reported increased incidence of spontaneous abortion, preterm labor, hypoxemia, and growth retardation with pancreatitis. There is an 11 to 38 percent perinatal mortality.

C. **Cause.**
   1. **Causative factors.** Reported causes of pancreatitis in pregnancy include biliary disease and passage of gallstones with obstruction of the ampulla or Vater (35 to 90 percent of cases), alcohol abuse, preeclampsia, tetracycline therapy, thiazide diuretic therapy, liver disease, hyperlipidemia, and hyperparathyroidism. *Physiological hyperlipidemia of pregnancy* may be due to hyperinsulinism, to decreased levels of apo-CII, or to an estrogen-induced increase in triglyceride synthesis and very low density lipoprotein secretion.
   2. **Predisposing factors.** Several physiologic alterations of pregnancy may predispose to pancreatitis, including:
      a. A possibly increased incidence of cholelithiasis due to progesterone-caused decreased gallbladder emptying and increased tone in the sphincter of Oddi
      b. Increased serum cholesterol and triglyceride levels in pregnancy, changing the composition of bile and favoring gallstone formation
      c. Increased pancreatic secretions in pregnancy
      d. Increased intraabdominal pressure, causing pancreatic ducts to rupture

D. **Pathogenesis and pathology.** Obstruction of the pancreatic duct may be the factor that causes pancreatitis, as it is almost always associated with gallstones in pregnancy. Other reported associations are hypertriglyceridemia, *Ascaris lumbricoides,* and alcoholism. The enzymes within the pancreas can cause damage by edema, inflammation, hemorrhage, and necrosis. Pancreatic pseudocysts and abscesses may result.

E. **Differential diagnosis**
   1. Preeclampsia
   2. Cholecystitis
   3. Hepatitis
   4. Duodenal ulcer
   5. Appendicitis
   6. Gastroenteritis
   7. Intestinal obstruction

F. **Diagnosis**
   1. **History and physical examination.** Common signs and symptoms are nausea, vomiting, and epigastric pain radiating to the back; less common signs and symptoms are jaundice, fever, pleuritic right-sided chest pain, ileus, and shock. Physical examination may be relatively unremarkable or may include discovery of epigastric left upper quadrant or

flank tenderness, flank ecchymosis (Grey-Turner's sign), fever, ascites, and periumbilical discoloration (Cullen's sign).

2. **Laboratory evaluation**
   a. **Serum amylase.** The serum amylase level may be elevated, especially if obtained early in the disease process. Serum amylase levels are > 200 U/100 ml 2 to 12 h after the onset of pain. A return to normal serum levels of amylase may occur by 48 h. There is no correlation between amylase levels and maternal or infant mortality. (Serum amylase activity varies widely during pregnancy and may be as high as 150 IU/L in normal pregnant women, although serum amylase isoenzyme activity remains unchanged.)
   b. **Serum lipase.** The serum lipase level is also increased in acute pancreatitis and may be a more specific test.
   c. **Serum calcium.** Hypocalcemia may occur with pancreatitis.
   d. **Urine amylase/creatinine clearance.** The urine amylase/creatinine clearance ratio is increased during acute pancreatitis. Urine amylase rises within 1 or 2 days of the onset of symptoms and remains elevated for up to 10 days.
   e. The amylase/creatinine clearance ratio, which is normally lower during pregnancy, remains elevated longer than the serum amylase/creatinine and urine amylase/creatinine ratios. It is useful in diagnosing pancreatitis in patients who present after a few days of clinical symptoms with a normal serum amylase level.

3. **Ultrasound examination.** Ultrasound may be helpful in visualization of the pancreas and biliary system. Gallstones, extrahepatic biliary obstruction, pancreatic masses, or pseudocysts may be visualized by ultrasound, thus aiding the determination of a causative or predisposing factor or disease complication.

G. **Management**
   1. **Supportive care.** Supportive measures are the mainstay of management of pancreatitis in pregnancy and include:
      a. **Nothing by mouth (NPO)** to suppress pancreatic secretions (dietary restriction of long chain fatty acids in hyperlipidemia-associated pancreatitis).
      b. **Nasogastric suction.**
      c. **Intravenous fluid therapy** to prevent hypovolemia and to correct electrolyte disturbances, hyperglycemia (with insulin), and hypocalcemia (with calcium gluconate).
      d. **Analgesics** (meperidine, 50 to 100 mg q3–4 h intramuscularly p.r.n. pain).
      e. **Antibiotics.** Ampicillin (0.5 to 2 g q6 h, usually intravenously) if there is a persistent fever. The length of administration of the antibiotic depends on the clinical response of the patient to therapy. Minimally, a sus-

tained afebrile response is sought before antibiotic therapy is discontinued.

f. **Treatment of any underlying disease** is very important, as any associated causative stimulus will be maintained until the underlying disease is brought under control.

g. **Parenteral hyperalimentation** is rarely necessary, although it may be required if a catabolic starvation state ensues when NPO/intravenous fluid therapy is continued for more than 10 days to 2 weeks.

h. **Plasma exchange,** used experimentally, has been reported to lower the serum triglyceride level and remove the precipitating cause of pancreatitis in hyperlipidemia-associated pancreatitis of pregnancy.

2. **Severe cases of pancreatitis may require peritoneal lavage** to reduce intraperitoneal irritation, and **surgical resection or drainage** may be needed for pseudocysts and abscesses. (Up to 30 percent of pseudocysts < 5 cm in diameter resolve spontaneously. Chronic pseudocysts [persisting > 6 weeks] > 5 cm in diameter rarely do.)

H. **Prognosis.** Pancreatitis is usually a self-limited disease. With conservative management, gallstones will invariably pass into the duodenum and pancreatitis will subside, permitting surgical treatment if necessary to be performed electively during the second trimester or in the postpartum period. The recurrence rate has been reported to be up to 52 percent compared with 20 percent in nonpregnant subjects.

VII. Appendicitis

A. **Incidence.** The incidence of appendicitis in pregnancy is 0.03 to 0.2 percent of pregnancies and 1/1500 deliveries (0.07 percent). There is no predisposition to appendicitis in pregnancy. The incidence is equal in all three trimesters. Appendicitis is the most common surgical emergency occurring during pregnancy.

B. **Morbidity and mortality.** Maternal mortality has been estimated to be as high as 1 to 2 percent. By gestational age, maternal mortality has been reported to be 1.9 percent in the first and second trimesters and 11.2 percent thereafter, compared with 0.27 percent for the general population. The increased mortality may be due to decreased localization of infection with the appendix high in the peritoneal cavity, the enlarged uterus reducing the efficacy of the omentum in isolating the appendix, and the possible prevention of adhesion formation by Braxton Hicks contractions. It is also suggested that the pregnancy-related increase in adrenocorticoids may suppress the normal response to inflammation. Finally, delay in diagnosis contributes to the higher mortality rate in pregnancy. Appendiceal perforation occurs in pregnancy and the puerperium with an incidence of 25 to 60 percent compared to 29 percent in the general population. Premature labor is probably the most common fetal complication (10 to 15 percent of cases). The overall fetal loss is

3 to 10 percent, but mortality is increased if perforation occurs (up to 70 percent).
C. **Pathogenesis and pathophysiology.** In the pathogensis of appendicitis the appendiceal lumen becomes occluded by lymphoid hyperplasia or by a fecalith. An infection then occurs in the appendix and acute appendicitis ensues. Distention of the appendix follows, causing pain, usually periumbilical in location. As the serosa becomes inflamed and contacts the peritoneum, the pain becomes more intensive locally. As the ischemia increases, perforation may occur, with resultant peritonitis.
D. **Differential diagnosis.** Other conditions in the differential diagnosis of appendicitis are ectopic pregnancy, salpingitis, ruptured corpus luteum or dermoid, adnexal torsion, round ligament pain, preterm labor, abruptio placentae, degenerating leiomyomata, and, less commonly, pneumonia, endometriosis of the appendix, and diseases of the bowel, urinary tract system, gallbladder, or pancreas. In a recent review of several series, the final diagnosis in 545 patients with a preoperative diagnosis of acute appendicitis during pregnancy was appendicitis in 73 percent, normal appendix in 21 percent, and other diagnoses in 6 percent.
E. **Diagnosis**
   1. **Signs and symptoms.** Signs and symptoms of acute appendicitis include nausea and vomiting, anorexia, periumbilical pain that localizes in the right lower quadrant about 50 percent of the time, low-grade fever, and leukocytosis. Guarding is found in 60 percent of patients and rebound in 70 percent, but their presence is less constant in late pregnancy. In one series, 85 percent of patients without rebound tenderness were found to have retrocecal appendices. **Bryan's sign** (pain elicited when the gravid uterus is shifted to the right side) has been reported to be a reliable physical finding. **Alder's sign** is said to be helpful in distinguishing intrauterine and extrauterine disease. The patient is turned on her left side from a supine position while maintaining pressure on the point of maximum tenderness. If the pain is lessened, it is intrauterine in origin; if it is fixed, it is extrauterine. The close proximity of the ureter to an inflamed appendix late in pregnancy may result in sterile pyuria.
   2. **Pregnancy complicating the diagnosis.** Pregnancy may make the diagnosis of appendicitis more difficult because of:
      a. Cephalad movement of the location of the appendix as pregnancy progresses
      b. Normal elevated white blood cell count in pregnancy
      c. Greater difficulty in performing a physical examination because of the presence of an enlarged uterus, lifting the abdominal wall away from the appendix, causing muscular laxity and diminished peritoneal signs
      d. Nausea, vomiting, constipation, abdominal discomfort, and urinary symptoms, which are common complaints in pregnancy

3. Other diagnostic measures
   a. **Laparoscopy** may be useful in the first trimester; however, the diagnosis can usually be made on the basis of clinical and laboratory assessment alone. (Technically, this becomes more difficult as pregnancy progresses.)
   b. **Culdocentesis** can confirm the presence of pus in the cul-de-sac from perforation of the appendix. This is not without risk in view of the soft, very vascular, enlarged uterus in the pelvis.
   c. **Ultrasonography.** A high degree of diagnostic accuracy for acute, nonperforating appendicitis and appendiceal mass has been reported with graded compression; however, its sensitivity in the presence of perforation is low. Ultrasonography is useful in excluding uterine and ovarian disorders from the differential diagnosis.

F. Management
   1. Appendectomy. Appendectomy is the treatment for appendicitis, whether or not associated with pregnancy. If performed on a pregnant patient, special attention should be paid to avoiding manipulation of the uterus during the surgery. Such manipulation may cause the onset of premature labor. If the patient is in active labor and delivery is imminent, the operation may be delayed for a short time, but immediate appendectomy is advised if prolonged labor is anticipated. The incision should be made at the point of maximum tenderness. A right, transverse, muscle-splitting incision superior to the fundus of the uterus has been used in many series, although a low midline incision and a right paramedian incision (when the diagnosis is uncertain) have also been reported. Cesarean delivery should be performed only for obstetric indications.
   2. Antibiotics. Antibiotics should be administered if the appendix is found to be ruptured at surgery. Antibiotics should be chosen to cover gram-negative rods and anaerobes (e.g., **cefoxitin,** 2 g IV q12 h, or **clindamycin,** 600 mg IV q6 h, and **gentamycin,** 60 to 80 mg IV q8 h). Whether to give antibiotics to the patient whose appendix is unruptured at the time of surgery is controversial.
   3. Tocolytics. If uterine irritability occurs before, during, or in the first few days after surgery, tocolytic agents should be administered. Whether to administer tocolytics prophylactically is controversial and is a decision that the clinician must make on an individual basis at the time of treatment (see Chapter 22).
   4. Prophylactic appendectomy at the time of elective cesarean section has been shown to be a safe procedure.

VIII. Extreme obesity. Morbidly obese women are at greater risk for hypertension, diabetes, large-for-gestational-age infants, and other peripartum complications.

A. **Jejunoileal bypass.** Jejunoileal bypass is an operative technique to reduce the active surface of the intestine for the purpose of weight reduction. To accomplish this, the proximal 35 cm of the jejunum is anastomosed to the terminal 10 cm of the ileum.

   1. **Morbidity.** Complications from jejunoileal bypass include abnormality of liver function and amino metabolism, electrolyte imbalance, vitamin deficiency, hypocalcemia, hypomagnesemia, nephrolithiasis, cholelithiasis, polyarthritis, and diarrhea. Fertility does not seem to be impaired. Premature labor and subsequent premature delivery and intrauterine growth retardation have been reported to be increased following jejunoileal bypass, especially during the period of greatest weight loss.

   2. Management. The complications of jejunoileal bypass may be decreased if pregnancy is delayed 1 to 2 years after the bypass surgery. Monitoring for fetal well-being may be indicated, depending on the obstetric situation. Parenteral nutritional supplementation may be necessary if gastrointestinal function is so poor that inadequate nutrition is provided during pregnancy.

B. **Gastroplasty.** Gastroplasty, which surgically reduces the stomach volume by 90 percent, is a safer alternative to intestinal bypass surgery since patients generally experience fewer metabolic and nutritional problems. Available data have led to the conclusion that neither the mother nor the fetus is at higher risk for complications if pregnancy occurs after the period of rapid postoperative weight loss. One study reported a decreased incidence of hypertension (from 46 to 9 percent) and a significant decline in mean birth weight (from 3604 to 3205 g). There was no significant difference in the incidence of prematurity, small-for-gestational-age babies, prolonged hospitalization of the newborn, or perinatal deaths.

IX. Inflammatory bowel disease

A. **Incidence.** Regional enteritis and ulcerative colitis are diseases that may affect young women of childbearing age. Regional enteritis occurs in approximately 0.02 percent and ulcerative colitis in 0.1 percent of the childbearing population.

B. **Morbidity and mortality. Regional enteritis** may lead to abdominal abscesses or intestinal obstruction. **Severe ulcerative colitis** may produce complications such as toxic megacolon, colonic perforation, and colonic stricture. A hemorrhage rate of 10 to 15 percent has been reported. Systemic manifestations may occur in almost any body part.

C. **Cause.** Inflammatory bowel disease seems to have a hereditary predisposition. An autoimmune process may be responsible for the disease state, but other causes that have been suggested are diet, infection, and abnormal blood flow to the bowel. The risk of inheriting inflammatory bowel disease has not been established; however, several reports suggest a polygenic influence with varying degrees of penetration (observed family incidence ranging from 5 to 35 percent). The familial occurrence is less for patients with ulcerative colitis than for Crohn's disease.

D. **Pathogenesis and pathophysiology**

1. **Regional enteritis.** Regional enteritis is usually a chronic condition characterized by inflammatory changes in the bowel, causing diarrhea and pain. Malabsorption of iron and vitamin B_{12} may occur if the terminal ileum is involved. The inflammation may extend transmurally, and enteroenteris fistulas can occur. The mucosa becomes "cobblestoned" in appearance, with sequential lesions.

   a. **Fertility.** Regional enteritis **may decrease fertility;** however, this conclusion is controversial. Early studies did not address the effect of birth control practices (previously, patients were cautioned against pregnancy), nutritional status before and after bowel surgery, the effect of severe perineal fistulas and decreased libido from a debilitated state on fertility, and fertility of the male partner.

   b. **Effect of pregnancy on regional enteritis.** Pregnancy does not cause an exacerbation of the disease. If the disease is active at conception, exacerbation of symptoms may occur during the pregnancy. (Approximately one-third will improve, one-third will remain unchanged, and one-third will deteriorate.) The first trimester or the puerperium is suggested as the most likely time for relapse.

   c. **Effect of enteritis on pregnancy.** Complications such as **spontaneous abortion** and **prematurity** may be increased when regional enteritis is active during pregnancy. The site of involvement does not appear to affect the pregnancy.

2. **Ulcerative colitis.** Ulcerative colitis is a more acute condition than regional enteritis and causes bloody, watery diarrhea. The bowel mucosa is friable, with small ulcerations. Usually the distal colon and rectum are affected.

   a. **Fertility.** Patients with ulcerative colitis do not appear to have a greater incidence of infertility.

   b. **Effect of pregnancy on ulcerative colitis.** Pregnancy does not usually cause exacerbation of the disease. The severity of ulcerative colitis during pregnancy depends on the disease activity at conception. In patients with active disease at the time of conception, approximately 50 percent will worsen, about 25 percent will improve, and about 25 percent will remain unchanged. The first trimester is a period of high risk for relapse. Studies also report the second trimester and the puerperium as times of high risk that may be related to changes in levels of corticosteroids. Disease activity has also been reported to be affected by psychological factors (e.g., the attitude toward pregnancy).

   c. **Effect of ulcerative colitis on pregnancy.** If the disease is severe, the fetal outcome may be compromised; increased rates of spontaneous abortion and prematurity have been reported. Total parenteral nutrition and better fetal monitoring may improve the prognosis for this group of patients. An initial attack during pregnancy is not more severe than in the nonpregnant state. Disease activity during one pregnancy is probably independent of that of subsequent pregnancies. Ileostomies have not been shown to affect fertility or the course of pregnancy. Patients with ileostomies are concerned about the change in abdominal shape, requiring a new appliance, fluid and electrolyte management during period of nausea and vomiting, and stomal ileal prolapse from increased abdominal pressure (usually when pregnancy occurs within less than a year of ileostomy placement).

E. **Diagnosis.** Diagnosis of inflammatory bowel disease is usually made prior to pregnancy. Often the diagnostic procedures used during pregnancy are for evaluation of exacerbations and complications. The **history and physical exam findings** suggest the disease; diarrhea, nausea, vomiting, and abdominal pain are the common presentations. **Microscopic examination of the stool for white cells, stool culture, sigmoidoscopy, colonoscopy,** and **biopsy** may also be necessary to assess disease activity. Although it is best to avoid irradiation when possible, **x-ray exams** should be performed if necessary to evaluate for bowel perforation or megacolon. (Double-contrast barium enema examination has been estimated to expose the fetus to .008 Gy (.8 rad), which is far below the .25 Gy (25 rads) reported to be associated with gross fetal abnormalities.)

F. **Management**

   1. **Regional enteritis.** The treatment of regional enteritis during pregnancy is similar to the standard treatment of the disease:

     a. Rest.

     b. High-calorie, high-protein, low-fat diet. Nutritional factors including serum albumin and total protein should be followed monthly in patients with active disease.

     c. Total parenteral nutrition and hyperalimentation is a treatment in severe cases.

     d. Antidiarrheal medication: diphenoxylate (Lomotil), 10 mL q6–8 h.

     e. Prednisone, 40 to 60 mg/d p.o., can be used for acute exacerbation, with the dose tapered gradually as the patient improves. The dose is then reduced to 5 to 10 mg q.d. over the following 2 to 6 months.

     f. Surgery is indicated for bowel obstruction, abscess or

fistulas, or for symptoms that do not respond to medical treatment.

g. Cesarean section should be considered if perirectal abscesses and fistulas are present or have been a complication in the past.

Note: Azathioprine, which is used in the standard treatment of regional enteritis, has not been proven safe for use in pregnancy, although normal deliveries have been reported in renal transplant patients using steroids and azathioprine. The congenital anomaly rate is less than 4 percent. The efficacy of prophylactic steroid use during the puerperium to prevent relapses has not been established.

2. **Ulcerative colitis.** The treatment of ulcerative colitis in pregnancy is similar to the standard treatment of the disease. The following measures are taken during an acute attack:

a. Bed rest.

b. Low-residue diet to rest the bowel.

c. A blood count during disease exacerbation.

d. Antidiarrheal medication with diphenoxylate (Lomotil), 10 mL q6–8 h. Toxic megacolon may be precipitated in severely ill patients.

e. Hospitalization with hyperalimentation or total parenteral nutrition may be necessary in severe cases.

f. Steroids: Prednisone, 40 to 80 mg/d p.o., or glucocorticoid enemas (50 mg hydrocortisone) may be used in resistant cases.

g. Sulfasalazine (Azulfidine), starting with 1 mg/d p.o. and increasing to 2 to 4 m/d in divided doses, has anti-inflammatory and immunosuppressive effects that are useful in alleviating acute exacerbations. Sulfasalazine interferes with folic acid absorption in the small bowel; therefore, patients taking sulfasalazine often require supplemental folic acid. Sulfasalazine crosses the placenta, and theoretically can displace unconjugated bilirubin from plasma albumin and cause kernicterus, but this rarely occurs. It reaches concentrations in breast milk of 45 percent of that of maternal serum and has not been demonstrated to be harmful in nursing infants.

h. Surgical treatment may be necessary for bowel obstruction or perforation, toxic megacolon, or hemorrhage.

BIBLIOGRAPHY

Biggs JFG. Treatment of gastrointestinal disorders of pregnancy. Drugs 1980; 29:70.

Burrow GN, Ferris TF, eds. Medical Complications During Pregnancy. 3rd ed. Philadelphia: WB Saunders; 1988.

Creasy RK, Resnik R, eds. Maternal Fetal Medicine Principles and Practice. 2nd ed. Philadelphia: WB Saunders; 1984.

Cunningham FG, MacDonald PC, Gant NF, eds. Williams Obstetrics. 18th ed. New York: Appleton; 1989.

Dunagan WC, Ridner ML, eds. Manual of Medical Therapeutics. 26th edition. Boston/Toronto: Little, Brown; 1989.

Gleicher N, ed. Principles of Medical Therapy in Pregnancy. 2nd ed. Norwalk: Appleton and Lange; 1992.

Miller JP. Medical disorders of pregnancy. Clin Obstet Gynecol 1977; 4:297.

Nausea and Vomiting/Hyperemesis Gravidarum

Depue RH, Bernstein L, Ross RK, et al. Hyperemesis gravidarum in relation to estradiol levels, pregnancy outcome, and other maternal factors: A seroepidemiologic study. Am J Obstet Gynecol 1987; 156:1137–1141.

Jarnfelt-Samsioe A. Nausea and vomiting in pregnancy: A review. Obstet Gynecol Survey 1987; 41:422–427.

Klebanolt MA, Kostowe PA, Kaslow R, Rhoads GG. Epidemiology of vomiting in early pregnancy. Obstet Gynecol 1985; 66:612–616.

Morim M, Nobuyuki A, Tamaki H, et al. Morning sickness and thyroid function in normal pregnancy. Obstet Gynecol 1988; 72:355.

Weigel RM, Weigel MM. Nausea and vomiting of early pregnancy and pregnancy outcome: A meta-analytical review. Br J Obstet Gynaecol 1989; 96:1312–1318.

Gastroesophageal Reflux

Desmond PV, Watson KJR. Metaclopramide—a review. Med J Aust 1986; 144:366–368.

Llauro JL, Runnebaum B, Zander J. Progesterone in human peripheral blood before, during and after labor. Am J Obstet Gynecol 1968; 101:867–873.

Van Thiel DH, Gavater JS, Joshi SN, et al. Heartburn of pregnancy. Gastroenterology 1977; 72:666–668.

Peptic Ulcer Disease

Monk JP, Clissold SP. Misoprostol: A preliminary review of the pharmacodynamic and pharinadokinetic properties, and therapeutic efficacy in the treatment of peptic ulcer disease. Drugs 1987; 33:1–30.

Pancreatitis

Block P, Kelly TR. Management of gallstone pancreatitis during pregnancy and the postpartum period. Surg Gynecol Obstet 1989; 168:426–428.

Corlett RC, Mishell Dr. Pancreatitis in pregnancy. Am J Obstet Gynecol 1972; 113:218–290.

Devore GR, Bracken M, Berkowitz RL. The amylase/creatinine clearance ratio in normal pregnancy and pregnancies complicated by pancreatitis, hyperemesis gravidarum and toxemia. Am J Obstet Gynecol 1980; 136:747–754.

Joupplla P, Mokkar R, Larmi TKI. Acute pancreatitis in pregnancy. Surg Gynecol Obstet 1974; 139:879–882.

McKay AJ. Pancreatitis, pregnancy and gallstone. Surg Gynecol Obstet 1979; 139:879–882.

McKay AJ. Pancreatitis, pregnancy and gallstones. Br J Obstet Gynaecol 1980; 87:47–50.

Ranson JHC, Rifkind KM, Roses DF. Prognostic signs and the role of operative management in acute pancreatitis. Surg Gynecol Obstet 1974; 139:69–81.

Strickland DM, Hauth JC, Widish J, et al. Amylase and isoamylase activities in serum of pregnant women. Obstet Gynecol 1984; 63:389–391.

Appendicitis

Babaknia A, Parsa H, Woodruff JD. Appendicitis during pregnancy. Obstet Gynecol 1977; 50:40–44.

Black WP. Acute appendicitis in pregnancy. Br Med J 1960; 1:1938–1941.

Frisenda R. Acute appendicitis during pregnancy. Am Surg 1979; 45:503.

Horowitz MD, Gomez GA, Santiesteban R, Burkett G. Acute appendicitis during pregnancy. Arch Surg 1985; 120:1362–1367.

Masters K, Levine BA, Gaskill HV, Sirinek KR. Diagnosing appendicitis during pregnancy. Am J 1984; 148:768–771.

Parsons AK, Sauer M, Parsons MT, et al. Appendectomy at time of cesarean section. Obstet Gynecol 1986; 68:479–482.

Puylaert JB, Rutgers PH, Lalisang RI, et al. A prospective study of ultrasonography in the diagnosis of appendicitis. N Engl J Med 1986; 317:666–669.

Jejunoileal Bypass

Wood JR. Influence of jejunoileal bypass on protein metabolism during pregnancy. Am J Obstet Gynecol 1978; 130:9–17.

Gastroplasty

Printen KJ, Scoh D. Pregnancy following gastric bypass for the treatment of morbid obesity. Am Surgeon 1982; 48:363–365.

Richards DS, Miller DK, Goodman GN. Pregnancy after gastric bypass for morbid obesity. J Reprod Med 1987; 32:172–176.

Inflammatory Bowel Disease

Fedorkow DM, Persaud D, Nimrod CA. Inflammatory bowel disease: A controlled study of late pregnancy outcome. Am J Obstet Gynecol 1989; 160:998–1001.

Hanan IM, Kirsner JB. Inflammatory bowel disease in the pregnant woman. Clinics in Perinatology 1985; 12:669–682.

Korelitz BI. Pregnancy, fertility and inflammatory bowel disease. Am J of Gastroenterology 1985; 80:365–370.

Miller JP. Inflammatory bowel disease in pregnancy: A review. J Roy Soc of Med 1986; 79:221–225.

Nilsen OH, Andreassen B, Bondesen S, Jarrum S. Pregnancy in ulcerative colitis. Scand J Gastroenterol 1985; 18:735–742.

Porter RJ, Stirrat GM. The effects of inflammatory bowel disease on pregnancy: A cease-controlled retrospective analysis. Br J Obstet Gynaecol 1986; 93:1124–1131.

CHAPTER 33

Hepatobiliary Diseases

Michael T. Parsons
Marcello Pietrantoni

Hepatobiliary disease in pregnancy often presents diagnostic dilemmas, as some of the biochemical parameters necessary for evaluation of hepatobiliary disease are altered in pregnancy.

Unchanged laboratory values. Serum aspartate aminotransferase (serum glutamic-oxaloacetic transaminase), alanine aminotransferase (serum glutamic-pyruvic transaminase), lactate dehydrogenase, bilirubin, and the prothrombin time are usually unchanged in pregnancy.

Altered laboratory values in pregnancy
1. **Increased:** total alkaline phosphatase, triglycerides, cholesterol, fibrinogen, transferrin, ceruloplasmin, bromsulphalein retention at 45 min.
2. **Decreased:** albumin levels.

I. **Hepatitis.** Hepatitis is the major cause of jaundice during pregnancy. The major forms of viral hepatitis are (1) hepatitis A virus (HAV), (2) hepatitis B virus (HBV), (3) hepatitis C virus (HCV) (parenterally transmitted non-A, non-B hepatitis), (4) hepatitis D virus (HDV), formally called the *delta agent,* and (5) hepatitis E virus (HEV) (previously known as *epidemic* or *water-borne non-A, non-B hepatitis*).
  A. **Incidence.** The overall incidence of hepatitis in the pregnant population is similar to that in the nonpregnant population (0.03 to 0.1 percent in North America). In pregnancy, less than 10 percent of cases are due to HAV, 75 to 80 percent to HBV, and the remainder to the other three.
  B. **Morbidity and mortality**
    1. **HAV** in pregnant patients has a mortality similar to that of the general population, less than 0.1 percent. A chronic carrier state occurs rarely, if ever, in HAV. Some reports indicate that the incidence of preterm labor may be increased. The risk of vertical transmission to the fetus is low due to the brief viremic period.
    2. **HBV** follows a course in the pregnant state similar to that in the nonpregnant state; mortality is less than 0.1 percent.

Patients with medical disorders are more likely to have a prolonged and severe course. Fulminant hepatitis is a severe complication with massive hepatic necrosis, encephalopathy, and coma but is rare. The carrier state occurs in 0.1 to 1 percent of cases and may include chronic active hepatitis. Long-time carriers of hepatitis B surface antigen (HBsAg) have an increased incidence of hepatocellular carcinoma. Third-trimester involvement may increase the chance of preterm birth. Transmission of the virus to the infant (vertical transmission), either in utero or at the time of delivery, places the infant at risk for acute hepatitis and its complications.

3. **HCV** has a course in pregnancy similar to that in the nonpregnant state. Although clinically HCV and HBV have similar courses, HCV is less severe, and up to two-thirds of patients have few or no symptoms. However, a greater percentage of HCV patients will progress to a chronic carrier state with fluctuating transaminase levels.

4. **HDV:** Acute infection may be associated with fulminant hepatitis, and chronic infection is frequently associated with a severe form of chronic hepatitis.

5. **HEV** is clinically similar to HAV, being self-limiting and mild, except in pregnant women, in whom mortality rates have been reported to reach 10 to 20 percent.

C. **Cause**
1. **HAV** is caused by a single-stranded, 27-nm RNA picornavirus, enterovirus type 72.
2. **HBV** is caused by a double-stranded, 44-nm DNA virus belonging to the hepadnaviridae. A 7-nm HBsAg is present on the outer portion, a 27-nm hepatitis B core antigen (HBcAg) is present on the surface of the core, and a hepatitis B e antigen (HBeAg) is contained in the core.
3. **HCV:** The genome of HCV, recently isolated, is a single-stranded RNA of approximately 10 000 nucleotides possibly related to the togaviridae or flaviviridae.
4. **HDV** is a defective RNA-containing particle that requires the presence of HBV (HBsAg) for infection and replication to occur.
5. **HEV** is caused by a single-stranded, linear RNA and possibly a member of the calciviridae.

D. **Pathogenesis and pathophysiology**
1. **HAV** is predominantly spread by fecal-oral transmission. Contamination of food and drinking water can lead to large outbreaks. Parenteral transmission is rare. The incubation period is approximately 15 to 50 days. Epidemics have been reported on large regional bases in child care centers.
2. **HBV** is most often spread by infected blood or serous fluid products via percutaneous or permucosal routes, including close physical contact with an infected person. The in-

cidence of acquired HBV increases with the number of sexual partners. The incubation period is 15 to 49 days, with resolution normally occurring in 6 months.

3. **HCV** is most often spread parenterally or by blood products and is found in 0.2 to 1.5 percent of random blood donors. HCV accounts for up to 95 percent of all current transfusion-associated hepatitis cases. Like HBV it may be spread by close physical contact with an infected person. The median incubation period is 50 days. A carrier state also exists, and chronic hepatitis may occur.

4. **HDV** is most often spread parenterally or by blood products, with most cases involving drug users. HDV may occur as a coinfection with HBV or superimposed upon an existing HBV infection.

5. **HEV** is most often spread by the fecal-oral route and is known to cause epidemic hepatitis in young adults in South Africa, North Africa, and Eastern Europe.

E. **Viral pathophysiology.** Viral hepatitis may result in a wide range of manifestations from asymptomatic illness to death. The prodromal period begins a few days to 2 weeks before jaundice (bilirubin > 4 mg/dL) appears. Symptoms that may arise include gastrointestinal upset with nausea and vomiting, fatigue, anorexia, headache, myalgia, arthralgia, pruritus, weight loss, and photophobia. A low-grade fever may be present. As these symptoms subside, jaundice and dark urine develop. The liver increases in size and becomes tender. Serum chemistry abnormalities include elevated serum transaminase levels, often above 1000 mU/mL. The serum albumin level also rises. The hepatic cells undergo necrosis and infiltration of mononucleocytes.

Most patients recover completely within 3 to 6 months. Less than 10 percent of patients with HBV develop a chronic infection with circulating HBsAg. A chronic infectious state also has been seen with HCV. Severe complications include a fulminant condition that progresses to hepatic failure and coma. This is uncommon in the United States. HEV is similar to HAV in that chronicity does not occur. But the clinical course of HEV is often more severe than that of HAV, especially in pregnant women, who have a much greater mortality rate.

One fetal complication is an increased incidence of prematurity. Another is the intrauterine transmission of HBV. In chronic HBsAg carriers (1 percent), the probability of fetal transmission is increased to 80 percent if the mother is positive for the e antigen (HBeAg), which in addition increases the fetus's chances of becoming a carrier. If the mother is HBeAg negative or develops the antibody (+ anti-HBE), the risk decreases. HBV, DNA, and DNA polymers are markers of active viral replication, which may be a better predictor of the fetal risk of hepatitis. The risk of vertical transmission is greater when acute HBV infection occurs in the third trimester. In addition, intrapartum or postpartum transmission of HAV, HBV, and possibly HCV from mother to infant may occur.

F. **Differential diagnosis.** Other disorders that may be confused with viral hepatitis include preeclampsia, hyperemesis gravidarum, cholestasis, acute fatty liver, alcohol abuse, drug use, gastrointestinal upset, and cholelithiasis.

G. **Diagnosis.** A history of nausea, vomiting, gastrointestinal upset, fatigue, anorexia, headache, photophobia, physical examination demonstrating jaundice, tender liver, and elevated laboratory values will raise the suspicion of hepatitis.

1. **HAV** can be detected early by anti-HAV antibody of the IgM class (5 months or less) and later by IgG.

2. **HBV** is established early by demonstrating HBsAg 30 to 50 days after exposure. HBcAg and HBeAg follow. Antibodies to HBcAg and HBeAg appear as the hepatitis B, c, and e antigens disappear. The appearance of the last antibody, HBsAb, indicates recovery from the infection or vaccination.

3. **HCV:** Immunoassays for anti-HCV antibodies are commercially available and routinely used in blood banking procedures.

4. **HDV** infection is diagnosed by serum anti-HDV antibodies and HDV antigen in liver biopsy specimens.

5. **HEV:** Serologic diagnosis is not yet available.

H. **Management**

1. **Treatment:** The treatment of hepatitis in pregnancy, as in the nonpregnant state, is mainly supportive. Adequate caloric and fluid intake is essential. Restriction of physical activity is needed during the acute illness. Hospitalization is not usually necessary unless dehydration or fulminant disease is present.

2. **Prevention**

a. **HAV:** This is prevented by the administration of immunoglobulin, 0.02 mL/kg IM, to individuals exposed to infected contacts. It should not be withheld from pregnant women.

b. **HBV.** It is now recommended that all pregnant women be screened for HBV by HBsAg at the first prenatal visit. Maternal identification and newborn prophylaxis can significantly reduce neonatal infection and life-threatening sequelae. Ideally, both the hepatitis B vaccine and the HBV immunoglobulin (HBIG, 5 mL) should be given within 48 hours of delivery to infants of HBsAg-positive women. High-risk infants whose mothers were HBsAg-positive and who demonstrated high serum HBV DNA levels were shown in one study to have decreased vertical transmission if they were delivered by cesarean section.

HBV recombinant vaccines are recommended for pregnant women who are at high risk for contracting

HBV. HBIG should be given to a susceptible pregnant woman within 48 h after exposure to HBV.

II. **Cholestasis of pregnancy**
   A. **Incidence.** The incidence of cholestasis of pregnancy (pruritus gravidarum) is less than 0.1 percent of all pregnancies. It is the second most common cause of jaundice in pregnancy. It usually manifests in the third trimester and usually recurs in subsequent pregnancies.
   B. **Morbidity and mortality.** Pregnant women with cholestasis suffer from pruritus and occasionally coagulation abnormalities due to decreased vitamin K absorption. Some studies suggest an increased incidence of preterm delivery and stillbirth. There is also an increase in the frequency and severity of postpartum hemorrhage.
   C. **Cause.** Increased sensitivity to estrogens has been suggested as a possible factor in cholestasis of pregnancy. Genetic studies show an autosomal dominant pattern of inheritance.
   D. **Pathogenesis and pathophysiology.** Histologic changes in the liver are those of cholestasis without hepatocellular damage (necrosis or inflammation). Bile plugs are present in the canaliculi.
   E. **Differential diagnosis.** The differential diagnosis of hepatitis in pregnancy includes biliary tract diseases (cholecystitis, cholelithiasis), drug reaction, preeclampsia, hepatitis, and acute fatty liver of pregnancy.
   F. **Diagnosis**
      1. **History:** The history consists of an onset of general pruritus, usually in the third trimester but sometimes appearing as early as the sixth week. Other features are fatigue, jaundice, insomnia, mental disturbances, steatorrhea, and dark urine. Symptoms remit after delivery.
      2. **Physical examination:** Signs of scratching may be visible on physical examination. Jaundice may be present.
      3. **Laboratory evaluation**
         a. Serum bile acid levels are elevated 10 to 100 times normal. This does not correlate with the degree of pruritus.
         b. Serum alkaline phosphatase levels are elevated up to 10 times normal for pregnancy.
         c. Bilirubin levels are elevated up to 5 mg/mL.
         d. Serum transaminase levels may range from normal to moderately elevated.
         e. Stool fat excretion may be abnormal.
   G. **Management**
      1. **Cholestyramine:** 4 g p.o., t.i.d. to increase the serum bile acid level.
      2. **Antipruritics:** diphenhydramine hydrochloride (Benadryl), 25 or 50 mg, p.o., q4–6 h, to a maximum dose of 300 to 400 mg/d, or hydroxyzine hydrochloride (Vistaril), 50 to 100 mg

IM, q4–6 h or 25 to 50 mg, p.o. q6 h as needed. Success is limited.

3. **Topical skin preparations** with lanolin base may reduce local symptoms from the disease or from scratching.

4. **Phenobarbital:** 90 mg/d h.s. with a 1-week trial. This induces hepatic microsomal enzymes and increases bile salt secretion and flow, and may be indicated when cholestyramine is not effective.

5. **Plasmapheresis** may provide relief for up to several weeks.

III. Acute fatty liver of pregnancy

A. **Incidence.** The incidence is reported to be less than 1/12 000 pregnancies. Patients with multiple gestations are at higher risk, and those with male fetuses are two to three times more likely to be affected.

B. **Morbidity and mortality.** Maternal mortality has been reported to be up to 80 percent, but this figure has been decreasing in recent years, approaching 30 percent. Fetal mortality is also extremely high.

C. **Cause.** The cause of acute fatty liver of pregnancy is unknown. One suspected mechanism is a hepatic mitochondrial defect.

D. **Pathogenesis and pathophysiology.** Histologic examination demonstrates a microvesicular fatty infiltrate (free fatty acids) in the hepatocytes (foamy hepatocytes). Oil red O is the specific fat stain used to detect these cells. Cellular necrosis is not usually present, and one-quarter of cases may show a mild chronic inflammation histologically. Similar disease has been described with tetracycline toxicity and Reye's syndrome in children.

E. **Differential diagnosis.** The major differential diagnosis is severe preeclampsia. Others are drug-induced liver failure, biliary tract disease, acute rupture of the liver, and viral hepatitis. It is important to suspect acute fatty liver of pregnancy early for optimal treatment.

F. **Diagnosis.** The combination of the history, physical examination, and laboratory studies should suggest acute fatty liver as a possible diagnosis. Being aware of the disease is a necessity since its rarity may cause the clinician to omit it from the differential diagnosis.

1. **History:** Tha patient usually develops this disease in the third trimester. Nausea, vomiting, headache, and epigastric or right upper quadrant pain are often the first symptoms.

2. **Physical examination:** Within a few days, jaundice, possible fever, preeclamptic signs, mental confusion, coma, and multiple organ failure can follow.

3. **Laboratory evaluation:** Abnormalities in laboratory values include mild to moderate increases in the levels of serum transaminase (300 to 500 IU), bilirubin (10 mg/dL), and alkaline phosphatase. Hypoglycemia, abnormal serum ammonia levels, elevated white blood cell count, prolonged prothrombin time, other evidence of disseminated in-

travascular coagulation, and elevated uric acid levels are common.

4. **Liver biopsy:** Biopsy of the liver is the definitive diagnostic measure, but the attendant risk of clotting abnormalities in a pregnant patient must be weighed on an individual basis. The use of fresh frozen plasma prior to biopsy may be helpful.

G. **Management.** Aggressive treatment must be rapidly undertaken to provide an optimal chance for survival of the mother and fetus. Treatment consists primarily of supportive care, which must be administered in an intensive care unit. Steps in intensive management include the following:

1. Correction of coagulopathies by component therapy (fresh frozen plasma, etc.). The prothrombin time should be maintained at < 15 seconds to prevent bleeding from the gastrointestinal and other systems.
2. Close monitoring of and correction of abnormalities of serum electrolytes and glucose is necessary.
3. Maintenance of an airway and respiratory support may be necessary.
4. Nutritional support including hyperalimentation is usually necessary.
5. Close monitoring of the hepatic, gastrointestinal, pancreatic, pulmonary, renal, hematologic, and central nervous systems is mandatory.
6. Delivery of the fetus may be helpful in shortening the disease state.

IV. **Cholelithiasis in pregnancy**
   A. **Incidence.** Despite isolated reports, there is no evidence that the incidence of cholelithiasis (gallstones) and its associated complications is higher in pregnancy than in the nonpregnant state (0.1 percent).
   B. **Morbidity and mortality.** If the disease is recognized and treated appropriately, the maternal and fetal outcome should not be compromised. However, if delays occur and biliary tract obstruction leads to pancreatitis, fetal mortality of 60 percent is reported.
   C. **Cause.** Gallstones are composed primarily of either cholesterol or calcium bilirubinate. The majority of gallstones in pregnant women are cholesterol.
   D. **Pathogenesis and pathophysiology**
      1. Gallstones are formed from supersaturation of bile with cholesterol, followed by crystallization and growth of the stone. Estrogens and/or progestins may increase the concentration of cholesterol in bile and increase stone formation.
      2. The net effect of pregnancy on stone formation and subsequent diseases is controversial.
         a. The biliary cholesterol saturation may be increased in pregnancy.

    b. The size of the fasting gallbladder is increased, and emptying takes longer because of the inhibitory action of progesterone.

    c. The bile ducts may be dilated, allowing easier passage of the stone.

E. Signs and symptoms. If a gallstone does form, **blockage of the cystic duct may cause biliary colic or cholecystitis.** If a stone blocks the common duct, pancreatitis may occur. **Jaundice** may be present. Biliary colic usually occurs within 2 h after meals. This results from blockage of the cystic duct. The **pain** may be steady or intermittent in the right subcostal or epigastric region and may radiate to other parts of the abdomen or upper back. **Nausea and vomiting** may occur. Inflammation of the gallbladder may produce **fever** and an **elevated white blood cell count.**

F. Differential diagnosis. All disorders that may cause upper abdominal pain and/or jaundice in pregnancy must be considered, including gastrointestinal upset, appendicitis, hepatitis, acute fatty liver of pregnancy, pancreatitis, cholestasis, and pregnancy-related conditions such as preeclampsia and abruptio placentae.

G. Diagnosis. Cholelithiasis is often asymptomatic and may be observed on routine obstetric ultrasound examination during pregnancy. When disease is suspected, ultrasound examination of the gallbladder should be performed to look for stones both within the gallbladder and blocking the ducts.

H. Management.

    1. Asymptomatic cholelithiasis. If asymptomatic gallstones are found on routine ultrasound examination, their presence should be noted but no treatment is necessary.

    2. Biliary colic. Biliary colic should be treated with nasogastric suction, hydration, analgesics, and antibiotics if indicated. If the condition does not improve or if pancreatitis develops, surgery is necessary for removal of the stone and possible cholecystectomy.

BIBLIOGRAPHY

American College of Obstetrics and Gynecologists, Committee on Obstetrics. Maternal and fetal medicine: Guidelines for hepatitis B virus screening and vaccination during pregnancy. No. 103, March 1992.

Berg B, Helm G, Petersohn L, et al. Cholestasis of pregnancy. Acta Obstet Gynecol Scand 1986; 65:107–113.

Biggs JFG. Treatment of gastrointestinal disorders of pregnancy. Drugs 1986; 29:70.

Burrow GN, Ferris TF, eds. Medical Complications During Pregnancy. 3rd ed. Philadelphia: WB Saunders; 1988.

Cohen M, Cohen H. Dealing with viral hepatitis during pregnancy. Contemp Ob/ Gyn 1983; 22:29–56.

Creasy RK, Resnik R, eds. Maternal Fetal Medicine Principles and Practice. 2nd ed. Philadelphia: WB Saunders; 1989.

Cunningham FG, MacDonald PC, Gant NF, eds. Williams Obstetrics. 18th ed. New York: Appleton-Century Crofts; 1989.

Dunagan WC, Ridner ML, eds. Manual of Medical Therapeutics. 26th ed. Boston: Little, Brown; 1989.

Gleicher N, ed. Principles of Medical Therapy in Pregnancy. 2nd ed. Norwalk: Appleton and Lange, 1992.

Kaplan M. Acute fatty liver of pregnancy. N Engl J Med 1985; 33:367–370.

Liddle C, Craig PI, Farrell GC. The A, B, C, D and E of viral hepatitis. New agents for old diseases. Aust NZ J Med 1990; 20:3–4.

McKay AJ. Pancreatitis, pregnancy and gallstones. Br J Obstet Gynecol 1980; 87:47.

Pastorek JG, Miller JM, Summers PR. The effect of hepatitis B antigenemia on pregnancy outcome. Am J Obstet Gynecol 1988; 158:486–489.

Rolfes DB, Ishak KG. Acute fatty liver of pregnancy: A clinicopathologic study of 35 cases. Hepatology 1985; 5:1149–1158.

Snydman DR. Hepatitis in pregnancy. N Engl J Med 1985; 33:1398–1401.

CHAPTER 34

Diabetes Mellitus

William N. Spellacy

I. **Incidence.** Before 1921, when insulin was not available as a therapy, very few patients with diabetes mellitus became pregnant. Most young diabetic women did not live to their reproductive age, and the few who did usually had amenorrhea and infertility due to their uncontrolled metabolic disease. In the few cases that did exist, there was usually a poor outcome. For example, in one study, approximately 25 percent of the mothers and about 50 percent of the infants died. In the years since insulin became available the disease has become a common complication of pregnancy, with frequency now of more than 5 percent. During the 1950s, the prognosis for the infant could be predicted by the White classification. This classification (A–T) is shown in Table 34.1. It is less useful today, for with modern management of the pregnant diabetic, the outcome has improved greatly and now is similar to that of women without this medical complication. This chapter will outline detection methods, maternal complications, infant complications, pregnancy management, contraception, and interpregnancy care.

II. **Morbidity and mortality**
   A. **Maternal morbidity and mortality**
   1. Maternal mortality is rare today and is usually the result of a diabetic vascular lesion (stroke or myocardial infarct) or of inappropriately treated ketoacidosis.
   2. Maternal morbidity is common in pregnant women with complicating diabetes mellitus, but the problems are short-term and manageable. There are no long-term sequelae resulting from the pregnancy (see Section VI).
   B. **Perinatal morbidity and mortality.** The most serious problems in pregnancy occur with the fetus and seem to be generally related to maternal hyperglycemia. They include spontaneous abortion, congenital anomalies, macrosomia, neonatal hypoglycemia, respiratory difficulties, and sudden perinatal death, as well as other problems (see Section VI).

III. **Cause.** Although many studies have been done in this area, the exact cause of all diabetes mellitus is unknown. Clearly, a genetic factor is

Table 34.1. White Classification of Diabetes in Pregnancy

Class A:	Gestational diabetes, onset in pregnancy
B:	Onset after age 20 years Duration less than 10 years No vascular disease
C:	Onset between ages 10 and 19 years Duration 10 to 19 years No vascular disease
D:	Onset before age 10 years Duration greater than 20 years Some vascular disease — retina, legs
E:	Pelvic arteriosclerosis demonstrated by x-ray
F:	Vascular nephritis
R:	Proliferative retinopathy
T:	Transplantation

Source: Modified from White P. Joslin's Diabetes Mellitus. 11th ed. Philadelphia: Lea & Febiger; 1971.

involved in some types of the disease, and specific human leukocyte antigen (HLA) types are associated. Other causes include infections, especially with viruses, and autoimmune problems.

IV. Pathogenesis/pathophysiology. While hyperglycemia is a laboratory marker of diabetes mellitus, its cause varies from lack of insulin production by pancreatic beta cells to delayed-release mechanisms by those cells. An accompanying systemic problem is accelerated atherogensis, with resulting disease in the arterial vascular system. The pregnancy problems are related both to the hyperglycemic effects and to the abnormal maternal vascular system.

V. Diagnosis. While some women begin gestation with a known diagnosis of diabetes, many are unaware of this problem. As a result, routine screening is advised for all pregnant women.
   A. Routine screening. It is well recognized that some women are at increased risk of having this disease. These include women with a close family history of diabetes, obese women, those with glucosuria in a fasting state, and those who have had infants who were macrosomic (birth weight > 4500 g), anomalous, or still-born for unexplained reasons. Despite the ability to identify this high-risk group, it is now recommended that **all pregnant women have a blood glucose screening test at the end of the second trimester of pregnancy (weeks 24 to 28).** The specific screen is to administer a 50-g oral glucose load and then to draw

a blood sample 1 hour afterward. A fasting state is not required for screening. **Normally the plasma level for glucose should be less than 140 mg/dL.** If it is higher, the screening test is positive and glucose tolerance testing is necessary. If the screen is negative but other factors suggest diabetes, testing may need to be repeated at other times in the pregnancy.

B. **Glucose tolerance test.** Women with a positive screening test need an oral glucose tolerance test to evaluate their carbohydrate metabolism unless the screening value is very high (> 250 mg/dL). This test should be done after 3 days of an adequate diet (150 g carbohydrate per day) and 10 h of fasting. The woman should remain seated during the test, and urine samples should not be obtained. The stimulus should be a 100-g oral glucose load, and blood samples should be drawn over 3 h. The upper limits of normal for each sample are listed in Table 34.2. If all of the values are below these four points, the patient is normal. If two or more values are elevated, the patient has diabetes. If one value is elevated, her condition is still suspicious and one should consider repeating the glucose tolerance test in 1 month.

C. **Maternal complications**
   1. **Hypoglycemia and hyperglycemia**
      a. **Low blood glucose** problems occur especially during the first half of pregnancy. This results most often from the woman's inability to consume and/or retain her meals due to the effects of high chorionic gonadotropin levels, and unless her insulin dose is reduced, she will be hypoglycemic. There is little evidence that these episodes are hazardous to the fetus.
      b. **Elevated blood glucose** is a significant risk factor for the fetus.
   2. **Insulin shifts.** For the insulin-dependent diabetic, the same insulin resistance of pregnancy occurs. The patient will usually need to increase her insulin dose by two to three times. If her insulin requirements decrease late in pregnancy, placental failure is often suggested and should be regarded seriously. Immediately after delivery the patient's

Table 34.2. Glucose Tolerance Tests in Pregnancy

TIME (H)	FASTING	1	2	3
Plasma glucose (mg/dL)	105	190	165	145
Blood glucose (mg/dL)	90	165	145	125

Source: Modified from O'Sullivan JB, Mahan CM. Criteria for the oral glucose tolerance test in pregnancy. Diabetes 1964; 13:279. Reprinted with permission. Copyright © 1964 by American Diabetes Association, Inc.

insulin needs revert back toward prepregnancy levels, so the dose should be decreased acutely.

3. **Glucosuria.** Large amounts of estrogen are produced by the placenta and fetus causing systemic vasodilation. In the kidney, this results in increased renal blood flow. Since glucose is transferred to glomerular urine by simple diffusion, filtration depends on both blood concentration and blood flow. The increased flow causes more glucose to be filtrated, exceeding the kidney tubules' ability to reabsorb it. As a result, all pregnant women demonstrate glucosuria, with an average excretion of about 300 mg/d. Diabetics with some hyperglycemia may excrete much greater amounts. Urine glucose levels during pregnancy are poorly correlated with blood concentrations, so they are of little use in managing the patient during pregnancy. Twenty-four-hour glucose excretion is a useful parameter of control and is a test that is recommended for management.

4. **Urinary tract infection.** In the diabetic with a tendency toward higher blood glucose substrates in the urine, invading bacteria are more likely to grow. As a result, urinary tract infections occur two times more frequently in these patients. They must have a urine culture done at the first prenatal visit, again at 32 to 34 weeks of gestation, and any time there are symptoms of infection such as increased frequency or dysuria. When bacteriuria occurs, it must be appropriately treated with antibiotics and the urine checked to ensure that it is sterile after the treatment.

5. **Hypertension.** The physiologic changes of pregnancy affect blood vessels and therefore blood pressure. The increased estrogen levels cause the liver to produce more of the protein angiotensinogen, which is converted to angiotensin II, causing vasospasm. The blood vessel endothelium produces increasing amounts of prostacyclin, which antagonizes the angiotensin II. As a result, blood pressure normally falls in midpregnancy. If the woman has abnormal blood vessels, as diabetics frequently do, she has normal high angiotensin II but low prostacyclin, which results in vasospasm and hypertension. The frequency of hypertension is increased more than two times in pregnant diabetics and increases the risks for both the mother and the fetus.

6. **Hydramnios.** Excess amniotic fluid usually includes amounts above 2000 mL. About 10 percent of diabetics have this problem.

7. **Retinopathy.** The severity of eye ground changes in pregnancy relates more to the duration of the disease than to the glucose control. While there is worsening of retinopathy in about 15 percent of patients during gestation, the most serious problems occur in women with proliferative retinopathy. If these lesions are untreated, they progress in about 85 percent of patients, and some women can premanently

lose vision. With laser coagulation, however, the lesions can be controlled. It is important for diabetic patients to have an ophthalmologic consultation early and serially during pregnancy so that appropriate detection and treatment can occur.

D. Fetal problems. The most serious problems with this complication of pregnancy occur in the fetus and generally seem to be related to maternal hyperglycemia.

1. **Spontaneous abortion.** In general, the spontaneous abortion rate for women with well-controlled diabetes mellitus is similar to that for women without the disease. However, if the blood glucose level is markedly elevated during the first trimester of pregnancy, the spontaneous abortion rate is significantly elevated as well. Thus good glucose control in early pregnancy is important.

2. **Congenital anomalies**

   a. **Associated anomalies.** It has been recognized for years that infants of diabetic mothers (IDMs) have about a threefold increased risk of anomalies. While sacral agenesis is a unique anomaly for this group, it is rare. More common anomalies are cardiac and limb deformities. When the gestational time of insult is studied, it is found that these anomalies occur between the third and sixth weeks of pregnancy. This becomes important in terms of prevention.

   b. **Hemoglobin A1C.** The cause of these anomalies can be explored with a new biochemical tool — hemoglobin A1C. When blood glucose levels become elevated above normal, some of the glucose couples with serum proteins. This also occurs with hemoglobin, where glucose covalently binds to valine on the beta chain. This linkage is irreversible, and the red blood cell is marked with this increased glycolysated hemoglobin for the remainder of its life, which is about 4 weeks. The glycolysated hemoglobin moves rapidly in electrophoresis and is termed *hemoglobin A1C*. One can then measure A1C and determine if hyperglycemia occurred in the prior month. When diabetic women are studied at the end of the first trimester, those with normal A1C levels (euglycemic) have no increased rate of anomalous infants, whereas those with high A1C levels have severalfold increased rate of anomalous infants. These data strongly suggest that hyperglycemia during weeks 3 to 6 causes fetal anomalies. A multicenter prospective study of glucose control in early pregnancy failed to confirm these suspicions. However, it is still recommended that good glucose control be maintained during the first trimester to prevent abortion and anomalies.

3. **Macrosomia.** The normal fetus utilizes the glucose that comes across the placenta by facilitated diffusion as its major

food for growth and development. When the mother's blood glucose levels are elevated, the increased glucose crosses the placenta and produces fetal hyperglycemia. The fetus in such a setting is "overfed" and grows large, with increased deposits of fat and glycogen. When the fetus exceeds 4500 g, it has macrosomia and is at significantly increased risk for birth trauma due mainly to shoulder dystocia. The IDM has larger shoulder measurements than similar-weight infants from nondiabetic women, which increases the risk of dystocia. These infants should be screened with ultrasound before vaginal delivery is attempted, and if extreme macrosomia is suspected, delivery is probably best accomplished by cesarean section.

4. **Neonatal hypoglycemia.** If the fetus is exposed to hyperglycemia, its production of insulin will increase. When it is delivered and the glucose supply is cut off but the insulin secretion persists, the infant can develop hypoglycemia, especially during the early hours of life. This can be serious since the central nervous system utilizes glucose as a major substrate. Prolonged hypoglycemia can produce brain dysfunction, so must be detected early and treated with parenteral glucose infusions.

5. **Respiratory difficulties.** Neonates from diabetic mothers of all ages tend to have a five- to sixfold increased frequency of respiratory distress syndrome (RDS). This may be due to fetal hyperglycemia and is poorly predicted by simple amniotic fluid surfactant tests like the lecithin/sphinomyelin (L/S) ratio or the shake test. The best predictor is the amniotic fluid phosphatidylglycerol level. Neonatal management includes exogenous surfactant, positive expiratory pressure respirators, oxygen, and humidity.

6. **Perinatal death.** Sudden fetal death, especially during episodes of severe maternal hyperglycemia, are common and are not well understood. General speculation is that poor oxygen release and hypoxia or fluid and electrolyte shifts are the causes. Control of maternal blood glucose levels is most important in reducing perinatal mortality.

7. **Other problems.** The IDM is prone to many other problems, including hypocalcemia, hyperbilirubinemia, polycythemia, and renal vein thrombosis. Careful neonatal evaluation and management are essential for these fragile infants. Later in life these children tend to be obese, and they have an increased risk of about 10 percent of developing diabetes mellitus.

VI. **Pregnancy management.** There are two key principles in the management of the diabetic mother in pregnancy: (1) control of maternal blood glucose levels and (2) early delivery in an appropriate site based on fetal heart testing and lung maturity. The details of this management program include the following:

A. **Insulin-dependent diabetes**
   1. **Frequent visits to the health care team.** In general these patients do not need prolonged hospitalization, but they do need to be seen frequently by the health care team. This may mean several visits per week. The team includes many health professionals, such as a maternal-fetal medicine subspecialist, obstetrician, neonatololgist, anesthesiologist, nutritionist, nurse, and social worker, as well as the patient.
   2. **Diet.** The patient will need about 300 calories per day more during her pregnancy than in the nonpregnant state. Thus her diet will be the number of calories per day that she consumes to maintain a normal weight when not pregnant plus 300. In general, this will be about 35 calories per kilogram of ideal body weight. It is critical that she consume the same number of calories every day at the same time of the day; otherwise, good glucose control will be impossible to achieve. She will need iron supplements in the second half of gestation, as do other pregnant women.
   3. **Glucose monitoring.** The best monitor of blood glucose control is blood glucose tests, and the patient can be taught to do these at home. She should do about four tests per day (fasting, before a meal, 1 h after a major meal, and at bedtime), and the results should be recorded and brought with her to every prenatal visit. Fasting glucose levels should be about 75 to 85 mg/dL, and 1-hour values should be about 120 to 140 mg/dL. If high levels occur, she must contact a team member immediately. In addition, she can bring a 24-h urine collection to each prenatal visit, where it can be quickly and inexpensively tested for glucose. With good glucose control, a sample will usually show only a trace to 1+ glucose (< 2 g/d). Monthly hemoglobin A1C levels are also helpful in monitoring glucose control. Hemoglobin A1C normally decreases as pregnancy progresses, to a low point at about 24 weeks of gestation.
   4. **Insulin dose.** Insulin, with a molecular weight of 6000, does not cross the placenta and therefore does not directly affect the fetus. The type of insulin used in treatment is less important than the amount. Patients need enough insulin to keep their blood glucose levels normal at all times, since glucose does cross the placenta and can harm the fetus. Insulin is usually administered by multiple injections per day of both long-acting and short-acting types. One method is to give two-thirds of the dose in the morning (two-thirds long-acting and one-third short-acting) and one-third in the evening (one-half long-acting and one half short-acting). Continuous subcutaneous infusion with portable pumps with the addition of small boluses of insulin before meals can also be used, but no better glucose control is achieved. It is expected that the insulin needs of the patient will increase two

to three times due to the pregnancy effects of "insulin resistance," and most of this change occurs between the 20th and 30th weeks of gestation. After the placenta is delivered, the dosage can be cut in half. Oral hypoglycemic agents are not recommended for use during pregnancy.

5. **Urine cultures.** As already discussed, the frequent maternal problems of urinary tract infections require urine cultures to be obtained at the first visit, at 32 to 34 weeks, and when symptoms or signs suggestive of infection such as albuminuria or dysuria occur. Positive cultures of ≥ 100 000 organisms per milliliter of urine should be treated with appropriate antibiotics.

6. **Ophthalmologic examination.** The eye grounds need to be evaluated early in pregnancy and at least once in each trimester. Some patients with extensive retinopathy or new visual symptoms need more frequent exams. Proliferative retinopathy can be treated with laser photocoagulation during the pregnancy.

7. **Fetal health assessments.** The well-being of the fetus needs to be monitored serially in these pregnancies. Generally, this starts between 30 and 32 weeks of gestation unless the woman also has hypertension, in which case earlier monitoring (at 26 to 28 weeks) is useful. Continuous electronic monitoring of the fetal heart rate is the method most commonly used today. Current data suggest that a contraction stress test done once per week is ideal and is probably more sensitive than a nonstress test (NST). Multiple NSTs per week are of no greater value than those conducted once a week.

8. **Fetal maturity assessment.** The IDM lung tends to be mature at about 38 weeks of gestation. The first tests are then planned for 37 weeks of gestation. One critical organ system whose maturity can be tested is the pulmonary system. Measurement of amniotic fluid phosphatidylglycerol is the best test for this population and has a lower false-positive rate than the L/S ratio. When amniocentesis is done, an aliquot of fluid can be sent for glucose testing, as it reflects the prior week of glucose control. If the fluid glucose value exceeds 25 mg/dL, fetal hyperglycemia has been present and more neonatal problems, including low Apgar scores, can be anticipated.

9. **Ultrasound.** Real-time ultrasound studies are helpful in these patients. Measurements in the first half of gestation help set the due date accurately and are useful in determining the date of the first amniocentesis. During pregnancy, estimates of fetal growth patterns and amniotic fluid volumes are helpful, as are studies for fetal anomalies. At the end of gestation, the ultrasound exam allows a safe amniocentesis to be performed by identifying easily accessible pools of fluid. Finally, assessment of fetal weight, utilizing abdominal cir-

cumference studies, will detect macrosomia so that elective cesarean section can be considered.

10. **Preterm labor.** The IDM tends to have more than the usual problems if delivered prematurely, so preterm labor in diabetic patients needs to be treated aggressively. Since the beta-mimetic tocolytic drugs like ritodrine raise blood glucose levels dramatically, the first-line tocolytic drug of choice for these patients is magnesium sulfate given by intravenous infusions. This is accompanied by bed rest and hydration.

11. **Delivery.** Delivery should occur at a site where an experienced team can handle all the perinatal problems. If spontaneous labor has not occurred by 39 to 40 weeks, induction of labor is usually indicated unless, it is obstetrically contraindicated or macrosomia exists. Tight glucose control during labor is important. Internal fetal heart rate monitoring during labor, when feasible, is important, and abnormal tracings may be studied further with fetal scalp blood pH tests.

B. **Ketoacidosis.** A very serious problem for both the mother and the fetus is ketoacidosis. It must be treated quickly and aggressively to reduce the sequelae, including death. Continuous intravenous infusion of insulin, restoration of hydration, and monitoring of pH and glucose are critical. In general, regular insulin should be infused intravenously at a rate of 25 U/h until the acidosis is reversed, and then 10 U/h should be given until the hyperglycemia is normalized. The fluid deficit of 3 to 6 L should be treated rapidly with 2 L of normal saline, and fluid then given according to the urine output. When the blood glucose level reaches 250 g/dL, glucose can be added to the infusion. Potassium replacement will be needed as the glucose is metabolized. Bicarbonate will be needed for severe acidosis (pH < 7.0).

C. **Gestational diabetes.** The normal insulin resistance of pregnancy produced by the hormones of the placenta causes pancreatic beta cells to hypertrophy and hyperfunction. If there is a subclinical abnormality in these cells there will be inadequate production of insulin and hyperglycemia will result. This condition is called *gestational diabetes* and will generally become subclinical after delivery. The pregnant woman with mildly elevated blood glucose values detected by glucose tolerance testing can usually be managed easily and is at low risk for fetal death. Blood glucose regulation is first attempted with dietary modification alone; if this is not adequate, insulin treatment may be necessary. If the fasting blood glucose values are elevated, these women will usually need insulin treatment. Women who are manageable with dietary modification alone do not need to measure the blood glucose at home but rather can have a fasting and a 1-hour postmeal glucose test done at their prenatal visit. A hemoglobin A1C level can also be measured the last 2 months of gestation. Generally these pregnancies are taken to term and labor is induced if it has not occurred by that time. The fetus may be monitored with weekly NSTs beginning at 38 weeks of gestation. The major fetal risk in gestational diabetes is macrosomia. This should be checked for with ultrasound before attempting vaginal delivery.

VII. Contraception. Women with diabetes mellitus should be encouraged to have their pregnancies early in their reproductive lives before serious vascular complications occur. Child spacing can best be done with barrier methods like the diaphragm with contraceptive cream. Intrauterine devices have also been used in diabetics, with no significant increase in pelvic infection. Since oral contraceptives may have an adverse effect on blood vessels, they are best avoided in this population. After the family is complete, sterilization should be offered.

VIII. Interpregnancy care. When the woman is planning for her next pregnancy, there are two things she should do. First, her blood glucose levels should be monitored and brought under tight control; otherwise, there may be unnecessary hyperglycemia during the early weeks of gestation. Second, she should take and record her basal body temperature so that the timing of ovulation is precise and therefore the gestational dating is accurate.

BIBLIOGRAPHY

Archimaut G, Belizan JM, Ross NA, et al. Glucose concentration in amniotic fluid: Its possible significance in diabetic pregnancy. Am J Obstet Gynecol 1974; 119:596.

Coustan DR, Nelson C, Carpenter MW, et al. Maternal age and screening for gestational diabetes: A population-based study. Obstet Gynecol 1989; 73:557.

Daughaday WH, Trivedi B, Winn HN, et al. Hypersomatotropism in pregnant women, as measured by a human liver radioreceptor assay. J Clin Endocrinol 1990; 70:215.

Garner PR, D'Alton ME, Dudley DK, et al. Preeclampsia in diabetic pregnancies. Am J Obstet Gynecol 1990; 163:505.

Miller E, Hare JW, Cloherty JP, et al. Elevated maternal hemoglobin A1C in early pregnancy and major congenital anomalies in infants of diabetic mothers. N Engl J Med 1981; 304:1331.

Mills JL, Baker L, Goldman AS. Malformations in infants of diabetic mothers occur before the seventh gestational week — implications for treatment. Diabetes 1979; 28:292.

Olofsson P, Sjoberg NO, Solum T, et al. Changing panorama of perinatal and infant mortality in diabetic pregnancy. Acta Obstet Gynecol Scand 1984; 63:467.

O'Sullivan JB, Mahan CM. Criteria for the oral glucose tolerance test in pregnancy. Diabetes 1964; 13:278.

O'Sullivan JB, Mahan CM, Charles D, et al. Screening criteria for high-risk gestational diabetic patients. Am J Obstet Gynecol 1973; 116:895.

Pedersen J. The Pregnant Diabetic and Her Newborn: Problems and Management. Baltimore: Williams & Wilkins; 1977.

Phelps RL, Honig GR, Green D, et al. Biphasic changes in hemoglobin A1C concentrations during normal human pregnancy. Am J Obstet Gynecol 1983; 147:651.

Spellacy WN. Diabetes mellitus complicating pregnancy. Mod Med 1969; 37:91.

Spellacy WN. Diabetes and pregnancy. In: Sciarra J, ed. gynecology and obstetrics. Vol 2. Hagerstown, Md: Harper and Row; 1978: chap 35.

Spellacy WN. Family planning and the diabetic mother. Semin Perinatol 1978; 2:395.

Spellacy WN. Buhi WC, Cohn JE, et al. Usefulness of rapid blood glucose measurements in obstetrics: Dextrostix/reflectance meter system. Obstet Gynecol 1973; 41:299.

Spellacy WN, Cruz AC, Buhi WC, et al. The acute effects of Ritodrine infusion on maternal metabolism: Measurements of levels of glucose, insulin, glucagon, triglycerides, cholesterol, placental lactogen and chorionic gonadotropin. Am J Obstet Gynecol 1978; 131:637.

Spellacy WN, Goetz FC. Plasma insulin in normal late pregancy. N Engl J Med 1963; 268:988.

Spellacy WN, Miller S, Winegar A, et al. Macrosomia — maternal characteristics and infant complications. Obstet Gynecol 1985; 66:158.

Stamler EF, Cruz ML, Mimouni F, et al. High infectious morbidity in pregnant women with insulin-dependent diabetes: An understated complications. Am J Obstet Gynecol 1990; 163:1217.

White P. Pregnancy complicating diabetes. Am J Med 1949; 7:609.

CHAPTER 35

Endocrine Disease

Jeffrey C. King

This chapter reviews the normal maternal endocrine adaptations to pregnancy as well as the effects of specific endocrine disorders, except diabetes mellitus, which is discussed in Chapter 34. Unrecognized or untreated maternal endocrine abnormalities are often incompatible with conception and successful pregnancy. When pregnancy does occur, there is no doubt that the added demands of pregnancy in the face of an altered endocrine milieu may adversely affect the developing fetus.

THYROID PHYSIOLOGY AND THE EVALUATION OF THYROID FUNCTION IN PREGNANCY

Thyroid dysfunction is relatively frequent in women of childbearing age. Because of the various endocrine effects of normal pregnancy on the gravida, the diagnosis and management of thyroid disorders in the pregnant women are quite challenging. Since the usual signs and symptoms of a hypermetabolic state (warm skin, palpitations, increased gland size, heat intolerance) often occur in normal pregnancy, the interpretation of thyroid function tests becomes critical in the diagnosis and management of pregnant patients with thyroid disorders.

During normal pregnancy, maternal thyroid function should remain normal. An increase in the serum concentrations of total thyroxine (T_4) and triiodothyronine (T_3) and a decrease in triiodothyronine resin uptake (T_3RU) occur as a result of hyperestrogenemia and estrogen-induced increases in thyroxine-binding globulin (TBG). Serum thyroid-stimulating hormone (TSH) is generally unchanged by pregnancy. The thyroid secretes at least two biologically active hormone: T_4 and T_3. Most of the circulating T_3 is formed as a result of peripheral conversion of T_4. Reverse T_3 (rT_3) is similarly formed by peripheral deiodination of T_4, but rT_3 does not appear to have biologic activity. The placenta is impermeable to the natural iodothyronines (T_4, T_3, and rT_3), as well as to TSH.

Since T_4 and T_3 are bound to TBG, serum values are often elevated; however, the active or free T_4 and T_3 are unchanged by pregnancy. Calculation of the free thyroxine index (FT_4I) and of the free triiodothyronine index (FT_3I) is easy, and their values correlate well with actual free T_4 and T_3 values.

$$FT_4I = T_4 \times \frac{T_3RU \text{ of the patient}}{T_3RU \text{ normal mean}}$$

$$FT_3I = T_3 \times \frac{T_3RU \text{ of the patient}}{T_3RU \text{ normal mean}}$$

An abnormally high FT_4I value is consistent with hyperthyroidism, and a low value suggests hypothyroidism. The main purpose of determining the FT_3I is to confirm the diagnosis of hyperthyroidism (Table 35.1).

Thyroid stimulating antibodies (TSab), which are present in 90 percent of patients with Graves' disease, cross the placenta and may produce fetal or neonatal hyperthyroidism. Various names have been given to these antibodies, including *long-acting thyroid stimulator (LATS,), LATS protector,* and *thyroid-stimulating immunoglobulin (TSI)*. Because the fetal thyroid begins to concentrate iodine at about 10 weeks' gestation, the use of either diagnostic or therapeutic radioactive iodine after this time is contraindicated.

Hyperthyroidism

I. **Incidence.** Approximately 0.2 percent of obstetric patients have hyperthyroidism.

II. **Morbidity and mortality**
   A. **Maternal.** Fertility is generally not affected by mild to moderate hyperthyroidism, and in the absence of thyroid storm the pregnant woman is at little increased risk from hyperthyroidism.

Table 35.1. Results of Thyroid Function Tests during Pregnancy

TEST	NONPREG-NANT NORMAL	PREGNANT NORMAL	PREGNANT HYPER-THYROID	PREGNANT HYPO-THYROID
Total T$_4$	Normal	Increased	Increased	Decreased
Free T$_4$	Normal	Normal	Increased	Decreased
FT$_4$I	Normal	Normal	Increased	Decreased
Total T$_3$	Normal	Slight increase	Normal to slight increase	Normal to slight decrease
FT$_3$I	Normal	Normal	Normal to increased	Normal to decreased
T$_3$RU	Normal	Decreased	Increased	Decreased
TSH	Normal	Normal	Normal to decreased	High
TSab	Negative	Negative	Often positive	Negative

B. Fetal. Some studies have indicated that the fetus is at increased risk for congenital malformations when the mother was hyperthyroid and untreated at conception (a risk of 6 percent) compared to fetuses whose mothers were euthyroid on therapy during the first trimester (a risk of 0.2 percent). The fetus is at a small increased risk of mortality but at a definite increased risk of low birth weight.

III. Cause. The most common cause of hyperthyroidism in pregnancy is **Graves' disease,** which accounts for 85 percent of cases. However, other causes that must be considered include acute and subacute thyroiditis, chronic lymphocytic thyroiditis (Hashimoto's disease), toxic nodular goiter, toxic adenoma, hydatidiform mole, and choriocarcinoma.

IV. Pathogenesis. The pathogenesis of **Graves' disease** is unknown. A viral infection (adenovirus, coxsackie virus, influenza virus, and echovirus) is suspected as the cause of **acute thyroiditis.** The pathophysiology of Hashimoto's disease is the production of serum antibodies to thyroglobulin and microsomal fractions of the thyroid gland.

V. Diagnosis
   A. Signs and symptoms. The classic signs and symptoms of hyperthyroidism include nervousness, palpitations, heat intolerance, weakness, weight loss, fatigue, diarrhea, tachycardia, hyperreflexia, tremor, eye signs (exophthalmos, lid lag, stare), and skin changes. Unfortunately, many of these signs and symptoms occur in normal pregnancy, making the diagnosis difficult. The strongest clues are persistent maternal tachycardia (pulse > 100 beats per min) and unexplained weight loss or failure to gain weight appropriately during pregnancy.
   B. Physical examination. The thyroid gland is usually diffusely enlarged (two to five times its normal size) in patients with hyperthyroidism. A thrill may be felt on palpation of the thyroid gland or a bruit may be heard when the gland is auscultated. Multinodular goiter or single adenoma is found in 10 percent of patients. Mild enlargement of one or both lateral lobes of the thyroid gland in association with pain, often radiating to the posterior auricular process, is found in patients with acute thyroiditis.
   C. Laboratory examination
   1. **T_4, T_3, T_3RU, FT_4I, and FT_3I** values are all elevated in hyperthyroidism. The diagnosis can be confirmed by finding an elevated free T_4 value. In patients who present with clinical signs of hyperthyroidism but whose thyroid studies are normal, T_3 and FT_3I values should be obtained to diagnose T_3 hyperthyroidism.
   2. Tests for **TSab** are useful to determine if the fetus is at risk for Graves' disease.

VI. Management. Antithyroid medication is the treatment of choice for most patients. Subtotal thyroidectomy is reserved for the patient who is allergic or resistant to antithyroid medications. However, drug resistance is usually due to poor patient compliance with medical therapy.

A. Medical management: Antithyroid medications. The goal of antithyroid medical therapy in pregnancy is to achieve a euthyroid or slightly hyperthyroid state in the mother and to avoid fetal hypothyroidism or hyperthyroidism.

  1. Graves' disease. Propylthioruracil (PTU) and methimazole (the thioureas) are the mainstay of drug therapy of Graves' disease. PTU crosses the placenta more slowly than methimazole (Tapazole) and blocks not only intrathyroid synthesis of T_4 but also peripheral conversion of T_4 to T_3. Therefore, of the two drugs, **PTU has become the drug of choice** for the treatment of Graves' disease in pregnant women. The disease is usually brought under control in 3 to 4 weeks when the drug is given at least twice a day. The **initial dose of PTU is 300 to 400 mg/d (in oral divided doses)** and **that of methimazole is 30 to 40 mg/d (in oral divided doses),** depending on the patient's symptoms. Most patients respond favorably to drug therapy with a decrease in pulse rate, weight gain, and improvement in thyroid function, and the amount of antithyroid drug can be reduced by half as soon as the thyroid test results return to near normal. The FT_4l is the first value to normalize, with the FT_3l lagging by a few weeks. Since the plasma half-life to T_4 is 7 days, laboratory assessment at intervals of less than 1 week is not indicated. Further reductions in dosage may be made every 2 weeks if improvement continues. After euthyroidism has been established and maintained for at least 4 to 6 weeks, antithyroid medications may be tapered and the patient followed clinically for evidence of relapse. Ideally, PTU should have been tapered to < 100 mg/d by term. With methimazole, the target by term is < 10 mg/d.

    a. Maternal complications of thioureas occur in 3 to 5 percent of patients. The most frequent problems are skin rash, pruritus, fever, and nausea. As there is little cross-reactivity, the alternate drug should be substituted at the equivalent dosage if side effects develop. Fortunately, granulocytopenia and agranulocytosis are rare (0.1 percent) complications. They are usually associated with sore throat and fever and occur after 1 to 2 months of therapy. Patients must be advised to discontinue their medication and to see their physician for a white blood cell count if these symptoms occur.

    b. Fetal effects. The fetus and neonate must be observed for the development of hypothyroidism or goiter. Ultrasound evaluation of the fetal neck diameter may prove diagnostic. During labor, assessment of neck flex-

ion may be helpful in evaluating fetal gland size. Obviously, thyroid function studies should be obtained for all neonates following delivery if the mother has been treated with thiourea medication.
   c. **Long-term maternal and fetal effects.** Long-term follow-up of both infants and mothers exposed to thioureas has not revealed any mental or physical deficits.
   d. **Use of thiourea medication during lactation.** Use of PTU during lactation is controversial. While the drug has been shown to enter breast milk, levels are very low. The use of normal PTU doses (200 to 300 mg/d) probably carries no significant risk to the neonate. **Methimazole** is secreted in higher concentrations in breast milk and is therefore **not recommended** for lactating mothers.
2. **Acute thyroiditis.** No antithyroid medication is advised for the treatment of the usually mild hyperthyroid symptoms of acute thyroiditis. Small doses of thioureas may be necessary in the treatment of Hashimoto's disease if the serum T_4 level is greater than 20 and the FT_4I level is elevated.

B. **Surgical management.** No prospective trials comparing the merits of surgical vs. medical treatment have been published. However, it is generally accepted that the risks of postoperative hypoparathyroidism, recurrent laryngeal nerve paralysis, preterm labor, and anesthetic mishaps make surgery a less attractive approach to therapy. Surgery may be indicated for the removal of a single hyperfunctioning thyroid nodule. There is no surgical therapy for hyperthyroidism due to acute thyroiditis, Hashimoto's disease, or toxic multinodular goiter. Obviously, evacuation of a hydatidiform mole and surgical removal or chemotherapy for choriocarcinoma is indicated in the face of hyperthyroidism. If surgical treatment of Graves' disease is decided upon, it should be performed during the second trimester if possible. Preoperative treatment with propylthiouracil, Lugol's solution, or saturated solution of potassium iodide should be considered to reduce the risk of thyroid storm.

Hypothyroidism

I. **Incidence.** Hypothyroidism is a rare condition associated with pregnancy and is more often associated with infertility.

II. **Morbidity and mortality.** If hypothyroidism is detected during pregnancy, it is usually very mild, since a severe lack of T_4 results in elevated prolactin and anovulation, and hence infertility. Pregnancies complicated by hypothyroidism may be associated with increased fetal loss, but apparently infants born of hypothyroid mothers show no physical or intellectual deficiencies.

III. Cause. The principal causes of hypothyroidism are chronic lymphocytic thyroiditis, previous I^{131} treatment of Graves' disease, and subtotal thyroidectomy.

IV. Diagnosis

    A. Signs and symptoms. Generally, patients with hypothyroidism often have nonspecific symptoms such as tiredness, lethargy, and weakness, as well as cold intolerance, constipation, and arthralgias.

    B. Physical examination. Patients with hypothyroidism often have dry, coarse skin, a slow pulse, and a delayed reflex relaxation phase. A goiter may be palpated. Hair loss at the lateral aspects of the eyebrows is often noted.

    C. Laboratory examination. The diagnosis of hypothyroidism is confirmed by the finding of low serum T_4 and FT_4I levels along with an elevated TSH.

V. Management. Therapy consists of thyroid replacement with **T_4 (Synthroid), 0.1 to 0.2 mg/d (orally in a single dose)** to achieve clinical and chemical euthyroidism. TSH values may take up to 8 weeks to return to normal after initiation of therapy, and the frequency with which the TSH level is measured to monitor therapy should be decided accordingly.

PARATHYROID DISEASE

The growth and development of the human fetus requires the accumulation of up to 30 g of calcium prior to delivery. Normally this calcium accumulation occurs without depletion of maternal plasma or bone. The maternal plasma level depends on complex interactions of peptide hormones (parathyroid and calcitonin) and sterol hormones (vitamin D and its metabolites) with various target tissues.

Calcium Metabolism in Pregnancy

The amount of calcium required by the fetus during pregnancy for skeletal development does not increase in a linear way throughout pregnancy but instead accelerates rapidly during the third trimester. In the absence of major changes in the mass of calcium in the skeleton, the extracellular calcium concentration is determined by the balance between calcium absorption from the gut and its excretion into the urine and feces. The maternal skeleton acts as a surface to provide about 300 mmol of calcium exchange between blood and bone per day. This exchange is regulated by parathyroid hormone (PTH), which shifts calcium into the blood, and by calcitonin, which inhibits this shift.

The placenta contains a calcium pump that maintains fetal levels at about 1 mEq/L higher than the maternal level. During pregnancy, maternal calcium levels are maintained within a relatively narrow range but show a slight downward trend. This change is believed to be an attempt to correct the calcium drop. While there is also a modest rise in calcitonin, the reason for this rise is unknown.

Hyperparathyroidism

I. **Incidence.** Hyperparathyroidism is an exceedingly rare condition complicating pregnancy. It is rarely encountered before puberty and is two to three times more common in females than in males.

II. **Morbidity and mortality.** Fertility is not affected, and labor and delivery are normal in hyperparathyroidism. However, the disease has a detrimental effect on the fetus, causing high morbidity and variable mortality. Low-birth-weight infants are more commonly born of hyperparathyroid mothers, and over 50 percent of gravidas with hyperparathyroidism deliver infants who develop neonatal tetany when the maternal supply of calcium is removed, with subsequent profound, prolonged neonatal hypocalcemia.

III. **Cause.** The cause of hyperparathyroidism is essentially unknown. In about 50 percent of cases it is caused by a single autonomous parathyroid adenoma. Other causes include hyperplasia of all four parathyroid glands and carcinoma of the parathyroid glands.

IV. **Diagnosis**
   A. **Signs and symptoms.** Patients with hyperparathyroidism are generally asymptomatic, although when symptoms are present, they may include polydipsia, polyuria, fatigue, constipation, nausea and vomiting, and nephrolithiasis. Profound hypercalcemia may result in stupor or coma.
   B. **Physical examination** is generally unremarkable, as palpable adenomas of the parathyroid gland are exceedingly uncommon.
   C. **Laboratory examination.** Laboratory findings include persistently elevated serum PTH and calcium levels (> 10 mg/dL), along with low serum phosphate levels. Tests of tubular readsorption of phosphate or urinary excretion of cyclic adenosine monophosphate may also be helpful.

V. **Management**
   A. **Maternal management.** The treatment of choice for hyperparathyroidism is surgical removal of the adenoma or hyperplastic parathyroid glands. This should be performed early enough during pregnancy so that maternal and fetal calcium levels return to normal and allow full recovery of the suppressed fetal parathyroids. When surgery is contraindicated, therapy with oral phosphate may be an effective alternative (24 ml of 1 M dibasic sodium phosphate q.i.d. to supply a total dose of 3 g of phosphate per day. Dibasic potassium phosphate may be combined with sodium phosphate if reduced sodium intake is required.)
      Severe hypercalcemia may require immediate therapy with large-volume administration of intravenous saline and Lasix to promote renal clearance of calcium.
   B. **Neonatal management.** The neonate should be evaluated com-

pletely following delivery. Prophylactic calcium administration may prevent neonatal tetany. Unfortunately, most cases of maternal hyperparathyroidism are detected postpartum after the occurrence of neonatal tetany.

Hypoparathyroidism

I. **Incidence.** Whether associated with pregnancy or not, hypoparathyroidism is even rarer than hyperparathyroidism.

II. **Morbidity and mortality.** Treated hypoparathyroidism has no deleterious effect on pregnancy or on the newborn. Offspring of mothers with untreated hypoparathyroidism may develop hyperparathyroidism. This disease of the neonate is self-limited; x-ray evidence of osteitis fibrosa cystica disappears within 4 months of birth.

III. **Cause.** The most common cause of hypoparathyroidism is iatrogenic, usually due to inadvertent removal or compromise of the blood supply during thyroid surgery. It is postulated that idiopathic hypoparathyroidism may be an autoimmune disorder.

IV. **Diagnosis**
   A. **Signs and symptoms.** Weakness, fatigue, paresthesias, muscle cramps, seizures, tetany, and psychiatric aberrations are common signs and symptoms of hypoparathyroidism. Rarely, laryngeal stridor or generalized convulsions may be seen. Maternal hyperventilation and alkalosis are the most common causes of maternal tetany during pregnancy.
   B. **Physical examination.** The elicitation of Chevostek's or Trousseau's sign is helpful in uncovering latent maternal tetany. The skin may be dry and scaly, and the nails may be brittle and have transverse ridges.
   C. **Laboratory examination.** Serum calcium and PTH levels are abnormally low and the phosphate level is elevated. Urinary calcium and phosphate excretion are both depressed.

V. **Management**
   A. **Antepartum management.** Generally, the hypoparathyroid patient is receiving vitamin D (10 000 to 100 000 IU/d) and calcium therapy (1.0 to 1.5 g/d) prior to pregnancy. Fortunately, no alternation of the regimen is necessary. Concentrations of calcium and phosphorus should be monitored monthly. The obstetric hypoparathyroid patient requires 2 g of elemental calcium or 24 g of calcium gluconate or 8 g of calcium lactate per day.
   B. **Intrapartum management.** Patients with hypoparathyroidism must be monitored carefully during labor, since hyperventilation may lead to alkalosis and tetany. Treatment with calcium glu-

conate during labor will maintain a normal serum level. The use of magnesium should be avoided if possible.

C. **Fetal effects and management.** The question of fetal congenital abnormalities as a result of therapy for hypoparathyroidism has been raised, since vitamin D crosses the placenta. However, no evidence has been found to link fetal malformations, particularly cardiovascular or craniofacial, to vitamin D usage.

D. **Breast-feeding** is undesirable for patients with hypoparathyroidism due to the calcium demands of lactation (400 mg/L of human milk) in addition to the normal daily calcium requirement.

ADRENAL DISEASE

The adrenal gland plays a central role in the metabolism of the human. Clinical and laboratory evaluations of the integrity of adrenal function are very difficult because signs and symptoms of dysfunction mimic those of normal pregnancy.

Physiology during Pregnancy

The weight of the maternal adrenal gland does not increase with pregnancy. While adrenocorticotropic hormone (ACTH) levels are apparently unchanged, the adrenal gland appears to be more responsive to stimulation. Plasma cortisol circulates as an unbound free form or is bound to corticosteroid-binding globulin (CBG). Plasma cortisol levels rise progressively during pregnancy and reach a plateau above the upper limits of normal during the second trimester. There is no loss of the normal diurnal rhythm.

The fetal adrenal grows rapidly and by the 16th week is larger than the fetal kidney. There are two zones in the fetal adrenal: the inner or fetal zone represents 80 percent of the cortex in utero, and the outer zone is destined to become the adult adrenal. Fetal adrenal function begins at approximately 8 weeks' gestation.

Adrenocorticol Insufficiency (Addison's Disease)

I. **Incidence.** Addison's disease is rare, with only a few hundred cases reported in association with pregnancy.

II. **Morbidity and mortality.** With diagnosis and treatment, the maternal and fetal prognosis is good in Addison's disease. The neonate should be watched for the rare condition of adrenal suppression secondary to maternal adrenal steroid replacement therapy. Patients with undiagnosed or untreated Addison's disease tolerate pregnancy well. However, they may present with acute adrenal insufficiency postpartum due to an inability to mount an adrenal response to the stress of delivery.

III. **Cause.** The cause of chronic adrenal insufficiency is most commonly associated with polyendocrine autoimmune disorders causing impairment of adrenal steroid synthesis, along with decreased function of other target organs. Other causes of hypoadrenalism are surgical adrenalectomy or secondary adrenal insufficiency from pituitary or hypothalmic dysfunction. **Acute adrenal insufficiency (addisonian crisis)** is usually due to abrupt termination of adrenal steroid medication given on a chronic basis. Additionally, it may occur following delivery or whenever the patient is unable to mount an appropriate adrenal response to stress.

IV. Diagnosis
    A. Signs and symptoms. Usually weakness, lassitude, mild nausea, increased pigmentation, and nondescript abdominal pain are seen in patients with chronic adrenocortical insufficiency. Weight loss and persistent nausea and vomiting should alert the physician to the possibility of adrenal insufficiency.
    B. Physical examination. Essentially no abnormalities are found in patients with Addison's disease on physical examination.
    C. Laboratory examination. Hyponatremia and hyperkalemia are common. Spontaneous hypoglycemia is often seen. Plasma cortisol concentrations may be in the normal range. The diagnosis is confirmed by the lack of rise in the plasma cortisol concentration after ACTH infusion.

V. Management of chronic adrenocortical insufficiency
    A. Antepartum management. For chronic adrenocortical insufficiency, the usual dosage of adrenal steroid replacement is **oral cortisone acetate, 25 mg each morning and 12.5 mg each evening.** Alternate treatment with 5.0 and 2.5 mg of **prednisone** for the respective day and night doses is acceptable. In addition to cortisone, patients with bilateral adrenalectomy require 0.1 mg of fluorocortisone per day because of its salt-retaining effect.
    B. Intrapartum management. During labor, patients with chronic adrenocortical insufficiency require good **hydration, 25 mg of cortisol hemisuccinate every 6 h, and 100 mg of cortisol at the time of delivery.** In patients with suspected addisonian crisis, ACTH and cortisol assays should be performed. Adrenal steroid replacement therapy is begun with 100 mg of hydrocortisone intravenously (IVPB), along with 5% dextrose and saline. During the first 24 h, 100 mg Solu-Cortef IVPB will ensure prompt recovery. Adequate fluids are essential in the patient with acute adrenal insufficiency to correct dehydration.

Cushing's Syndrome
 I. Incidence. Cushing's syndrome is rarely encountered in association with pregnancy.

 II. Morbidity and mortality. There is a high incidence of preterm birth (50 percent), and a 25 percent fetal loss rate in Cushing's syndrome.

III. Cause. The most likely cause of Cushing's syndrome is a small pituitary adenoma. The possibility of an adrenal tumor, including adrenal carcinoma, should be considered.

IV. Diagnosis
  A. **Signs and symptoms.** Increased hirsutism and acne are particularly common in Cushing's syndrome.
  B. **Physical examination.** Moon face, buffalo hump, and broad purple abdominal striae are often seen.
  C. **Laboratory examination.** Cushing's syndrome is characterized by elevated plasma cortisol values without diurnal variation. A 24-h urine collection for free cortisol provides evidence of increased cortisol secretion. This 24-h urine collection for free cortisol should be followed by a serum ACTH level measurement to determine if the cortisol feedback mechanisms are intact. Adrenal and/or sella turcica computed tomography (CT) examination may be necessary to confirm a suspected adrenal tumor.

V. Management. If the cause of Cushing's syndrome is a pituitary adenoma, its surgical removal during the second trimester is indicated. If an adrenal tumor is the cause, immediate surgical excision is the primary therapy. There is no medical management for Cushing's syndrome.

Congenital Adrenal Hyperplasia (CAH)

21-HYDROXYLASE DEFICIENCY

I. Incidence. Women treated inadequately for 21-hydroxylase deficiency rarely become pregnant, and puberty does not occur in untreated patients with a severe defect. When treated adequately, 60 percent of patients become pregnant if they so desire. Approximately 90 percent of patients with CAH have partial or complete deficiency of the 21-hydroxylase enzyme.

II. Morbidity and mortality. Cesarean section rates are higher for patients with 21-hydroxylase deficiency due to premature closure of the epiphysis or abnormal external genitalia. Spontaneous abortion occurs in 20 percent of pregnancies complicated by CAH in the mother. An increased androgen level results in virilization of the fetus and ambiguous genitalia in female infants. Most children of CAH mothers are otherwise normal, depending on the genotype of the father.

III. Cause. The disorder is inherited as an autosomal recessive trait.

IV. Diagnosis
  A. **Signs and symptoms.** Most untreated patients with 21-hydroxylase deficiency are infertile and have irregular menses

due to ovarian inactivity as a result of inhibition of pituitary gonadotropins by increased adrenal androgen and estrogen.

B. Physical examination. A small pelvis is common, but the other findings are usually normal.

C. Laboratory findings. Typical laboratory findings include low normal or decreased plasma cortisol values, increased plasma dehydroepiandrosterone and 17-hydroxyprogesterone levels, and abnormally high urinary pregnanetriol levels. In 33 percent of patients, hyponatremia is noted due to a decrease in aldosterone production and resultant sodium loss. Prenatal fetal diagnosis has become possible. Elevated amniotic fluid 17-hydroxyprogesterone is also suggestive of 21-hydroxylase deficiency in the fetus.

V. Management

A. Maternal management. In the antepartum period, replacement involves therapy with **cortisone acetate or prednisone** and the addition of fluorocortisone acetate for patients with sodium depletion. The dosage should be adjusted to restore normal serum and urinary levels. The usual oral daily maintenance dose of 37.5 mg of cortisone or 7.5 mg of prednisone (plus 0.1 mg fluorocortisone when necessary) need not be altered by pregnancy. However, the stress of labor and delivery merits an increased steroid dose, as described for Addison's disease (see Sections V.A and V.B).

B. Fetal management. Following delivery, every neonate must be examined for signs of adrenal insufficiency. In the female fetus, masculinization results in clitoral enlargement. The male fetus may show genital enlargement that is not initially regarded as abnormal.

11B-HYDROXYLASE DEFICIENCY

I. Incidence. 11B-hydroxylase deficiency is an extremely rare form of CAH; therefore, coexistent pregnancy is very rare.

II. Morbidity and mortality. The morbidity and mortality associated with 11B-hydroxylase deficiency are essentially the same as for 21-hydroxylase deficiency (see section II in the discussion of 21-hydroxylase deficiency).

III. Cause. The disorder is inherited as an autosomal recessive trait.

IV. Diagnosis.

A. Signs and symptoms. Infertility is common in women with the disorder.

B. Physical examination. Typical findings are hypertension due to increased 11-deoxycorticosterone (DOC) and virilization due to excessive androgens.

C. **Laboratory examination.** In women with the disorder, aldosterone levels are decreased; 11-deoxycortisol and DOC levels and total urinary 17-ketosteroids are increased. Prenatal fetal diagnosis is possible due to an elevated level of 11-deoxycortisol in amniotic fluid.

V. **Management.** Therapy for 11B-hydroxylase deficiency consists of replacement doses of cortisone acetate or prednisone, as for 21-hydroxylase deficiency (see Section V in the discussion of 21-hydroxylase deficiency). Fluorocortisone is not necessary due to the high levels of DOC, which is a salt-retaining hormone.

PITUITARY DISEASE

Integrity of the pituitary gland is essential for conception; thus, pregnancy is uncommon in women with pituitary abnormalities. In the normal woman, there is a twofold to threefold enlargement of the pituitary gland during pregnancy due to an increase in the size and number of lactotrophs. Pituitary gonadotropin levels are low due to increased estrogens during normal pregnancy.

Hypopituitarism

I. **Incidence.** Hypopituitarism is exceedingly rare, whether associated or unassociated with pregnancy.

II. **Morbidity and mortality.** If replacement therapy is given, morbidity and mortality are essentially nil.

III. **Cause.** Postpartum pituitary necrosis (Sheehan's syndrome) and post-transsphenoidal surgery are the most common causes of hypopituitarism. Idiopathic hypopituitarism has no apparent abnormality of the central nervous system or peripheral target glands. Pituitary necrosis may also occur in pregnant diabetics characterized by deep midline headaches and a decreased insulin requirement. Maternal death is seen in over 50 percent of these diabetic patients.

IV. **Diagnosis**
A. **Signs and symptoms.** Hypopituitarism is difficult to diagnose during pregnancy because its symptoms—nausea and vomiting, fatigue, lassitude, weakness, and headache—are common in normal pregnancy. Failure of lactation and rapid breast involution are the earliest postpartum signs of hypopituitarism. Because postpartum fatigue and lassitude are common in patients with hypopituitarism, many are mistakenly treated for postpartum depression. Menses are scanty or absent in patients with hypopituitarism.
B. **Physical examination.** Axillary and pubic hair is sparse, and decreased skin pigmentation due to inhibited melanin production is seen in patients with hypopituitarism.

    C. Laboratory examination. Serum T$_4$ and TSH levels should be measured to distinguish between primary hypothyroidism and pituitary-hypothalamic hypothyroidism. Secondary adrenal insufficiency is suspected when fasting glucose levels are below 60 mg/dL; suspected adrenal insufficiency can be assessed by comparing fasting and 8 P.M. cortisol values with normal pregnancy cortisol values.

V. Management. Medical management of hypopituitarism involves replacement of adrenal corticosteroids and thyroid hormone. Fluorocortisone therapy is not necessary.

Diabetes Insipidus (DI)

I. Incidence. DI is extremely rare.

II. Morbidity and mortality. DI causes no impairment in fertility, and pregnancy is unaffected.

III. Cause. Most cases of DI occur as a result of trauma or tumor that has damaged the hypothalamic-hypophyseal region. Idiopathic DI is seen in about 33 percent of patients. Less than 1 percent of patients have an autosomal dominant hereditary form of the disease. Recently, DI associated with preeclampsia has been increasingly described.

IV. Diagnosis
    A. Signs and symptoms. Polyuria and polydipsia, with a urine specific gravity of less than 1.005, are the hallmark symptoms of DI.
    B. Physical examination. No abnormalities are found in patients with DI on physical examination.
    C. Laboratory examination. The diagnosis is made by the demonstration of increasing serum osmolality in the face of low urine osmolality when the patient is deprived of water. These osmolar changes are corrected after treatment with vasopressin.

V. Management. The rare patient with DI should be referred to an endocrinologist for medical management, which consists of parenteral vasopressin. There has been great variability in the drug of choice and the therapeutic dose. Recently, L-deamina-8-d-arginine vasopressin (DDAVP) has become the drug of choice, since it can be given intranasally and is reliable and since patients do not develop drug intolerance.

Pituitary Tumors and Pregnancy

I. Incidence. An increasing number of pregnant women with pituitary tumors are being seen as a result of the successful medical treatment of prolactinomas with bromocriptine.

II. Diagnosis

A. **Signs and symptoms.** Pituitary tumors are generally diagnosed prior to pregnancy due to infertility, galactorrhea, and elevated prolactin values.

B. **Physical examination.** Extension of tumor growth may result in visual field defects, detected by visual field examination or as a result of patient complaints of altered vision.

C. **Diagnostic studies.** Serial prolactin determination is unnecessary, and regular visual field testing is not cost effective. Sellar CT or magnetic resonance imaging (MRI) studies should be obtained if visual field deficits, persistent headaches, or blurred vision occurs.

III. Management. Microadenoma without neurologic or visual symptoms is not a contraindication to pregnancy or induction of ovulation.

A. **Prepregnancy management.** Macroadenomas should be treated surgically prior to pregnancy to prevent the complications of expansion during pregnancy. Bromocriptine should be stopped when pregnancy is confirmed; however, congenital abnormalities do not appear to be increased in fetuses exposed to this medication.

B. **Management during pregnancy.** Attention to physical findings is essential to uncover progression of tumor growth. If visual field deficits occur, reinstitution of bromocriptine is generally recommended, with transsphenoidal hypophysectomy reserved as a therapeutic alternative for severe cases or those unresponsive to bromocriptine. If the patient is close to term, the pregnancy should be terminated by induction of labor.

C. **Management postpartum.** Breast-feeding remains controversial, but it is suspected that the risk of tumor growth induced by nursing is considerably lower than that induced by pregnancy itself. Thus, there is no reason to discourage nursing in women with microadenomas. Women with macroadenomas may also nurse, but they should be followed closely for the possibility of tumor enlargement.

BIBLIOGRAPHY

Burrow GN. The management of thyrotoxicosis in pregnancy. N Engl J Med 1985; 303:562.

Carr BR, Parker CRP Jr, Madden JD, et al. Maternal plasma adrenocorticotropin and cortisol relationships throughout human pregnancy. Am J Obstet Gynecol 1981; 139:416.

Cheron RG. Neonatal thyroid function after propylthiouracil. N Engl J Med 1981; 304:525.

Clark D, Seeds JW, Cefalo RC. Hyperparathyroid crisis and pregnancy. Am J Obstet Gynecol 1981; 170:840.

Cunningham FG. Maternal and fetal thyroid physiology: Function and pathology. In: Wallach EE, ed. Philadelphia: Postgraduate Obstetrics and Gynecology; 1983; 3:1–8.

Hughes IA, Laurence KM. Antenatal diagnosis of congenital adrenal hyperplasia. Lancet 1979; 2:7.

Mestman JH. Diagnosis and management of hyperthyroidism in pregnancy. In: Leventhal JM, ed. Current Problems in Obstetrics and Gynecology, Vol IV, No 10. Chicago: Year Book Medical Publishers; 1981:5–50.

Molitch ME. Pregnancy and the hyperprolactinemic woman. N Engl J Med 1985; 312:1364.

Montoro M, Collea JV, Faiser D, et al. Successful outcome of pregnancy in women with hypothyroidism. Ann Intern Med 1981; 94:31.

Pitkin RM, Reynolds WA, Williams GA, et al. Calcium metabolism in normal pregnancy: A longitudinal study. Am J Obstet Gynecol 1979; 133:781.

Ramsy I. Thyrotoxicosis in pregnancy. Clin Endocrinol 1983; 18:73.

Ruiz-Velasco V, Tolis G. Pregnancy in hyperprolactinemic women. Fertil Steril 1984; 41:793.

CHAPTER 36

Hematologic Disease

Nina Boe

ANEMIA IN PREGNANCY

All pregnant patients should be evaluated for anemia as part of routine prenatal care, as approximately one-half of these patients have anemia. Definitions vary; Kitay has defined normal values for hemoglobin and hematocrit in pregnancy (Table 36.1). The incidence of anemia also varies somewhat according to race, location, nutrition, and socioeconomic status. Certainly, any patient with a hematocrit < 30 percent and/or hemoglobin < 10 g/dL has a clinically significant anemia that should be evaluated.

The term *physiologic anemia of pregnancy* is a misnomer. Plasma volume increases, on average, 1000 mL in pregnancy. The red blood cell mass increases by 300 mL. The resulting "anemia" is actually a reflection of the 3 : 1 ratio of plasma volume increase to red blood cell volume increase. A relative anemia is present, rather than a true anemia, with decreased red blood cells and diminished oxygen-carrying capacity.

In evaluating these patients, the family/personal history can be helpful in cases of inherited diseases. Patients who are black or of Asian or Mediterranean ancestry should be tested for hemoglobinopathies. Symptoms, if present, are usually indistinguishable from common complaints of pregnancy (lethargy, fatigue, mild shortness of breath). Physical findings (skeletal abnormalities, splenomegaly, jaundice, and petechiae) are helpful if present. Patients with a chronic disease state should be able to relate that history.

Laboratory evaluation starts with red blood cell indices and a reticulocyte count (see Fig. 36.1). From that point, only a few additional tests will be needed to clarify the cause of the anemia. It is also helpful to think in terms of the mechanism of anemia when pursuing a diagnosis. Is the production of erythrocytes decreased, are normal cells being produced, is destruction of the erythrocytes increased, or is some combination of these conditions in effect? A thorough and systematic approach will reveal the cause of the anemia and allow appropriate management plans and treatment to be instituted. A listing of normal values for laboratory tests in pregnancy is provided in Table 36.2.

Table 36.1. Normal Hemoglobin/Hematocrit (Hgb/Hct) Values in Pregnancy

		Hgb (g/dL)	Hct (%)
First trimester	(12 weeks)	12.5	38.3
Second trimester	(24 weeks)	11–12	34–39
Third trimester	(36 weeks)	11	34–39

Source: Adapted from Kitay DZ, ed. Hematologic Problems in Pregnancy. Oradell, NJ: Medical Economics Books; 1987.

NUTRITIONAL DEFICIENCIES

I. **Iron deficiency anemia**
   Definition. Iron deficiency anemia is the most common cause of anemia in pregnant women. It is caused by insufficient iron intake to meet the demands of pregnancy.
   A. **Incidence.** Iron deficiency anemia is the cause of approximately 75 percent of the anemias identified during pregnancy.
   B. **Diagnosis.** Hypochromic, microcytic erythrocytes are seen on the peripheral smear. Laboratory values include a mean corpuscular volume (MCV) < 80 fL, mean corpuscular hemoglobin concentration (MCHC) < 30 percent, iron level < 50 μg/dL, and transferrin saturation ≤ 15 percent.
   C. **Morbidity and mortality**
      1. Pregnancy imposes an increased demand for iron on the patient. Many patients are predisposed to iron deficiency as a result of poor nutrition and frequent pregnancies (< 1 year apart).
      2. Estimates of the total amount of iron required for a singleton pregnancy range from 1000 to 1200 mg. Of this, increased maternal hemoglobin (Hgb) in the red blood cell mass accounts for 450 to 500 mg; the fetus and placenta need 300 to 360 mg; blood loss at delivery will take 190 to 230 mg; and 190 to 200 mg will be lost by excretion from the gastrointestinal tract, urine, and desquamated skin cells.
      3. Maternal iron stores (~ 300 mg) are insufficient to meet this demand, so iron supplementation is necessary. Intestinal absorption of iron increases each trimester, from 10 percent initially, to 25 percent in the second trimester, to 30 percent in the third trimester.
      4. Patients with mild iron deficiency anemia are asymptomatic. With mild to moderate anemia, patients may complain of fatigue and malaise and become more irritable. When iron

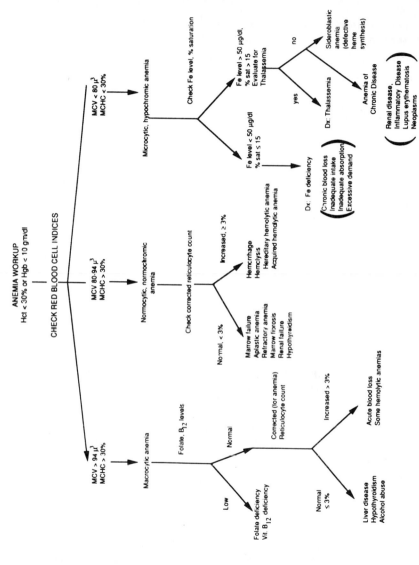

FIGURE 36.1. Diagnostic workup for anemia.

459

Table 36.2. Laboratory Tests in Pregnancy

TEST	NONPREGNANT ADULT FEMALE	PREGNANCY
Hemoglobin	12–16 g/dL	10–13 g/dL
Hematocrit	37–45%	30–39%
RBC	4.2–5.4 million/mm^3	3.8–4.4 million/mm^3
WBC	4.7–10.6 (1000/mm^3	6–16 (1000/mm^3)
MCV	80–100 fL	70–90 fL
MCH	27–34 pg/cell	23–31 pg/cell
MCHC	32–35 g/dL/RBC	32–35 g/dL/RBC
Reticulocyte count	0.5–1.0%	1.0–2.0%
Corrected reticulocyte count*	< 3%	< 3%
Serum iron	50–110 μg/dL	30–100 μg/dL
Total iron-binding capacity (TIBC)	250–300 μg/dL	280–400 μg/dL
Transferrin saturation (% sat)†	25–35%	15–30%
Serum folate	4–16 ng/mL	4–10 ng/mL
Serum vitamin B$_{12}$	70–85 ng/dL	70–500 ng/dL
Activated partial thromboplastin time	25–35 s	25–35 s
Partial thromboplastin time	60–85 s	60–85 s
Prothrombin time	11–15 s	11–15 s
Fibrinogen	200–400 mg/dL	200–600 mg/dL
Bleeding time	2–7 min	2–7 min

*Corrected reticulocyte count = $\dfrac{\text{patient hct}}{\text{normal pregnancy hct (36\%)}}$ × reticulocyte count

†% sat = $\dfrac{\text{serum iron}}{\text{TIBC}}$

Source: Adapted from Kitay DZ, ed. Hematologic Problems in Pregnancy. Oradell, NJ: Medical Economics Books; 1987:16, 404–405.

deficiency is severe enough to cause tissue iron deficiency, patients will note headaches, paresthesias, and burning of the tongue. Some will develop pica of various types: geophagia (dirt), pagophagia (ice), and amylophagia (starch). Pagophagia is specific for iron deficiency anemia.

5. The fetus rarely suffers from maternal iron deficiency because it preferentially receives iron, at the expense of the mother, if maternal supplies are inadequate. Only in severe iron deficiency anemia (hemoglobin < 6.5 g/dL) are fetal effects reported (intrauterine growth retardation [IUGR] and stillbirths).

D. **Differential diagnosis.** It is important to consider other causes of microcytic hypochromic anemia. Anemia of chronic disease (such as renal disease, chronic inflammatory bowel disease, rheumatoid arthritis, systemic lupus erythematosus, and neoplasms) should not be overlooked. Heterozygous thalassemia is the other important diagnosis to consider. In addition, it is certainly possible for an individual to have both a thalassemia trait and some degree of iron deficiency.

E. **Management in pregnancy**
1. Prophylactic iron supplementation with ferrous sulfate or ferrous fumarate, one 325-mg tablet daily, should be prescribed. Even with good nutrition, maternal iron stores are insufficient to meet the increased demands for iron in pregnancy without supplementation. Patients who are iron deficient will need to take iron supplements two to three times a day, depending on the severity of the anemia.
2. Absorption is increased by an acidic environment; taking the iron with ascorbic acid will promote absorption. Patients will frequently complain of nausea, dyspepsia, and constipation. They should be warned that iron will cause dark and black stools.
3. Laboratory values should be rechecked in 3 to 4 weeks after initiating treatment.
4. Patients who are unable to tolerate oral iron preparations may be given intramuscular or intravenous iron preparations. Their use should be restricted to patients who have moderate to severe iron deficiency **and** who have failed on oral iron therapy, have a contraindication to oral administration of iron, or have a malabsorption syndrome.
5. Rarely, patients with severe anemia are given blood transfusions to correct their anemia rapidly. This might be done in a patient prior to cesarean section delivery or another surgical procedure.

II. Megaloblastic anemia: Folate deficiency

Definition. Megaloblastic anemia is a macrocytic anemia caused by deficiency of folate or of vitamin B_{12}.

A. **Incidence.** Folate deficiency severe enough to cause

megaloblastic anemia is reported to occur in 25 percent of pregnant women.

B. Pathophysiology

1. The normal adult daily requirement for folate is 50 to 100 μg. Pregnancy increases the requirement to 150 to 350 μg/d. If maternal folate stores are low, the fetus will remove enough folate efficiently from her circulation to maintain normal fetal levels even as the mother becomes severely anemic. Inadequate dietary intake of animal protein, fruits, and leafy green vegetables is the most common cause of folate deficiency.

2. Deficiency can also result from impaired absorption. Hyperemesis, delayed gastric emptying, and slower intestinal absorption are direct consequences of the pregnant state that may contribute to folate deficiency. Patients with malabsorption syndromes (e.g., sprue) will have increased folate requirements.

3. Certain medications have an adverse effect on folate absorption and metabolism (diphenylhydantoin, ethanol, nitrofurantoin, pyrimethamine, methotrexate, and trimethroprim). Patients will also need more folate if they develop an infection, have a multiple gestation, or have a chronic hemolytic anemia.

4. Folate is an essential nutrient. On the molecular level, it functions as a coenzyme (tetrahydrofolic acid) in the synthesis of thymidylate, which is used in DNA synthesis. Hematopoietic cells are strikingly affected, having a smaller nucleus (impaired nuclear DNA synthesis and mitosis) with a large cytoplasm, giving an overall macrocytic appearance. These erythrocytes have a reduced oxygen-carrying capacity. Their survival is shortened due to hemolysis in the reticuloendothelial system.

   Other cell lines are also affected (leukocytes and platelets), and leukopenia and thrombocytopenia may develop.

C. Diagnosis. Red blood cell indices show macrocytosis (MCV > 94) and a normal MCHC. The peripheral smear will reveal macrocytic erythrocytes and neutrophils with five or more lobes in their nuclei. Serum folate levels < 4 ng/mL and erythrocyte folate activity < 20 ng/mL are diagnostic.

D. Management in pregnancy

1. Pregnant patients should be given folate supplementation, 1 mg/d prophylactically, to meet the increased demands of pregnancy.

2. Patients who are diagnosed with folate deficiency will benefit from a divided dosage schedule. Absorption of folate from the upper gastrointestinal tract is slow, only 10 to 20 μg every 6 to 8 h. Maximal absorption can be achieved by administering one-half of a 1-mg tablet two to four times a day.

3. Folate can be given parenterally if necessary (e.g., to

patients with severe malabsorption syndromes or those who have had surgical resection of the upper small intestine).

4. Patients with multiple gestations, malabsorption syndromes, known hemoglobinopathies, chronic hemolytic anemias, or those who are on diphenylhydantoin or on antimetabolites that affect folate, should probably be put on the divided dosage schedule. A history of a previous pregnancy with folate deficiency is an indication for folate supplementation.

5. The role of good nutrition in preventing folate deficiency should be emphasized, and intake of leafy green vegetables, fruits, and animal protein encouraged.

6. Iron deficiency frequently accompanies folate deficiency. Although serum iron levels may appear high initially when folate deficiency is diagnosed, this is due to the ineffective erythropoiesis. Correction of the folate deficiency with subsequent normalization of the erythropoietic process will rapidly use up the available iron in hemoglobin synthesis. Further correction of the anemia would then be limited by iron availability; thus iron supplementation is helpful.

7. Folate levels, a complete blood count (CBC) with red blood cell indices, and a reticulocyte count should be checked 1 week after starting treatment. The reticulocyte count should be increased (if it is not, the patient may be iron deficient), and all other parameters should show some improvement.

8. Megaloblastic anemia is also caused by vitamin B_{12} deficiency. Because it occurs rarely (1/6000 to 1/8000 pregnancies), most authors focus on folate deficiency. Folate supplementation will correct red blood cell indices even if the underlying cause is vitamin B_{12} deficiency. Untreated vitamin B_{12} deficiency will cause neurologic deficits in motor and sensory functions involving the posterolateral column. Given the seriousness of untreated vitamin B_{12} deficiency and the ease of ascertaining the blood level, both folate and vitamin B_{12} levels should be checked when evaluating megaloblastic anemia.

9. Recent studies have shown a possible link with low folate levels and neural tube defects. Patients who have had one child with a neural tube defect are now being advised to start folate supplementation **prior** to conception of the next pregnancy.

III. Megaloblastic anemia: Vitamin B_{12} deficiency

Definition. Megaloblastic anemia is a macrocytic anemia caused by deficiency of vitamin B_{12} or of folate.

A. **Incidence.** This is a rare complication of pregnancy, reported in 1/6000 to 1/8000 pregnancies. It usually affects people over 40 years of age. Younger black women are often affected. A higher incidence is also found in Scandinavians.

B. **Pathophysiology**
1. Vitamin B_{12} deficiency ultimately impairs DNA synthesis. It

functions as an important coenzyme to the methyltransferase enzyme involved in conversion of methylmalonyl coenzyme A (CoA) to succinyl CoA and in the conversion of homocysteine to methionine. The methyltransferase also converts N^5-methyl-FH_4 to FH_4, which is subsequently used as a folate coenzyme in the thymidylate synthetase reaction. The entire pathway slows down, with accumulation of the methyl folate compound (N^5-methyl-FH_4). This deprives thymidylate synthetase of its folate coenzyme and interferes with DNA synthesis.

2. The normal adult female has vitamin B_{12} stores of 3000 μg. It would take 3 to 4 years to deplete that reserve fully if intake of vitamin B_{12} was stopped. During pregnancy the fetus will need 50 μg of vitamin B_{12}, which is transferred transplacentally from the mother to the fetus. Normal maternal serum levels of 70 to 500 ng/dL may trend downward to 80 to 120 ng/dL as pregnancy progresses. Intrinsic factor is necessary for absorption of vitamin B_{12}. Intrinsic factor is produced by the gastric mucosa; vitamin B_{12} and intrinsic factor are absorbed in the terminal ileum. Patients with a history of gastric or intestinal surgery are thus at risk for vitamin B_{12} deficiency.

3. Tropical sprue, pancreatic disease, Crohn's disease, or ulcerative colitis, which cause malabsorption, are rare causes of B_{12} deficiency.

4. Animal protein is the only dietary source of vitamin B_{12}. A strict vegetarian diet, followed for 3 to 4 years, would deplete body reserves and cause vitamin B_{12} deficiency. This can be avoided if vegetarians supplement their diet with milk, eggs, or vitamin B_{12} tablets (1 μg/d).

5. Patients with significant vitamin B_{12} deficiency may have infertility problems. If the deficiency is not treated, patients may develop progressive megaloblastic anemia, glossitis, elevated lactate dehydrogenase (LDH), and serious neurologic problems.

6. It is important to note that a megaloblastic anemia caused by vitamin B_{12} deficiency, but treated with folate, will show correction of red blood cell indices and partial improvement of anemia and symptoms. However, neurologic symptoms may present acutely if not present already, and in those who have neurologic involvement, it will not improve and will probably progress unless treatment with vitamin B_{12} is instituted.

7. Like folate deficiency, vitamin B_{12} deficiency adversely affects bone marrow cellular maturation. Erythroid cells are macrocytic, neutrophils are hypersegmented, and hemolytic anemia, thrombocytopenia, and leukopenia may develop in severely deficient states. Iron deficiency may also be present.

C. **Diagnosis.**

1. The peripheral smear will reveal macrocytic erythrocytes

and neutrophils with hypersegmented nuclei. A serum vitamin B_{12} level < 70 ng/dL is diagnostic of deficiency. Folate levels are elevated unless concurrent folate deficiency is present.
2. Methylmalonic aciduria (> 3.5 mg/24-h urine collection) is indicative of vitamin B_{12} deficiency, except in individuals who have it as a result of an inborn error of metabolism.
D. **Management in pregnancy**
   1. Treatment consists of vitamin B_{12} injections sufficient to meet the daily requirement and restore maternal stores to normal. Several regimens exist. One example is 1 mg IM daily for 2 weeks followed by 1 mg twice a week for 4 weeks, then 1 mg once a month for life.
   2. Symptoms usually improve in 48 to 72 h. Reticulocytosis will be seen as normal hematopoiesis is reestablished. Hypokalemia has been reported to occur due to rapid uptake of potassium by young erythrocytes. As with folate deficiency, iron levels may appear to be normal or increased initially and then may be rapidly consumed in the erythorpoietic process. An underlying iron deficiency should be suspected if the reticulocyte count does not rise in the first week after treatment. The hematocrit should start rising within 10 days.
   3. Patients with a severe megaloblastic anemia can be treated empirically with both folate and vitamin B_{12}, after levels are drawn, without waiting for the results. Vitamin B_{12} is nontoxic, and excess amounts will be excreted renally.

HEMOLYTIC ANEMIAS: HEREDITARY

I. **Hereditary spherocytosis**
Definition. Hereditary spherocytosis is an autosomal dominant inherited disorder caused by a defect in the erythrocyte membrane. The erythrocytes have a characteristic spherocytic shape on peripheral smear.
A. **Incidence and inheritance**
   1. Hereditary spherocytosis is the most common hereditary hemolytic anemia. It is seen most frequently among persons of Northern European extraction. A British study found an incidence of 1/3000 to 1/5000.
   2. It is inherited in an autosomal dominant fashion. Spontaneous mutations are rare. A case of recessive inheritance has been identified, but autosomal dominance is the usual mode of inheritance.
B. **Morbidity and mortality**
   1. Pregnancy is thought to exacerbate the disease process, stimulating an increased frequency of hemolytic crises. Infections and traumatic events are also precipitating factors.
   2. **Hemolytic crises** are characterized by abdominal pain,

tachycardia, emesis, fever, and (sometimes) clinically apparent jaundice. Physical examination is notable for isolated splenomegaly, found in over 70 percent of affected patients.

3. Patients may also have a purely **aplastic crisis,** although this is rare. A strong association with viral infections has been noted in these crises. These patients are less symptomatic than in the hemolytic crisis, even though the hematocrit drops significantly.

4. The red blood cell in hereditary spherocytosis has a **life span** only 10 percent of the usual 120 days of normally shaped erythrocytes. The spherocytes are rapidly destroyed by the spleen. The oxygen-carrying capacity of the spherocytes is normal.

5. In addition, patients with hereditary spherocytosis are at increased risk for **gout** and **gallbladder disease.** The accelerated destruction of erythrocytes leads to increased metabolism of the hemoglobin, and pigment calculi may develop.

6. Characteristic **radiologic changes** have been described in the skull and maxillary bone. Erythroid hyperplasia of the bone marrow fills and expands the cancellous bone and changes the trabecular architecture.

   In the skull, widening of the diploic space in the frontal and parietal regions is characteristic. Sometimes radiating trabeculae of bone extending at right angles to the inner and outer tables are seen. This is the classic "hair on end" appearance. In the maxillary sinuses, thickening of the bony walls due to marrow hyperplasia can limit the size of the sinus air spaces. Enlargement of the maxillary bone may cause malocclusion and overbite.

C. **Cause.** At the molecular level, a deficiency of spectrin, which is a protein subunit of the erythrocyte cell membrane, causes the structural deformity that results in the spherocytic shape of the erythrocyte. The degree of spectrin deficiency present is thought to correlate with the severity of the disease.

D. **Diagnosis**

1. Family history or a hemolytic episode should instigate a diagnostic workup (Fig. 36.1). Examination of the peripheral blood smear will reveal variable numbers of spherocytes, along with normal erythrocytes. Increased numbers of reticulocytes are also present. Other laboratory values are as noted in Table 36.3.

2. Spherocytes have increased **osmotic fragility.** When placed in subphysiologic sodium chloride, spherocytes will lyse at higher concentrations than do normal cells. The spherocytes do not tolerate lower osmotic concentrations of physiologic normal saline and lyse sooner than normal cells would as the osmotic concentration decreases from normal. A newer test, the acidified glycerol lysis test, is based on the classic test just described but is thought to be more specific.

3. Erythrocyte osmotic fragility correlates very well with the

Table 36.3. Laboratory Tests in Hereditary Spherocytosis

Hematocrit	Decreased
MCV	Decreased to normal
MCH	Normal
MCHC	Normal to increased
Reticulocyte count	Increased
TIBC	Low to normal
Iron	Normal to increased
Bilirubin	Increased
Indirect coombs test	Negative
Peripheral smear	Spherocytes

Source: Adapted from Kitay DZ, ed. Hematologic Problems in Pregnancy. Oradell, NJ. Medical Economics Books; 1987:154.

results of **radioimmunoassay for red cell spectrin.** This may well become the diagnostic test of choice and may replace tests of erythrocyte osmotic fragility for hereditary spherocytosis.

E. **Management**

1. **Supportive care** is the usual mainstay of treatment in both acute hemolytic crises and aplastic crises. Analgesics and antipyretics should be used to treat symptoms. Transfusions should be used in the event of significant pain or anemia (hematocrit < 25 to 30 percent). Bone marrow suppression is reported to resolve within 1 week in most patients given supportive care.

2. **Splenectomy** is recommended by some as a treatment for hereditary spherocytosis. With the spleen removed, the spherocytes approach a normal life span, as they are not constantly being removed from the circulation by a spleen that perceives them as abnormal.

   The timing of splenectomy, if performed, is variable, depending on the stage of pregnancy when hereditary spherocytosis is diagnosed. If a crisis occurring in the second trimester leads to the diagnosis, the patient should be stabilized with transfusions and supportive care, with splenectomy performed subsequently. If the patient has a crisis in the third trimester, she should be treated as in the second trimester. However, splenectomy should be deferred until the postpartum period to avoid the risks of major abdominal surgery in a gravid patient and the high risk of instigating preterm labor.

Spenectomy is not indicated in all cases. Many people have a milder form of hereditary spherocytosis, probably due to variable penetrance of this autosomal dominant condition, and may not need a splenectomy.

3. All patients with hereditary spherocytosis should have dietary **folic acid supplementation.** Folic acid deficiency may or may not play a role in triggering hemolytic crises, but folic acid requirements are increased in all chronic hemolytic syndromes. Iron replacement is unnecessary in most cases due to the accelerated absorption found in patients with a chronic anemic process.

4. The infant of the patient with hereditary spherocytosis, if affected, is at high risk for neonatal jaundice due to hyperbilirubinemia from the accelerated destruction of spherocytes. ABO incompatibility is an alternative cause of jaundice. Splenectomy is not recommended in children under 5 to 6 years of age due to the risk of bacterial infections caused by encapsulated organisms.

II. Glucose-6-phosphate dehydrogenase (G6PD) deficiency

Definition. G6PD is an enzyme in the pentose phosphate (hexose monophosphate) shunt that generates nicotinamide-adenine dinucleotide phosphate (NADPH) (Table 36.4). NADPH is needed to maintain reduced hemoglobin and degrade peroxides in the red blood cell. If insufficient G6PD is available, the red blood cell is affected on many levels: low energy production, accumulation of peroxides leading to cell injury, hemoglobin degeneration, membrane destabilization, and cell lysis.

A. **Incidence and inheritance**

1. This is the most common red blood cell enzyme deficiency causing hemolytic anemia, with over 100 million people affected worldwide.

Table 36.4. G6PD Enzyme Types

G6PD.B	Normal enzyme—normal activity
G6PD.A	Normal variant—normal activity, increased electrophoretic mobility
G6PD.A(−)	Abnormal—common in American and African blacks
G6PD.Mediterranean	Abnormal—common in Italians, Greeks, Sardinians, and Sephardic Jews
G6PD.Canton	Abnormal—present in Oriental populations

Source: Adapted from Kitay DZ, ed. Hematologic Problems in Pregnancy. Oradell, NJ: Medical Economics Books; 1987:143.

2. It is inherited as an X-linked recessive condition. Reported frequencies show that 10 percent of males are hemizygous, 20 percent of females are heterozygous, and 1 to 2 percent of females are homozygous. Blacks are affected most frequently, with 13 percent of black males affected and 25 percent of black females known to be carriers.

B. **Morbidity and mortality.** Hemolysis of red blood cells is stimulated by pregnancy, exposure to oxidizing agents, bacterial or viral infection, fever, and certain foods (e.g., fava beans) (Table 36.5). Hemoglobinuria occurs, and in some cases the patient is at risk of renal shutdown. Some studies report an increased risk of urinary tract infections, low birthweight infants and spontaneous abortions. A few cases of hydrops fetalis have been reported in hemizygous male fetuses.

C. **Diagnosis**

1. A personal or family history of hemolytic anemia, or membership in certain ethnic (Sephardic Jews), geographic

Table 36.5. Some Potential Inciting Agents of Hemolysis in G6PD Deficiency

Drugs and chemicals
Acetylsalicyclic acid
Acetophenetidin
p-Aminosalicyclic acid
Aminopyrine
Ascorbic acid (megadoses)
Chloramphenicol
Chloroquine
Dimercaprol (BAL)
Fava beans
Methylene blue
Nalidixic acid
Naphthalene (moth balls)
Nitrofurantoins
Pamaquine
Phenylhydrazine
Primaquine
Probenecid
Quinidine
Quinine
Sulfas
Tolbutamide
Vitamin K (water soluble)

Other causes
Viral infections
Infectious mononucleosis
Bacterial pneumonias

Source: Adapted from Kitay DZ, ed. Hematologic Problems in Pregnancy. Oradell, NJ: Medical Economics Books; 1987:144.

(Mediterranean, Africa), or racial groups (blacks, Orientals), are indicators of risk that warrant diagnostic testing.

2. The peripheral smear during a hemolytic episode will show spherocytes, poikilocytes, nucleated red blood cells, cell fragments, and Heinz bodies (clumps of denatured hemoglobin).

3. Laboratory tests include a screening dye reduction test (to measure enzyme content) and a methemoglobin test.

D. Management

1. Pregnant women who have G6PD deficiency should avoid any agents known to be oxidants (see Table 36.5).

2. A daily dose of 1 mg of folic acid to supplement the diet is recommended in all patients with hemolytic anemia. Pregnancy increases the daily requirement for folic acid by three- to sevenfold above the nonpregnant state. Iron supplementation should not be given unless indicated by testing.

3. Patients in hemolytic crisis should be given supportive care and transfusions as indicated. Intravenous fluid hydration should be provided to assist in resolution of the hemoglobinuria. Most important, the agent or stimulus of the crisis must be withdrawn.

E. Prevention. Patients should be given lists of drugs to avoid and counseled to avoid these medications if they plan to breast-feed. Babies with G6PD deficiency could have a hemolytic crisis and neonatal jaundice if exposed to an oxidant via the mother's breast milk.

III. Pyruvate kinase deficiency

Definition. Pyruvate kinase deficiency is caused by deficiency of the enzyme pyruvate kinase, which catalyzes conversion of phosphenol pyruvate to pyruvate, which produces 1 mole of adenosine triphosphate (ATP). (Deficiency of the enzyme results in a red blood cell with insufficient energy-producing compounds and leads to shortened red blood cell survival.) Spontaneous hemolysis occurs.

A. Incidence and inheritance

1. Pyruvate kinase deficiency is the second most common red blood cell enzyme deficiency causing hemolytic anemia.

2. It is inherited as an autosomal recessive trait; affected individuals are homozygous (heterozygotes are not affected). People with a Northern European background are more frequently affected. A German study found an incidence of 1/10 000 for homozygous individuals and a 1/50 to 1/100 incidence of the carrier state.

B. Morbidity and mortality. Pyruvate kinase deficiency is frequently diagnosed in childhood due to jaundice and anemia. No precipitating factors have been identified as causing hemolytic crises (except for a report linking oral contraceptive use to anemia in one patient). These patients are at increased risk of cholelithiasis, similar to the risk of patients with spherocytosis.

The mode of clinical presentation is reported to be quite variable. Splenomegaly is common.

C. **Diagnosis**
1. Patients with **hemolytic anemia** who do not have spherocytosis or G6PD deficiency should have a workup for pyruvate kinase deficiency.
2. Peripheral smears are notable for **macrocytosis** and increased **reticulocytes.** Hematocrits range from 17 to 37 percent. A fluorescent spot test for pyruvate deficiency is available.

D. **Management**
1. Pregnancy is not known to exacerbate pyruvate kinase deficiency. As with other chronic hemolytic anemias, **folic acid supplementation** is indicated on the basis of the underlying disease, as well as for the increased demands of pregnancy. Iron should be given only as indicated by the results of testing, since absorption is usually enhanced in chronic anemic states. **Crises** should be managed by providing supportive care, treating inciting factors such as infections, and giving transfusions as indicated by the maternal condition.
2. **Splenectomy** does not have as beneficial an effect in pyruvate kinase deficiency as it does in hereditary spherocytosis. The life span of the red blood cell is only moderately extended. For this reason, splenectomy is not done unless patients develop a need for frequent transfusions. Every attempt should be made to put off splenectomy until the age of 5 to 6 years in children because of the significant risk of bacterial infections due to encapsulated organisms.

HEMOGLOBINOPATHIES

Hemoglobin is the oxygen-transporting molecule found in red blood cells. Each molecule has two pairs of polypeptide chains, with a heme moiety on each chain. Normal adult hemoglobin (hemoglobin A) has two α-globin chains and two β-globin chains. A mutation will affect α-globin chains or β-globin chains, but not both. (The α-globin gene is on chromosome 16 and the β-globin gene is on chromosome 11.)

Hemoglobinopathies, or production of abnormal hemoglobins, are usually due to point mutations that cause a single amino acid substitution in an α- or β-globin chain. Most of the clinically significant hemoglobinopathies are caused by β-globin chain mutations. The tertiary structure of the molecule is dictated by the polypeptide sequence. Interference with the tertiary structure of the molecule, secondary to a mutation affecting the polypeptide globin chain, will alter the ability of the molecule to perform its function of oxygen transport.

I. **Sickle cell anemia**
Definition. Sickle cell disease is caused by hemoglobin S. Both β-globin genes code for hemoglobin S, in which valine is substituted for glutamic acid at the sixth position in the β chain.

A. **Incidence and inheritance**
   1. Sickle cell trait (hemoglobin AS) occurs in 1/12 black Americans. It is a heterozygous state in which one β globin gene is affected. Both hemoglobin A and hemoglobin S are produced; they are inherited in an autosomal codominant manner.
   2. Sickle cell anemia is a homozygous state in which both β genes have the mutation for hemoglobin S. It occurs in 1/500 to 1/708 patients. Inheritance is autosomal recessive. Each parent must have sickle cell trait (hemoglobin AS), and the risk of each child having homozygous hemoglobin SS (sickle cell disease) is 1 in 4.
   3. Blacks are not the only ethnic group affected; people from the Mediterranean area, Turkey, Saudi Arabia, and India are also at risk for sickle cell disease.
B. **Morbidity and mortality**
   1. Patients with sickle cell trait have one normal globin β gene and one β^S globin gene; they produce hemoglobin AS. Approximately 60 percent of the hemoglobin is hemoglobin A, and 40 percent is hemoglobin S.
   2. Sickle cell trait is not usually associated with an increased medical risk. Decreased perfusion of the renal papillae, causing hematuria, has been reported in sickle trait patients. Another rare finding reported in patients with sickle cell trait is splenic infarction after extended exposure to low oxygen concentrations.
   3. A clinically significant finding in this group of patients is that urinary tract infections (UTIs) and asymptomatic bacteriuria are found twice as often as in patients without sickle cell trait.
   4. Sickle cell disease causes severe problems in affected individuals. *Sickling* refers to the characteristic sickle shape assumed by red blood cells under conditions of low oxygen tension. The hemoglobin S becomes relatively insoluble in the deoxygenated state, and clumps of the hemoglobin form fibers that deform the erythrocyte.

      The sickled cells block the microcirculation and cause local hypoxia, pain, and microinfarction. A self-perpetuating cycle, the sickle cell crisis cycle, is set up. It can be precipitated by hypoxia, acidosis, dehydration, physical stress, trauma, and infection.

      Sickling damages the erythrocyte, which is removed by the reticuloendothelial system, resulting in a chronic hemolytic anemia. Sickle cells may be present in the circulation for only 5 to 10 days.
   5. Sickle cell crises have several typical forms of presentation. The *chest syndrome* consists of fever, cough, pleuritic chest pains, and infiltrates on chest x-rays. Antibiotics are usually prescribed. The extremities *(hand-foot syndrome)*, joints, and skeleton may be painfully affected. Osteomyelitis (es-

pecially *Salmonella* osteomyelitis) is frequently seen in sickle cell patients. Patients may have symptoms of a UTI or kidney stone (fever, pain, hematuria) that are actually caused by renal papillary necrosis due to a sickle crisis. Pyelonephritis is seen more often. Abdominal pain may represent a crisis or is equally likely to be due to one of the many causes of an acute abdomen. Abdominal pain in a patient with sickle cell disease is a diagnostic dilemma. It is always challenging to try to differentiate between infarction and infection. The mainstays of treatment are oxygen, intravenous hydration, and analgesics.

6. On physical examination, patients are often jaundiced and underweight, with cardiomegaly accompanied by a heart murmur and hepatomegaly. Splenomegaly is not seen in adults. Their spleens are small to normal in size as a result of multiple crises, with microinfarction and fibrosis.

7. Characteristic radiologic changes are seen in patients with sickle cell disease. They are similar to the changes seen in patients with Cooley's anemia (homozygous β-thalassemia major). Anemia leads to erythroid hyperplasia of the bone marrow, which causes decreased bone density. Bone infarction in the epiphyses is common. Osteomyelitis may be seen in any bone. Pathologic fractures may be seen in thinner bones as a result of infarction and infection. The spine has a characteristic vertebral contour with localized central depressions of the disc surfaces. Compression deformities are also seen.

C. **Diagnosis**

1. The sickle cell preparation (screening test) is positive. Sickle cells are seen on the peripheral smear. Patients have a normochromic, normocytic, hemolytic anemia. The reticulocyte count is high. Hemoglobin electrophoresis will reveal the specific type of hemoglobinopathy.

2. Patients and their partners who are at risk on the basis of family history or ethnic background should be offered testing.

D. **Management in pregnancy**

1. Pregnant patients with sickle cell disease (hemoglobin SS) should be managed as high-risk patients with close supervision, frequent follow-up, and an awareness of the multiple associated risks to the patient and her fetus (see Table 36.6).

2. Preconception planning with sickle cell patients would allow administration of pneumococcal vaccine. Genetic counseling and prenatal diagnosis using DNA analysis are available and should be offered to couples whose fetus is at risk. Chorionic villus sampling can be performed at 9 to 12 weeks of gestation. Amniocentesis for amniocytes can be done at 16 to 18 weeks.

3. Folate supplementation, 1 mg/d, is recommended for all chronic hemolytic states. Iron supplementation, if indicated

Table 36.6. **Pregnancy-Associated Risks in Sickle Cell Disease Patients**

Spontaneous abortion	14.8%
Stillbirth	18.5%
Neonatal demise	6.9%
Infections	Increased 50–67%
Cholelithiasis	25–30%
Preeclampsia	~ 33%
IUGR	Increased
Preterm birth	10–55%
Multiple gestation	Increased
Sickle cell crisis	Increased

Source: Modified from Kitay DZ, ed. Hematologic Problems in Pregnancy. Oradell, NJ: Medical Economics Books; 1987:121 and Gabbe SG, Niebyl JR, Simpson JL, eds. Obstetrics: Normal and Problem Pregnancies. 2nd ed. New York: Churchill Livingstone; 1991:1140.

by testing, is advised. Many sickle cell patients have normal iron stores.

4. Screening urine cultures should be obtained at the first prenatal visit and repeated on a monthly basis, as these patients have an increased incidence of asymptomatic bacteriuria, UTIs, and pyelonephritis.

5. Fetal surveillance (nonstress test [NST] and biophysical profile [BPP]) should be initiated at 28 to 32 weeks. Serial ultrasound examinations to document adequate intrauterine growth should be performed.

6. The role of exchange transfusions in pregnancy is very controversial. Some physicians offer it prophylactically on a routine basis to all sickle cell patients. Others wait, observe the patient's clinical course, and transfuse only if a crisis occurs. Studies have found both improvement in the outcome of pregnancy **with** transfusions and no significant differences **without** transfusions. Certain patients are at higher risk and would probably benefit from transfusions: those with crises in pregnancy, those with a prior perinatal death, those who have twins, and those who have had a significant infection in pregnancy (e.g., pyelonephritis, osteomyelitis, or pneumococcal pneumonia).

7. The benefits of partial exchange transfusion are replacement of hemoglobin S with hemoglobin A, improved oxygen-carrying capacity, and suppression of hemoglobin S synthesis. The risks include transfusion reaction; possible exposure to hepatitis B, hepatitis C, and human immunodeficiency

virus (HIV); development of erythrocyte antibodies; and potential cardiovascular overload.

8. It has been recommended that patients have their first partial exchange transfusion at 28 weeks. Subsequent transfusions should be done at 36 to 38 weeks, or if the hematocrit is < 25 percent and the hemoglobin A < 20 percent, or for a crisis. The goal of partial exchange transfusion is to replace hemoglobin S with hemoglobin A; over 40 percent of the blood should be hemoglobin A when the transfusion is completed.

9. In labor, patients should have matched blood available and should be put on oxygen. Intravenous fluids must be titrated to prevent both dehydration and cardiac overload. The mode of delivery should be governed by obstetric indications only. Pregnancy should not be prolonged past 40 weeks.

10. Postpartum, the patient should still be followed closely for signs of infection or crisis. Pulmonary emboli and cerebral infarction are reported to occur most frequently in the puerperium.

11. Acute sequestration, with a sudden severe drop in the hematocrit, may occur near delivery, during labor and delivery, or postpartum. Maternal blood should be available for transfusion if the hematocrit falls rapidly or is < 20 percent.

II. Hemoglobin SC disease

Definition. Hemoglobin SC disease is caused by mutations in the β-globin chains, similar to sickle cell disease. These patients are double heterozygotes in that each β-globin gene has a different mutation. One β-globin gene has valine substituted for glutamic acid at the sixth position to make hemoglobin S. The other β-globin gene has lysine substituted for valine at the sixth position to make hemoglobin C.

A. **Incidence and inheritance.** Sickle cell-hemoglobin C disease, or hemoglobin SC disease, is inherited in an autosomal recessive fashion. It occurs in 1/600 to 1/757 patients.

B. **Morbidity and mortality**

1. The pathophysiology of the sickling is the same as in sickle cell disease. Although these patients have high-risk pregnancies, the morbidity and mortality are not as high as in sickle cell disease. Similarities are present in the increased incidence of spontaneous abortion, stillbirths, preterm births, preeclampsia, and neonatal deaths. Differences exist in the degree of hemolytic anemia (milder for hemoglobin SC), fewer crises in pregnancy for sickle cell SC, and time of diagnosis. Hemoglobin SC patients may not even have their first crisis until they are pregnant.

2. Another important difference is the severity of the crisis event. Patients with hemoglobin SC usually have severe

bone pain indicative of bone marrow infarction. Emboli of fat and/or marrow may cause pulmonary infarction, respiratory distress, and acute respiratory insufficiency. Embolization to the central nervous system (CNS) may cause neurologic changes, seizures, and coma.

3. Other clinical findings particular to hemoglobin SC disease include proliferative retinopathy and avascular necrosis of the femoral heads. As in sickle cell disease and sickle cell β thalassemia, adults with hemoglobin SC may experience the splenic sequestration syndrome (splenomegaly, rapid drop in hematocrit during a crisis, and mild thrombocytopenia).

C. **Diagnosis.** Diagnostic criteria and methods of diagnosis are the same as for sickle cell disease. Electrophoresis will reveal the banding patterns of hemoglobin S and hemoglobin C.

D. **Management in pregnancy.** Principles of management in pregnancy are the same as those for sickle cell disease. Partial exchange transfusions are indicated for patients with the risk factors mentioned previously and for patients in crisis. Although the hemolytic anemia is not as severe as in sickle cell disease, the vaso-occlusive crises in hemoglobin SC patients may have more damaging sequelae (pulmonary infarction and CNS involvement) that would justify prophylactic partial exchange transfusions.

III. **Sickle cell β thalassemia**

Definition. Sickle cell β thalassemia is a milder form of sickle cell disease in which one β-globin gene codes for hemoglobin S and the other for β thalassemia (decreased synthesis of the β chain for hemoglobin A).

A. **Incidence and inheritance.** The incidence is 1/1672. The inheritance is autosomal recessive.

B. **Morbidity and mortality**

1. The severity of clinical involvement is dependent upon which β thalassemia allele is inherited. The β^0 allele does not produce any hemoglobin A; these patients have a clinical picture similar to that of a sickle cell disease patient. The β^+ allele allows some production of hemoglobin A. Patients usually have elevated amounts of hemoglobin A_2 and hemoglobin F.

2. Anemia may be mild to moderate. The splenic sequestration syndrome (splenomegaly, splenic crisis, and mild thrombocytopenia) is seen in adults as well as children. Perinatal morbidity and mortality are similar to those of patients with hemoglobin SC disease; maternal morbidity is also similar.

C. **Diagnosis.** Diagnostic criteria and methods are the same as for sickle cell disease. Electrophoresis will show hemoglobin S and β thalassemia.

D. **Management in pregnancy.** Management principles in pregnancy are the same as for sickle cell disease. Fewer partial exchange transfusions may be needed in these patients. In the event of a splenic sequestration syndrome, a partial exchange transfusion should be done.

IV. **Other hemoglobinopathies**

1. Patients who have hemoglobin C trait (hemoglobin A/C) or hemoglobin C-β thalassemia (hemoglobin C/β) usually do well in pregnancy. A few women with homozygous hemoglobin C disease will require transfusions (if the hematocrit is $\leq$ 20 percent).

2. Hemoglobin E is usually found in Southeast Asian patients. The glutamic acid at the 26th position on the β globin chain is replaced by lysine. Homozygous hemoglobin E is reportedly well tolerated in pregnancy, with patients having only mild anemia. Hemoglobin E-β thalassemia is associated with severe anemia, and patients may require transfusions.

3. Hemoglobin D trait and homozygous hemoglobin D are clinically benign. Sickle cell-hemoglobin D may be asymptomatic or may cause a mild hemolytic anemia.

4. Other hemoglobinopathies that are reported to do well in pregnancy are hemoglobins G and O.

THALASSEMIAS

I. **α Thalassemias**

Definition. Patients with α thalassemia have structurally normal hemoglobin but abnormal production of α-globin chains.

A. **Incidence/inheritance.** Thalassemias are inherited as an autosomal recessive trait. α Thalassemia is widely distributed in specific geographic areas: the Mediterranean, the Middle East, and parts of Africa, Asia, and India. The highest incidence is found in Southeast Asia.

B. **Cause**

1. The gene coding for α-chain synthesis is located on chromosome 16. Two identical α genes are present on the chromosome; a normal genotype is written ($\alpha\alpha/\alpha\alpha$). Decreased synthesis of α chains is caused by gene deletion. The severity of clinical disease correlates with the degree of diminished production of α chains, which in turn correlates with the number of genes deleted.

2. Decreased production of normal amounts of hemoglobin leads to a microcytic, hypochromic anemia. The excess β chains will precipitate out in the red blood cell (Heinz bodies) and be removed by reticuloendothelial cells. In the process, the red blood cell membrane is damaged and will be removed by the spleen, contributing further to the anemia.

C. **Morbidity and mortality.** Patients with α thalassemia have differing outcomes related to how many copies of the gene are deleted and how much α globin is produced (Table 36.7).

Table 36.7. α Thalassemias

CLASSIFICATION	GENES	NO. OF GENES DELETED	α-CHAIN PRODUCTION	HEMOGLOBIN	CLINICAL OUTCOME
Homozygous (Barts)	$(\_\_/\_\_)$	4	0%	80% Hgb Barts (γ_4) 20% Hgb H (β_4)	Hydrops, IUGR, pregnancy-induced hypertension, stillbirth
Heterozygous Hemoglobin H disease	$(\_\_/\_\alpha)$	3	25%	Hgb Bart (γ_4) Hgb H (β_4) Hgb A $(\alpha_2\beta_2)$	Hemolytic anemia, transfusion dependent, usually dies in childhood
Heterozygous		2		Hgb A $(\alpha_2\beta_2)$	Minimal to moderate hypochromic, microcytic anemia
α_1 Thalassemia minor (usually found in Orientals)	$(\_\_/\alpha\alpha)$		50%		
α_2 Thalassemia minor (usually found in blacks)	$(\_\alpha/\_\alpha)$		50%		
Silent carrier state (α Thalassemia-2)	$(\_\alpha/\alpha\alpha)$	1	75%	Hgb A $(\alpha_2\beta_2)$	No clinical abnormality
Normal	$(\alpha\alpha/\alpha\alpha)$	None	100%	Hgb A $(\alpha_2\beta_2)$	Normal

Source: Modified from Eden RD, Boehm FH, eds. Assessment and Care of the Fetus: Physiological, Clinical, and Medicolegal Principles. Norwalk, CT: Appleton & Lange; 1990:747.

1. **Homozygous α thalassemia,** in which all four copies of the gene are deleted, results in fetal death in utero or death shortly after birth. The normal fetal hemoglobin, hemoglobin F, contains two α-globin chains and two γ chains. In the absence of α chains, hemoglobin Bart's, a tetramer of γ chains, makes up the majority of hemoglobin for the fetus. It has a high oxygen affinity but does not release the oxygen well. The fetus will develop hydrops fetalis. The homozygous deletion is found mainly in Southeast Asians. The heterozygous state, in which two deletions of the gene are found, can be expressed as two possible genotypes (α__/ α__ or αα/__ __). Southeast Asians are more likely to have the (αα/__ __) genotype, and if two heterozygotes have children, there is a 25 percent chance of the fetus having the (__ __/__ __) genotype.

2. **Deletion of three genes,** known as *hemoglobin H disease,* causes patients to become transfusion dependent due to hemolytic anemia. The available hemoglobins are hemoglobin H (a tetramer of β chains), hemoglobin Bart's (a tetramer of γ chains), and very small amounts of hemoglobin A (due to the small amount of α chains produced by their single copy of the α gene). The abnormal hemoglobin H and hemoglobin Bart's precipitate in the red blood cells, forming Heinz bodies. Hemolytic anemia results as these cells are removed by the reticuloendothelial system. Death usually occurs in childhood.

3. **Heterozygous disease,** in which two copies of the gene are deleted, is usually fairly well tolerated. These patients have a hypochromic, microcytic anemia. Southeast Asians usually have the genotype (__ __/αα), known as α_1 *thalassemia minor.* Blacks usually have the genotype (α__/α__), known as α_2 *thalassemia minor.*

4. **Deletion of a single** copy of the α gene (__α/αα) produces a silent carrier state with no clinical abnormality. This is also known as α *thalassemia 2.*

D. **Diagnosis**

1. Patients at risk based on family history or ethnic background (Orientals, blacks, Indians, those of Mediterranean origin) should be evaluated. Some patients will present with a microcytic hypochromic anemia, which on evaluation leads to the diagnosis of thalassemia (Fig. 36.2).

2. All patients found to have thalassemia should be offered **evaluation of their partner** to assess the risk to the fetus. The partner should have a CBC with indices and hemoglobin electrophoresis. If he is heterozygous, or a carrier, or has α thalassemia himself, genetic counseling of the couple should be done.

3. **Antenatal diagnosis** of thalassemia and hemoglobinopathies can be done using amniocentesis to obtain fetal cells. The cells are cultured, and the number of α genes present in the

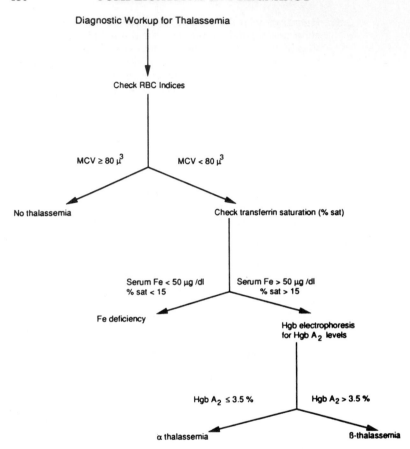

FIGURE 36.2. Diagnostic workup for thalassemia. (Adapted from Kitay DZ, ed. Hematologic Problems in Pregnancy. Oradell, NJ: Medical Economics Books; 1987.)

cellular genome is measured with molecular hybridization. Another method uses restriction endonucleases to map the DNA obtained from amniotic cells in order to assess the number of α genes deleted.

E. **Management in pregnancy**
   1. The patient whose fetus has homozygous α thalassemia should be counseled as to the poor prognosis, i.e., death in utero or shortly after birth. She is at increased risk of preeclampsia; therefore, the option of termination should be offered.
   2. Patients who have hemoglobin H disease usually do not live long enough to reproduce. Those who do will likely require frequent transfusions. Maternal and fetal surveillance should be intensified.

3. Patients who have α thalassemia minor will have a microcytic, hypochromic anemia but are reported to do well in pregnancy.
4. All of the above patients should receive folate supplementation and increased fetal surveillance.
5. Patients who have only a single α-gene deletion are clinically normal and would be expected to have a good pregnancy outcome.

II. β Thalassemias

Definition. Patients with β thalassemia have structurally normal hemoglobin but decreased synthesis of β-globin chains. A microcytic, hypochromic anemia results.

A. **Incidence and inheritance.** Thalassemias are inherited as an autosomal recessive trait. Patients with thalassemia are usually of Mediterranean, Middle Eastern, African, Indian, or Asian origin.

B. **Cause**
1. In contrast to α thalassemia, gene deletions are rarely a cause of β thalassemia. Rather, the cause is usually **point mutations** that can cause defective mRNA synthesis, nonfunctional mRNA, and coding mutations that also affect splicing. Over 80 different point mutations have been described, affecting every step in the production of β globin. The genes coding for β, δ, and γ globins are located on chromosome 11.
2. Since fetal hemoglobin (hemoglobin F—two α chains, two γ chains) is unaffected by β thalassemia, the fetus with β thalassemia will not present with problems until after birth, when it is several months old, when β-globin production should be rising as γ chain production falls to minimal levels. Levels of hemoglobin A₂ are elevated (two α chains, two δ chains) in β thalassemia.
3. Decreased β globin synthesis causes a relative overproduction of α-globin chains. The extra α globin precipitates out in red blood cells (Heinz bodies). The damaged red blood cell membranes often leads to hemolysis.

C. **Morbidity and mortality**
1. The **homozygous form** of β thalassemia, also known as β *thalassemia major* or *Cooley's anemia,* produces the most severe effects. With no β globin produced, no hemoglobin A is produced, and the majority of hemoglobin is hemoglobin F and hemoglobin A₂. Infants are diagnosed with severe anemia and failure to thrive, at ages 1 to 4 months, as their fetal hemoglobin production falls. These individuals are transfusion dependent and often die in childhood. Females who reach reproductive age are frequently sterile (Table 36.8).

Characteristic facial and skeletal changes are seen. Erythroid hyperplasia of the bone marrow expands the cancellous bone and causes changes in the trabecular archi-

Table 36.8. β Thalassemias

CLASSIFICATION	GLOBIN ALLELES	HEMOGLOBIN	CLINICAL OUTCOME
Homozygous			
Thalassemia major	$\beta^{\circ}\beta^{\circ}$	No Hgb A, Hgb F ↑ (Cooley's anemia)	Transfusion dependent, usually die in childhood
	$\beta^{+}\beta^{\circ}$	Some Hgb A, Hgb F ↑	Moderate anemia
	$\beta^{\circ}\beta^{\circ}$	No Hgb A, 100% Hgb F (hereditary persistence of fetal hemoglobin)	Moderate anemia
Heterozygous			
Thalassemia minor	$\beta^{\circ}\beta$	Hgb A$_2$ > 3.5%, Hgb F 2–5%; remainder is Hgb A	Microcytic, hypochromic anemia (most common form of β thalassemia)
	$\beta^{+}\beta$	Majority is Hgb A; normal amounts of Hgb A$_2$ and Hgb F	Mild anemia (diagnosed by family pedigree)
Normal	$\beta\beta$	Normal Hgb A ($\alpha_2\beta_2$)	Normal

Source: Modified from Eden RD, Boehm FH, eds. Assessment and Care of the Fetus: Physiological, Clinical, and Medicolegal Principles. Norwalk, CT: Appleton & Lange; 1990:747.

tecture. The thalassemic facies is one of prominent maxillary bones and protrusion of the upper jaw. Malocclusion and overbite are seen. In the skull, the diploic space in the frontal and parietal regions is widened. The classic "hair on end" appearance of a skull x-ray is due to radiating trabeculae of bone that extend at right angles to the inner and outer tables of the skull. Peripheral skeletal changes include widening of the shafts of the metacarpals, metatarsals, and phalanges.

Other problems include gallstones, risk of iron overload from transfusions, and risks from blood products.

Some patients with homozygous disease will have only moderate anemia. One group of patients may produce small amounts of β globin and larger than average amounts of hemoglobin F. Another group of patients are known to have moderate anemia; 100 percent of their hemoglobin is hemoglobin F. These individuals have hereditary persistence of fetal hemoglobin, i.e., their γ globin gene did not switch off at the usual time in early infancy.

2. The term **thalassemia intermedia** is applied to patients with heterozygous β thalassemia who have significant anemia and splenomegaly. These patients may require transfusions in pregnancy.

3. **Heterozygous β thalassemia,** or *thalassemia minor,* is characterized by one normal β-globin allele and one abnormal β-globin allele ($\beta°$, β^+, or $\beta^\pm$). A mild hypochromic, microcytic anemia is present, which is unaffected by iron supplementation. These patients may be asymptomatic.

   Carriers who have one β thalassemia allele and one normal allele ($\beta° \beta$) are the most common. Their hemoglobin A_2 is elevated over 3.5 percent, and their hemoglobin F is increased at 2 to 5 percent.

   Carriers who have one β thalassemia allele that is β^+ or $\beta^\pm$, along with a single normal allele, have only mild anemia. Their hemoglobin A_2 and hemoglobin F levels are normal. These alleles allow some production of β-globin chains and thus some normal hemoglobin A.

D. **Diagnosis.** Patients who give a family history, have an affected child, or are members of the ethnic group(s) at risk should be evaluated. Iron levels will be normal; red blood cell indices will show a microcytic, hypochromic anemia. Hemoglobin electrophoresis will confirm the diagnosis.

E. **Management in pregnancy**

1. General considerations in pregnancy include folate supplementation (increased demand in pregnancy, increased erythrocyte turnover) and increased maternal and fetal surveillance.

2. Patients with β thalassemia should have their partner assessed to determine if he has any hemoglobinopathy, since this is an inherited disease.

   Couples at risk should be offered prenatal diagnosis. Amniocentesis is done to obtain fetal cells. DNA analysis with restriction endonucleases will reveal a diagnosis in the majority of cases.

3. Patients with β thalassemia major (Cooley's anemia) rarely become pregnant, but those who do become severely anemic, may develop heart failure, and will need transfusions. These patients are at risk for spontaneous abortion, IUGR, and preterm labor. Multiple transfusions are known to improve patient survival and pregnancy outcome. Bedrest may be helpful. Iron overload is a potential problem. Splenectomy may be necessary for patients who need frequent transfusions or who have significant splenomegaly. Splenectomy is best done in the second trimester if it is necessary during pregnancy. It should be avoided in the third trimester if possible, as major abdominal surgery is difficult in a gravid patient and could precipitate preterm labor. Subsequently, these patients will be more susceptible to infections caused by encapsulated organisms.

4. Patients with β thalassemia intermedia may develop severe enough anemia to require transfusions in pregnancy.

5. β thalassemia minor patients usually do well in pregnancy and have a good outcome.

THROMBOCYTOPENIA IN PREGNANCY

Thrombocytopenia has many causes, usually involving decreased production, increased consumption, or sequestration. Severe vitamin B_{12} or folate deficiency will cause defective platelet maturation. A careful history regarding the patient's medications may reveal the causative agent in drug-induced thrombocytopenia (Table 36.9). Viral infections and sepsis lead to increased consumption of platelets. Thrombocytopenia may be the initial presentation of patients who have or who will develop systemic lupus erythematosus. Severe hemorrhage, disseminated intravascular coagulation, the HELLP syndrome (hemolysis, elevated liver enzymes, low platelets), and thrombotic thrombocytopenic purpura are other causes of thrombocytopenia to be considered in the differential diagnosis.

Table 36.9. Drugs Implicated in Thrombocytopenia or Abnormal Platelet Function

Antiinflammatory Agents	*Immune-Mediated Destruction*
Aspirin	Chlorothiazides
Ibuprofen	Chlorpropamide
Indomethacin	Diazepam
Mefenamic acid	Diphenylhydantoin
	Gold salts
Antibiotics	Quinidine
Ampicillin	Quinine
Penicillin G	Sulfisoxazole
Gentamicin	
Carbenicillin	*Others*
Nitrofurantoin	Acetaminophen
	Aminopyrine
Cardiovascular Drugs	Antihistamines
Dipyrimadole	Chloropromazine
Propranolol	Cimetidine
Theophylline	Glyceryl guaiacolate
	Furosemide
Cytoxic Drugs	Heparin
Nitrogen mustard	Heroin
Cyclophosphamide	Penicillamine
5-Fluorouracil	Phenylbutazone
Methotrexate	Procaine
	Sulfonamides
	Tolbutamide

Sources: Adapted from Creasy RK, Resnik R, eds. Maternal-Fetal Medicine: Principles and Practices. 2nd ed. Philadelphia, PA: WB Saunders; 1989:908 and Kitay DZ, ed. Hematologic Problems in Pregnancy. Oradell, NJ: Medical Economics Books; 1987:276.

The diagnosis of immune thrombocytopenia should considered if all of the above causes are ruled out. The diagnosis is confirmed by demonstration of platelet-directed autoantibodies.

I. Immune thrombocytopenic purpura

Definition. Immune thrombocytopenic purpura (ITP) is an autoimmune disorder in which the body manufactures antibodies directed against antigens found on platelets and megakaryocytes.

Patients may have an acute or a chronic form (Table 36.10). The acute form will not be addressed here, as pregnant patients usually have the chronic form.

A. Incidence. Females are affected three times more often than males. Whites are affected more frequently than blacks. The usual time of onset is between 20 and 40 years of age. The incidence in pregnancy is 1–2/1000 cases.

B. Cause. Antiplatelet antibodies, usually of the IgG class, are responsible for destruction of the platelets. The reticuloendothelial system (spleen, bone marrow, and liver) removes the antibody-coated platelets, causing thrombocytopenia.

C. Diagnosis
1. Patients with a platelet count < 100 000/mm^3 have thrombocytopenia. Many tests are available for identifying antiplatelet antibodies. A sensitive test is the direct assay of platelet-associated IgG and C$_3$ with radioactively labeled IgG antisera.
2. A radiolabeled monoclonal antibody to the Fc portion of IgG is in development and will probably become the diagnostic test of choice in the future.

D. Morbidity/mortality
1. The initial presentation is variable but usually involves some

Table 36.10. ITP

	ACUTE	CHRONIC
Age at onset	2–6 years (usually); rarely adults	20–40 years
Female : male ratio	1 : 1	3 : 1
Disease course	≤ 6 months (avg. 4–6 weeks)	Months to years
Inciting illness	Viral infection	Rarely
Spontaneous remission	80% within 6 months	Uncommon
Thrombocytopenia	< 20 000 platelets/mm^3	30 000–80 000 platelets/mm^3

Source: Adapted from Kitay DZ, ed. Hematologic Problems in Pregnancy. Oradell, NJ: Medical Economics Books; 1987:290.

degree of either bruising or excessive bleeding. It can occur after a traumatic injury or spontaneously. Commonly reported presentations include petechiae, ecchymosis, epistaxis, gingival bleeding, hematomas, menorrhagia, and hematuria. Significant bleeding does not usually occur until the platelet count is $< 30\ 000/mm^3$. Oral mucous membrane involvement with hemorrhagic bullae signifies severe thrombocytopenia, $< 5000/mm^3$. These patients are at high risk of intracranial hemorrhage and need immediate treatment. Mortality is < 5 percent in treated patients.

2. Treatment with **corticosteroids** (e.g., prednisone, 1.0 to 1.5 mg/kg/d) for several weeks is successful in most patients. The dose is tapered to the minimum amount required to maintain a clinically normal state with no spontaneous bleeding or petechiae.

3. Patients unresponsive to corticosteroids are candidates for **splenectomy**. The benefits are two-fold:
   a. Removal of the site of platelet destruction
   b. Decreased antibody production
   This will increase the platelet count in 75 percent of patients.

4. **Immunosuppression** with cytotoxic drugs (azathioprine, cyclophosphamide, vincristine, and vinblastine) has been used in patients treated unsuccessfully with steroids and/or splenectomy. These drugs are contraindicated in pregnancy.

5. **Intravenous γ globin** therapy (400 mg/kg for 5 days) and **plasmapheresis** will elevate the platelet count. The effect is transient, however, and these two therapies seem to be most useful in optimizing the patient's platelet count prior to surgical procedures (cesarean section, splenectomy). Platelet counts need to be $\geq 50\ 000/mm^3$ for surgical procedures.

6. **Platelet transfusions** are not effective, as the platelets are rapidly destroyed. The normal platelet usually is present in the circulation for 7 to 12 days; platelets of patients with ITP last for periods ranging from minutes to 2 to 3 days.

E. **Management in pregnancy**
   1. The **fetus** of a mother with ITP is also at risk, since maternal IgG platelet antibodies cross the placenta and attack the fetal platelets, causing fetal thrombocytopenia. Even if the mother's condition has been stabilized by the use of corticosteroids or splenectomy, her antiplatelet antibodies remain and may cause problems for the fetus.
   2. Considerable controversy exists regarding the optimal mode of delivery, vaginal or cesarean, in patients with ITP.
      a. The fetus with a platelet count $< 50\ 000/mm^3$ is at risk for intracranial hemorrhage. Cesarean delivery may decrease this risk. The problem is to determine which fetus has significant thrombocytopenia. Maternal platelet counts, maternal platelet antibody levels, prior maternal splenectomy, and maternal corticosteroid treatment do

not correlate with the fetal platelet count. Fetal scalp sampling for platelet count may be inaccurate.

b. Two useful factors identified by Samuels et al. are a maternal history of ITP and an elevated titer of indirect circulating antiplatelet IgG. A mother who has both of these risk factors has a fetus with a significant chance of severe thrombocytopenia. These mothers should have percutaneous umbilical blood sampling performed to determine the fetal platelet count. A fetus with a platelet count $> 50\ 000/mm^3$ can deliver vaginally. A fetus with a platelet count $< 50\ 000/mm^3$ should be delivered by cesarean section. The fetal blood sampling should be performed in a center with immediate access to an operating room, or in an operating room, as fetal bradycardia necessitating cesarean delivery is a known complication.

c. In centers where this technique is not available, it would be reasonable to deliver such an infant by cesarean section if the mother has both of the aforementioned risk factors.

3. In spite of these attempts to decrease fetal morbidity and mortality by minimizing the trauma of labor and delivery, it should be recognized that a significant number of fetal deaths occur even before the onset of labor.

4. Delivery-related trauma, such as episiotomies and lacerations, should be minimized. Fetal scalp electrodes should not be used. The maternal platelet count needs to be $> 50\ 000/mm^3$ if cesarean delivery is done, and postpartum hemorrhage is frequently seen if the platelet count is $< 100\ 000/mm^3$. Aggressive use of pitocin, Methergine, or other agents such as Prostin $F_2\alpha$ to help the uterus contract will minimize uterine bleeding.

5. Neonates who are not thrombocytopenic at birth may become so in the first 3 to 4 weeks after birth. The platelet count is usually lowest at 4 to 6 days after delivery and then gradually improves. Small amounts of platelet antibodies have been found in breast milk. Whether this precludes breast-feeding is controversial.

II. Isoimmune thrombocytopenia

Definition. Isoimmune thrombocytopenia is the platelet equivalent of Rh disease. The mother forms platelet antibodies directed against fetal platelet antigens that her platelets do not have. The maternal antibodies cross the placenta and react with fetal platelets, causing their destruction, and fetal thrombocytopenia.

A. **Incidence.** This disease occurs in 1/5000 pregnancies.

B. **Diagnosis.** If a mother has already had an infant with isoimmune thrombocytopenia, each subsequent pregnancy should be considered at risk and evaluated. Maternal platelet antibodies such as anti-PLA 1 and anti-BAK will frequently be identified.

C. **Morbidity/mortality.** The fetus is at risk for intracranial hemorrhage and death. One study reported a 20 to 35 percent incidence of intracranial hemorrhage. Mortality rates are reportedly high in firstborn infants (24 percent) but decrease to 5 percent in the next pregnancy due to recognition of, and preparation for, this problem.

D. **Management in pregnancy.** Early treatment with corticosteroids, intensified maternal and fetal surveillance, and liberal use of cesarean delivery are factors in the improved survival rate. Treating mothers with intravenous immunoglobin may be preventive (1 g/kg/week). Percutaneous umbilical blood sampling (PUBS) can be done to assess the fetal platelet count. If it is low, maternal platelets can be transfused into the fetus. Alternatively, maternal platelets can be given after the infant is born, or an exchange transfusion can be done.

III. **Thrombotic thrombocytopenic purpura and hemolytic uremic syndrome**

Definition. Thrombotic thrombocytopenic purpura (TTP) is diagnosed when hemolytic anemia, thrombocytopenia, neurologic abnormalities, renal dysfunction, and fever are present together. Hemolytic uremic syndrome (HUS) consists of hemolytic anemia, thrombocytopenia, renal failure, fever, and sometimes neurologic abnormalities. These two syndromes, both with significant morbidity and mortality, may be clinically indistinguishable.

A. **Incidence.** TTP is diagnosed more often in women than in men (female : male ratio is 3 : 2) and usually occurs in the twenties and thirties, although people of all ages may be affected. HUS is a disorder seen primarily in childhood, although adult cases are also described. Both occur rarely in pregnancy.

B. **Pathophysiology**
   1. The cause of TTP and HUS is unknown. Without therapy, patient mortality is high (50 to 90 percent). It may be idiopathic or associated with neoplastic conditions, infections, autoimmune diseases, oral contraceptive use, and drug allergies. It may present during pregnancy and in the puerperium. It has also been described as *peripartal renal failure, postpartum renal failure with microangiopathic hemolytic anemia,* and *postpartum nephrosclerosis.*
   2. These syndromes have in common microvascular injury caused by increased platelet aggregation. The characteristic histologic appearance is microthrombi in arterioles and capillaries composed of hyaline material with platelets and fibrin. These microthrombi in the circulatory system will damage erythrocytes, leading to microangiopathic hemolytic anemia. Renal and neurologic abnormalities result when this process continues to the point of significant vascular blockage with ischemia.
   3. Patients with TTP usually present with neurologic changes, malaise, fatigue, abdominal pain, fever, jaundice, and

abnormal bleeding. Neurologic changes can be mild to severe (headache, visual changes, cranial nerve palsies, syncope, paralysis, organic brain syndrome, seizures, and coma). Physical examination is notable for ecchymoses, purpura, pallor, and neurologic changes, which may or may not persist.

4. Laboratory evaluation will reveal moderate to severe anemia and thrombocytopenia, hematuria, elevated LDH, indirect bilirubin, blood urea nitrogen (BUN), and creatinine. The peripheral smear shows microangiopathic hemolysis, with schistocytes, reticulocytes, and nucleated red blood cells.

5. HUS is seen in both adults and children. The childhood form is usually preceded by a viral or bacterial gastrointestinal illness with diarrhea; subsequently, fever, bleeding, abdominal pain, thrombocytopenia, microangiopathic hemolytic anemia, and renal failure will develop. Although renal hypertension, oliguria, and severe renal failure are frequently seen, 90 percent of patients will recover with normal renal function. The microvascular lesions are seen only in the kidneys, and neurologic changes are usually not present.

   The adult form has a much higher morbidity and mortality. It is seen more often in the postpartum period. Patients have microangiopathic hemolytic anemia, thrombocytopenia, bleeding, and renal failure.

6. It is very difficult to distinguish between TTP and HUS in adults due to the similarity of their clinical presentation. However, patients with HUS are more likely to have had an antecedent gastrointestinal illness, less likely to have neurologic involvement, more likely to have profound anemia and thrombocytopenia, and more likely to have early onset, severe renal failure with hypertension.

7. Current treatment with plasmapheresis, blood transfusions, and supportive care has increased survival to 90 percent. In addition, antiplatelet agents (aspirin, 600 to 1200 mg daily, and dipyridamole, 400 to 600 mg daily) are beneficial. Platelet transfusions should **not** be given. Plasmapheresis should be done every other day until platelets are in the normal range and neurologic symptoms resolve. Patients treated in this manner usually recover in about a week. Patients are at risk for relapse; aspirin and dipyridamole therapy should be prescribed for an additional 6 to 12 months after the initial episode.

8. It is thought that the increased platelet aggregation in TTP-HUS may be related to an abnormality in the prostacyclin-thromboxane A_2 balance. Prostacyclin inhibits platelet aggregation, and thromboxane A_2 is its antagonist; both are found in plasma. A deficiency of one or an excess of the other is a possible explanation for this syndrome and explains why plasmapheresis leads to improvement. Plas-

mapheresis restores the usual balance of these factors or of any other possible plasma factor involved.

C. **Diagnosis.** HUS-TTP is diagnosed when a patient has hemolytic anemia, thrombocytopenia, neurologic abnormalities, renal dysfunction, and fever.

The peripheral smear will show microangiopathic hemolysis, with schistocytes, reticulocytes, and nucleated red blood cells.

D. **Management in pregnancy**
    1. One of the most difficult diagnostic dilemmas is trying to determine if a pregnant patient with the above findings has preeclampsia with the HELLP syndrome, or if she has HUS-TTP. The course of HUS-TTP is unaffected by pregnancy. In contrast, for patients with preeclampsia and HELLP syndrome, delivery is the indicated treatment. Patients start to recover once they are delivered.

        Therefore, patients near term should be delivered. If delivery does not effect improvement, patients should be treated as though they have HUS-TTP. Those who present early in pregnancy should be treated with plasmapheresis, transfusions, and antiplatelet medications if the diagnosis of preeclampsia with HELLP syndrome is ruled out.

        Patients with HUS-TTP are more likely to have fever and purpuric skin changes (although a patient with HELLP syndrome would also have fever is she developed chorioamnionitis or endometritis).

        Those patients whose diagnosis remains unclear, and who are still early in pregnancy, need to be carefully assessed and evaluated; as the clinical picture becomes clearer, treatment can be instituted.
    2. Skin biopsy has been proposed as a diagnostic aid in this situation. Unfortunately, the classic histologic picture is found only 50 percent of the time. Thus skin biopsy is helpful only if it is positive.

HEREDITARY COAGULATION DEFECTS

I. **Hemophilia A**
    Definition. Hemophilia A is an X-linked recessive disorder with low factor VIII coagulant activity. Patients bleed abnormally because of a functional defect in factor VIII.

    A. **Incidence and inheritance.** Hemophilia affects 10–20/100 000 males. Affected (hemizygous) males have inherited an abnormal X chromosome (from their mother). Females are rarely affected. For a female to have hemophilia A, two abnormal X chromosomes must be present. Weiner has outlined the six possible situations in which a female may have hemophilia.
        1. Chance lyonization of sufficient X chromosomes carrying the normal gene, resulting in absent/reduced coagulant activity

2. Daughter of a hemophiliac male and a female carrier
3. Monosomy X
4. Wrong diagnosis; the patient has Von Willebrand's disease
5. Spontaneous mutation of the normal X chromosome at the zygote stage of a carrier fetus
6. Autosomal dominant hemophilia; only one well-documented kindred to date

It is theorized that a high spontaneous mutation rate contributes to the incidence of hemophilia since many patients report no family history or other affected family members. Hemophilia A is more common than hemophilia B; 85 percent of hemophiliacs have hemophilia A. Sons of female hemophiliacs will all be hemophiliacs. Daughters will all be carriers. Fifty percent of a carrier's sons will be hemophiliacs. Fifty percent of her daughters will also be carriers.

B. **Morbidity and mortality.** Carriers are not clinically affected. Hemophiliacs can be classified as mild, moderate, or severe. Mild hemophiliacs will have significant bleeding from injury or surgery. Moderate hemophiliacs will have significant bleeding from minor trauma. Severe hemophiliacs will have spontaneous bleeding into the skin, viscera, and joints. Hemathroses, hematuria, epistaxis, and mucous membrane bleeding occur frequently. Death usually occurs from intracranial hemorrhage.

C. **Cause.** Hemophilia A is caused by low factor VIII coagulant activity. The factor VIII complex has two parts: the larger component, Von Willebrand factor (F VIII:RCoF), carries with it factor VIII–related antigen (FVIII:RA); the smaller component contains the site of coagulant activity (FVIII:C). The coagulant protein is present in normal amounts but is functionally abnormal, so that the coagulant activity is decreased. Factor VIII:C levels are a measure of coagulant activity.

D. **Diagnosis.** Laboratory findings include decreased levels of factor VIII coagulant activity, prolonged partial thromboplastin time (PTT), and normal prothrombin time (PT). As factor VIII coagulant activity decreases, the patient's chances of a hemorrhagic episode increases (Table 36.11).

E. **Management of pregnancy**
1. **Genetic counseling** should be offered to women at risk of delivering an affected male fetus (carriers, women who have hemophilia, women with a family history). Prenatal diagnosis to determine the fetal sex can be done by chorionic villus sampling, genetic amniocentesis, or PUBS. The latter can also obtain blood to assess fetal factor VIII. Ultrasound examination will also reveal the fetal sex.
2. Pregnancies in females with hemophilia have not been well studied. Coagulation factors are known to increase in pregnancy. However, it would be good preparation to have cryoprecipitate and fresh frozen plasma available when a hemophiliac patient is delivering. The mode of delivery should be based on the obstetric indications. Medications

Table 36.11. Relationship of Factor VIII or Factor IX Level to Disease Severity

DISEASE SEVERITY	LEVEL
Mild	> 5%
Moderate	1–5%
Severe	< 1%
Carriers	50%

Source: Adapted from Gleicher N, ed. Principles of Medical Therapy in Pregnancy. New York: Plenum Medical Book; 1985:1022–1023.

that affect platelet function or coagulation should be avoided. Intramuscular injections should not be given if another route of administration is available. Fetal scalp electrodes should not be applied. Delivery should be as atraumatic as possible, trying to prevent lacerations and an episiotomy. Postpartum, uterine massage and uterotonics should be used aggressively to achieve prompt uterine contraction to minimize blood loss. Until the hematologic status of the male infant is known, circumcision should be deferred.

3. Carriers for hemophilia are seen much more frequently for delivery than actual hemophiliacs. Some authors recommend testing the level of factor VIII in these patients. Patients with levels < 30 percent should receive cryoprecipitate (cryoprecipitated antihemophiliac factor) for delivery. Levels that are < 50 percent in patients who need cesarean delivery should be increased to > 80 percent prior to surgery. Postoperatively, cryoprecipitate should be continued to keep levels > 30 to 40 percent for several days.

The number of bags of cryoprecipitate needed can be calculated from the following formula:

$$\frac{\text{Factor VIII level (in \%)} \times \text{plasma volume (mL)}}{80 \text{ (average no. of factor VIII units/bag)}} = \text{no. of bags of cryoprecipitate}$$

II. Hemophilia B
Definition. Hemophilia B, also known as *Christmas disease,* is caused by deficiency of factor IX.
  A. **Incidence and inheritance.** Hemophilia B is a similar to hemophilia A in that it is an X-linked recessive trait. Its prevalence is only 1–3/100 000. The genetic distribution is similar to that of hemophilia A. Hemizygous males are affected, where-

as two abnormal X chromosomes are required for females to be affected.

B. Morbidity and mortality. Clinically, patients with hemophilia B have the same disease manifestations as those with hemophilia A, ranging from mild to severe. Fifteen percent of all hemophiliacs have hemophilia B.

C. Diagnosis. Laboratory testing reveals prolonged bleeding time, prolonged PTT, and sometimes prolonged PT. Factor IX levels will predict the severity of disease.

D. Management in pregnancy

1. As with hemophilia A, cases of pregnancy in hemophilia B are rare and not well studied. Levels of coagulation factors rise during pregnancy. Plasma should be available for transfusion in the event of hemorrhage (cryoprecipitate has insufficient factor IX to be useful). Concentrates of factor IX, prepared from a large pool of donors, have a high risk of causing hepatitis B.

2. In managing the labor and delivery of a patient with hemophilia B, follow the same principles as with hemophilia A. Be prepared for plasma transfusion and/or plasmapheresis. Medications that affect platelet function or coagulation should be avoided. Intramuscular injections should not be given if another route of administration is available. Fetal scalp electrodes should not be applied. Delivery should be as atraumatic as possible, trying to prevent lacerations and an episiotomy. Until the hematologic status of the male infant is known, circumcision should be deferred.

3. Prenatal diagnosis is available and should be offered to women with the disease, with a family history, or with an affected family member. Fetal blood can be collected via PUBS.

III. Von Willebrand's disease

Definition. Von Willebrand's disease is an inherited defect of coagulation in which von Willebrand factor (also known as the *ristocetin cofactor*) portion of the factor VIII complex is abnormal.

Type I (classic) von Willebrand's disease: quantitative decrease in von Willebrand factor

Type IIA von Willebrand's disease: absence of large and intermediate-sized multimers of von Willebrand factor for both plasma and platelets

Type IIB von Willebrand's disease: absence of multimers from plasma only

A. Incidence and inheritance. Von Willebrand's disease has a prevalence of 1/10 000 and is the most common hereditary coagulopathy. The usual mode of inheritance is autosomal dominant, although an autosomal recessive pattern has also been identified.

B. **Morbidity and mortality.** The clinical presentation is almost always due to bleeding or hemorrhage. Patients may present with easy bruising, mucosal hemorrhage, menorrhagia, postpartum hemorrhage, intraoperative hemorrhage, or unexpected bleeding from trauma.

C. **Cause.** Von Willebrand factor is the large component of the factor VIII complex that is crucial for platelet aggregation and clot formation at the site of a vascular injury. It is made by platelets and by endothelium.

D. **Diagnosis.** A family history or clinical evidence of bleeding may prompt evaluation. Laboratory evaluation reveals a prolonged bleeding time, prolonged PTT, a low factor VIII level, and abnormal platelet adhesion.

E. **Management**
   1. In most patients, levels of factor VIII and von Willebrand factor increase significantly during pregnancy, sometimes to normal levels. Bleeding time usually improves as pregnancy progresses.
   2. At the time of delivery, the factor VIII level should be checked; if it is > 50 percent of normal and the bleeding time is normal, then postpartum hemorrhage is less likely. However, late postpartum hemorrhage remains a concern, as factor VIII levels return to baseline 2 to 3 days postpartum.
   3. In the patient whose factor VIII level is not > 50 percent of normal at delivery, factor VIII-rich cryoprecipitate or fresh frozen plasma should be given. For the patient who requires a cesarean delivery, prophylactic cryoprecipitate or fresh frozen plasma should be given prior to surgery unless the bleeding time is normal and the factor VIII is 80 percent of normal. Some advocate aggressive treatment with cryoprecipitate (15 to 20 U b.i.d. for the first 2 to 3 days, then 8 to 10 U b.i.d. for the next 4 to 5 days). However, this exposes the patient to a large quantity of blood products with their attendant risks. Nevertheless, in view of the significant risk of delayed postpartum hemorrhage faced by patients with von Willebrand's disease, many would agree that treatment for a full week postpartum is warranted.
   4. Anticipation and preparation for the delivery of a patient with von Willebrand's disease will facilitate a good outcome. A team approach involving the patient, physician, nurses, blood bank, delivery room, and operating room personnel will benefit all concerned.
   5. Patients should not receive any drugs affecting platelet function. Intramuscular injections are contraindicated. Episiotomies and lacerations during delivery should be avoided if possible.
   6. Prenatal diagnosis is now possible via chorionic villus biopsy with DNA analysis. In cases where both parents have the

disorder and offspring are at risk for the more severe bleeding disorder associated with homozygous disease, this is an option the parents may want to consider. Some authors suggest cesarean delivery of a fetus whose mother has severe disease.

The fetus of a mother with von Willebrand's disease should be treated as though it too has the disease until a diagnosis is made after delivery. Fetal scalp electrodes should not be used. Delivery of the baby, whether vaginally or by cesarean section, should be as atraumatic as possible. No circumcision should be done until the baby's status is known.

IV. **Antithrombin III deficiency**
Definition. Antithrombin III (AT III) deficiency is the most common clotting disorder in women and is caused by insufficient amounts of the regulatory protein that inhibits thrombin, factor Xa, and other serine proteases.
  A. **Incidence and inheritance.** The incidence is 1/2000 people. The disease is inherited in an autosomal dominant pattern.
  B. **Morbidity and mortality.** Studies have shown that 40 to 70 percent of affected persons will at some point develop a deep vein thrombosis. Often this occurs before age 40. Even patients without AT III deficiency will have significant decreases in their AT III levels in the presence of mild infection, preeclampsia, and thrombosis.
  C. **Cause.** AT III has an important role in the physiology of blood coagulation. As a serine protease inhibitor, it regulates the amount of fibrin generated by activated factors XII, XI, X, and IX and thrombin. Heparin binds to AT III and causes acceleration of the rate of formation of enzyme inhibitor complexes. This explains why patients with AT III deficiency require larger than expected amounts of heparin for anticoagulation. The presence of AT III is required for heparin to work.
  D. **Diagnosis.** Patients who have a family history of AT III deficiency or who have a thrombotic event should be tested. Measurement of AT III activity in these patients usually reveals levels 25 to 50 percent of normal. The diagnosis should be suspected in patients on heparin therapy who require larger than expected levels of heparin to achieve adequate anticoagulation.
  E. **Management in pregnancy**
    1. Pregnancy itself is a hypercoaguable state. The pregnant patient who also has AT III deficiency is at very high risk of a thrombotic event. Studies have reported an incidence of 66 to 75 percent of thrombosis in these patients. Patients with a history of thrombosis are at high risk for recurrence.
    2. **Prophylactic anticoagulation** with heparin should be given as soon as the diagnosis of pregnancy is confirmed. The amount of heparin required will be significantly higher than usual to achieve anticoagulation due to the resistance to heparin mediated by the low AT III activity. One study

showed that if AT III activity is 40 to 50 percent of normal, 20 000 to 45 000 U of heparin per 24 hours will be necessary (e.g., 15 000 U s.q. q8 h). Heparin therapy should continue until 4 weeks postpartum. The patient's heparin level should be adjusted to keep the PTT prolonged 1.5 times normal for prophylaxis.

3. If the patient has an acute thrombotic event during pregnancy, the heparin level should be sufficient to prolong the PTT to 1.5 to 2.0 times normal. It is to be expected that as the pregnancy progresses, the amount of heparin required may increase. For this reason, PTT should be followed at least weekly.

4. Prolonged heparin therapy carries with it the risks of overcompensating, with resultant bleeding episodes, thrombocytopenia, and osteoporosis. In the patient with AT III deficiency, however, the benefits of anticoagulation seem to outweigh the risks.

5. If available, AT III concentrate should be given during labor and delivery to keep AT III levels ≥ 80 percent normal.

V. Protein S and protein C deficiencies

Definition: Protein C is a vitamin K–dependent protein whose active form inactivates factors Va and VIIIa, inhibiting coagulation. It also facilitates thrombolysis by stimulating endothelial cells to produce plasminogen activator. Calcium, protein S, and phospholipids are required for these actions. Protein S is a vitamin K–dependent protein that functions as a cofactor of protein C. Deficiency of either of these proteins leads to a hypercoagulable state.

A. **Incidence.** Deficiencies of either protein S or protein C are thought to occur more frequently than AT III deficiency (1/2000) but are not well studied. Both are inherited as autosomal dominant traits.

B. **Morbidity and mortality**
1. Patients are usually heterozygous and have only 50 percent of the normal level of protein S or protein C. Protein C deficiency is seen in 8 percent of patients whose first episode of thromboembolism occurs before age 40. Patients often have their first thrombosis in their early twenties and give a history of recurrent thromboembolism. The family history is usually notable for thrombotic events and recurrences.

2. Homozygous protein C deficiency is rarely seen. It may cause death in affected neonates due to systemic intravascular coagulation.

3. Patients with a thromboembolism are treated initially with heparin and then with oral anticoagulants. Unfortunately, coumadin antagonizes vitamin K, which will inactivate not only protein S and protein C, but also the other vitamin K–dependant clotting factors. Coumadin may also cause skin necrosis in protein C–deficient patients.

C. **Diagnosis.** A family history of thromboembolism or pulmonary embolus, or a history of a thromboembolic event in the patient, should prompt investigation into the reason for a hypercoaguable state. Patients should be tested for AT III, protein S, and protein C deficiencies. If these levels are normal, rare causes such as dysfibrinogenemia or dysplasminogenemia should be considered.

D. **Management in pregnancy**
1. Pregnancy is a hypercoaguable state; some clotting factors are known to be increased (fibrinogen [factor I], factors VII, VIII, X, XII), while others are decreased (factors XI, XIII), and still others are variably reported as either unchanged or increased (factors II, V, IX). Protein S is reportedly decreased in pregnancy.
2. Patients who are known to be protein S or protein C deficient should be maintained on therapeutic heparin throughout pregnancy. Requirements will usually increase as the pregnancy progresses. This is due to the increased plasma volume, increased renal clearance, and placental heparinase.

BIBLIOGRAPHY

Creasy RK, Resnik R, eds. Maternal-Fetal Medicine: Principles and Practices. 2nd ed. Philadelphia, PA: WB Saunders; 1989.

Cunningham FG, McDonald PC, Gant NF, eds. Williams Obstetrics, 18th ed. Norwalk, CT: Appleton & Lange; 1989.

Eden RD, Boehm FH, eds. Assessment and Care of the Fetus: Physiological, Clinical, and Medicolegal Principles. Norwalk, CT: Appleton & Lange; 1990.

Gabbe SG, Niebyl JR, Simpson JL, eds. Obstetrics: Normal and Problem Pregnancies. 2nd ed. New York: Churchill Livingstone; 1991.

Gleicher N, ed. Principles of Medical Therapy in Pregnancy. New York: Plenum Medical Book Company; 1985.

Kitay DZ, ed. Hematologic Problems in Pregnancy. Oradell, NJ: Medical Economics Books; 1987.

Morrison JC, Schneider JM, Whybrew WD, et al. Prophylactic transfusions in pregnant patients with sickle hemoglobinopathies: Benefit vs. risk. Obstet Gynecol 1980; 56:274.

Samuels P, Bussel JB, Braitmen LE, et al. Estimation of the risk of thrombocytopenia in the offspring of pregnant women with presumed immune thrombocytopenia purpura. N Engl J Med 1990; 323:229.

Thompson MW, McInnes RR, Willard HF, eds. Thompson & Thompson: Genetics in Medicine. 5th ed. Philadelphia, PA: WB Saunders; 1991.

Weiner CP. Treatment of coagulation and fibrinolytic disorders. In: Kitay DZ, ed. Hematologic Problems in Pregnancy. Oradell, NJ: Medical Economics Book; 1987.

CHAPTER 37

Immunologic Disease

Milo B. Sampson
Joaquin Santolaya

The cause of **immunologic diseases,** which are also called *rheumatic* or *autoimmune diseases,* is unknown. However, mechanisms that cause the humoral or cellular components of the body's immune system to respond to the self-antigens of the body to produce disease may be involved. Many of these diseases preferentially occur in women in the childbearing years and can affect the outcome of pregnancy because most autoimmune diseases produce IgG antibodies that cross the placenta. **Systemic lupus erythematosus** is the most important of these diseases discussed in this chapter, although **rheumatoid arthritis, scleroderma, polymyositis,** and **dermatomyositis** will also be described.

SYSTEMIC LUPUS ERYTHEMATOSUS

I. **Incidence.** Systemic lupus erythematosus (SLE) preferentially affects women of childbearing age (90 percent of cases) and has an increased incidence in blacks compared to whites and Orientals. The incidence is 1/400 overall, with a genetic component, as evidenced by family and twin studies and by the increased frequency of HLA-DR2 and DR3 in patients. From 9 to 21 percent of patients first present with the disease in pregnancy. SLE occurs in 1/1660 pregnancies.

II. **Morbidity and mortality.** Thirty years ago, patients with SLE lived for only a few years after diagnosis. Earlier diagnosis using antinuclear antibody (ANA) tests and the introduction of steroids (1975) and antiinflammatory agents have extended life more than 10 years for 90 percent of patients. When diffuse proliferative glomerulonephritis or central nervous system involvement is present, the prognosis is poorer. Patients with only skin involvement have an excellent prognosis, but 15 percent will still develop mild SLE. The use of steroids, dialysis, and renal transplantation has decreased deaths from SLE caused by uremia and central nervous system disease but has increased the incidence of serious fungal and bacterial infections.

III. Cause. SLE, like all autoimmune diseases, occurs when, for unknown reasons, cell-mediated and humoral components of the immune system produce antibodies to the body's antigens.

IV. Pathogenesis and pathophysiology
   A. **Autoimmune disease effects.** Damage to the body results from
      autoimmune reactions throughout the body. Specific organs are
      often especially involved. For example, antibodies to DNA,
      nucleoproteins, histones, and nuclear ribonucleoproteins are
      found in glomerular and vascular basement membranes in the
      kidney. Systemically, T and B lymphocytes are decreased and a
      fall in T cells parallels increased disease activity.
   B. **Effects on the fetus and neonate**
      1. Twenty percent of fetuses are **small for gestational age
         (SGA),** perhaps due to transplacental immune complexes
         found early in pregnancy that can persist for up to 2 weeks
         postpartum. **Congenital heart block** with endocardial fibro-
         elastosis is probably due to soluble ribonucleoprotein anti-
         gen Ro(SS-A). **Cutaneous lesions** can occur, which resolve
         within 12 months of delivery. Other congenital anomalies
         are not increased. Lupus anticoagulant factor, an autoanti-
         body acquired by some patients with SLE, has been associ-
         ated with increased abortion and stillbirth. Use of cortico-
         steroids and low-dose aspirin appears to improve the out-
         come in these cases.
      2. The **spontaneous abortion** rate is high (21 percent), as is
         prematurity (17 to 37 percent) and **stillbirth** (12 to 30 per-
         cent), all of which increase in active disease. In renal dis-
         ease, when the serum creatinine is > 1.5 mg/dL, fetal loss is
         50 percent, which increases to 80 percent if there is also
         significant proteinuria.

V. Differential diagnosis. Since many organs can be affected in a
   variable manner by the autoimmune process, the signs and symptoms
   of the disease may mimic those of a vast variety of diseases. However, some systems are commonly affected:
   A. **Dermatologic manifestations** occur in 70 to 80 percent, **renal
      disease** in > 40 percent, **hematologic abnormalities** in > 50
      percent, and **cardiovascular disease** in 30 to 50 percent of
      patients.
   B. **Preeclampsia and SLE nephritis.** These two conditions are dif-
      ficult to differentiate. ANA are not found in preeclampsia, and
      early onset of symptoms at 27 to 30 weeks with severe hyperten-
      sion, renal involvement, anemia, thrombocytopenia, coagula-
      tion defects, and circulating antibody complexes suggests SLE.

VI. Diagnosis of SLE
   A. **Signs and symptoms**
      1. Fever
      2. Migratory arthralgias

      3. Rash on hands and face

      4. Fatigue and malaise

      5. Weight loss and anorexia

      6. Irregular or heavy menses

B. Physical examination

      1. Pain upon movement or palpation in fingers, hands, wrists, knees, and ankles, without swelling

      2. Tachycardia without congestive heart failure or tamponade

      3. Pleuritic friction rub

      4. Psychosis similar to steroid psychosis

      5. Paralytic ileus and enlarged liver

      6. Enlarged, nontender lymph nodes

C. Laboratory examination and diagnostic procedures

      1. Anemia. Normochromic, normocytic anemia with red blood cell autoagglutination, positive Coombs test, leukopenia, and thrombocytopenia are present.

      2. Urinalysis. The urine sediment has red and white cell casts with proteinuria and an elevated erythrocyte sedimentation rate.

      3. Biologic false-positive syphilis tests may precede the symptoms of SLE by years, and autoantibodies that react with red and white blood cells, platelets, and B and T lympocytes are present. The lupus erythematosus (LE) cell is not always present. More sensitive tests that detect ANA are used. Directly detected DNA antibodies are present in active disease, especially nephritis. Complement is usually depressed, reflecting fixation to immune complexes. Complement levels do not accurately predict disease activity.

D. Diagnostic criteria. Four or more of the following 10 manifestations are necessary for diagnosis (99 percent specific):

      1. Malar rash

      2. Discoid lupus

      3. Photosensitivity

      4. Oral ulcers

      5. Arthritis

      6. Presence of anti-DNA, anti-Sm, or LE cells

      7. Proteinurea (0.5 g/d or cellular casts)

      8. Pleuritis or percarditis

      9. Psychosis or seizures

      10. Hemolytic anemia (11 g/dL), leukopenia (4500/mm), or thrombocytopenia (100 000/cm)

VII. Management

A. Antepartum care

      1. Steroid therapy. Patients should be treated with corticosteroids, as in the nonpregnant state.

        a. **Prednisone.** Give 20 to 40 mg/d orally for minor flares and 40 to 80 mg/d when there is central nervous system involvement or vasculitis. **Short-acting steroid prep-**

arations, i.e., prednisone (Deltasone, Meticorten) or methylprednisolone (Medrol, Solu-Medrol), are used.

b. **Side effects of glucocorticoids.** All glucocorticoids have similar side effects related to dosage and administration, including hypoadrenalism, decreased resistance to infection, changes in physical appearance, depression and psychosis, hyperglycemia, electrolyte abnormalities, myopathies, and osteopenia responsive to vitamin D.

2. **Immunosuppressive therapy.** Azathioprine (Imuran) is felt to be a better agent than **cyclophosphamide** (Cytoxan) because up to 40 percent of babies born after the use of the latter agent have had low birth weight, whereas no anomalies have been reported with azathioprine. Azathioprine, 1.0 to 2.5 mg/kg/d, may be used in uncontrolled, life-threatening disease uncontrolled by steroids.

3. **Plasmapheresis and dialysis** are not now used in the management of SLE.

4. **Fetal surveillance** should be started before fetal viability. This includes an initial ultrasound examination with follow-up scans, nonstress tests beginning at 28 weeks, biophysical profiles, and Doppler velocimetry studies if fetal compromise is suspected.

   Thrombocytopenia and **proteinuria** occur more often in pregnancy, while the incidence of pleuritis and pericarditis decreases. When maternal platelet antibodies are present, the fetus may be thrombocytopenic. Percutaneous umbilical blood sampling (PUBS) may be done before labor and fetal scalp sampling early in labor for platelets. Aspirin can induce bleeding with circulatory anticoagulants, and infection can be increased by steroids.

   Thrombotic thrombocytopenic purpura is a serious pregnancy complication in SLE patients with low complement levels. Delivery or termination, depending on the gestational age, improves this condition.

5. **Clinical considerations.** SLE exacerbations occur when the third (C3) or fourth (C4) complement components or total hemolytic component (CH50) fall. If these components fall or the patient develops nephropathy for the first time, glucocorticoids should be started at the lowest dose that stabilizes the patient.

6. **Cardiolipins and lupus anticoagulant.** Elevated cardiolipin antibodies and lupus anticoagulant levels have been associated with poor pregnancy outcomes. Use of prednisone and low-dose aspirin (80 mg/d) may improve the outcome by inhibiting thromboxane synthesis without affecting prostacyclin synthesis.

B. **Intrapartum care**
   1. **Management of patients on steroid therapy.** During labor, surgery, or an acute medical illness, patients on steroid

therapy should be given extra doses of steroids, usually hydrocortisone, 100 to 150 mg IV or IM q8 h, which are maintained for 24 h after the acute event. This regimen should be continued throughout the first postpartum day to avoid hypoadrenalism. Patients not on steroids do not require postpartum of postabortion steroids since flares are not increased by these events.

C. **Postpartum care**
   1. **Contraception.** If further fertility is desired, barrier methods of birth control should be used, since oral contraceptives have been associated with disease exacerbation and intrauterine contraceptive devices with infection.
   2. Cervical dysplasia is increased in immunosuppressed patients such as those with SLE. Careful evaluation with Pap smears and colposcopy as indicated is important.

VIII. **Prognosis.** In general, patients with severe SLE do not become pregnant, although pregnancy itself has no long-term effect on SLE. Two-thirds of patients with inactive disease at the beginning of pregnancy remain quiescent, whereas one-half of patients with active disease in early pregnancy have exacerbations. From 18 to 25 percent of patients develop preeclampsia. Prematurity and fetal wastage, including spontaneous abortion, are also increased.

RHEUMATOID ARTHRITIS

I. **Incidence.** The incidence of this disease is 0.35 percent using the revised New York diagnostic criteria (1966), with a 3 : 1 female : male ratio. There is a fourfold increase of disease in relatives, suggesting a genetic predisposition. The peak incidence is in the forties, and the diseae occurs from the third to the seventh decade of life.

II. **Morbidity and mortality.** Ten percent of patients are incapacitated within 10 to 15 years after the onset of the disease; 15 percent are in remission, and the others have a variable course. Symptoms improve during pregnancy, with relapse usually occurring in the first postpartum month. The long-term outcome of rheumatoid arthritis is unaffected by pregnancy.

III. **Cause**
   A. **Antigen response.** The disease may represent an aberrant response to an unknown antigen (possibly from a microbial infection) in a genetically susceptible individual. Dense lymphocyte collections are seen in the synovial membranes. Rheumatoid factor (IgM and IgG antibodies against the Fc region of IgG) and ANA, antilymphocyte, and antigranulocyte autoantibodies are synthesized in the synovial membrane.
   B. **Association with the HLA-DR4 locus.** The HLA-DR4 locus is associated with seropositive rheumatoid arthritis. Thus, sus-

ceptibility to the disease is inherited and is associated with gene products of this major histocompatibility system.

IV. **Pathogenesis and pathophysiology.** Rheumatoid arthritis is a chronic systemic disease with (usually) symmetric inflammation of peripheral joints. The hematologic, pulmonary, neurologic, and cardiovascular systems may also be affected. The proximal interphalangeal (PIP), metacarpophalangeal (MCP), wrist, elbow, ankle, and cervical spines are most often involved; the distal interphalangeal (DIP) joints are less often affected. Extraarticular factors such as nodules occur with high rheumatoid factor levels, immune complexes, and joint involvement. Rheumatoid nodules occur in 20 percent of patients, and pulmonary granulomas occur in smokers. Other nodule sites are the myocardium, heart valves, coronary arteries, and aortic root. Vasculitis, Felty's syndrome, and Sjogren's syndrome can occur.

V. **Differential diagnosis.** Septic arthritis, gout, pseudogout, and ankylosing spondylitis must be differentiated from this disease. Calcium pyrophosphate occurs in the synovial fluid of pseudogout. Gout and ankylosing spondylitis have a predilection for males. Uric acid is elevated in gout, which also usually has a hereditary pattern.

VI. **Diagnosis**
   A. **Signs and symptoms.** The symptoms of rheumatoid arthritis are insidious and include fatigue, weight loss, malaise, and anorexia. Other symptoms are fever, vasomotor instability (including Raynaud's phenomenon), swelling, and morning stiffness (the severity of which is a measure of disease activity).
   B. The **New York diagnostic criteria** (1966) require the presence of **two** or more of the following criteria for diagnosis:
      1. History of joint pain involving three or more limb joints, but joints that occur in groups (i.e., PIP or MCP on one side) count as a single joint.
      2. Swelling, limitation of movement, subluxation, or ankylosis of at least three limb joints (excluding the DIP, PIP, first metacarpals, hips, and first MIP), with symmetry of at least one joint pair. There must be involvement of one hand, wrist, or foot.
      3. X-ray characteristics of erosive arthritis in the hand, wrist, or foot.
      4. Positive serologic test results for rheumatoid factor.
   C. **Laboratory examinations and diagnostic procedures.** The erythrocyte sedimentation rate reflects disease activity, as does C-reactive protein and serum haptoglobin. The latex fixation test for rheumatoid factor is positive in 70 percent of patients. Synovial fluid contains specific IgG antibodies. Rheumatoid factor and assays of urates and calcium pyrophosphate dihydrate may diagnose gout and pseudogout, which can mimic rheumatoid arthritis. HLA-B27 is associated with ankylosing spondylitis and

Reiter's syndrome. Mild anemia with decreased iron and iron binding are common, and a few patients have eosinophilia.

VII. Management. The management of rheumatoid arthritis in the pregnant patient is similar to that in the nonpregnant state, with the exception of certain drugs that may be harmful to the fetus. **Rest, exercise, heat, and physical therapy together with salicylate therapy** are the mainstays of treatment.

   A. **Salicylates** act as prostaglandin inhibitors in inflamed tissue to stabilize lysozomes and suppress B and T lymphocytes. The average requirement for the drug of choice in pregnancy **(acetylsalicyclic acid)** is 3.6 to 4.0 grains/d in divided oral doses. Gastrointestinal irritation is avoided with enteric-coated preparations.

   B. **Nonsteroidal antiinflammatory agents** should not be used in pregnancy.

   C. **Immunosuppressives** such as azathioprine (Imuran) should be reserved for extremely ill patients and should probably not be used in pregnancy otherwise. Azathioprine (initial dosage of 3 to 5 mg/kg with an oral maintenance dosage of 1 to 3 mg/kg/d) seems safer than cyclophosphamide (Cytoxan), which should not be used in pregnancy.

   D. **Corticosteroids** are reserved for patients who do not respond to conventional therapy. Prednisone ($\leq$ 10 mg/d orally) is most commonly used and is considered safe, although it is rarely used since patients improve during pregnancy.

   E. **Intraarticular steroids** are effective in controlling local joint inflammation. Beneficial effects last for days to months and may forestall the use of systemic steroids. Doses vary from 2 to 5 mg in a finger to 37.5 mg in a knee.

   F. **Gold compounds.** The action of gold compounds is unknown, but they are valuable therapeutically, although bone marrow suppression can occur (rarely). There is little information on usage in pregnancy, and gold treatment should probably be delayed until after pregnancy.

   G. **Antimalarials** are not used during pregnancy since they cause chromosome changes and fetal retinopathy.

   H. **Penicillamine** is a chelating agent used in pregnant patients with Wilson's disease. There is no information on fetal effects, although the drug does cross the placenta.

   I. **Orthopedic surgery** may be useful in some cases but is best done after pregnancy.

   J. **Plasmapheresis** yields results that last for weeks, but it is not used in pregnancy since it reduces antibody levels.

   K. **Radiation therapy** therapy is sometimes effective but is not used in pregnancy.

VIII. Prognosis. Rheumatoid factors do not cross the placenta, so there is no direct effect of rheumatoid arthritis on the fetus. The long-term outcome of rheumatoid arthritis is unaffected by pregnancy.

SCLERODERMA (SYSTEMIC SCLEROSIS)

I. Incidence. Scleroderma is rare, with only five new cases per million population each year. The diagnosis is usually made between 35 and 55 years of age. The disease is three times more common in females than in males.

II. Morbidity and mortality. Pregnancy occurring in a patient with rapidly progressive scleroderma with renal or cardiac involvement can be life-threatening, although the disease occurs infrequently in pregnancy and more often after the childbearing years. Abortion, prematurity, and perinatal mortality are increased, but infants do not have the stigmata of maternal disease. Blacks and males may have a worse prognosis than whites and females.

III. Cause. The cause of scleroderma is unknown.

IV. Pathogenesis and pathophysiology. Scleroderma results in fibrosis of collagen, which affects the microvascular system, leading to vascular insufficiency. The skin and various internal organs, including the muscles, gastrointestinal (GI) tract, heart, lungs, kidneys, and, rarely, the nervous system, are affected.

V. Differential diagnosis. Scleroderma begins insidiously and often may be diagnosed as undifferentiated connective tissue disease. Progression is usually slow, and severe cutaneous and visceral involvement rarely occurs before 6 months.

VI. Diagnosis
   A. Signs and symptoms. Scleroderma often presents as polyarthritis with edematous hands. Raynaud's phenomenon, followed by thickened, taut skin, may precede or follow visceral involvement. Other diagnostic clues are:
   1. Tortuosity, dilatation, and diminished nail bed capillaries.
   2. Pitting scars below the nails.
   3. Pulmonary fibrosis or change in GI motility. Weakness, weight loss, stiffness and aching, arthritis, and diffuse edema of the hands occur.
   B. Physical exam. The disease progresses to produce taut, thickened, edematous skin in the hands, with joint immobilization and contractures. The hair is thin, and the face is smooth and waxy. Joint deformity and shrinkage of the mouth occur. Dry crackles at the lung bases are found with pulmonary involvement, and myocardial ischemia with replacement of cardiac muscle by fibrous tissue occurs. Microangiopathic hemolysis may give a warning of progressive renal disease. Trigeminal neuropathy is occasionally seen.
   C. Laboratory examination and diagnostic procedures. An elevated erythrocyte sedimentation rate and mild anemia are seen. From

30 to 50 percent of patients have hypergammaglobulinemia, up to 35 percent have rheumatoid factor, and 40 to 80 percent have ANA. X-rays may reveal loss of soft tissue of the terminal phalanges. Upper GI examination reveals a dilated esophagus in over one-half of patients, and small bowel films demonstrate segmental atony. Pulmonary studies show a dense reticular honeycomb pattern in the lower lungs.

VII. Management. The most important goal is to preserve function of the hands. Therapy includes exercise and treatment of infection. Erythromycin (E-mycin, Erythrocin), 0.5 g/d orally in two or three divided doses, is used to treat malabsorption in the upper intestine, and antacids are given to prevent esophagitis. Thiazide diuretics, beta blockers, and peripheral vasodilators such as phenoxybenzamine, reserpine, prazosin, calcium channel blockers, and ganglionic blockers have been used, as well as Captopril for severe hypertension. Captopril and other angiotensin converting enzyme (ACE) inhibitors are actually contraindicated in pregnancy. Most of these agents have not been tried in pregnancy and should be avoided. Steroids are used when pulmonary fibrosis occurs, but they are not effective in softening the hands. Systemic sclerosis with major organ involvement is detrimental to pregnancy, and toxemia is common. Progressive cardiac or renal decompensation is an indication for immediate pregnancy termination.

VIII. Prognosis. The course of the disease is variable. Patients with pulmonary, cardiac, or renal involvement may progress rapidly to death, while those with skin and esophageal involvement have nearly normal life expectancies.

POLYMYOSITIS AND DERMATOMYOSITIS

I. Incidence. The incidence is 7/1 million population. Bimodal peak ages of onset are 10 to 14 and 50 years. There is a 2 : 1 female : male ratio.

II. Morbidity and mortality. There is probably increased perinatal wastage and low birth weight, although pregnancy itself has little effect on the disease.

III. Cause. Polymyositis and dermatomyositis are inflammatory disorders that affect primarily striated muscles of the limb girdle, neck, and pharynx. The cause is unknown, although cell-mediated immunity may be important.

IV. Pathogenesis and pathophysiology. Degeneration of muscle fibers with necrosis, atrophy, and fibrosis are seen. Dermal edema occurs, but the basement membrane does not stain for immunoglobulin.

V. Differential diagnosis. Polymyositis is an inflammatory skeletal muscle disease that may overlap with other connective tissue diseases. However, 70 percent of patients will have proximal muscle weakness. Polymyositis can be mimicked by a number of diseases including thyroid disease. McArdle's syndrome, renal tubular acidosis, trichinosis, toxoplasmosis, hypereosinophilia, diabetes, and polymyalgia rheumatica.

VI. Diagnosis
   A. Signs and symptoms
   1. Weakness of proximal muscles is the complaint in 70 percent of patients. It begins in the hip girdle and proximal leg and extends to the shoulder, proximal arm, and neck muscles. Arthralgias occur in 25 percent of patients. Dysphagia occurs secondary to weak striated muscle. Congestive heart failure and pneumonia are rare.
   2. Five criteria have been proposed. With four present, there is definite disease.
      a. Symmetric proximal muscle weakness, with or without dysphagia or respiratory muscle weakness
      b. Elevated serum muscle enzymes
      c. Electromyographic (EMG) anomalies
      d. Muscle biopsy showing degeneration, regeneration, necrosis, phagocytosis, and interstitial mononuclear infiltrates
      e. Rash of dermatomyositis
   B. Physical examination. In addition to variable muscle weakness and wasting, a rash is present on the forehead, neck, shoulders, arms, and trunk in one-third of patients. A heliotrope rash of the upper eyelids and face is occasionally seen.
   C. Laboratory examination and diagnostic procedures. Muscle enzymes (creatinine phosphokinase), transaminases (serum glutamic-oxaloacetic transaminase, serum glutamic-pyruvic transaminase), and lactic dehydrogenase are elevated intermittently. There is a mild anemia. EMGs are abnormal. Muscle biopsy shows degeneration, necrosis, phagocytosis, and mononuclear infiltrate.

VII. Management. Prednisone, 50 to 100 mg/d, is the drug of choice. Enzyme levels should return to normal in 2 months. Exacerbations occur with premature tapering, and maintenance therapy may be necessary for years. Methotrexate or azathiopine may be useful in treatment failures. Drugs are given in the same manner as described in the section on SLE.

VIII. Prognosis. Pregnancy has little effect on the disease. Five-year survival with steroid therapy is 80 percent, but is lower when an underlying malignancy is present (usually breast, ovary or stomach).

BIBLIOGRAPHY

Ballou SP, Morby JJ, Koshner I. Pregnancy and systemic sclerosis. Arthritis Rheum 1984; 27:295.

Dixit R, Krieg AM, Atkinson JP. Thrombotic thrombocytopenic purpura developing during pregnancy in a C2 deficient patient with a history of systemic lupus erythematosus. Arthritis Rheum 1985; 28:341.

Grimes DA, LeBott SA, Grimes KR, et al. Systemis lupus erythematosus and reproductive function: A case control study. Am J Obstet Gynecol 1985; 153:179.

Haystett JP, Lynn RI. Effect of pregnancy in patients with lupus nephropathy. Kidney Int 1980; 18:207.

Infante-Rivard C, David M, Gauthier R, et al. Lupus anticoagulants, anticardiolipin antibodies, and fetal loss. N Engl J Med 1991; 325:1063.

Lockshin MD. Pregnancy associated with systemic lupus erythematosus. Semin Perinatol 1990; 14:130.

Lockshin MD, Harpel PCM, Druzin ML, et al. Lupus pregnancy. Arthritis Rheum 1985; 28:58.

Lockshin MD, Remitz E, Druzin ML, et al. Lupus pregnancy. Case-control prospective study demonstrating absence of lupus exacerbation during or after pregnancy. Am J Med 1984; 77:893.

Lockwood CDJ, Romero R, Feinberg RF, et al. The prevalence and biologic significance of lupus anticoagulant and anticardiolipin antibodies in a general obstetric population. Am J Obstet Gynecol 1989; 161:369.

Loizous M, Byron MA, Englert HJ, et al. Association of quantitative anticardiolipin antibody levels with fetal loss and time of loss in systemic lupus erythematosus. WJ Med 68:525, 1988.

Lubbe WT, Palmer SJ, Butler WS, et al. Fetal survival after prednisone suppression of maternal lupus anticoagulant. Lancet 1983; 1:1361.

McCarty DJ. Arthritis and Allied Conditions. 10th ed. Philadelphia: Lea and Febiger; 1985:551.

Mor-Yusef S, Navott D, Bobriowitz R, et al. Collagen disease in pregnancy. Obstet Gynecol Surv 1984; 39:67.

Pattison NS, McKay EJ, Liggins GC, et al. Antecardiolipin antibodies: Their presence as a marker for lupus anticoagulant in pregnancy NZ Med J 1987; 100:61.

Pitkin RM. Polyarteritis nodosa. Clin Obstet Gynecol 1983; 26:579.

Schwartz RS. Immunologic and genetic aspects of systemic lupus erythematosus. Kidney Int 1981; 19:471.

Scott J, Maddison PS, Taylor PU, et al. Connective-tissue disease, antibodies to ribonucleoprotein and congenital heart block. N Engl J Med 1984; 309:209.

Syrop CW, Vanner MW. Systemic lupus erythematosus. Clin Obstet Gynecol 1983; 267:547.

Thurrman GB. Rheumatoid arthritis. Clin Obstet Gynecol 1983; 26:558.

Urowitz MB, Gladman DD. Rheumatic disease in pregnancy. In: Burrow GN, Ferris TF, eds. Medical Complications During Pregnancy. 3rd ed. Philadelphia: WB Saunders; 1988:499.

Walsh SW. Low-dose aspirin: Treatment for the imbalance of increased thromboxane and decreased prostacyclin in preeclampsia. Am J Perinatol 1989; 6:124.

Wyngaarden JB, Smith LA. Part XVII. Connective Tissue Diseases. Cecil's Textbook of Medicine. 16th ed. Philadelphia: WB Saunders; 1982:1823.

CHAPTER 38

Neurologic Diseases

Aldo D. Khoury
Baha M. Sibai

Neurologic disorders are relatively rare during pregnancy. The overall incidence is less than 1 percent, with seizure disorders being the most common. The majority of pregnant patients with neurologic diseases are usually diagnosed prior to pregnancy. Certain neurologic diseases, however, may have their onset for the first time during pregnancy or are more likely to be encountered in the pregnant patient. These may include certain seizure disorders, cerebrovascular accidents, Guillain-Barré syndrome, Bell's palsy, and herniation of an intervertebral disk.

A third group of neurologic disorders are related to pregnancy. They include eclampsia, peripheral nerve compression syndrome, and chorea gravidarum.

I. **General consideration.** Regardless of the relationship between a neurologic disorder and pregnancy, certain basic points must be kept in mind in the evaluation and management of neurologic diseases during pregnancy.

   A. **Physiologic changes related to pregnancy.** Certain physiologic changes during pregnancy will influence the course of some diseases, as well as the dose of medication being used to treat them. The rise in plasma volume coupled with the decrease in gastrointestinal motility and absorption, decreased protein binding, enhanced hepatic metabolism, and increased glomerular filtration rate leads to more rapid substance clearance. All of the above factors may lead to subtherapeutic plasma concentrations of drugs used in pregnancy. This situation is reversed in the postpartum period over 4 to 6 weeks, leading to overdosage of medications and their toxic effects.

   B. **Diagnosis of neurologic diseases in pregnancy.** Pregnancy imposes few restrictions on diagnostic procedures to be used in the evaluation of neurologic disorders. Radiation exposure to the fetus should be minimized. An abdominal shield should be used when possible; hence myelography, fluroscopy, and x-rays of the thoracolumbar spine should be restricted as much as possible. Newer techniques such as magnetic resonance imaging (MRI) appear to be safe during pregnancy.

II. Seizure disorders. These are among the more common complications of pregnancy. They include eclampsia and epilepsy. Since eclampsia is discussed in Chapter 29, this discussion will be restricted to epilepsy.
  A. **Cause**
    1. Epileptic seizures are disorders caused by abnormal electrical activities of the brain, the characteristics of which are recurrent, chronic, paroxysmal changes in neurologic function. They may be manifested by sensory, cognitive, and emotional episodes or may be convulsive when accompanied by motor manifestations.
    2. Epilepsy may result from a neurologic injury or a structural brain lesion, or it can occur as part of a systemic illnesses. When neither a neurologic nor a structural dysfunction is elicited, the seizures are considered idiopathic. The incidence of epilepsy is 0.3 to 0.5 percent. Classification of seizures is based on physical manifestation and frequency and is outlined in Table 38.1.
  B. **Incidence.** The incidence of epilepsy in pregnancy is 0.3 to 0.5 percent.
  C. **Pathophysiology.** There is a direct relationship between the hormonal milieu and the seizure threshold. Estrogens activate seizure foci, while progesterones decrease the activity. This may explain the occurrence of convulsions, in some cases, only

Table 38.1. Classification of Epileptic Seizures

1 Partial or focal seizures
   a. Simple partial seizures (with motor, sensory, autonomic, or psychic signs)
   b. Complex partial seizures (psychomotor or temporal lobe)
   c. Secondary generalized partial seizures

2 Primary generalized seizures
   a. Tonic-clonic (grand mal)
   b. Tonic
   c. Absence (petit mal)
   d. Atypical absence
   e. Myoclonic
   f. Atonic

3 Status epilepticus
   a. Tonic-clonic status
   b. Absence status

4 Recurrence patterns
   a. Sporadic
   b. Cyclic
   c. Reflex (photomyoclonic, somatosensory, musicogenic, reading epilepsy)

during pregnancy (i.e., gestational epilepsy), or the increase in their frequency during menstruation (i.e., menstrual epilepsy). However, in the majority of women, oral contraceptive use does not seem to worsen epilepsy. Progesterone-mediated hyperventilation that leads to respiratory alkalosis may also increase susceptibility to seizures.

1. **The effect of pregnancy on epilepsy** is variable; 50 percent of the patients show no change, 40 to 45 percent have increased frequency of seizures, and 5 to 10 percent show decreased frequency.

   It is noted that prepregnancy seizure frequencies are the best predictor of future courses of attacks. Epileptic women who prior to pregnancy had more than one seizure per month, especially if they were on optimal anticonvulsant therapy, can almost always expect an increase in the frequency of the attacks. The longer the interval between seizures, the better the prognosis.

   Only 25 percent of patients who have been seizure-free for more than 9 months prior to their pregnancy can expect worsening of the disease. Fluid and electrolyte imbalances, excessive weight gain, and water retention may lead to poor seizure control. Insomnia, especially late in pregnancy, can provoke seizures in spite of therapeutic levels of anticonvulsants.

2. **Effect of epilepsy on pregnancy:** Several maternal-fetal and neonatal adverse effects have been reported to increase in epileptics.

   a. **Maternal effects** include increased antepartum bleeding (which may be related to the use of anticonvulsant drugs and not to maternal epilepsy per se), increased premature labor, increased incidence of preeclampsia, and increased rate of cesarean section.

   b. **Fetal effects.** Fetal asphyxia, along with perinatal mortality, is increased. The incidence of stillbirth is higher (often at term). The cause does not seem to be related to either maternal seizures or high level of anticonvulsant drugs. However, a recent report from Finland comparing the outcome of pregnancy in 150 epileptic women to that in 150 matched control subjects revealed no differences regarding any of the above complications.

   c. **Neonatal effects** include decreased head circumference, an increased incidence of malformation, and an increased incidence of intrauterine growth retardation. Additionally, an increased incidence of seizure disorders is noted in the offspring of epileptic mothers (1/30).

D. **Diagnosis**

1. For new-onset seizure disorders occurring during pregnancy, a thorough and detailed history should be obtained, including the use of drugs or medication (consider with-

drawal of alcohol, barbiturates, and other sedatives), any history of psychological disorders, diabetes, use of insulin, and a history of head trauma.

2. Detailed neurologic and general examinations are essential in looking for cardiac lesions, neurologic disorders, and lateralizing deficits. An electroencephalogram (EEG) is utilized to determine the cause of seizures, their differential diagnosis, and their classification. Other adjunctive studies in seizure evaluation are lumbar puncture, which is still employed when infections or subarachnoid hemorrhages are suspected, skull x-rays, and arteriograms if needed.

3. Routine blood studies should be done to evaluate the metabolic status of various electrolytes (sodium, magnesium, calcium, glucose, creatinine, and blood urea nitrogen), as well as the levels of various drugs and medications to rule out toxicity or withdrawal. Arterial blood gases are also an integral part of the metabolic status evaluation. Biochemical abnormalities should be corrected and their cause determined.

E. **Management.** The goal is to keep the expectant mother seizure-free while trying to identify the cause if the seizure is being diagnosed for the first time.

1. For patients presenting with isolated seizures, management consists of the following:

   a. Supportive measures protect the patient from self-inflicted injuries by using a tongue pad to avoid tongue swallowing and biting. Aspiration is provided by turning the patient on her left side and suctioning the secretion. Oxygen should be administered and respiratory support provided if needed.

   b. Medical therapy consists of administration of anticonvulsant drugs to prevent further seizures. Treatment should involve the fewest drugs (mono-therapy is recommended if at all possible) in the smallest amounts needed to control the convulsions. In patients with pre-existing epilepsy on therapy, blood levels of anticonvulsant drugs should be measured.

   Epileptic patients receiving anticonvulsant drugs have an increased incidence of fetal congenital anomalies (6 to 10 percent, three to four times the general population rate). The teratogenicity of anticonvulsant medication is associated with an elevated level of the toxic intermediary oxidative metabolites (epoxides) that are normally eliminated by the enzyme epoxide hydrolase. Anticonvulsants associated with teratogenicity are listed in Table 38.2.

   Most anitconvulsant medications cause bone marrow suppression and depression of vitamin K–dependent clotting factors. Supplemental folate and neonatal administration of vitamin K are indicated.

Table 38.2. Effects of Commonly-Used Anticonvulsants in Pregnancy

DRUG	CATEGORY	ASSOCIATED ANOMALIES
Trimethadione	D	Trimethadione syndrome: pre- and postnatal growth failure, mental retardation, and craniofacial, limb, and cardiac malformations
Valproic acid	D	Face-heart-limb syndrome and lumbosacral spina bifida
Phenytoin	D	Fetal hydantoin syndrome: microcephaly, facial clefts and dysmorphism, limb malformations, distal phalangeal and nail hypoplasia, folic acid and vitamin K dependent, deficiency of clotting factors
Carbamazepine	C	Fetal hydantoin-like syndrome
Phenobarbital	D	Cleft lip and palate, cardiac malformation, and hemorrhagic disease of the newborn
Clonazepam	C	Neonatal depression and apnea

2. **Generalized status epilepticus** is defined as repeated or continuous seizures lasting for about 30 or more minutes. Fortunately, the incidence is very rare, occurring in about 1 percent of epileptics. The cause is usually noncompliance with the therapeutic regimen during pregnancy and an unrecognized increase in the apparent clearance of phenytoin. It may occur secondary to cerebral anoxia, head trauma, or metabolic or electrolyte disorders. Status epilepticus is a life-threatening emergency. If left untreated, it will result in permanent brain damage and a maternal mortality of 30 percent, while fetal mortality may reach 50 percent. Pregnancy has no bearing on the protocols of treating status epilepticus.
   a. Immediate **treatment** for status epilepticus consists of securing the airway, protecting the patient from self-inflicted harm, and establishing parenteral access. Therefore, an indwelling venous catheter should be inserted and blood obtained for metabolic evaluation, as suggested previously.
   b. An indwelling Foley catheter should be placed and respiration, blood pressure, and EKG are monitored.
   c. **Medical therapy** includes intravenous administration of a 50-mL 50% dextrose solution even when hypoglycemia is a remote possibility. Thiamine, 100 mg, is given intramuscularly while infusing diazepam intravenously at a rate of 2 mg/min until seizures stop or a total of 20 mg has been given. Phenytoin is infused at a rate of 50

mg/min for a total dose of 18 mg per kilogram of body weight.

d. If seizures persist, the patient is intubated to support respiration and a short-acting barbituate (amobarbital) is given at a rate of 50 mg/min for a total dose of 250 mg. If seizures continue despite the above medications, general anesthesia is induced with halothane and a neuromuscular blocker. It is important to keep in mind that supportive measures, as listed previously, should be instituted along with the above medications.

III. **Cerebrovascular accidents**

A. **Cerebrovascular accidents** may occur secondary to several abnormalities, including vasculopathy (such as aneurysms or vascular malformations), cerebral embolism, or cerebral venous thrombosis.

B. In general, the **incidence** is 4.1/100 000 under age 35 and 25.7/100 000 at ages 35 to 44. Overall, pregnancy increases the risk of ischemic infarction 13-fold over the expected rate for young women.

C. **Clinical presentation** and findings are varied. Cerebrovascular accidents are usually sudden in onset, and may present as headache and visual disturbance, convulsions, alterations of consciousness, or hemiplegia. They are often associated with fluctuations in blood pressure and neck rigidity.

D. **Diagnosis** is accomplished after a thorough evaluation of the patient utilizing skull x-rays and computed tomography (CT) scans of the head. Conventional arterial angiography can also be done. Recently, intraarterial digital subtraction angiography has emerged as the safest high-resolution technology for examining the cerebral vessels.

E. **Specific lesions**

1. **Vascular aneurysms ("berry" aneurysms)** are saccular aneurysms occurring in the circle of Willis. Their most common site is at the angle of bifurcation of the vessels or in the proximal course of their branches. The next most common location is the bifurcation of the internal carotid arteries. Less common locations include the anastomotic area of the vertebral arteries as they form the basilar artery, the intracranial portion of the vertebral arteries, and the internal carotid artery before its division.

a. These aneurysms are **caused** by congenital defects in the media elastica of the vessel walls and are usually seen at 30 to 35 years. They may be associated with polycystic kidney disease and coarctation of the aorta. Though the underlying defect is congenital, the mechanism by which they rupture is controversial.

b. **Diagnosis.** Congenital aneurysms are clinically silent, but they may cause focal neurologic deficits by virtue of size compression until rupture occurs, causing a variety of neurologic deficits. CT scans and angiography are of great diagnostic value; EEGs are less helpful.

c. During pregnancy they show an increased tendency to **rupture and bleed** in each trimester, especially the third. Though rare during labor, this tendency increases again postpartum. This seems to indicate that the hemodynamic changes of pregnancy are more important in promoting rupture than is the stress of labor.

d. **Treatment** consists of surgical clipping under critical conditions (hypothermia, hyperventilation, hypotension, and corticosteroid use). These patients can deliver vaginally if bearing down is avoided, using epidural anesthesia and forceps to shorten the second stage of labor. If an aneurysm bleeds in the third trimester or in patients with a recent bleed who go into labor, a cesarean section should be performed.

e. The fetal **prognosis** is very good, even under the critical conditions, mentioned above, needed for surgery.

2. **Vascular malformations (arteriovenous shunts)** result from developmental defects of vessel formation, leading to arteriovenous communication without intervening capillaries. They differ in size and shape. They may compress or distort the adjacent cerebral tissue, with resultant gliosis due to mechanical and ischemic factors.

a. Usually they are seen in the 20- to 25-year age group.

b. **Signs and symptoms** are similar to those of space-occupying lesions (headache, focal deficits, and subarachnoid hemorrhage) since most arteriovenous malformations are supratentorial (usually in the middle cerebral artery territory).

c. **Diagnosis** is made by CT scan and arteriography.

d. During pregnancy they tend to bleed early in gestation (16 to 24 weeks) and during labor.

e. **Treatment,** as in vascular aneurysms, is surgical. Other options, especially for inoperable cases, include embolization and proton beam therapy. Vaginal delivery is possible if lesions were surgically corrected, with the recommended use of epidural anesthesia and forceps. Cesarean section is indicated in untreated patients and in those who bleed after 36 weeks' gestation.

f. The fetal and maternal **prognosis** is good in surgically treated patients.

3. **Cerebral embolism** is the most common cause of stroke during pregnancy. There is an **increased incidence with age,** while pregnancy increases the incidence by three- to fourfold. The most common sites are the middle cerebral artery (involved in 35 percent of cases) and the internal carotid artery (involved in 20 percent of cases). About 25 percent will have no demonstrable lesion by arteriography.

a. **Predisposing factors** include cardiac disease (mitral stenosis with atrial fibrillation or cardiomyopathy with mural thrombi), cerebral vasculitis, thrombotic thrombocytopenic purpura, polycythemia, and sickle cell disease.

b. **Diagnosis** is made by searching for the source of the emboli and identifying the cause. Evaluation of the heart by echocardiography, evaluation of central peripheral blood vessels, and identification of underlying systemic diseases should be done thoroughly. Neurodiagnostic evaluation with EEG, a CT scan of the brain, and arteriography should be done as indicated.

c. No specific stage of pregnancy is associated with an increased risk.

d. **Treatment** is usually supportive, and rehabilitative care is provided if no underlying cause is identified. Anticoagulation is not needed in patients with a small, stable infarct as documented by CT scan. Dexamethasone may be used to treat cerebral edema if present; the usual dose is 10 mg intravenously followed by 4 mg every 6 h for 36 to 48 h.

e. The **prognosis** is usually good, and 80 percent of neurologic function will return to normal within 6 weeks after a stroke.

4. **Cerebral venous thrombosis** is very rare, with a frequency of 1/30 000 deliveries.

a. It usually occurs in the postpartum period (3 days to 3 weeks after delivery), with 80 percent of cases developing during the second or third week postpartum. The **cause** is still unknown; it has been associated with coexistent phlebitis in the legs and pelvis. The cortical veins and sagittal sinus are the most frequent sites.

b. The cardinal **diagnostic findings** are headache, convulsions, and focal neurologic deficits. The seizures are usually focal, and hemiparesis is the most common focal neurologic sign. The headache may be unilateral or bilateral. The **differential diagnosis** includes late-onset postpartum eclampsia, cerebral embolism, intracerebral hemorrhage, and hypertensive encephalopathy. Lumbar puncture reveals clear fluid with mild elevation of cerebrospinal fluid pressure and proteins. CT scan will show the presence of an infarct, and arteriography is definitive.

c. **Management** consists of controlling convulsions, general supportive measures, and treatment of cerebral edema with steroids. Anticoagulation is not indicated except in patients with progressive neurologic deficits in the absence of central nervous system bleeding.

d. The **prognosis** is usually good, with spontaneous resumption of neurologic function in the majority of cases within a few weeks. However, mortality is high in patients with massive infarction.

IV. Myasthenia gravis

A. The **cause** is autoimmune, due to circulating antibodies to acetylcholine receptors. About 60 percent of cases have associated enlargement of the thymus.

B. The **incidence** is about 1/20 000 patients, and the disease is more common in females than in males.

C. **Clinical findings** include weakness and easy fatigability of muscles with repeated use. Ocular, facial, and bulbar muscles are frequently involved, resulting in difficulties in swallowing and speaking. The course of the disease during pregnancy is variable, with a tendency toward exacerbation during the postpartum period.

D. **Treatment** consists of anticholineesterases with either neostigmine, 15 mg q.i.d, or pyridostigmine, 60 mg q.i.d. During labor the medication should be given parenterally. Epidural analgesia to be used during labor with vaginal delivery should be anticipated.

  1. It is important to avoid the use of neuromuscular blocking agents, which might produce a myasthenic crisis. Such drugs include magnesium sulfate, aminoglycosides, curare, ether, and chloroform. The disease may be differentiated from myasthenic crisis by evaluating the response to a 1-mg injection of edrophonium (Tensilon). If symptoms worsen, then the crisis is due to overdosage of medications; if symptoms improve, then it is a myasthenic crisis.

  2. Patients are usually at risk for myasthenic crisis during the first week postpartum. All medications should be resumed immediately after delivery, and patients should be observed closely during the first postpartum week.

E. **Neonatal effects.** About 10 percent of infants will develop transient myasthenic symptoms due to placental transfer of maternal antibodies. Symptoms will appear during the first 2 days in the form of hypotonia, impaired neural reflex, poor sucking, and crying. The symptoms resolve spontaneously within a week.

V. Multiple sclerosis

A. **Multiple sclerosis** is an autoimmune disease of myelin, involving central nervous system (CNS) white matter and resulting in patchy demyelination characterized by relapses and spontaneous remissions. The **cause** is unknown (slow-acting viruses and immunology have been implicated).

B. The **incidence** is 1–7/10 000, and the disease is more common in whites than in blacks and American Indians.

C. The age of **onset** is 20 to 40 years, with a male : female ratio of 1 : 2. The older the individual is at the age of onset, the more likely the course is to be progressive.

  1. Precipitating factors include infections, injury, trauma, and emotional upset, but the evidence remains anecdotal.

  2. Clinical symptoms include diverse findings, such as weakness in the lower extremities, difficulties with coordination, paresthesias, visual symptoms, and loss of urinary and bowel control. Rarely, gray matter symptoms such as convulsions occur.

    3. The course during pregnancy is variable. There appears to be no effect on the pregnancy. The relapse rate in the first 3 months postpartum is nearly three times that of age-matched, nonpregnant patients.

D. **Diagnosis** is mainly clinical, based on the neurologic history (at least two episodes of neurologic deficit).

    1. Lumbar puncture may reveal increased IgG in cerebrospinal fluid (CSF) (>15 percent of total protein). Mainly oligoclonal bands of IgG are present.

    2. An MRI scan shows multiple white matter lesions.

    3. Auditory and visual evoked responses are usually abnormal, and in the absence of visual and auditory complaints, the diagnosis of multiple sclerosis is more favorable.

E. **Treatment** is mainly supportive.

    1. Acute excerbations of optic neuritis may be treated with a short course of either ACTH or prednisone (60 mg/d for 10 days). Immunosuppressive therapy (azathioprine or cyclophosphamide) is used as a last resort. Plasmapheresis and interferon have equivocal results.

    2. In cases of uninhibited hyperreflexive bladder, Pro-Banthine (propantheline bromide), 15 to 30 mg/d, or Ditropan (oxybutynin chloride), 5 mg/d, should be given.

    3. Spinal anesthesia should be avoided since it is associated with cases of exacerbation. Experience with epidural anesthesia is limited, but the results are favorable. Regional and general anesthesia can be administered. Forceps are used to shorten the second stage of labor and the period of exhaustion. Cesarean section is done for obstetric indications only.

F. The **prognosis** is variable. Average life expectancy is 15 to 25 years after the onset of symptoms. The child of a mother with multiple sclerosis has a 3 percent lifetime risk of developing the disease compared to a 0.1 to 0.5 percent lifetime risk for the general population.

VI. Pseudotumor cerebri (PC). PC, usually known as *benign intracranial hypertension,* is defined as increased intracranial pressure **not** caused by an intracranial space-occupying lesion, hydrocephalus, or infection.

A. The disease is extremely rare, with a female : male ratio of 3 : 1. The highest **incidence** is at ages 20 to 30. Ninety percent of patients are obese (greater than 20 percent of ideal body weight), and are usually alert and healthy.

B. Although the **cause** is unknown, PC is associated with thrombosis of the transverse venous sinus and of the sagittal sinus, chronic pulmonary diseases (e.g., emphysema), endocrinopathies, hypo- and hypervitaminosis A, vitamin D deficiency, certain medications (indomethacin, oral contraceptives, sulfa, tetracyclines, nitrofurantoin, and nalidixic acid), and anemia, particularly iron deficiency anemia (especially common in overweight young women).

C. **Pathophysiology.** Several mechanisms have been employed to explain PC, including:
   1. Increased intracranial blood volume.
   2. Hyperstimulation of CSF by the choroid plexus (estrogen/prolactin imbalance theory).
   3. Cerebral edema (primary or vasogenic).
   4. Reduced CSF absorption, which is usually self-limiting. Clinical findings include headache (95 percent), papilledema (100 percent), blurred vision (73 percent), diplopia (14.6 percent), and nausea and vomiting.
D. **Diagnosis** is made mainly by exclusion. Ophthalmolgic examination reveals papilledema, and CT scan shows no evidence of a space-occupying lesion. Lumbar puncture reveals elevated CSF pressure and normal CSF composition.
E. **Management** includes pain relief (analgesics), bed rest, weight reduction (limit weight gain to 9 kg), diuretics (acetazolamide, furosemide) and corticosteroids. Occasionally, lumbar punctures to reduce intracranial pressure may be needed. Surgical treatment (lumbar peritoneal shunt, ventricular shunt, and suboccipital decompression) is reserved for severe refractory disease. During labor, use low forceps or vacuum extraction to shorten the second stage (maternal pushing efforts may lead to increased intracranial pressure). Cesarean section should be reserved for obstetric indication. PC shows no effect on pregnancy. Patients should have a normal labor and delivery course. PC commonly begins in the first half of pregnancy (mean onset at 14 weeks) and may be self-limited, with headache and papilledema disappearing in 1 to 3 months. The majority of patients recover completely after delivery. If the disease is not controlled even with treatment, it may lead to optic atrophy and blindness; therefore therapeutic abortion is indicated.

VII. **Spinal cord injuries.** Spinal cord injuries (paraplegia) are usually due to trauma prior to or during pregnancy. Fertility is usually preserved.
   A. Complications include urinary tract infections, bed sores, anemia, rapid or precipitous labor, and the syndrome of autonomic hyperreflexia.
      1. Autonomic hyperreflexia is a syndrome common in patients with lesions above T_6, manifested by sudden severe paroxysmal systolic and diastolic hypertension, anxiety, perspiration, facial flushing, nasal congestion, intense throbbing headache, and tachycardia. Reflex bradycardia may occur if baroreceptor and vagus nerves are intact. Cardiac arrhythmias, dilated pupils, flushing, and diaphoresis above the lesion may occur.

2. Autonomic hyperreflexia is caused by spinal reflex of splanchnic sympathetic and parasympathetic outflow without CNS inhibition. Precipitating factors include painful stimuli; bladder, rectal, or cervical distention; and uterine contractions and manipulations. The syndrome is most common during labor.

B. **Management** consists of preventive and supportive measures in the form of physiotherapy, suppressive therapy with antibiotics to prevent urinary tract infections, treatment of anemia with iron supplements, and avoidance of factors that precipitate autonomic hyperreflexia. Epidural analgesia is very helpful due to its interruption of the reflex arc. Antihypertensive therapy, if necessary, consists of 5 to 10 mg of intravenous hydralazine. Repeated intravenous bolus doses or continuous infusions to control severe hypertension, ganglionic blocking agents, nitroglycerin, and nitroprusside may be used in refractory hypertension.

VIII. Tumors

A. **Pituitary tumors.** Pit“tary tumors are most frequent, and are more prone to be symptomatic during pregnancy. Bromocriptine may be used to treat prolactinomas prior to and during pregnancy to avoid rapid growth.

B. **Cerebral tumors.** Clinical symptoms are diverse, depending on the type and location of the tumor. Manifestations are usually multiple, with insidious onset and slow progression. The usual findings are headache, personality changes, focal neurologic deficits, nausea, vomiting, focal convulsions, and abnormal speech. Meningiomas, angiomas, and neurofibromas tend to grow rapidly during pregnancy.

Treatment depends the type, size, and location of the tumor. Astrocytomas are associated with high maternal and fetal mortality. Surgical intervention is indicated for rapidly expanding tumors and posterior fossa tumors. Cerebral edema should be treated with dexamethasone. Termination of pregnancy is indicated if rapid expansion of the tumor is threatening the life of the mother.

C. **Spinal cord tumors** are very rare during pregnancy. They may be extramedullary or intramedullary. Extramedullary tumors result in compression symptoms with various sensory and motor defects, depending on the nerve roots involved. Anigomas and hemangiomas tend to increase during pregnancy and are more likely to bleed or thrombose. Treatment is surgical if the tumor is diagnosed early in pregnancy. If the patient is at term, allow delivery and consider surgery afterward. Radiotherapy should be postponed until after delivery.

IX. Guillain-Barré syndrome. This is an idiopathic, inflammatory, demyelinating polyneuropathy. It is extremely rare during pregnancy.

A. The **cause** is unknown, but the syndrome is preceded by infect-

ion in 50 percent of cases (usually respiratory or gastrointestinal) 1 to 3 weeks before the onset of symptoms.
B. **Findings** include acute onset of motor deficits in the form of weakness in extremities and bilateral facial weakness. Proximal muscles usually lose power before distal onset. The disease may involve respiratory muscles, leading to paralysis. Sensory symptoms of pain, numbness, paresthesia, and "glove and stocking" hypaesthesia are often found.
C. **Diagnosis** is clinical, along with evaluation of proteins in CSF (usually elevated) and a leukocyte count <10 cells per cubic millimeter.
D. **Differential diagnosis** includes diphtheria, botulism, porphyria, and poisoning with lead, arsenic, or triethyl cresyl phosphate.
E. **Treatment** is supportive, along with prevention of complications, as with multiple sclerosis. Steroids may be used, but their benefit is not well established. Plasmapheresis is effective for some patients if started within 7 days of onset.
F. **Prognosis.** Recovery may be spontaneous, and vaginal delivery should be anticipated. The fetus is not affected.

X. **Bell's palsy** is a neuropathy affecting the facial nerve (cranial nerve VII).
A. The **cause** is unknown, but it has been associated with a viral agent (herpes simplex virus), diabetic mononeuropathies, and interstitial edema.
B. The **incidence** is 2–5/10 000, with an apparently increased median during pregnancy. It is usually seen during last trimester and the first 2 weeks postpartum.
C. **Symptoms** include paralysis of facial muscles and loss of taste in the anterior two-thirds of the tongue. Pain is not prominent. Its presence in severe forms should raise the possibility of otitis media, skull fractures, or herpes zoster infection of the geniculate ganglion (the Ramsay Hunt syndrome). The course during pregnancy is unchanged.
D. **Treatment** is with prednisone, 40 mg/d × 10 days.
E. **Prognosis** is good, with spontaneous recovery anticipated.

XI. **Herniation of intervertebral discs** occurs rarely during pregnancy, with an incidence of 1/10 000.
A. **Predisposing** factors include relaxation of spinal joints, accentuation of lumbar lordosis, and wearing high-heeled shoes.
B. The most common **site** of involvement is the fifth lumbar and first sacral roots.
C. **Clinical findings** consist of low back pain that radiates down to the leg with hypesthesia along the anterior or lateral aspect of the leg, depending on the nerve root involved. The ankle jerk may be decreased or absent.
D. **Diagnosis** is based on the history, clinical findings, and electromyography.
E. **Treatment** is usually conservative, with bed rest, physical ther-

apy, application of local heat, and analgesics. If these fail, surgery with laminectomy may be performed after the first trimester. Injection of chymopapain into a disc is not recommended during pregnancy.

XII. Conditions related to pregnancy
A. Compression neuropathies
1. Carpal tunnel syndrome
   a. Caused by compression of the median nerve at the wrist
   b. Clinical findings: pain and tingling in the thumb, index, middle fingers, and radial aspect of the ring finger
   c. Symptoms get worse at night, especially the tingling sensation
   d. Transient form seen mainly during pregnancy secondary to fluid retention
   e. Treatment: dorsal split with wrist in flexion and diuretics
   f. Local injection of steroids may be useful
   g. Prognosis: symptoms usually resolve after delivery. Surgery is rarely indicated unless there is marked neurologic impairment.

2. **Femoral nerve neuropathy**
   a. Caused by injury to the femoral nerve at the time of pelvic surgery or cesarean section
   b. Clinical findings: weakness of the quadriceps and sartorius muscles and sensory loss along the anteromedial aspect of the thigh. The knee jerk may be decreased or absent.
   c. Treatment: physical therapy
   d. Prognosis: usually good, with spontaneous recovery within 1 to 3 months

3. **Lumbosacral cord neuropathy**
   a. Caused by injury secondary to prolonged labor or midforceps rotations
   b. Clinical findings: foot drop, with weakness of dorsiflexion and aversion of the foot
   c. Management: supportive, with a good prognosis

4. **Obturator neuropathy**
   a. Caused by injury from the fetal head or high forceps application
   b. Clinical findings: pain in the groin and upper thigh, with weakness or abduction of the thigh
   c. Management: physical therapy, with spontaneous recovery

5. **Peroneal neuropathy**
   a. Caused by poorly positioned leg holders
   b. Clinical findings: foot drop and numbness along the lateral aspect of the leg and dorsum of the foot
   c. Management: conservative, with spontaneous recovery within 3 months

B. Chorea gravidarum is an increasingly rare disease.
1. The cause is associated with rheumatic fever, resulting in subclinical damage to the basal ganglia.
2. Clinical findings: purposeless, nonrepetitive movements of extremities and facial muscles. It is seen most commonly during the first pregnancy, with 20 percent of patients having recurrent chorea in subsequent pregnancies. About 50 percent of attacks occur in the first trimester and 30 percent in second trimester.
3. Treatment consists of bed rest with careful feeding. Chlorpromazine or haloperidol may be needed to treat the movement. Give 2 to 6 mg/d for mild cases; more severe cases may require 20 mg/d.
4. Prognosis: usually self-limiting, with resolution of symptoms late in pregnancy or postpartum.

BIBLIOGRAPHY

Barno A, Freeman DWL. Maternal deaths due to spontaneous subarachnoid hemorrhage. Am J Obstet Gynecol 1976; 125:384.

Bellur SN. Neurologic disorders in pregnancy. In: Gleicher N, ed. Principles of Medical Therapy in Pregnancy. New York: Plenum; 1985:916–932.

Dalessio DJ. Neurologic disease. In: Burrow GN, Ferris TF, eds. Medical Complications During Pregnancy. Philadelphia: WB Saunders; 1982:435–473.

Dalessio DJ. Seizure disorders and pregnancy. N Engl J Med 1985; 312:559.

Donaldson JO. Stroke. Clinic Obstet Gynecol 1981; 24:825.

Duttino L Jr, Freeman RK. Seizure disorders of pregnancy. Contemp Ob/Gyn 1985; 25:620.

Hilesmaa VK, Bardi A, Teramo K. Obstetric outcome in women with epilepsy. Am J Obstet Gynecol 1985; 152:499.

Hopkins A. Neurological disorders. Clin Obstet Gynecol 1977; 4:418.

McGregor JA, Meeuwsen J. Autonomic hyper-reflexia: A mortal danger for spinal cord damaged women in labor. Am J Obstet Gynecol 1985; 151:330.

Rubinson JL, Hall CS, Sedzimer CB. Arteriovenous malformations, aneurysms, and pregnancy. J Neurosurg 1974; 41:63.

Tuttleman RM, Gleicher N. Central nervous system hemorrhage complicating pregnancy. Obstet Gynecol 1981; 58:651.

CHAPTER 39

Dermatologic Disease

Iris K. Aronson
Barbara N. Halaska

During pregnancy, a variety of changes in the skin may occur. These skin changes are best understood by separating them into three categories: (1) common, nonspecific, endocrine-related skin changes that occur in pregnancy, (2) skin disease unique to pregnancy, and (3) preexisting skin disease affected by pregnancy.

COMMON SKIN CHANGES THAT OCCUR IN PREGNANCY

I. **Hyperpigmentation.** Beginning in the second trimester, some form of hyperpigmentation occurs in up to 90 percent of pregnant women and is more apparent in brunettes and darker-skinned individuals than in blondes. Facial hyperpigmentation, which is known as **melasma** or the **mask of pregnancy,** is a most noticeable and disturbing type of hyperpigmentation and may be a cosmetic problem for some women. Serum levels of estrogen, progesterone, and melanocyte-stimulating hormone (MSH) are increased in pregnancy. These increases are thought to be related to such hyperpigmentation. Exposure to the sun is a major causative factor in melasma. In addition to pregnancy, melasma may be induced by oral contraceptives and cosmetics, as well as by hepatic disease. In melasma there is an increase in the number and activity of melanocytes secondary to ultraviolet (UV) light activation. Hyperpigmentation of **light brown color** is due to increased melanin in the epidermis. An **ashen gray or blue color** is due to melanin contained within dermal macrophages. A **deep brown color** indicates melanin of mixed type (epidermal and dermal).

   A. **Clinical features.** Clinically, melasma consists of discrete, hyperpigmented macules on the face in a centrofacial pattern (most common), a malar pattern, or a mandibular pattern. Pigmentation can be light or dark brown, ashen gray or blue, depending on the amount and distribution of the melanin. Melasma may be confused with hyperpigmentation that may occur after inflammation of the skin — postinflammatory hyperpigmentation. Phototoxicity reactions to cosmetics must be considered in the differential diagnosis of melasma, as well as systemic treatment with certain medications that are known to cause hyperpigmentation — gold, silver, copper, bismuth, arsenic, iron, and quinacrine. In the pregnant woman, the increased melanogenesis also results in darkening of the areolae, linea alba, and genital skin.

B. Management

1. **Decreasing exposure to sunlight.** In summer, patients should use a broad-spectrum sunscreen, screening both UV-B and UV-A light. High sun protection factor (SPF) sunscreens (45 or higher) containing either para-aminobenzoic acid (PABA) esters or cinnamates **and** bensophenones are recommended. In addition, the use of makeup base with a high-SPF sunscreen is helpful. The alternative, of course, is to avoid any sun exposure. Postpartum continued use of broad-spectrum sunscreens is necessary to avoid recurrence. Melasma increases with sun exposure during pregnancy. Post partum, the melasma may completely disappear or regress significantly in the majority of individuals.

2. **Depigmenting agents.** For those individuals with residual melasma, depigmenting agents may be useful. The predominantly epidermal type (brown color) responds to depigmenting agents, but the dermal type (ashen gray or blue color) responds very little to treatment. Depigmenting formulations containing 2 to 4 percent hydroquinone, such as Eldopaque cream or Melanex solution, applied only to the affected area b.i.d., may be tried for 6 to 8 weeks. Fifteen percent azelaic acid in a cream base is another depigmenting agent that may be effective. Broad-spectrum sunscreens used during and after depigmenting agent therapy is necessary to avoid recurrence of melasma.

II. **Changes in hair distribution in pregnancy:** Hirsutism and postpartum telogen effluvium. During pregnancy, the normal hair cycle is altered; the proportion of anagen (growing) hair to telogen (resting) hair is increased, leading to the appearance of hirsutism. Postpartum return to the normal cycle may lead to temporary thinning of hair (telogen effluvium).

A. **Clinical features.** The diagnosis of mild or marked hirsutism or of telogen effluvium is made on inspection.

1. **Hirsutism.** Mild degrees of hirsutism are relatively common, whereas marked hirsutism is very uncommon (0.001 percent of pregnant women). **Mild hirsutism** is associated with endocrine changes in pregnancy, probably those resulting from placental endocrine activity. Mild hirsutism is found on the face and occasionally on the arms, legs, and back. **Marked hirsutism,** however (especially in the presence of acne and other signs of virilization), may be associated with virilizing tumors.

2. **Postpartum telogen effluvium.** Diffuse hair thinning is common in the postpartum period. **Telogen effluvium** (diffuse

thinning of hair) is a common but very disturbing event following delivery. On the scalp, the normal conversion of active growing hair (anagen) to resting hair (telogen) is slowed during pregnancy, leading to thicker hair growth. Postpartum, a higher percentage of hair changes from growing to resting hair. These resting hairs are then shed, leading to thinner hair in the postpartum period.

B. Management

1. **Hirsutism.** Mild hirsutism does not usually require treatment, since it disappears by 6 months postpartum. Patients with marked hirsutism should be evaluated for the presence of a virilizing tumor.

2. **Postpartum telogen effluvium.** There is no treatment for postpartum telogen effluvium other than reassurance. Scalp hair returns to its normal growth pattern within 6 months postpartum.

III. Striae. Striae occur in 90 percent of pregnant women. Two factors that are involved in the cause of striae are stretching or distention (which can also occur without inducing striae) and hormonal factors, including adrenocortical steroids and/or placental estrogen. Histologically, fresh striae display breakage, retraction and curling of elastic fibers, and dilation of blood vessels.

A. Diagnosis. Striae appear as atrophic linear bands on the skin that are pink to purple in color. They develop on the abdomen, breasts, thighs, or inguinal area.

B. Management. There is no therapy to prevent striae. Postpartum, the color of striae fades to a less apparent white color, but the striae persist permanently.

IV. Vascular changes. Some form of cutaneous vascular change occurs in 70 percent of pregnant women. These changes consist primarily of increased vascular permeability and proliferation and are thought to be related to high levels of circulating hormones.

A. Vascular spiders. Vascular spiders consist of a central red vessel with radiating, tortuous branches resembling a spider. They appear on the face, neck, chest, and upper extremities between the second and ninth months. The majority of spider angiomas disappear by 3 months postpartum. The remaining spiders may be lightly cauterized or treated with cryotherapy.

B. Palmar erythema. Palmar erythema may be seen early in pregnancy (the second month). The erythema may be localized to the midpalmar, hypothenar, and thenar areas or it may be diffuse, with a splotchy appearance. Palmar erythema fades postpartum. Systemic lupus erythematosus or other collagen vascular diseases and cirrhosis of the liver may also cause palmar erythema.

C. Vascular proliferation. Small capillary hemangiomas develop on the head and neck areas in an estimated 2 percent of pregnant women. The majority of these lesions will involute spontaneously after delivery.

D. **Edema.** Some evidence of increased vascular permeability occurs in 50 percent of pregnant women. Edema of the face, eyelids, and extremities, particularly the ankles and hands, is commonly seen in pregnancy and must be differentiated from the edema of cardiac, renal, or hepatic origin.

V. **Common cutaneous tumors during pregnancy.** Cutaneous tumors may first appear or increase in size during pregnancy. The most common tumors seen are pyogenic granulomas and skin tags.
A. **Pyogenic granuloma of pregnancy.** Pyogenic granuloma of pregnancy is an oral lesion with an alleged incidence of 1 to 2 percent. It usually appears between the second and fifth months. Pyogenic granuloma of pregnancy is associated with hormonal changes in pregnancy.
B. **Molluscum gravidarum (skin tags).** Molluscum gravidarum, or skin tags, are common in pregnancy.
1. **Diagnosis.** Skin tags consist of small, skin-colored or slightly hyperpigmented, soft, pedunculated lesions appearing on the sides of the neck, anterior chest, and axillary area, typically in the second half of pregnancy.
2. **Management.** The lesions may disappear spontaneously postpartum. If they are irritated or cosmetically unacceptable, they may be removed by cutting them level with the skin surface, by electrodesiccation, or by freezing.

DERMATOSES UNIQUE TO PREGNANCY

I. **Pruritus gravidarum**
A. **Incidence.** Pruritus gravidarum is a mild, anicteric form of recurrent cholestatis of pregnancy. Its reported incidence varies from 0.02 to 2.4 percent. A higher incidence is reported in some countries (e.g., Scandinavia, 3 percent and some groups (e.g., Chilean Indians, 14 percent).
B. **Maternal morbidity and complications.** Maternal morbidity involves severe, uncomfortable pruritus during gestation and an increased incidence of postpartum hemorrhage. The pruritus subsides after delivery. Postpartum hemorrhage is associated with this condition and is explained by inadequate absorption of vitamin K due to decreased levels of bile salts that promote absorption of the vitamin. The pruritus of pruritus gravidarum appears to be related to the dihydroxy bile acids or other components of bile in skin. Studies have shown that the application of dihydroxy acids to keratin-stripped human skin induces pruritus. These mediators stimulate nerve endings to induce the sensation of pruritus.
C. **Fetal complications.** Although the risk of complications for the individual fetus is not proportional to the severity of maternal cholestasis, there is a higher incidence of complications with higher bilirubin and serum cholic acid levels. There is an increased risk of intrauterine or neonatal death, intrauterine fetal

distress as determined by meconium-stained amniotic fluid, premature deliveries, and low-birth-weight babies.

D. **Differential diagnosis.** Itchiness in pregnancy is common (17 percent of pregnant women) and may also be due to atopic or contact dermatitis, drug-induced eruptions, urticaria, scabies, pediculosis, or candida infections.

E. **Diagnosis.** Pruritus gravidarum begins in the second half of pregnancy, most commonly in the last trimester. Itching may be localized to certain areas initially but later becomes generalized. There are no primary skin lesions, and excoriations produced by scratching are the only cutaneous manifestations. Pruritus of cholestasis disappears rapidly postpartum, but it may reappear in subsequent pregnancies.

F. **Management.** Relief from pruritus of hepatic cholestasis is a difficult goal. The main agent currently in use is **oral cholestyramine resin** (4 g orally, one to three times daily), which may induce side effects such as constipation, abdominal discomfort, nausea, vomiting, diarrhea, steatorrhea, and vitamin deficiency (especially of vitamin K). Phototherapy is a promising modality for pruritus of hepatic cholestasis that has not been fully studied in pregnancy.

II. **Papular eruptions during pregnancy.** The diagnosis of papular eruption during pregnancy is marked by controversy due to the suggestion that there are two types of papular eruption, one of them benign (**prurigo gestationis**), the other associated with high fetal mortality (**Spangler's papular dermatitis of pregnancy [PDP]**). The controversy stems from the fact that no series of patients subsequent to Spangler's have corroborated his findings of high fetal mortality (27 percent). In addition, the clinical evidence that differentiated the two disorders was that in PDP the papular lesions were not grouped and were distributed more widely than in prurigo gestationis. The separation of these disorders on this clinical basis has been questioned, and until further evidence is available, we believe that all pregnancies with papular eruptions should be carefully evaluated and the maternal and fetal status monitored.

A. **Incidence.** The incidence of prurigo gestationis is reported as 1/300 pregnancies, while that of PDP is reported as 1/2500 pregnancies. Both are described as occurring at any time during pregnancy.

B. **Morbidity and mortality**
1. **Maternal morbidity and mortality.** Maternal morbidity in both prurigo gestationis and PDP is limited to discomfort caused by the pruritus. There is no mortality.
2. **Fetal morbidity and mortality**
   a. **Prurigo gestationis.** None
   b. **PDP.** Based on calculations of fetal deaths in previous pregnancies, Spangler calculated a mortality rate of 27 percent. No data were given on which fetal deaths were stillbirths and which were spontaneous abortions. We

agree with Holmes and Black, who feel that it is unwise to draw any definite conclusions with regard to fetal prognosis from Spangler's cases.

C. **Cause and pathogenesis**
  1. **Prurigo gestationis.** Unknown.
  2. **PDP** Spangler attributed PDP to abnormal placental function or hypersensitivity to placental tissue. Evidence for this view included persistence of disease when placental fragments were retained postpartum, positive skin results to placental extracts, and elevated urinary chorionic gonadotropin levels.

D. **Differential diagnosis.** Scabies, cholestasis of pregnancy, dermatitis herpetiformis

E. **Diagnosis**
  1. **Signs and symptoms**
     a. **Prurigo gestationis.** Small (1 to 3 mm), itchy papules that are rapidly and severely excoriated are seen. The lesions are grouped on the extensor surfaces of limbs, with a distal or proximal distribution. The upper trunk may also be involved.
     b. **PDP.** Small (3 to 5 mm), almost urticarialike papules, often excoriated, are seen. However, unlike prurigo gestationis, the lesions are widely scattered, without grouping or a predilection for any area.
  2. **Laboratory examination**
     a. **Prurigo gestationis.** None have been described or conducted.
     b. **PDP.** The following laboratory findings were described by Spangler, although they have not been subsequently reported: (1) markedly elevated levels of urinary chorionic gonadotropin, ranging from 25 000 to 500 000 IU; (2) reduced plasma cortisol; (3) low urinary estriol levels. These biochemical investigations have not been described in prurigo gestationis, nor have they been repeated in other groups of patients with PDP.

F. **Management**
  1. **Topical corticosteroids.** Topical corticosteroids are used to reduce pruritus and inflammatin (e.g., 1% hydrocortisone creams and ointments b.i.d.). When necessary because of severe symptoms, short-term usage of triamcinolone 0.1% ointments is useful on a b.i.d. regimen.
  2. **Systemic antihistamines.** Systemic antihistamines (Chlor-Trimeton, q6 h or q.h.s., may be used to treat pruritus).
  3. Assessment of the intrauterine environment and fetal well-being is indicated (see Chapter 16).

III. **Herpes gestationis (HG)** is an autoimmune disease process that has **absolutely no relation** to herpes simplex virus.
  A. **Incidence.** Reports of the incidence of HG vary from 1/3000 to

1/60 000 deliveries. It has been reported in association with hydatiform mole and choriocarcinoma.

B. Morbidity and mortality

1. **Maternal morbidity.** Maternal morbidity involves pruritus, discomfort, and complications associated with blistering eruptions.

2. **Fetal morbidity and mortality.** One study showed an increased risk of stillbirth (7.7 percent compared with 1.3 percent in the general population) and prematurity (23 percent compared with 5 percent), while another recent study of 24 patients with HG showed no maternal mortality and no stillbirths or neonatal deaths but an increased incidence of small-for-dates babies. A few infants have been reported to be affected by blistering lesions at birth that resolved spontaneously within a few weeks.

C. Cause and pathogenesis. The specific cause is unknown, but HG is regarded as an autoimmune process. Patients with HG appear to have a high frequency of human leukocyte antigen (HLA) haplotypes A1/B8 and DR3/DR4, and these are markers of high immune responsiveness associated with a number of autoimmune diseases. HG may be triggered when women with a genetic predisposition to increased immune responsiveness are exposed to antigens derived from their sexual partners (via the fetus). Women with HG frequently have anti-HLA antibodies directed against the fathers' HLA antigens. Direct immunofluorescence of skin lesions demonstrate a bandlike deposit of the third component of complement (C_3), and in some IgG, at the basement membrane zone (BMZ). A circulating serum factor called *herpes gestationis factor* is present, which fixes C_3 at the BMZ of human skin in in vitro complement-binding studies. This factor has been shown to be an IgG molecule capable of crossing the placenta and activating both the classic and alternate complement pathways in the deposition of C_3 at the BMZ. Hormonal factors also play a role in HG, as evidenced by recurrence in subsequent pregnancies, premenstrual exacerbations when the disease has persisted postpartum, and reactivation of HG with oral contraceptive use (but **not** **without** prior pregnancy).

D. Diagnosis

1. **Differential diagnosis**

   a. **Herpes gestationis must be differentiated from pruritic urticarial papules and plaques of pregnancy (PUPPP.).** The distributions of PUPPP and HG are similar, with papules beginning on the abdomen and arms prior to becoming generalized. In many HG patients, the papular lesions precede the bullous component by over a month, and in the prebullous stage, differentiation of HG from PUPPP is very difficult. Some patients with HG may develop no bullae at all in their first pregnancy. Vesicles also occur in both HG and PUPPP, but those in

PUPPP are never larger than 1 or 2 mm, whereas they grow larger in HG.

b. **HG must also be differentiated from diseases that occur coincidentally during pregnancy,** including erythema multiforme, bullous pemphigoid, pemphigus, dermatitis herpetiformis, and bullous drug-induced eruptions.

2. **Signs and symptoms.** HG may begin any time between 2 weeks' gestation and 1 week postpartum. A prodrome, if present, may consist of fever, malaise, headache, and nausea. Pruritus and/or a burning sensation may precede the eruption by a few days. In almost 90 percent of cases, the eruption begins around the umbilicus and then spreads to the abdomen and thighs. The back, breasts, palms, and soles are frequently affected, and the face and scalp are occasionally involved. The morphology of the lesions includes urticarial erythematous papules, urticarial plaques, target lesions, polycyclic erythema, vesicles, and bullae. The course of the disorder involves exacerbations and remissions, with postpartum exacerbations (75 percent) being very common. The average postpartum duration is 60 weeks. Postpartum premenstrual flareups may occur for up to 18 months. Recurrence occurs with subsequent pregnancies and may also appear with the use of oral contraceptives.

3. **Laboratory examination and diagnostic procedures.** There may be leukocytosis with eosinophilia. Direct immunofluorescence examination of perilesional skin demonstrates C_3 deposition at the BMZ in all patients and IgG deposition in 25 percent of patients. Indirect immunofluorescence demonstrates a circulating "HG factor" that fixes complement at the BMZ.

E. **Management**

1. **Mild cases** may be treated with topical steroids and antihistamines (triamcinolone 0.1% cream or ointment, b.i.d. to q.i.d., and Chlor-Trimeton 4 mg q6 h p.r.n.).

2. Severely affected patients for whom topical steroids offer no relief may be treated with systemic steroids, such as 30 to 40 mg prednisone per day.

3. The pregnancy should be followed closely, as in any high-risk pregnancy, including weekly nonstress tests after 30 weeks.

IV. **Pruritic urticarial papules and plaques of pregnancy (PUPPP)** (other names: *toxic erythema of pregnancy* [*TEP*], *polymorphous eruption of pregnancy* [*PEP*]. The incidence described for PUPPP ranges from 1/120 to 1/240. PUPPP has not been associated with either increased maternal or fetal risks. Its cause is unknown. In particular, there is no evidence of an antibody-mediated immunologic basis, as in HG.

A. **Diagnosis**
 1. **Signs and symptoms**
    a. **PUPPP.** PUPPP is a clinical diagnosis when the skin lesions generally begin on the abdomen (often in the striae) and later spread to the thighs, buttocks, and arms. It is a disease seen most commonly but not exclusively in the third trimester, and the associated pruritus is often severe. Clinically, the skin lesions of PUPPP range from erythematous, urticarial papules and plaques to slightly raised, erythematous patches that may be discrete or confluent, surmounted by tiny papules or blisters of 1 mm that may be excoriated and crusted. In urticarial lesions, crusting is generally absent. Some patients have mainly the urticarial form of the dermatitis, others have mainly the erythematous patches with papules and tiny blisters, and still others have combinations of the two.
 2. **Laboratory evaluation of PUPPP.** There are no laboratory abnormalities in PUPPP. The histologic findings are nonspecific. Light microscopy usually reveals only a nonspecific, perivascular, lymphohistocytic infiltrate with some eosinophils and, in certain cases, epidermal edema. Immunofluorescence staining has been consistently negative for antibody directed at the BMZ. It is necessary to distinguish PUPPP from the early urticarial stage of HG. Direct immunofluorescence examination of a skin biopsy specimen will readily differentiate between the two: PUPPP lacks the C_3 deposition at the BMZ consistently seen in HG.
B. **Management.** The goal of therapy for PUPPP is to make the mother comfortable. The eruptions may resolve prepartum (in some), but the average duration is 1 to 2 weeks postpartum. Few cases persist for more than 3 weeks.
 1. Some patients may obtain adequate relief from pruritus with **emollients** alone.
 2. Most patients require topical applications of intermediate-potency **steroid creams and ointments** such as triamcinolone, 0.1% b.i.d., or lower-potency 1% hydrocortisone ointment t.i.d.
 3. In addition, many patients benefit from oral antihistamines such as Chlor-Trimeton, 4 mg q6 h p.r.n.
 4. Although there are no known fetal complications, we recommend monitoring of fetal well-being (see Chapter 16).

PREEXISTING SKIN LESIONS AFFECTED BY PREGNANCY

I. **Melanocytic nevi and malignant melanoma.** Melanocytic nevi are present in virtually all individuals. Malignant melanoma has an incidence of approximately 1.5 percent of all malignancies.
A. **Diagnosis**
 1. **Diagnostic problems.** Clinical problems arise because pig-

mented nevi may enlarge or become darker during pregnancy and previously unpigmented nevi may develop pigmentation. Diagnostic problems may arise since, during pregnancy, histologic examination of nevi may reveal larger melanocytes, an increase in pigment, and even occasional atypical cells in lesions that are not malignant. There are no data to indicate, however, that nevi undergo malignant transformation with greater frequency during pregnancy.

2. **Differentiation of benign nevi from malignant melanoma.** Benign nevi undergoing benign changes in pregnancy must be differentiated from early malignant melanoma arising de novo or in preexisting nevi. The clinical characteristics of early malignant melanoma include (a) asymmetry of the lesion, (b) irregular borders, (c) variegated color, ranging from tan and brown to blue and black, and sometimes intermingled with red and white (benign pigmented lesions are generally more uniform in color), (d) diameter generally greater than 6 mm; any sudden or continuing increase in size should be investigated, and (e) additional symptoms or signs associated with development of melanoma in a preexisting nevus, including erythema, pain, itching, bleeding, ulceration, diffusion of pigment into surrounding skin, changes in the consistency and surface characteristics such as scaliness or oozing, or the appearance of a bump or nodule.

B. **Management.** There no conclusive evidence to prove that transformation of a nevus to a melanoma is seen with greater frequency in pregnancy, but circumstantial evidence suggests that hormonal factors may influence the behavior of melanoma (i.e., stimulation of melanocytes, detection of estrogen receptors on benign nevi in patients with melanoma and in some melanomas).

1. **New lesions or changing lesions.** Lesions that develop any of the suspicious changes noted above should be referred to a dermatologist for evaluation and biopsy, and a complete excisional biopsy in indicated. If a diagnosis of malignant melanoma is made, treatment should be prompt and adequate, including resection of the primary lesion (complete excision of the lesion with adequate margins) along with the dissection of clinically involved regional lymph nodes.

2. **Melanoma.** The effect of pregnancy on the behavior of existing melanoma is in dispute, with some authors suggesting that there is and others claiming that there is no evidence that pregnancy adversely affects the prognosis of the melanoma. Endocrine manipulation by termination of pregnancy, oophorectomy, adrenalectomy, or hopophysectomy does not influence the course of disease and the 5-year survival rate.

BIBLIOGRAPHY

Elder DE, Gueryy D IV. On widths of margins in excisions of primary malignant melanoma. Am J Dermatopathol 1984; 6(suppl):131–133.

Garden JM, Ostrow D, Roenigk HH Jr. Pruritus in hepatic cholestasis: Pathogenesis and therapy. Arch Dermatol 1985; 121:1415–1419.

Holmes RC, Black MM. The specific dermatoses of pregnancy: A reappraisal with special emphasis on a proposed simplified clinical classification. Clin Exp Dermatol 1982; 7:65–73.

Holmes RC, Black MM. The specific dermatoses of pregnancy. J Am Acad Dermatol 1983; 8:405–412.

Holmes RC, Black MM, Dann J, et al. A comparative study of toxic erythema of pregnancy and herpes gestationis. Br J Dermatol 1982; 106:499–510.

Johnston WG, Baskett TF. Obstetric cholestasis: A 14 year review. Am J Obstet Gynecol 1979; 133:299–301.

Reid R, Ivey KJ, Rencoret RH, et al. Fetal complications of obstetric cholestasis. Br Med J 1976; 1:870–872.

Sanchez NP, Pathak MA, Sato S, et al. Melasma: A clinical, light microscopic, ultrastructural, and immunofluorescence study. J Am Acad Dermatol 1981; 4:698–710.

Shiu MH, Schottenfield D, MacLean B, et al. Adverse effects of pregnancy on melanoma. Cancer 1976; 37:181–187.

Spangler AS, Reddy W, Bardawil WA, et al. Papular dermatitis of pregnancy, a new clinical entity. JAMA 1962; 181:577–581.

Winton GB, Lewis CW. Dermatoses of pregnancy. J Am Acad Dermatol 1982; 6:977–998.

CHAPTER 40

Cancer

Gary H. Lipscomb

Cancer complicates approximately 1 out of every 1000 pregnancies. The most common malignancies seen in pregnancy, in order of frequency of occurrence, are cervical cancer, breast cancer, melanoma, ovarian cancer, leukemia/lymphoma, and colorectal cancer. As with any life-threatening illness occurring in pregnancy, fetal well-being often must be balanced against optimal maternal therapy. Other issues that must be addressed by both the clinician and the patient include the effect of pregnancy on the malignancy, the need for pregnancy termination, the timing of therapy, and the possibility of fetal metastasis.

I. **Cervical carcinoma**
   A. **Incidence.** Carcinoma of the cervix, which complicates 1 out of every 1000 to 2500 deliveries, is the most common malignancy encountered in the pregnant patient.
   B. **Pathophysiology.** A woman's risk of developing cervical carcinoma and its precursor is highly correlated with the number of her male sexual partners, as well as the number of sexual partners her male partner has had. Numerous causative agents, including human smegma and herpes simplex virus, have previously been suggested to be responsible for the venereal transmission of cervical cancer. Current studies indicate a strong association between human papilloma virus (HPV) infection and subsequent development of cervical carcinoma.

   HPV types 6, 11, 16, 18, 31, and 32 commonly infect the human genital tract. HPV types 6 and 11 are associated with development of genital condylomata, but not with invasive cervical cancer. HPV types 16, 18, 31, and 32 are associated with the development of cervical carcinoma. Although HPV infection appears to be essential for the development of cervical cancer and its precursors, other factors such as smoking, herpes virus infection, or other carcinogens may be required for full oncogenic expression of the HPV virus.
   C. **Diagnosis.** Prompt diagnosis and treatment of this disease is essential, as cervical carcinoma is potentially curable if treatment is obtained early. Unfortunately, pregnancy often delays the diagnosis of cervical carcinoma.

1. Vaginal bleeding, the most common symptom of cervical carcinoma in both the pregnant and nonpregnant patient, is often attributed to the pregnancy, and a complete investigation is not performed.

2. Since preinvasive and early cervical carcinomas are usually asymptomatic, all pregnant patients should be screened at their first prenatal visit for these lesions. The Pap smear remains the screening tool of choice for detection of both cervical dysplasia and carcinoma.

   a. Approximately 3 percent of all pregnant women will have abnormal cervical cytologic findings.

   b. Patients with an abnormal Pap smear should be further evaluated with **colposcopic examination** of the cervix. Any abnormal area found during colposcopy should be biopsied. An **endocervical curettage,** which is normally an essential part of the colposcopic evaluation, is contraindicated in the pregnant patient. **Biopsy** may be deferred until the postpartum period if the transformation zone is clearly seen and there are no abnormal areas or only areas of minimally white epithelium that are clearly not invasive. The decision not to perform a biopsy should be made only by an experienced colposcopist after a careful review of the colposcopic findings and Pap smear indicates minimal disease.

D. Treatment

1. Treatment of biopsy-proven **cervical dysplasia** should be delayed until 6 weeks postpartum. Prior to therapy, a repeat colposcopic examination with endocervical curettage should be performed. This examination is necessary both to evaluate the endocervical canal fully and because cervical dysplasia may resolve postpartum, probably due to tissue necrosis and sloughing following delivery.

2. Carcinoma-in-situ should be followed by an experienced colposcopist, with repeat colposcopic examination of the cervix every 6 weeks until delivery. Any vascular changes suggestive of invasion require repeat biopsy. Treatment may be safely postponed until the puerperium if colposcopy and/or biopsy fail to detect any evidence of invasion.

3. Microinvasion, defined as invasion less than 3 mm deep without lymphatic or vascular involvement, is the only absolute indication for conization of the cervix in pregnancy.

   a. Conization is necessary to differentiate true microinvasion, for which treatment may be safely delayed until the postpartum period, from invasive cancer, which may require immediate intervention.

   b. Conization should be delayed until the second trimester to avoid the increased risk of miscarriage associated with surgical procedures in the first trimester.

   c. Patients with microinvasion on cone biopsy should be allowed to continue the pregnancy to term. Cesarean section is not indicated and should be performed for obstetric indications only.

(1) If the depth of invasion on the cone specimen is less than 1 mm, conization is considered to be curative and no further treatment is required.

(2) For patients with invasion less than 3 mm but greater than 1 mm deep, postpartum hysterectomy has traditionally been recommended, although this has been questioned. Thus, in patients with microinvasion who strongly desire future pregnancy, conization alone may be adequate.

4. **Invasive disease**

a. Delay of treatment until the postpartum period is controversial in patients with a single focus of invasion 3 to 5 mm deep and no lymphatic or vascular invasion. While many authorities advocate prompt treatment, others argue that 5-year survival is not affected by delay until fetal lung maturity. In these cases, the decision on when to institute therapy should be made with a gynecologic oncologist after extensive patient counseling. A radical hysterectomy is indicated for final therapy.

b. In those patients in whom the carcinoma involves the lymphatic or vascular spaces, or exceeds 5 mm in depth of invasion, the treatment depends upon the gestational age.

(1) At < 24 weeks, the treatment is the same as that of the nonpregnant patient with the identical stage. Either radical hysterectomy or radiation therapy is appropriate for a IB lesion, while radiation therapy is indicated for more advanced lesions.

(2) If pregnancy is > 24 weeks, treatment is delayed until fetal lung maturity. Delivery is by cesarean section. Radical hysterectomy may be performed in conjunction with cesarean section. Alternatively, radiation therapy may be initiated as soon as the incision heals, usually 2 weeks postoperatively.

E. **Prognosis.** The prognosis for invasive squamous cell carcinoma of the cervix in pregnancy compares favorably to that of similar-stage nonpregnant women of the same age. Previous reports indicating a lower 5-year survival rate in pregnant women in general, reflects the fact that pregnant women often present at a more advanced stage. In one study by Nisher, the disease-free survival rate for patients with cervical cancer associated with pregnancy was 93.3 percent for stage 1A, 68.2 percent for stage 1B, 54.5 percent for stage II, and 37.5 percent for stage III.

II. **Breast cancer**

A. **Incidence.** Second only to carcinoma of the cervix, breast carcinoma is frequently encountered in pregnancy. The incidence of this cancer in pregnancy is estimated to be 0.3/1000 pregnancies.

B. Pathophysiology. The effect of pregnancy on the growth and spread of breast carcinoma is disputed. Factors in pregnancy that could adversely affect this malignancy include the increased vascularity and lymphatic drainage of the pregnant breast, increased estrogen and prolactin stimulation, and depression of the immune system due to increased glucocorticoid production.

1. Despite these potential concerns, the limited data available in the literature suggest that, stage for stage, the survival rate of patients with breast cancer is unchanged by pregnancy.

2. However, pregnant patients tend to present with more advanced disease than nonpregnant patients, resulting in an overall decreased survival rate. This may suggest an acceleration of the disease process in the preclinical period in susceptible individuals.

C. Diagnosis. Breast examination at the time of the first prenatal visit provides an opportunity for the detection of breast cancer early in pregnancy. Needle aspiration of a cystic mass will distinguish a cyst or galactocele from a solid tumor. Bloody fluid obtained by aspiration should be sent for cytologic examination and biopsy performed for definitive diagnosis. Biopsy, under local anesthesia if possible, should also be performed on all solid masses. Mammography is seldom helpful in pregnancy due to the increased radiographic density of the pregnant breast.

D. Treatment
1. **Hormonal considerations**
   a. Despite the theoretical advantage of removing hormonal stimulation, an increased survival rate for patients with localized breast carcinoma has not been documented following therapeutic termination of pregnancy. Since the treatment of localized disease is not compromised by pregnancy, therapeutic termination is no longer routinely recommended.
   b. Unlike local disease, the value of hormonal ablation in **disseminated breast carcinoma** is well accepted.
      (1) Oophorectomy alone will produce a remission in 50 percent of patients with metastatic disease occurring during pregnancy. Thus, appropriate therapy for the premenopausal woman with disseminated breast carcinoma often requires surgical castration.
      (2) In early pregnancy, therapeutic abortion in addition to castration is necessary to prevent hormonal stimulation of the carcinoma.
      (3) In more advanced pregnancy, a short delay in treatment while waiting for fetal lung maturity may be appropriate.
      (4) In all cases, the urgency of palliation and the

patient's wishes must be considered in making any decision regarding pregnancy termination.

2. **Chemotherapy** after the first trimester has been used in the pregnant patient with advanced disease who refuses termination. The alkalating agents, 5-flurouracil, and vinca alkaloids appear relatively safe for the fetus after the first trimester. Except in such circumstances, chemotherapy should be avoided in the pregnant woman with breast cancer at this time. However, recent reports indicating improved survival in premenopausal women when chemotherapy was used as an adjuvant therapy may soon alter this recommendation.

E. **Prognosis.** The effect of future pregnancy on survival after therapy for breast carcinoma is unknown.

1. Retrospective studies suggest that future pregnancy does not affect the incidence of recurrence or the overall survival rate.

2. Patients contemplating future pregnancy should be advised to wait at least 3 years following completion of therapy prior to attempting conception. Additionally, a metastatic survey including mammography of the opposite breast and chest x-ray, as well as bone and liver scans, should be performed prior to pregnancy to rule out occult recurrence. If conception is successful, close follow-up during pregnancy is essential.

III. **Melanoma**
   A. **Incidence.** The incidence of melanoma in pregnancy is 0.1/1000 pregnancies.
   B. **Pathophysiology.** Malignant melanoma may be one of the few malignancies adversely affected by pregnancy.
      1. **Estrogen receptors** have been isolated in melanoma cells, suggesting that the lesion may be hormonally active.
      2. Additionally, **melanocyte-stimulating hormone** is known to be increased in pregnancy. Induction or exacerbation of melanoma by these and other factors associated with pregnancy has been proposed.
      3. Partial or complete **regression** of melanoma **postpartum,** as well as recurrence in subsequent pregnancies, support this hypothesis.
   C. **Prognosis.** The effect of pregnancy on 5-year survival is uncertain. Reports of more rapid spread and decreased survival are contradicted by other studies that have found no difference in overall survival compared to nonpregnant women. Although these reports are based on small numbers, it seems prudent to advise patients with a history of malignant melanoma to avoid pregnancy for at least 3 years. It is during this period that patients are at the highest risk for recurrence. This recommendation must also be individualized and based on the size, depth of invasion, and evidence of dissemination of the initial lesion.

IV. Ovarian cancer

A. **Incidence.** Ovarian carcinoma, normally a disease of older women, occurs infrequently in pregnancy. The incidence of ovarian carcinoma in pregnancy is estimated to be 1/8000 to 1/20 000 deliveries.

B. **Pathophysiology.** Ovarian carcinomas are broadly classified according to the tissue from which they originate. Epithelial tumors develop from the coelomic epithelium overlying the ovary. Germ cell tumors arise from the primitive germ cells, and gonadal stromal tumors differentiate from the ovarian mesenchyme or primitive stroma.

Although knowledge of the cause of ovarian cancer is limited, several risk factors have been identified. Individuals with long periods of uninterrupted ovulation have an increased risk of developing ovarian epithelial carcinoma. Conversely, pregnancy, anovulation, and use of oral contraceptives have a protective effect. Other risk factors include previous breast cancer and a familial history of ovarian carcinoma.

C. **Diagnosis.** Ovarian carcinoma must always be considered in the differential diagnosis of an adnexal mass in a pregnant patient.

1. The differential diagnosis includes pelvic kidney, pedunculated uterine fibroid, ectopic pregnancy, functional cyst, and a congenital abnormality such as a rudimentary uterine horn. A pelvic ultrasound examination may be able to diagnose these conditions without surgery or potentially dangerous radiation to the fetus.

2. Most adnexal masses in pregnancy are functional follicular or corpus luteum cysts. Although generally less than 5 cm in diameter, functional cysts may reach large proportions.

3. An adnexal mass that persists after the 16th week of pregnancy requires surgical exploration and removal. This recommendation is based upon two facts:
   a. The majority of functional cysts will regress by this time.
   b. The risk of fetal wastage as a result of anesthesia and surgery is minimized after the first trimester.

4. Surgical intervention may be required earlier than 16 weeks if the mass undergoes torsion or rupture. Approximately 10 to 15 percent of all adnexal masses in pregnancy will undergo torsion, with 60 percent occurring prior to 16 weeks of gestation as the uterus rises rapidly out of the pelvis and most of the remainder occurring in the postpartum period as the uterus involutes. Sudden lower abdominal pain accompanied by nausea, vomiting, and rebound tenderness should alert the clinician to this possibility.

5. Solid ovarian neoplasms have a higher risk of malignancy and should be evaluated more aggressively.

D. **Treatment.** Successful treatment requires early diagnosis and expedient surgical management. Excessive delay, due to fear or fetal wastage, is more dangerous than the imagined fetal risk.

1. If an ovarian carcinoma is discovered at the time of surgical exploration, accurate staging is necessary to plan therapy. Peritoneal cytology, as well as biopsies of suspected metastatic lesions, both diaphragmatic surfaces, the omentum, and the upper and lower pelvic gutters, are required to stage ovarian carcinoma properly. Ideally, periaortic and pelvic lymph node biopsies should also be performed.

2. Epithelial carcinoma, such as serous or mucinous cystadenoma, is rarely encountered in the patient under 40 years of age. When an epithelial cancer is found in the pregnant patient, it is usually of low malignant potential or stage 1A. Stage 1A epithelial cancers may be safely treated with unilateral salpingo-oophorectomy alone. Patients with lesions beyond stage 1A are more appropriately treated with total hysterectomy and bilateral salpingo-oophorectomy.

3. Germ cell tumors are more common in the early reproductive-age patient than either epithelial or stromal tumors.
   a. Malignant teratomas, dysgerminomas, endodermal sinus tumors, and embryonal carcinomas can be managed with unilateral salpingo-oophorectomy in stage 1A.
   b. Except for dysgerminomas, adjuvant chemotherapy is necessary for all malignant germ cell tumors.
   c. Continuation of the pregnancy without adjuvant chemotherapy is recommended for dysgerminomas due to their relative lack of sensitivity to chemotherapy, as well as the good prognosis with surgery in stage 1 disease. Although 10 percent of patients with dysgerminoma treated conservatively will have recurrent disease, 75 percent of these recurrences will be cured with subsequent radiation therapy.

4. Stromal cell tumors, such as granulosa or Sertoli-Leydig tumors, are infrequent in the pregnant patient. The low malignant potential of these tumors dictates conservative management in the young reproductive-age woman.

V. **Colorectal cancer**
   A. **Incidence.** Eight percent of colorectal carcinoma occurs in women younger than age 40 and two percent in women younger than age 30. The incidence of colorectal carcinoma in pregnancy is estimated to be 0.01/1000 pregnancies.
   B. **Pathophysiology.** Pregnancy does not appear to have an adverse effect on colon cancer, nor does the carcinoma appear to be injurious to the pregnancy. Overall, patient survival is influenced only by the stage and grade of the tumor.
   C. **Diagnosis.** The most common symptoms of colon cancer in pregnancy are abdominal pain, nausea and vomiting, constipation, abdominal distention, rectal bleeding, and fever. Anemia unresponsive to iron therapy requires evaluation for gastrointestinal loss. Delay in diagnosis is a significant problem, as many of

these symptoms are frequently encountered in normal pregnancies.
D. Treatment
1. If the lesion is detected early in the first or second trimester and is operable, surgical resection without disruption of the pregnancy should be attempted. Abdominoperineal resection is usually performed for rectal lesions and anterior resection for rectosigmoid lesions. Successful vaginal deliveries have been reported after both procedures.
2. In the third trimester, induction of labor or cesarean section at the time of fetal lung maturity is indicated. Vaginal delivery is not contraindicated except in cases of anterior rectal wall carcinoma, as profuse bleeding may result or labor may become obstructed. If vaginal delivery is successful, operative resection should be delayed for a few weeks until the uterus has undergone involution. In the postpartum patient, prophylactic oophorectomy to prevent later ovarian metastasis should be considered at the time of resection.
3. When the lesion is inoperable, fetal well-being becomes paramount. Surgery should be performed only as a palliative measure. Chemotherapy, usually with 5-flurouracil, should be delayed until after the first trimester.

VI. Leukemia/lymphoma. Leukemia and lymphoma commonly affect young people. Not surprisingly, the initial diagnosis may occur during a pregnancy. Since these diseases may be cured or controlled for long periods of time with appropriate chemotherapy and/or radiation therapy, aggressive initial therapy is indicated. Lymphoma in pregnancy consists primarily of Hodgkin's disease. The mainstay of therapy for early-stage disease is radiotherapy, while advanced disease is treated with combination chemotherapy such as MOPP (nitrogen mustard, vincristine, procarbazine, and prednisone). Bulky disease is usually treated with a combination of both. With the exception of patients in the third trimester of pregnancy, the aggressive radiotherapy and chemotherapy needed to treat Hodgkin's disease properly requires termination of pregnancy. The physician must, of course, consider the patient's wishes should termination be refused.

VII. Metastatic disease to the fetus and placenta. Metastatic disease to the fetus or placenta is uncommon, with fewer than 50 cases reported. The most common metastatic lesions of either the fetus or placenta are melanoma, breast cancer, and leukemia/lymphoma. In one review of 24 cases, malignant melanoma was found in 11 and breast cancer in 4. Malignant melanoma is also the most likely cancer to metastasize to the fetus itself. In eight instances of fetal metastasis, malignant melanoma was responsible for seven of the eight cases, with lymphosarcoma accounting for the remaining case.

BIBLIOGRAPHY

Albain K. Adjuvant chemotherapy and endocrine therapy for node-positive and node-negative breast carcinoma. Clin Obstet Gynecol 1989; 32:835.

Allen H, Nisker J. Cancer in Pregnancy: Therapeutic Guidelines. Mt Kisco, NY: Future; 1986.

Barber H, Brunschwig A. Gynecologic cancer complicating pregnancy. Am J Obstet Gynecol 1963; 85:156.

Barry R, Diamond H, Craver L. Influence of pregnancy on the course of Hodgkins disease. Am J Obstet Gynecol 1962; 84:445.

Booth R. Ovarian tumors in pregnancy. Obstet Gynecol 1963; 21:189.

Breslow A. Thickness, cross-sectional areas and depth of invasion in the prognosis of cutaneous melanoma. Ann Surg 1970; 172:902.

Catanzarite V, Ferguson J. Acute leukemia in pregnancy: A review of the management and outcome. Obstet Gynecol Surv 1984; 39:663.

Creasman W, Rutledge F, Fletcher G. Carcinoma of the cervix associated with pregnancy. Obstet Gynecol 1970; 36:495.

Disaia P, Creasman W. Clinical Gynecologic Oncology. 3rd ed. St. Louis: CV Mosby; 1989:511.

Fisher R, Neifield J, Lipman M. Oestrogen receptors in human malignant melanoma. Lancet 1976; 2:337.

Grimes W, Bartholomew R, Colvin F, et al. Ovarian cysts in pregnancy. Am J Obstet Gynecol 1954; 68:594.

Hendleman L, Menstel A. Multiple carcinomatosis of the colon complicating pregnancy. Obstet Gynecol 1958; 11:119.

Herbst A, Ulfedert H, Poskanzer D. Adenocarcinoma of the vagina: Association with maternal stilbestrol therapy with tumor appearance in young women. N Engl J Med 1971; 248:878.

Hill J, Shiraz K, Talledo O. Colonic cancer in pregnancy. South Med J 1984;77:375.

Holleb A, Farrow J. The relation of carcinoma of the breast and pregnancy in 283 patients. Surg Obstet Gynecol 1962; 115:62.

Karlen J, Akbar A, Cook W. Dysgerminoma associated with pregnancy. Obstet Gynecol 1979; 53:330.

Koren G, Weiner L, Lisher M, et al. Cancer in pregnancy: Identification of unanswered questions on maternal and fetal risks. Obstet Gynecol Surv 1990; 45:509.

McGowan L. Cancer and pregnancy. Obstet Gynecol Surv 1964; 19:285.

Nicolson H. Cytotoxic drugs in pregnancy. J Obstet Gynaecol Br Commonw 1968; 75:307.

Pack G, Scharnagel L. The prognosis for malignant melanoma in the pregnant woman. Cancer 1951; 4:324.

Parente J, Amsel M, Lerner R, et al. Breast cancer associated with pregnancy. Obstet Gynecol 1988; 71:861.

Peters M, Meakin J. The influence of pregnancy in carcinoma of the breast. In: Ariel I, ed. Progress in Clinical Cancer. New York: Grune and Stratton; 1965:471.

Potter J, Schoeneman M. Metastasis of maternal causes to the placenta and fetus. Cancer 1970; 25:380.

Reintgen D, McCarty K, Vollmer R, et al. Malignant melanoma and pregnancy. Cancer 1985; 55:1340.

Reyoso E, Shepherd F, Messner H, et al. Acute leukemia during pregnancy: The Toronto Leukemia Study Group experience with long term follow-up of children exposed in utero to chemotherapeutic agents. J Clin Oncol 1987; 5:1098.

Rothman L, Cohen C, Asterloa J. Placental and fetal involvement by maternal malignancy. A report of rectal carcinoma and review of the literature. Am J Obstet Gynecol 1973; 116:1023.

Schardein J. Cancer Chemotherapeutic Agents. New York: Marcel Decker; 1988:467.

Smith R, Randall P. Melanoma during pregnancy. Obstet Gynecol 1969; 34:825.

Sokal J, Lessman E. The effect of cancer chemotherapeutic agents on the human fetus. JAMA 1960; 172:1765.

Stewart H. Case of malignant melanoma and pregnancy. Br Med J 1955; 1:647.

Summer W. Spontaneous regression of melanoma: Report of a case. Cancer 1953; 6:1040.

Sweet D, Kinzie J. Consequences of radiotherapy and antineoplastic therapy for the fetus. J Reprod Med 1976; 17:241.

Vorrhis B, Cruikshank D. Colon carcinoma complicating pregnancy — a report of two cases. J Reprod Med 1989; 34:923.

CHAPTER 41

Psychological and Psychiatric Diseases in Pregnancy

Henry Lahmeyer

PREGNANCY-ASSOCIATED MENTAL ILLNESS

Women are nearly twice as likely to suffer from mental illness during their reproductive years as men. Most of this excess is accounted for by depression, although women are twice as likely to suffer from anxiety disorders as well. It is not certain that women suffer excessively from mental illness perinatally, but it is clear that in the first month postpartum there is an increased risk of mental illness. The obstetrician is faced with a dilemma, however. Emotions run high during the perinatal period. The patient must be assisted in managing these strong emotions, and the good clinician must sort out these normal reactions from pathologic events.

I. **First trimester**
   A. **Adjustment in the family unit**
      1. The greatest adjustment occurs in the primiparous family. The expectant mother's role will expand radically from companion and lover to include the role of mother. If the baby is unwanted, intense ambivalence and anxiety now occur. Should the pregnancy be terminated? What will friends and family think? Does the father love me? Will he leave if I have the baby or vice versa? The teenage or immature patient has great difficulty with these decisions. The immature woman becomes confused with these monumental choices.
      2. The physician may need to act as the calm, neutral parent, but should also not be afraid to express opinions if they are empathic rather than arising strictly out of personal values.
   B. **Lethargy and tiredness.** These symptoms are common in the first trimester and may be trying for the anxious patient and spouse, who view them as signs of laziness or, worse, neglect of the spouse.

C. **Food preferences, nausea, and vomiting**
   1. The pregnant woman develops a voracious appetite. However, nausea and vomiting can also occur during the first trimester. Specific food cravings are legendary, such as cravings for pickles and ice cream. Cravings for ice, cornstarch, and clay may indicate iron deficiency. These dramatic changes are usually a problem to the woman who previously had either mild or significant weight conflicts— either anorexic or bulimic tendencies. These diseases are achieving somewhat of an epidemic status today, so that weight gain among the health club set is no trivial matter. Vomiting can even be viewed as beneficial to some women as a method of weight control. Many women have acquired considerable skill in self-deception regarding food habits and weight, so that the obstetrician must ask specific questions about diet and keep careful records of weight.
   2. Many women routinely take drugs to control weight. Specific advice should be given regarding the prohibition of these drugs, since many people consider over-the-counter drugs harmless.

D. **Hyperemesis gravidarum**
   1. Hyperemesis gravidarum has been ascribed psychologically to an attempt to expel the pregnancy. Although hormonal changes play a role, **anxiety** and **ambivalence** about mothering can contribute. Medically, the condition can become serious, as electrolyte imbalance and weight loss develop.
   2. **Management.** Initially the physician must rule out medical reasons for hyperemesis such as twins, a molar pregnancy, or pancreatitis. In the absence of these conditions, the obstetrician should meet with the patient and spouse to determine the sources of **marital tension, financial stresses, and emotional stresses** currently and in the past for the expectant mother. A first occurrence in a multigravida alerts the physician to psychological stresses or biological risk factors. In addition to close monitoring of the patient's medical status, with intervention as needed, psychiatric referral is often indicated, especially in severe or intractable cases. **Referral** will more likely be successful if the patient is told that psychiatric treatment is useful as an adjunct to medical management and monitoring. Hypnosis and behavioral therapy will be useful in reducing anxiety and actual vomiting, regardless of the diagnosis. A psychiatrist should interview the patient to establish the diagnosis prior to instituting any treatment. The psychiatrist should then recommend either psychotherapy, hypnosis, behavioral therapy, or a combination of these therapies.

E. **Abortion**
   1. Abortions, either spontaneous or induced, are associated with psychological sequelae. If unrecognized and unad-

dressed, these may cause long-term problems for the patient and her family. Planned first-trimester elective abortions are often associated with fewer psychological sequelae than childbirth, stillbirth later in pregnancy, and neonatal demise.

2. Counseling is important to help the patient make the best decision in cases of elective termination and to deal with possible feelings of guilt in cases of spontaneous loss. The patient should be encouraged to involve the members of her support system in all cases of pregnancy loss.

3. It is especially important to identify patients with extreme anxiety or guilt about abortion, especially induced abortion, so that intensive follow-up counseling can be arranged. **Risk factors** associated with negative postabortion reactions include young age, unmarried, Catholic or fundamental religious faith, and poor social support.

II. **Second trimester**

A. This period is usually a relatively quiescent one psychologically. Distress during this period is therefore ominous. **Sleep disturbances, appetite disturbances, anxiety, and depression** indicate that the issues of the first trimester have not been resolved psychologically or that medically the pregnancy is not progressing properly. Psychiatric symptoms in the second trimester therefore require an additional psychological inventory and careful medical monitoring.

   1. **Preeclampsia** can present late in the second trimester and usually occurs with **anxiety, irritability, sleep disturbance, and headache,** often before the classic symptoms of edema, proteinuria, and hypertension emerge.

   2. **Depression** is one of the more common problems in the second trimester. This may be manifested as insomnia, anorexia, weight loss, sadness, suicidal thoughts, decreased interest in family members, low energy, or excessive guilt.

   3. **Anxiety** is the other common problem in the second trimester. Symptoms include the need to keep active by pacing, a sense of panic, headaches, and tremulousness. Autonomic symptoms include tachycardia, diarrhea, diaphoresis, tachypnea, and dry mouth.

   4. The physician must determine if these symptoms are due to the stress of pregnancy, other stresses, or a chronic neurotic problem. Office counseling may help resolve the more immediate stresses.

B. **Psychotropic medications** are safer when given in the second than in the first trimester but should be avoided if possible, since neurologic maturation is still an active process.

C. Anxiety about amniocentesis is a special concern in this trimester. Anxiety about the outcome is usually intense. Precipitation of mental illness is possible in the vulnerable patient with a history of mental illness, particularly if the results are ominous.

The obstetrician must be prepared for a thorough airing of grief if the results are abnormal. The stress of amniocentesis is great for all women, but especially for older women, for whom abnormal results may mean that they will have no more children or that they will have to try to squeeze in another pregnancy, assuming that they can become pregnant. The clinician should be the one to break the news. He or she should set aside enough time for all questions. The shock may be great enough that subsequent counseling is usually required. A woman who does not improve in 6 to 8 weeks may need psychiatric referral. The clinician should actively use his or her personal and professional experience in these counseling sessions, giving empathic advice but allowing the patient to express anger and remain quiet.

III. **Third trimester**
   A. **Physical and emotional discomfort** reemerge during this period. Increased girth leads to dyspnea, slowed mobility, poor sleep, and uneven appetite. Muscle aches, cramps, and peripheral edema are common. Changes in girth, hair color, and skin tone all lead to distress about **body image. Sexual functioning** is difficult. As delivery nears, the expectant mother's concern draws inward often to the exclusion of the father. He thus can become less able to deal with her mounting anxiety and anticipation. Other emotional issues during the third trimester that may prompt **regression** in the pregnant mother center on the fear of fetal deformity, of her own disfigurement, and of the loss of her own childhood with imminent motherhood.
   B. Preeclampsia can present with **anxiety, headache, and irritability.**
   C. **Third-trimester anxiety** may be associated with prolonged or precipitous labor. **Prenatal classes** are invaluable during this period to fulfill some of the functions that in years past a woman's mother and extended family played. Frequent contact with the obstetrician occurs during the third trimester but may need to be increased even further if anxiety escalates. If anxiety does not improve, **lorazepam** (Ativan), 1 to 2 mg/d day (or another short half-life benzodiazepine) for anxiety or 1 to 2 mg p.r.n. for sleep is safe. Do not put the patient on a regular schedule of medication, and try to discontinue lorazepam 1 to 2 days before labor. The **short half-life** benzodiazepine will minimize the risk of neonatal sedation. Side effects of lorazepam are minimal, but excessive sedation can occur.
   D. **Fetal death**
      1. A significant **grief reaction** is almost universal after stillbirth or if the infant dies soon after birth. Grief can lead to true depression, where guilt and self-deprecation are prominent in a woman previously vulnerable to depression, or in a woman who was ambivalent about the child, or in a woman with some of the risk factors mentioned for abortion associated depression, particularly a **poor support system.**

2. Management
   a. The physician should ease the patient's grief by allowing her to talk about her feelings, her fear of future pregnancies, and her anger at fate and herself. The physician should be aware, however, that the **anger** that is so common during this period will sometimes be directed to him or her. It is important to understand that this anger usually is not directed personally at the physician. Acceptance of the upset is important; try not to react. If grief is prolonged for 6 weeks or more, or becomes worse, **depression** may be developing. The reasons for the depression should be sought. If the reasons are vague or if guilt and remorse are excessive, psychiatric referral is indicated. Antidepressants can be useful if a depressive syndrome has developed.
   b. It should be noted that nurses and other staff also often become depressed after fetal death, especially when legal issues complicate the professional-patient relationship.
 E. Prematurity. When an infant is born prematurely, parents often have considerable fear, guilt, and worry. They will usually be intimidated by the intensive care unit and hesitant to get involved in the infant's care. The **medical team** may often covertly discourage involvement as well. It is important to inform the parents about the possible causes of the infant's distress and the long-term prognosis as the parents become receptive to this information. If the infant is at high risk, the parents should be told the risks and asked how much contact they would like to have with the infant. They may choose to have little contact until the danger is over, as an intuitive attempt to minimize bonding until infant viability is assured. Parents of premature infants with a better prognosis should be encouraged to have contact with the infant to enhance bonding and to help them overcome their natural reluctance to interfere with the professional staff.

IV. Postpartum period
 A. Variations in bonding. Surprisingly, many women report negative or neutral reactions to their newborns; very few women are initially overjoyed. This may be because of exhaustion, overly high expectations, revulsion over the infant's physical appearance, disappointment over the gender of the newborn, or a biological reluctance to bond with the infant until viability is assured. Only severe bonding problems need attention in the hospital. These are manifested by:
 1. Lack of desire to have the infant visit
 2. Lack of attention to the infant's needs or safety
 3. Hostility or aggression toward the infant
 4. Extreme withdrawal while the infant is present
 These bonding failures can indicate severe depression or postpartum psychosis.

Minor bonding problems should be noted and followed up in well-baby pediatric visits.

B. **Normal psychological stresses**
   1. **Mood lability** in the postpartum period is almost universal. Emotions range from fear to joy to depression—especially tearfulness—very quickly. This lability can alarm those who are unprepared.
   2. **Fatigue** and **exhaustion** can cause many women to opt for bottle feeding. Support from family and medical personnel is needed to help the patient make an objective choice. Support is also needed so that bonding can proceed optimally. An exhausted mother must recover before she can perform her nurturing functions.
   3. **Anorexia** is very common in the first 3 days postpartum and does not indicate depression.
   4. **Hypersomnia** is also normal, although if it persists for weeks, it may indicate depression.

PSYCHIATRIC DISEASE COMPLICATED BY PREGNANCY

Psychiatric disease normally is devastating to the individual, although her suffering can sometimes be in silence, but perinatally this luxury is not available. The family always suffers, and the newborn can suffer inordinately if intervention is not available.

I. **Psychiatric illness presenting in several forms in pregnancy**
   A. **Schizophrenia.** Typically these patients have delusions, often of paranoid quality; often auditory hallucinations; thought disorder with looseness of association or idiosyncratic thinking; inappropriate, flat, or bizarre affect; or feelings of being controlled externally or thought broadcasting.
   B. **Depression.** This is the most common disorder during the perinatal period. Most importantly, these patients experience depressed mood, lowered self-esteem, loss of interest in self and others, often suicidal thoughts, insomnia, anorexia, sadness, crying, low energy, and unreasonable guilt or remorse.
   C. **Manic-depressive psychosis.** In this condition, patients experience depressive episodes but frequently the opposite—mania. Frequently encountered manic symptoms include euphoria or agitation, hyperactivity, loss of sleep, and pressured speech. Delusions of grandiosity can also occur, along with increased libido, spending sprees, and frequently disorganized, poorly considered behavior.
   D. **Anxiety disorders.** Anxiety presents in two forms.
      1. **Tonic anxiety** is a high level of chronic tension manifested by subjective tension, shakiness, jumpiness, headaches, and other somatic complaints.
      2. **Panic attacks or anxiety attacks** occur sporadically, with or without precipitants, and are characterized by episodes of subjective fear and panic and autonomic nervous system

manifestations, including storms of tachycardia, hyperventilation, diaphoresis, dizziness and vertigo, and blushing.

E. **Postpartum "blues."** This syndrome is a form of mild depression usually characterized by an egoalien feeling of depression, frequent crying, and fleeting inexplicable feelings of being unloved, unable to care for the newborn, and so on.

F. **Drug and alcohol abuse.** Heroin, cocaine, and alcohol abuse are common disorders in the general population and complicate pregnancy, requiring special management during pregnancy.

II. **Incidence.** Psychosis occurs in approximately 0.5–1 percent of pregnancies. If there is a history of psychosis during pregnancy, the incidence may be as high as 50 percent or more. During pregnancy, the incidence is similar to that of nonpregnant women. However, postpartum, the incidence is 5 to 10 times normal in the first postpartum month for serious mental illness. Postpartum blues that occur during the first 5 days postpartum may affect 50 to 70 percent of women.

III. **Morbidity and mortality.** The prognosis is generally good for postpartum psychoses and is particularly good for postpartum blues, but preexisting mental illness that recurs during pregnancy has an outlook similar to that of mental illness occurring at other times, with the added problem that psychotropic drugs may be less aggressively administered because of fetal effects.

A. **Suicide.** Depressed and psychotic patients are at risk for suicide. The obstetrician should know the major risk factors for suicide. These are described in Table 41.1. If it is possible that the patient might be suicidal, the physician must inquire about her thoughts and plans.

B. **Infanticide.** A psychotic, delusional, confused mother is at definite risk for infanticide. Psychotic mothers should not have unsupervised contact with their newborn. Contact should be monitored by a nurse familiar with the patient and by a family member, if possible. Observations of bonding can be made then. Some psychotic mothers progress with bonding; others do not. If progress is not being made, it may be wise to arrange alternative care for the infant while the patient's psychosis resolves.

Table 41.1. Risk Factors for Suicide

Claims of being suicidal and of having a plan
Previous suicide attempt
Presence of depression or psychosis
History of drug use
Recent suicide attempt and unresolved precipitating issues
Feelings of hopelessness or of being trapped in an impossible circumstance

C. **Sudden death.** Sudden, unexplained death can occur in the perinatally psychotic woman. The delirious and confused psychotic patient may be suffering from embolic or infectious disease and must be carefully evaluated and monitored.
D. **Loss of maternal bonding.** Bonding begins during pregnancy. This is attenuated in the anxious, depressed, or psychotic expectant mother. However, bonding suffers most during the postpartum period.

IV. **Infant distress.** Infants born to alcoholic or drug-using mothers are often premature, small for gestational age, and suffer withdrawal symptoms, excessive respiratory distress, and developmental delays. Mothers taking antipsychotics and antidepressants also produce infants with more distress than usual. Usually withdrawal symptoms occur, although their severity is less than with drugs of addiction.

V. **Cause**
A. **Schizophrenia.** The cause is unknown, although familial links are clear. The majority of cases, however, occur sporadically.
B. **Depression.** Women have a twofold higher incidence than men. Strong familial trends have been established, especially for manic-depressive illness. A perinatal-neonatal death almost always results in depression. The first month postpartum is associated with such a high rate of depression that hormonal changes must play a role. Psychological adjustment to the newborn may also be a factor.
C. **Postpartum blues.** The nearly universal occurrence of this condition points to biological causes, but specificity is lacking. Again, cortisol, estrogen, progesterone, or prolactin may play a role.
D. **Postpartum psychosis.** Several factors are associated with this condition, although the causality is unclear.
   1. If there has been a previous postpartum psychosis, it frequently recurs with each pregnancy. This is particularly true of postpartum mania.
   2. Cesarean section is associated with some increase in the occurrence of psychosis.
   3. Poor or nonexistent social supports are associated with perinatal mental illness. Interestingly, simply being unwed is not associated with mental illness if supports are good.
   4. Anxiety and depression in the last trimester tend to predict postpartum distress.
E. **Alcohol and drug addiction**
   1. Alcoholism show the existence of clear genetic links. The widespread availability of alcohol also contributes to the high incidence of alcoholism. Modeling by parents is also probably a factor.
   2. Familial factors are less evident in drug addiction than in alcoholism. Availability of drugs and certain psychopathologic conditions predispose to addiction.

VI. Differential diagnosis
  A. Common problems
    1. In the immediate postpartum period, the major challenge is to differentiate tearfulness and exhaustion from the more serious depression. If tearfulness escalates into diminished self-esteem, insomnia, and self-destructive thoughts, then depression is developing. If the patient develops fluctuating consciousness, psychosis may be developing.
    2. Anxiety during labor and delivery can be mild or serious. Escalating anxiety can make delivery dangerous and must be treated, but it usually remits spontaneously postpartum.
  B. Less common problems
    1. Psychosis is less likely to develop than depression or anxiety.
    2. Unusually high anxiety can indicate drug withdrawal or cocaine or hallucinogen use.
    3. Conversion disorder is unusual but can present as pseudocyesis (false pregnancy) or the reverse by denying the pregnancy.
    4. Pseudoseizures can mimic eclampsia. Usually those presenting with pseudoseizures have previously experienced eclampsia or have a close relative who had the syndrome.
    5. Toxic delirium is less common today than previously, but the presence of fever and an abnormal pulse and blood pressure, as well as abnormal physical and cognitive mental status, are consistent with delirium.

VII. Diagnosis
  A. History. In addition to the clinical picture previously described, the clinician must quickly obtain a collateral history from the family and nursing staff about symptoms of poor judgment, fluctuating consciousness, tearfulness, loss of appetite, and insomnia, as well as mother-infant interactions during the postpartum period. A history of drug addiction often also requires collateral sources of information.
  B. Physical examination is necessary to determine whether the cause is organic or psychiatric.
    1. Elevated blood pressure classically denotes preeclampsia. However, insomia and mental status changes also occur in this condition. Elevated temperature, blood pressure, and pulse accompany other forms of toxic delirium.
    2. Examination for blood loss is necessary.
    3. Pulmonary embolism can cause dyspnea and panic. A previously neurotic patient can also develop these symptoms, so the clinician must carefully assess dyspnea.
  C. Laboratory examination and diagnostic procedures. Psychiatric illness of unknown cause requires a thorough laboratory evaluation, including:
    1. Complete blood count and differential
    2. Blood chemistry assessments, including electrolytes
    3. Chest x-ray

4. Urinalysis
5. Other tests as indicated

VIII. Management
A. Schizophrenia
1. Generally schizophrenia must be managed with medication and psychological support, usually in the psychiatric setting. Treatment should be done in conjunction with a psychiatrist.
2. **Psychotropic medication.**
   a. Major tranquilizers can be used during the latter half of pregnancy and, if symptoms are severe, in the first trimester, since teratogenicity of antipsychotics is not confirmed. Fetal side effects of psychotropic drugs are not of concern until childbirth, when fetal tremors, restlessness, and rigidity may occur, as well as respiratory distress. The dosage can be tapered 10 to 15 days prior to anticipated labor. One should use a sufficient dosage to control psychotic symptoms but not fog the patient's thinking.
   b. Drugs and dosage
      (1) Give haloperidol (Haldol), 2 to 4 mg, initially. This can be increased to 10 to 20 mg/d as needed. The drug should be given regularly once initiated. If it must be given intramuscularly, approximately one-third of the dosage will be needed.
      (2) Give trifluoperazine (Stelazine), 5 to 10 mg initially. A high dosage would be 30 to 50 mg.
      (3) Give thioridazine (Mellaril), 100 to 200 mg initially. A high dose would be 500 to 600 mg. This drug produces fewer extrapyramidal side effects and is more sedating but cannot be given intramuscularly.
   c. Toxic reactions
      (1) Bone marrow suppression can occur but is rare.
      (2) Malignant hyperthermia, characterized by high fever, blood pressure, and pulse is rare.
      (3) Both toxic reactions require immediate discontinuance of the drug and medical referral.
   d. Side effects
      (1) Orthostatic hypotension can occur, particularly with Mellaril. The dosage can be reduced or Haldol substituted.
      (2) Anticholinergic effects—dry mouth, blurred vision, urinary retention, constipation — may occur.
      (3) Extrapyramidal effects: acute dystonia is most common. This occurs early in therapy and can be treated by lowering the dosage of the major tranquilizer or by adding benztropine (Cogentin), 1 to 2 mg b.i.d., for 7 days before the dose is tapered.

B. Manic-depression (bipolar) psychoses

  1. Lithium management. Many of these patients are on maintenance lithium carbonate therapy. This should be suspended during the first trimester, or longer, if at all possible. The medication may be reinstated during the second trimester, if needed, and then discontinued near term to avoid neonatal effects such as cyanosis, goiter, hypoglycemia, hypotonia, and, rarely, diabetes insipidus. The risk of mania in the puerperium is high, so lithium should be reinstated after delivery. If lithium is needed, breast-feeding should not be advised. Antipsychotics such as haloperidol, 10 to 20 mg/d, may be needed for manic control.

  2. Dosage. Patients previously on lithium carbonate can be given previously effective dosages, which can range from 300 mg b.i.d. to 1800 mg/d. The dosage is variable and is adjusted to achieve blood levels of 0.4 to 1.0 mEq/L for prophylaxis and 0.6 to 1.2 mEq/L for acute manic management.

  3. Contraindications

  a. Unreliable or alcoholic patients because high blood levels can lead to severe toxicity initiated by nausea, vomiting and diarrhea, followed by disorientation, coma, and death.   •

  b. Hypothyroidism.

  c. Significant renal disease.

  d. Atrioventricular cardiac conduction problems.

  e. Patients on concurrent diuretics. This is a relative contraindication, but patients on diuretics need renal consultation and very careful monitoring.

  4. Side effects. Side effects early in treatment are generally confined to the gastrointestinal tract (irritation and nausea). Therapeutic blood levels are associated with few psychiatric side effects.

C. Depression

  1. Management for suicide. Suicidal ideas are usually manageable if the patient does not have a plan, does not have command hallucinations telling her to die, or does not have a history of suicide attempts. The clinician should explore the reasons why the patient wants to die and can try to problem-solve with the patient and family. The family should almost always be involved in this crisis to provide active support and solve problems. They need to share the burden of risk with the physician. Suicidal ideation that does not remit may be related to clinical depression (see Table 41.1). Nortriptyline (Pamelor) should be initiated, giving 25 mg the first night and 50 mg the second night, increased to 75 mg by days 4 to 5, and then increased 25 mg at 4-day intervals until a 125-mg daily dose is achieved. If significant side effects such as bothersome orthostatic hypotension, dry mouth, urinary retention, or blurred vision occur, the dosage should be reduced by 25 mg until the symptoms resolve. Significant side effects or lack of a clinical response in 2 to 4 weeks may indicate high or low blood levels. Weekly blood levels should be obtained to achieve levels of 50 to 150 ng/mL. Fluoxetine (Prozac) is a good alternative. Most patients respond to 20 mg daily. Occasionally, 40 to 60 mg is needed if no response occurs in 4 to 6 weeks. Persistent side effects of increased anxiety require careful monitoring in about 10 percent of patients. If suicidal thoughts do not resolve quickly, a psychiatric consultation should be obtained to determine if the patient can be managed on the obstetric service or requires transferral to a psychiatric unit.

   2. **Psychotropic drugs**
      a. Tricyclic antidepressants should be avoided in the first trimester if possible, even though the teratogenic risk is very low. Neonatal effects include tachycardia and hyperhidrosis, which may last for up to 1 week after delivery.
      b. Antipsychotics such as haloperidol, 5 to 20 mg/d, may be needed for unresponsive psychotic, agitated, or highly suicidal patients. Once the psychotic symptoms are controlled, antidepressants can be added as needed according to the guidelines in Section VIII.B. The risk of thrombophlebitis is increased in these patients, and symptoms should be monitored.

   D. **Postpartum blues.** Most cases are resolve in 3 to 7 days as exhaustion and pain from labor subside. Bonding to the child seems to replace the depression. Family support, in the form of assisting the patient with the newborn and allowing her to sleep, is important.

IX. **Anxiety during labor and delivery.** Extreme anxiety is often a direct result of pain and fear of mutilation or fetal distress.
   A. **Management.** Prenatal classes and a birth plan are helpful. If the patient is well practiced and trusts those around her, she will more likely follow instructions during painful periods.
   B. **Psychotropic drugs.** If analgesics and psychological support fail and anxiety becomes uncontrollable, give halperidol, 2 mg IM every 30 min, until anxiety is controlled. The baby will not be excessively sleepy but may develop tremor or dystonia for a day or two.

X. **Postpartum psychosis**
   A. **Management**
      1. **Psychiatric consultation** is usually needed when:
         a. The patient's behavior is clearly bizarre.
         b. The patient is clearly suicidal.
         c. The patient is unable to care for her infant.

  2. **Psychiatric hospitalization** is needed when:
   a. Behavior is bizarre or the patient is felt to be potentially violent toward herself or the infant.
   b. Aggressive antipsychotic therapy with Haldol or Stelazine is ineffective (see Section VIII.A.2.b).
  3. **Family intervention**
   a. Social service consultation is usually helpful.
   b. The family must be told that postpartum disturbances are serious, relatively common, not the patient's fault, and usually have a good prognosis.
   c. They should be told that the infant will need alternative care until the mother is able to relate to and care for it. Siblings also will need alternative care.
   d. It is sometimes helpful to have the infant also hospitalized on the psychiatric unit so that bonding is not completely disrupted. Not all psychiatric units can do this.
 B. Psychotropic drugs
  1. **Psychotic depression.** As mentioned previously, antipsychotics are titrated until psychotic symptoms are controlled. Then tricyclic antidepressants can be added as described. Monoamine oxidase inhibitors are sometimes needed; obstetricians should obtain a psychiatric consultation before using them.
  2. **Undifferentiated psychoses** may respond to haloperidol, 5 to 20 mg/d, but electroconvulsive therapy is occasionally needed.

XI. Prognosis. The prognosis for perinatal mental illness is generally good. Postpartum events tend to recur only during subsequent pregnancies. Schizophrenia arising early in pregnancy has a poor prognosis but is no different from that of schizophrenia occurring at other times. Postpartum blues almost always remit, as does extreme anxiety during labor and delivery. Manic-depressive psychosis occurring early in pregnancy has a worse prognosis than postpartum events.

BIBLIOGRAPHY

Anath J. Side effects of fetus and infant of psychotropic drug use during pregnancy. Int Pharmacopsychiatry 1976; 11:246–260.

Brockington IF, Kumar R. Motherhood and Mental Illness. London: Academic Press; 1982.

Brown WA. Psychological Care During Pregnancy and the Postpartum Period. New York: Raven Press; 1979.

Lahmeyer HW, Jackson C. Affective disorders and mental illness during the puerperium. In: Val E, Gaviria M, Flaherty J, eds. Affective Disorders: Diagnosis and Treatment in Clinical Practice. Chicago: Year Book Medical Publishers; 1982.

Protheroe C. Puerperal psychosis: A long term study 1917–1961. Br J Psychiatry 1969; 115:9–30.

CHAPTER 42

Dental and Oral Diseases

Trusten P. Lee

Prenatal care should include attention to the patient's dental needs. The physician should stress the importance of good personal oral hygiene, along with professional prophylaxis and general dental care, to optimize the patient's oral comfort during the pregnancy. The physician can also confidently dispel the prevailing myths linking pregnancy to the loss of teeth, decalcification of teeth, and general decline in dental health.

DENTAL COMPLICATIONS OF PREGNANCY

I. **Pregnancy gingivitis and periodontitis**
   A. **Incidence.** Over 80 percent of pregnant women exhibit gingival inflammation. Pocketing of the gingiva around the dentition is present in approximately 25 percent. These figures are consistent with the incidence of periodontal disease in the general population, affecting 9 out of 10 adults. Though pregnancy has not been shown to cause gingivitis and periodontitis, it does exaggerate the symptoms, heightening the patient's awareness of the preexisting condition.
   B. **Morbidity.** When left untreated, gingivitis and periodontitis may cause tissue swelling, bleeding of the gingiva, and tenderness. Pus may develop, and tooth mobility and bone loss may increase. Shortly before delivery, conditions often improve and then stabilize.
   C. **Cause.** Changes in the progesterone and estrogen levels are thought to cause the vascular changes related to the tissue's exaggerated responses to local factors. Laxity in oral hygiene care, that is, inadequate brushing and flossing, also adds to the tissue's increased susceptibility.
   D. **Pathogenesis and pathophysiology.** Gingivitis and periodontitis are reactions of the gum tissue to tartar and colonized bacteria surrounding the dentition. There is no specific form of gingivitis or periodontitis associated with pregnancy. Rather, the increased incidence of tissue inflammation is linked to the hormonal changes inherent in normal pregnancy. Tissue changes may

occur as early as the second month, but most frequently occur toward the end of the first trimester and may continue until delivery.
E. **Diagnosis.** Gums will appear red, swollen, and hyperplastic, and may bleed easily upon brushing or probing. Pockets of ≥ 4 mL may form around the teeth, and bad breath and pus may be present. Increased tooth mobility may also be noted. Prominent bulbous interdental papillae may be apparent in general areas. A visual examination can indicate the presence of gingivitis. Severity of progression can be confirmed with radiographs and by physical probing and measuring of periodontal pockets.
F. **Management**
1. Hormone-related gingivitis will generally resolve without treatment, although the comfort of the patient may suggest temporary treatment in the interim.
2. Treatment of gingivitis consists of professional prophylaxis as indicated and a meticulous home hygiene regimen based on proper brushing and flossing techniques. Additionally, periodontal treatment may include regular professional dentition scalings during the second trimester. With severe cases of deep pocketing, gum reduction surgery may be necessary, although this treatment may be postponed until after delivery.
3. Vitamin supplements have not been found to be effective in treating these conditions.
G. **Prognosis.** An excellent prognosis is expected with proper hygienic care. Even without care, the condition may improve shortly before delivery. Proper home care will prevent and control almost all cases of pregnancy gingivitis.

II. **Pregnancy tumor (pyogenic granuloma, granuloma gravidarum, angiogranuloma)**
A. **Incidence.** Less than 1 percent of pregnant women develop these fibrous masses.
B. **Cause.** Growth of pregnancy tumors can be triggered by a local irritant. Generally, the causes of these granulomas are the same as those causing pregnancy gingivitis.
C. **Pathogenesis and pathophysiology.** The pregnancy tumor is a highly vascular mass and resembles gingival enlargement. The lesion may consist of lymphocytes, plasma cells, and histiocytes. The lesions may develop anywhere on the gingiva and are usually localized. In severe cases, large pregnancy tumors may ulcerate the gingival surface. These masses may develop at any time during the pregnancy but are most common after the first trimester. Unless the masses are too fibrous to permit regression, the granuloma sometimes will diminish in size after delivery; however, it rarely disappears completely.
D. **Diagnosis.** The pregnancy tumor may appear pink to deep red in color. It resembles a soft, pedunculated, or sessile enlargement and is prone to bleeding. Quite often, it develops interdentally.

The examination of pregnancy tumors should be similar to the pregnancy gingivitis and periodontitis examination.
   E. **Management.** Conservative treatment is first indicated, that is, prophylaxis and oral hygiene instruction. If necessary, debridement of involved pockets may be suggested. Finally, if the gingival condition cannot be resolved, excision should be considered.
   F. **Prognosis.** The prognosis for pregnancy tumor is excellent, provided that the patient continues to use diligent oral hygiene.

III. **Decay (caries)**
   A. **Incidence.** Over 70 percent of pregnant women exhibit dental caries in various stages of bacterial advancement. This figure also reflects the caries rate of nonpregnant women of corresponding age groups, indicating that pregnancy has no substantial effect on the rate of formation or advancement of dental caries.
   B. **Mortality and morbidity.** No concern about mortality is warranted in the medically uncomplicated patient. The pregnant patient may expect to develop caries and to continue dentition deterioration due to existing caries at the same rate experienced immediately prior to pregnancy unless a change in diet or dental hygiene is instituted.
   C. **Cause.** Caries is caused by organic acids secreted by the enzymes of bacterial plaque acting on carbohydrates. The acids demineralize surface enamel, allowing invasion of the dentin.
   D. **Pathogenesis and pathophysiology.** Caries is an infectious disease that promotes localized destruction of the teeth, beginning with the external surface and progressing to internal tissues. Unchecked, caries can cause infection and destruction of the vital pulp matter. Although there exists a clinical impression that pregnancy initiates increased caries, studies show that dental caries formed during pregnancy are solely due to local factors.
   E. **Diagnosis.** Irregularities in tooth surfaces may indicate caries. Other symptoms include sensitivity to hot, cold, or sweets. Various levels of discomfort may accompany this disease. Visual examination of the tooth surface will detect the most obvious caries, that is, those that are large, prominent, or advanced. Though early caries are best detected by radiographic examination, a thorough radiographic examination should be postponed until after delivery, although radiographs may be taken if needed to deal with advanced lesions.
   F. **Management.** Initial treatment of caries requires removal of bacteria, currently accomplished by mechanical removal of the affected enamel or dentin. The prepared cavity is then filled with an amalgam or composite mixture. This filling material will adapt to fill the cavity recesses and will allow carving to restore tooth contours. The filling mixture is then hardened according to appropriate procedures.
   Advanced caries disease may require cast restorations to re-

store tooth structures damaged by decay. The most advanced stage of caries endangers the vital pulp tissues of the tooth. Suggested treatments include endodontic therapy or removal of the tooth.

G. **Prognosis.** Although it is possible for the decay associated with caries to arrest naturally, it is more probable that the disease will advance destructively without treatment. When treated appropriately, the prognosis is excellent. The filling or cast restoration must, however, be observed regularly and maintained to preserve its integrity.

IV. **Decalcification.** No histologic, chemical, or radiologic evidence exists to support the theory that pregnancy initiates decalcification of the mother's teeth to provide minerals to the fetus' developing dentition. Since enamel is avascular, calcium loss cannot occur. Also, once formed, teeth do not engage in calcium metabolism. Therefore, supplemental fluoride in prenatal diets for the prevention of decalcification is needless. Some etching may be caused by excessive emesis, but this is extremely rare.

DENTAL TREATMENT OF THE PRENATAL PATIENT

I. **Timing of treatment.** Most professionals agree that essential care can be provided at any point in the pregnancy. Stressful elective procedures are best postponed until after delivery. Timeliness of care is most important to protect the crucial developing stages of the fetus and to provide for the mother's comfort. Because organogenesis is completed by the onset of the second trimester, and because the mother is not yet susceptible to supine postural hypertension, breathing problems, leg swelling, and other problems associated with her physical enlargement, the second trimester is the best time to pursue necessary care.

II. **Treatment protocol**
A. **Examination.** Dental care should start as early as possible to enhance successful treatment and avoid the need for extensive or traumatic procedures later in the pregnancy. A complete medical and dental history should be taken and a visual examination performed.
B. **Radiographs.** Because of possible radiation exposure to the developing fetus, radiographs should be limited to the affected teeth. A lead apron or shield should be used to protect the mother's abdomen and reproductive organs.
C. **Oral hygiene.** To avoid the many periodontal complications associated with pregnancy's increased hormone levels, the prenatal patient should receive oral hygiene instructions and regular dental prophylaxis (every 4 to 6 months).
D. **Medical advisor.** Before beginning treatment, the patient's medical advisor should be contacted to discuss the patient's

medical history, dental conditions, and planned treatment management.
E. **Medications.** Proper use of antibiotics and pain-controlling agents is less detrimental to the fetus than the problems that can result from denial of the indicated medication. In all cases, drugs should be prescribed only with the full support of the physician.
  1. Tetracycline produces enamel pigmentation of hypoplasia in the fetus' primary teeth when administered during calcification of the developing dentition, approximately at 4 months' gestation. Calcification of permanent teeth at about 9 months' gestation is another time in which the developing dentition is susceptible to tetracycline staining. Thus, tetracycline should be avoided in pregnancy.
  2. Lidocaine (2%) with epinephrine (1 : 100 000) is the most acceptable choice for a local anesthetic. It gives 60 to 90 min pulpal anesthesia and 3 to 4 h of soft tissue anesthesia.
  3. Tissue retraction cord impregnated with epinephrine should not be used during any dental treatment.

BIBLIOGRAPHY

Drinkard CR, Deaton TG, Bawden JW. Enamal fluoride in nursing rats with mothers drinking water with high fluoride concentrations. J Dent Res 1985; 64:877–880.

Gier RE, Janes DR. Dental management of the pregnant patient. Dent Clin North Am 1983; 27:419–428.

Littner MM, Kaffe I, Tamse A, et al. Management of the pregnant patient. Quintessence Int 1984; 2:253–257.

Nathional Health and Medical Research Council. Guidelines for dental treatment: Dentistry and pregnancy. Aust Den J 1984; 29:265–266.

Ramazzotto LJ, Curro FA, Paterson JA, et al. Toxicological assessment of lidocaine in the pregnant rat. J Dent Res 1985; 64:1214–1218.

Safety of antimicrobial drugs in pregnancy. Med Lett 1985; 27:93–95.

CHAPTER 43

Obstetric Emergencies

Sharon T. Phelan
David C. Shaver

I. **Shoulder dystocia**
   A. **Incidence**
      1. The general incidence is 0.2 to 0.4 percent of all deliveries. However, the occurrence is only 0.16 percent if the mode of delivery is spontaneous vaginal delivery versus 4.7 percent if midforceps are used.
      2. One-third of shoulder dystocias occur in pregnancies of 42 weeks' gestation. This may be a reflection of the larger fetal size. It has been noted that in fetuses of nondiabetic mothers that weigh 4500 g, there is up to a 23 percent incidence of shoulder dystocia. This figure is increased if the mother is diabetic.
   B. **Morbidity and mortality**
      1. Fetal injuries include fractured clavicle, dislocated shoulder, and brachial plexus injury. There is a 39 percent injury rate, with as much as a 10 percent chance of long-term neurologic disability. It is important to realize that most iatrogenic brachial plexus injuries occur during the initial efforts to release the shoulders. The downward or twisting traction on the head when the shoulders are locked can lead to a brachial plexus injury on the side of the anterior shoulder. By contrast, spontaneous injury to the brachial plexus tends to occur on the side of the posterior shoulder. In cases of severe dystocia, asphyxia may cause death (up to 7 percent) or severe neurologic compromise (up to 30 percent).
      2. Maternal trauma is primarily soft tissue trauma from the large epistiotomy and from vaginal manipulations. There is a risk of uterine rupture if excessive fundal pressure is used. Finally, due to the combination of a large infant and extensive manipulation, there can be uterine atony with a postpartum hemorrhage.
   C. **Cause**
      1. In shoulder dystocia, the anterior shoulder rotates anteriorly following the delivery of the vertex, but because of the

relative disproportion of the shoulder to the pelvis, the anterior shoulder rotates to a position above and behind the symphysis pubis. Rather than being delivered by the anterior rotation, it becomes impacted above the symphysis.

2. There are other causes of dystocia after the birth of the head that are not related to true shoulder dystocia. These include a short umbilical cord, abdominal or thoracic enlargement (i.e., tumor), locked or conjoined twins, and uterine constriction ring.

D. **Pathogenesis**
   1. Risk factors include anything that would cause a relatively "borderline pelvis," such as a large infant (for whatever reason) or a small pelvis.
      a. A small pelvis may be related to small stature or nongynecoid pelvis.
      b. Numerous factors may cause a relatively macrosomic infant, including maternal diabetes, excessive maternal weight gain, postdates, advanced maternal age, increased parity, or maternal obesity. The presence of maternal glucose intolerance and/or fetal weight of 4000 g predicts three-fourths of all cases of shoulder dystocia.

E. **Diagnosis**
   1. A prolonged second stage, excessive molding, and failure of the fetus to descend with adequate maternal effort should alert the obstetrician to a situation that has an increased risk of shoulder dystocia. Thus, before an operative vaginal delivery, one should critically assess the risks of dystocia.
   2. Shoulder dystocia should be assumed when, after delivery of the fetal head, there occurs a recoil of the head against the perineum, failure of spontaneous restitution of the head, and normal traction from below and pressure from above fail to deliver the child.

F. **General principles**
   1. The best management is **prevention** by critically evaluating the risk of dystocia before the use of forceps in a secondary descent disorder. It has been suggested that in any delivery at increased risk of shoulder dystocia, one should forgo suctioning the infant after delivery of the head and proceed immediately to delivery of the shoulders. This may prevent the shoulders from completing their rotation into an anterior-posterior lie.
   2. The most important factor when confronted with shoulder dystocia is to approach the problem in a methodical, logical way. Avoidance of panic and excessive traction on the fetal head will obviate many fetal injuries. It must be remembered that the decine of pH due to asphyxia is 0.2 U/5 min. In addition, fundal pressure is contraindicated, since this will only add to impaction of the fetal shoulders and may result in maternal injury.

G. Management — specific procedures

1. Be sure that there is an **adequate episiotomy** and that the bladder is empty. Some advocate trying the McRoberts maneuver before cutting an episiotomy. If this maneuver does not work, then a generous episiotomy is clearly indicated. A mediolateral episiotomy should be considered.

2. The **McRobert's maneuver** consists of sharp flexion of the mother's thighs against her abdomen. This straightens the sacrum relative to the lumbar spine with cephalad rotation of the symphysis (Fig. 43.1). The inlet is brought into the plan perpendicular to the maximum maternal expulsive force. This, with firm **suprapubic** (not fundal) pressure, may allow delivery of the anterior shoulder (Fig. 43.2).

3. While these maneuvers are being attempted, additional assistance including anesthesia should be summoned.

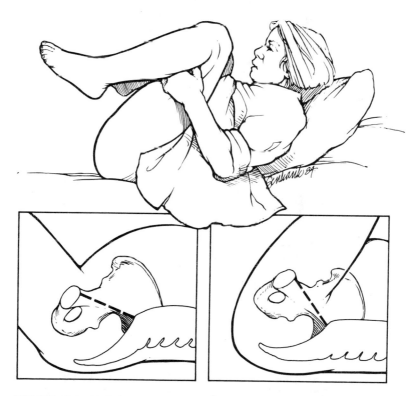

FIGURE 43.1. McRobert's maneuver: Sharp ventral rotation of both maternal hips brings the pelvic inlet and outlet into a more vertical alignment, facilitating delivery of the fetal shoulders. (From Gabbe SG, Niebyl JR, Simpson JL. Obstetrics: Normal and Problem Pregnancies. New York: Churchill Livingstone; 1986:481. Reprinted with permission.)

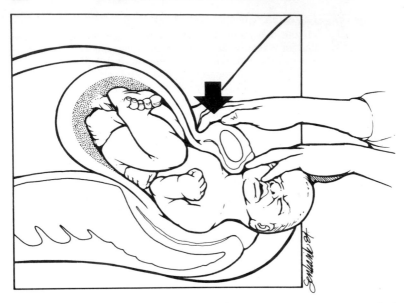

FIGURE 43.2 Moderate suprapubic pressure may disimpact the anterior fetal shoulder. (From Gabbe SG, Niebyl JR, Simpson JL. Obstetrics: Normal and Problem Pregnancies. New York: Churchill Livingstone; 1986:479. Reprinted with permission.)

4. A modified Woods Screw procedure can be tried (Fig. 43.3). This involves placing pressure on the posterior aspect of the posterior shoulder in an attempt to rotate the shoulders to an oblique lie, which may afford more room. This may work with mild dystocias but is less successful with severe cases. If the posterior shoulder cannot be reached, this is an omnious sign for successful vaginal delivery. By this point, if the patient does not have effective regional anesthesia, one should consider general anesthesia if available.

5. If the infant is still trapped, attempts should be directed to delivering the posterior shoulder. (If this cannot be felt, one should proceed to a cephalic replacement.) The practitioner's hand is placed in the vagina, the fetal elbow is flexed, and the forearm is grasped and pulled out. The posterior shoulder becomes engaged in the pelvis, and delivery should be possible. If not, the infant is rotated 180°, thereby resulting in delivery of the anterior shoulder. This procedure carries a high risk of humeral or clavicle fractures (Fig. 43.4).

6. If none of the above maneuvers are successful, a cephalic replacement (Zavanelli maneuver) with cesarean delivery is indicated. The practitioner's palm is applied to the fetal vertex, flexing the head and pushing it up to the level of the

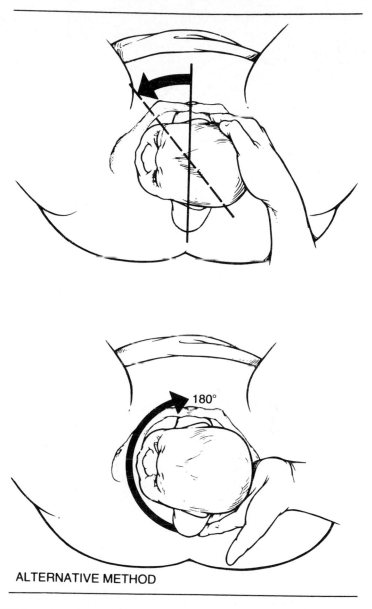

ALTERNATIVE METHOD

FIGURE 43.3. Pressure placed on the posterior aspect of the fetal shoulder may rotate the shoulder to an oblique lie and disimpact the anterior shoulder. (From Gabbe SG, Niebyl JR, Simpson JL. Obstetrics: Normal and Problem Pregnancies. New York: Churchill Livingstone; 1986:480. Reprinted with permission.)

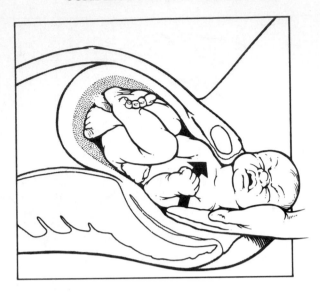

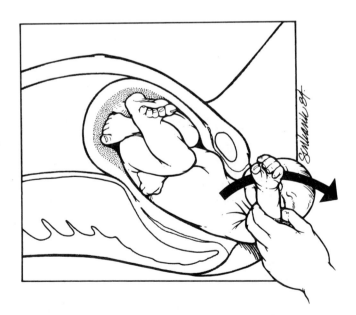

FIGURE 43.4 The posterior arm is delivered by inserting a hand into the posterior vagina and ventrally rotating the arm of the shoulder with delivery over the perineum. (From Gabbe SG, Niebyl JR, Simpson JL. Obstetrics: Normal and Problem Pregnancies. New York: Churchill Livingstone; 1986:480. Reprinted with permission.)

ischial spines. This may require general anesthesia or a tocolytic agent and an assistant to maintain the elevated position while a cesarean section is accomplished.

7. After delivery of the infant and the placenta, the mother must be carefully evaluated for vaginal or uterine trauma and uterine atony.

II. Cord prolapse

A. **Incidence.** Cord prolapse occurs in 0.18 percent of deliveries (range, 0.14 to 0.61 percent), with over 95 percent occurring within the hospital.

A. **Morbidity and mortality.** Maternal morbidity and mortality are related to complications from the emergent cesarean section used to deliver the largest proportion of these infants. Fetal morbidity and mortality are related to the delay from occurrence of the prolapse to delivery and the degree of circulatory compromise and hypoxia incurred by the fetus.

C. **Cause.** Risk factors are any situations that compromise or prevent good application of a presenting part to the lower uterine segment at the time of rupture of the membranes.

1. Multiparity, prematurity, multiple gestation, and hydramnios all increase the risk of malpresentation or floating presentation.

2. Malpresentation is clearly a risk, with a breech presentation as a group having a risk of 1/40 of cord prolapse and a transverse lie having relative risk of 1/20, in contrast to a vertex presentation, which has a risk of 1/714.

3. Iatrogenic prolapse can occur secondary to obstetric interventions such as artificial rupture of membranes, placement of forceps or a scalp electrode, or obtaining fetal scalp blood for pH. With each of these maneuvers, the presenting part may be elevated out of the pelvis.

4. Placental problems, including marginal previa that partially fill the lower uterine segment, prevent good application of the presenting part.

D. **Pathogenesis/pathophysiology.** The failure of the presenting part to occlude adequately to the lower uterine segment allows the cord to slip past the presenting part. The cord, in turn, becomes occluded with further progression of labor as the presenting part descends. Some have proposed that fetuses with poor cord turgor are at greater risk of prolapse.

E. **Differential diagnosis**

1. If the cord is palpable, there is no differential diagnosis. However, in cases of occult prolapse, other causes of cord compression need to be considered.

2. Diagnosis is based on palpation or visualization of the cord. Variable decelerations or prolonged bradycardia consistent with cord compression, with no other cause, may represent an occult prolapse.

F. **Management**
   1. Since an expeditious delivery is the main form of management, the majority of mothers have an emergent cesarean section.
   2. In situations where delivery must be delayed, the following procedure may help avoid fetal compromise until delivery. This should be done if the fetus is alive and greater than 26 weeks' gestation.
      a. The bladder is filled rapidly with 500 to 700 mL of sterile saline, using a No. 16 or 18 French Foley catheter.
      b. A tocolytic is administered intravenously and titrated by contractions and symptoms (ritrodrine, 50 mg in 500 mL at a rate of 2.5 to 4.0 mL/min).
      c. If the cord has prolapsed out of the vagina, it is gently returned and the introitus closed with a wet, warm gauze tampon.
      d. With this management, it is unnecessary to elevate the presenting part manually. Fifty-one cases managed this way have been reported, with a mean prolapse to delivery interval of 36 min (range, 15 to 80 min). The mean 5-min Apgar score was 9.5, and only three were less than 7. All infants did well postpartum.

III. **Amniotic fluid embolism (AFE)**
   A. **Incidence.** The incidence is approximately 1/40 000 pregnancies.
   B. **Morbidity and mortality.** AFE accounts for 4 to 10 percent of all obstetric maternal deaths. Up to 80 percent of the women with AFE die, with 25 to 50 percent dying within the first hour. Fetal mortality is only 40 percent, since many of these cases occur during delivery and the infant can be saved.
   C. **Cause.** Obstetric events are associated with AFE, although the actual cause is still unknown.
      1. Patients with an increased risk of AFE include those with high parity (88 percent of women with an AFE are multiparous), advanced maternal age (mean age, 32), or a macrosomic fetus, or those who have experienced blunt abdominal trauma.
      2. Procedures that have been associated with AFE include third-trimester amniocentesis, insertion of a uterine pressure catheter, the use of oxytocin (22 percent of the cases), and abortion. The last includes primarily saline-induced abortions, but there have been reports of emboli during suction curettage of a missed abortion in the second trimester.
      3. Labor events that may increase the risk of AFE include tumultuous labor (28 percent of the cases), uterine rupture, abruption, and uterine or cervical tears.
      4. Meconium staining appears to make the fluid more lethal.
   D. **Pathogenesis.** The clinical development of AFE is a biphasic process.

1. The initial response of the pulmonary vasculature to pathologic amniotic fluid and debris of fetal origin is intensive vasospasm. This, in turn, produces severe pulmonary hypertension and profound hypoxia. This reaction is transient, lasting for less than 60 min.
2. If the initial response is survived, then there is a secondary phase of hemodynamic compromise due to left ventricular failure and normal right ventricular function. In addition, there is a component of noncardiogenic pulmonary edema.
3. Finally, the AFE can activate the complement system, which in turn initiates the coagulation system, causing disseminated intravascular coagulation (DIC).

E. Differential diagnosis
1. The differential diagnosis includes any precipitous event that would cause cardiovascular collapse and hypoxia (Table 43.1).
2. The diagnosis must be made quickly, since most patients die within the first hour.
    a. The only symptom the patient may complain of prior to collapse is sudden dyspnea.
    b. The clinical signs of cyanosis, hypotension with cardiovascular collapse and cardiac arrest, shock, and coma will quickly follow. From 10 to 20 percent of the victims of AFE will have seizures. One may find bibasilar rates or pink, frothy sputum.
    c. If the patients survive the first hour, 40 to 50 percent develop coagulopathy. This is compounded by uterine hemorrhage from uterine atony.
    d. To confirm the diagnosis, aspiration of blood from the central circulation via a catheter and histologic confirmation of the presence of fetal squamous material is necessary, along with the proper clinical presentation.
    e. Laboratory findings may help to confirm the clinical suspicions, assuming that the patient survives long enough for these evaluations to be performed.

TABLE 43.1. Events to Be Considered in the Differential Diagnosis of AFE

Anesthesia reaction

Aspiration pneumonia

Eclampsia

Myocardial infarction

Septic shock

Uterine rupture

Venous or air embolism

(1) Central pressure monitoring will show increased pulmonary capillary wedge pressure (PCWP), pulmonary artery pressure, and central venous pressure. There is decreased cardiac output due to left ventricular dysfunction and, in turn, hypotension. There also appears to be decreased systemic vascular resistance, compounding the hypotension and poor cardiac output.

(2) An electrocardiogram will show right heart strain and tachycardia.

(3) A chest x-ray will show engorged pulmonary vessels, pulmonary edema, and bilateral infiltrates (70 percent).

(4) A lung scan may confirm a ventilation-perfusion defect.

(5) Arterial blood gases will show decreased P_{O_2} and increased P_{CO_2} with decreased pH due to a mixed respiratory-metabolic acidosis.

(6) Clotting studies show increased fibrinogen and fibrin split products, with a prolonged prothrombin time, a prolonged partial thromboplastin time, and decreased platelets.

F. Management. Management focuses on aggressive life support through the biphasic response. Given this, the principles of ABCD of resuscitation pertain: airway, breathing, circulation, and delivery.

1. Oxygenation must be ensured. This involves obtaining a secure airway, effective ventilation, and supplementary oxygen.

2. The maintenance of cardiac output and blood pressure is crucial. Two large-bore intravenous (IV) line should be started immediately. Then isotonic crystalloids (normal saline or lactated Ringer's solution) should be administered at a rate determined by the patient's sensorium, blood pressure, and urine output (> 50 mL/h), and PCWP (> 14 mmHg). Other forms of diagnostic and therapeutic access must be secured, including a Foley catheter, an arterial line, and potentially a pulmonary line. With central line placement, one must remember that DIC may occur, with the resultant risk of hematoma formation. The use of pressor agents such as dopamine may be needed to maintain blood pressure.

3. One must anticipate and treat DIC with red blood cells, platelets, and fresh frozen plasma as needed. There is insufficient data to warrant routine heparin or aminocaproic acid use. In cases of severe DIC unresponsive to replacement management, one should consider heparin use.

4. Surveillance of uterine atony with resultant hemorrhage is important due to the myometrial depressant effects of AFE.

IV. **Acute uterine inversion**
  A. **Incidence.** Although acute uterine inversion may vary at different locations, the incidence is generally reported to be about 1/2000 to 1/2500 deliveries.
  B. **Morbidity and mortality.** In older studies, maternal morbidity ranged from 15 to 25 percent. With current management methods and blood banking, maternal death from the associated postpartum hemorrhage is rare.
  C. **Pathogenesis and pathophysiology.** Due to the rarity of this event and the inability to predict its occurrence, controlled studies on its true pathogenesis have not been done. However, a number of apparent risk factors have been identified.
     1. Uterine atony may predispose to inversion.
     2. Since the fundal region of the uterus has the least support, any excessive traction on the mucosal surface of the fundus may serve as a nidus for an inversion. Undue traction on the umbilical cord may increase this risk. Although this has been a commonly quoted cause of inversion, the association is difficult to confirm.
     3. Any problem that interferes with normal placental separation increases the risk of inversion. Therefore an abnormal uterine configuration or accreta are risk factors.
  D. **Diagnosis.** In the case of a complete inversion, the diagnosis is easy since the uterus extends out of the introitus. In cases of partial inversion, the first indication is commonly a significant postpartum hemorrhage with associated pain and rapidly developing shock. The bimanual exam may reveal the uterus protruding through the cervix (2° inversion) or a uterus that seems too small for an immediated postpartum uterus (a partial inversion).
  E. **Management.** The primary objective is to replace the uterus and then the vascular volume losses.
     1. If pitocin is being infused, it should be stopped immediately.
     2. Since this can rapidly result in hypovolemic shock, additional assistance including anesthesia should be requested immediately.
     3. One should try to replace the uterus immediately. If the placenta is still attached, it should initially be left in place. The uterus should be replaced in the reverse order in which it was inverted.
     4. While uterine replacement is being attempted, a large-bore line should be started, with blood obtained for type and crossmatch for 4 U and a complete blood count. Isotonic saline solutions should be used (normal saline or Ringer's lactate), with the rate determined by the clinical situation.
     5. If one is unable to replace the uterus, administer
        a. MgSO$_4$, 2 to 4 g IV at a rate of 1 g/min or
        b. Terbutaline, 0.25 mg IV.
     6. If one is still unable to replace the uterus, the placenta

should be removed to debulk the volume of uterine mass and reattempt uterine replacement.

7. The hydrostatic (O'Sullivan) technique may then be attempted if manual replacement is unsuccessful. Briefly, this consists of replacement of the uterus in the vagina. A large-bore catheter is inserted in the vagina, and a receptacle filled with saline is then attached and elevated several feet above the level of the introitus (e.g., enema bag and tubing). The uterus is then replaced by direct pressure on the fundus combined with dilatation of the cervical ring due to lateral pressure on the vagina.

8. If one still is unable to replace the uterus, general anesthesia with a halothane-type agent can be employed as the uterine relaxant. This also prepares the patient for exploratory laparotomy and operative replacement of the uterus, which is the last option.

9. Once the uterus is replaced, the placenta should be removed manually if it is still attached and the uterus held in place until oxytocin or methergine produces appropriate uterine tone.

10. These patients may experience reinversion during the immediate postpartum period, so close surveillance is indicated.

11. Postpartum management needs to address two concerns: infection and blood loss. Although prophylactic antibiotics have not proven to be useful, one should consider using them, since aseptic technique is usually impossible in these emergencies. A better estimate of blood loss at delivery can be provided by taking the predelivery hematocrit, subtracting the predischarge hematocrit, and multiplying by 150 mL. This figure should be added to the number of milliliters of blood replacement to determine the final estimated blood loss.

V. Cardiac arrest

A. Incidence

1. Although the incidence of cardiac arrest in pregnancy is unknown, it is becoming less common, as maternal mortality in general has declined over recent years. Currently, maternal mortality is < 10/100 000.

2. As maternal medical care has improved, the incidence of maternal deaths secondary to chronic medical problem has decreased, and acute events have thus become more important as precipitating events for cardiac arrest and subsequent maternal death.

B. Morbidity and mortality

1. **Maternal survival** and the long-term prognosis following cardiopulmonary resuscitation are unknown. However, since most cases are secondary to acute events, successful resuscitation is thought to be associated with a favorable

long-term outcome. Limited reports in the medical literature suggest that if initial efforts are unsuccessful, prompt delivery of the fetus (within 5 min) is associated with an improvement in resuscitative efforts and in the subsequent maternal outcome.

2. **Fetal survival** following maternal cardiopulmonary arrest is well established. References to neonatal survival as the result of postmortem cesarean section have appeared throughout the ages. As the cause of maternal cardiac arrest has changed, the survival rate has increased. Additionally, fetal survival and subsequent outcome are related to the timing of delivery following cardiac arrest. Prompt delivery is associated with an improved neurologic outcome (Table 43.2). Virtually all cardiac arrests occurring during the third trimester may be associated with fetal survival.

C. **Cause.** The contributing factors leading to cardiac arrest are different in the obstetric patient than in the nonpregnant one.

1. Cardiac arrest in nonpregnant women of childbearing age is very rare, and frequently is due to either congenital or acquired (e.g., cardiomyopathy) heart disease.

2. The causes of cardiac arrest in pregnancy have changed over time due to improved medical care in general and a lower incidence of women with a chronic medical problem of childbearing age. As a result, most cases of cardiac arrest are related to acute events such as anesthetic complications, pulmonary embolism, trauma, drug intoxication, and hemorrhagic and septic shock. The presence of preexisting medical complications, however, increases the risk.

3. Sudden cardiac arrest is classically separated into arrhythmic events and circulatory collapse. Acute deaths typically result from arrhythmia, with ventricular fibrillation as the

Table 43.2. Outcome of Surviving Infants Delivered by Postmortem Cesarean Section Based on Time Interval from Delivery to Maternal Death

TIME INTERVAL (MIN)	NO. OF PATIENTS/OUTCOME
0–5	42 (normal outcome)
6–10	7 (normal outcome) 1 (mild neurologic sequelae)
11–15	6 (normal outcome) 1 (severe neurologic sequelae)
16–20	1 (severe neurologic sequelae)
21+	2 (severe neurologic sequelae) 1 (normal outcome)

Source: Katz et al. 1986; 68:574.

final event. In contrast, circulatory failure usually occurs in patients with a longer duration of illness, with underlying medical problems such as renal disease, cancer, or sepsis.

D. Diagnosis. By definition cardiac arrest is abrupt. Loss of consciousness is uniform, although mentation may be present during the onset. Therefore, acute loss of consciousness with absence of spontaneous respiration and a palpable pulse will be found. Electrocardiographic monitoring will usually reveal ventricular fibrillation (often preceded by ventricular tachycardia) or asystole.

E. Management

1. Although rare occurrences of spontaneous resolution of cardiac arrests have been described, death can be presumed to occur within minutes if intervention is not undertaken.

2. The initial response is to establish whether or not cardiac arrest has occurred. In monitored patients, the electrocardiogram will reveal the presence of arrhythmia. In unmonitored patients, it must be determined whether a pulse is present or if the patient is conscious or arousable. The presence of gasping or stridor may indicate aspiration of a foreign body, which could be relieved by performing the Heimlich maneuver.

3. Once the diagnosis of cardiac arrest is confirmed, basic life support or cardiopulmonary resuscitation (CPR) is begun. The purpose of CPR is to maintain tissue perfusion until definitive therapy is successful. After establishing unresponsiveness, a call for help should be initiated and the patient should be positioned on a flat, firm surface. The uterus should then be displaced laterally, either manually or by placing a wedge under the right hip.

4. The principles of basic life support emphasize the ABC approach to resuscitation. In pregnancy, a fourth component, delivery (D) is added (Table 43.3).

5. The rationales for prompt delivery are many. Since CPR generally can be expected to generate only about 30 percent of normal cardiac output, and since obstruction of the vena cava by the gravid uterus will decrease this amount further, delivery should be associated with a more successful outcome, as suggested by anecdotal reports. Additionally, rapid delivery should decrease the likelihood of both fetal death and perinatal hypoxia, with a better neonatal outcome. Currently, the recommendation is to proceed with perimortem cesarean section within 4 min if CPR is unsuccessful. However, if a longer period of time has elapsed since maternal collapse, and if the fetus is still alive and viable, a cesarean section should be performed, since successful neonatal outcomes have been reported and the beneficial maternal effects of delivery would still be anticipated.

Table 43.3. Basic Life Support in Pregnancy

Establish unresponsiveness.
Call for help and give the location.
Position the patient on a firm, flat surface and displace the uterus.
Proceed with the ABCDs of CPR.
1. Airway
   a. Open the airway with the head tilt and chin lift maneuver.
2. Breathing
   a. Administer two breaths by mouth-to-mouth resuscitation or Ambu bag.
3. Circulation
   a. Begin chest compressions, depressing the sternum 3 to 5 cm, at a rate of 80/min.
   b. Administer 15 chest compressions and then two breaths for one-person CPR.
   c. Administer five chest compressions followed by one breath for two-person CPR.
      Reasses for the pulse every four cycles.
4. Delivery
   a. Perform perimorterm cesarean section in 4 min if CPR is unsuccessful.
   b. Do not worry about a sterile field, draping, and so on.
   c. Continue CPR after the infant is delivered.

BIBLIOGRAPHY

Acker DB, Sachs BP, Friedman EA. Risk factors for shoulder dystocia. Obstet Gynecol 1985; 66:762–768.

Brar H, Greenspoon J, Platt U, et al. Acute puerperal uterine inversion — new approach to management. J Reprod Med 1989; 34:173–177.

Clark S. Amniotic fluid embolism. Female Patient 1989; 14:49–61.

Harris B. Shoulder dystocia. Female Patient 1990; 15:69–76.

Katz VL, Dotters DJ, Droegemueller W. Perimortem cesarean delivery. Obstet Gynecol 1986; 68:571–576.

Katz Z, Shoham Z, Lancet M, et al. Management of labor with umbilical cord prolapse: A 5-year study. Obstet Gynecol 1988; 72:278–281.

Kooning P, Paul R, Campbell C. Umbilical cord prolapse: A contemporary look. J Reprod Med 1990; 35:690–692.

Lee RV, Rodgers BD, White LM, et al. Cardiopulmonary resuscitation of pregnant women. Am J Med 1986; 81:311–318.

Levy H, Meier P, Makowski E. Umbilical cord prolapse. Obstet Gynecol 1984; 64:499–502.

O'Leary JA, Leonetti HB. Shoulder dystocia: Prevention and treatment. AJOG 1990; 162:5–9.

Price T, Baker V, Cefalo R. Amniotic fluid embolism. Three case reports with a review of the literature. Ob Gyn Survey 1985; 40:462–475.

Shah-Hosseine R, Evrard J. Puerperal uterine inversion. Obstet Gynecol 1989; 73:567–570.

Appendix A

Immunization during Pregnancy

Immunization during Pregnancy

IMMUNO-BIOLOGIC AGENT	RISK FROM DISEASE TO PREGNANT WOMAN	RISK FROM DISEASE TO FETUS OR NEONATE	TYPE OF IMMUNIZING AGENT	RISK FROM IMMUNIZING AGENT TO FETUS	INDICATIONS FOR IMMUNIZATION DURING PREGNANCY	DOSE SCHEDULE*	COMMENTS
			LIVE VIRUS VACCINES				
Measles	Significant morbidity, low mortality; not altered by pregnancy	Significant increase in abortion rate; may cause malformations	Live attenuated virus vaccine	None confirmed	Contraindicated (see immune globulins)	Single dose SC, preferably as measles-mumps-rubella†	Vaccination of susceptible women should be part of postpartum care
Mumps	Low morbidity and mortality; not altered by pregnancy	Probable increased rate of abortion in first trimester	Live attenuated virus vaccine	None confirmed	Contraindicated	Single dose SC, preferably as measles-mumps-rubella	Vaccination of susceptible women should be part of postpartum care

Disease	Effect of pregnancy on disease	Effect on fetus or neonate	Type of immunizing agent	Risk from immunizing agent to fetus	Indications for vaccination during pregnancy	Dose schedule	Comments
Poliomyelitis	No increased incidence in pregnancy, but may be more severe if it does occur	Anoxic fetal damage reported; 50% mortality in neonatal disease	Live attenuated virus (oral polio vaccine [OPV]) and enhanced-potency inactivated virus (e-IPV) vaccine‡	None confirmed	Not routinely recommended for women in U.S., except persons at increased risk of exposure	*Primary:* 2 doses of e-IPV SC at 4–8-week intervals and a 3rd dose 6–12 months after the 2nd dose. *Immediate protection:* 1 dose OPV orally (in outbreak setting)	Vaccine indicated for susceptible pregnant women traveling in endemic areas or in other high-risk situations
Rubella	Low morbidity and mortality; not altered by pregnancy	High rate of abortion and congenital rubella syndrome	Live attenuated virus vaccine	None confirmed	Contraindicated	Single dose SC, preferably as measles-mumps-rubella	Teratogenicity of vaccine is theoretic, not confirmed to date; vaccination of susceptible women should be part of postpartum care
Yellow fever	Significant morbidity and mortality; not altered by pregnancy	Unknown	Live attenuated virus vaccine	Unknown	Contraindicated except if exposure is unavoidable	Single dose SC	Postponement of travel preferable to vaccination, if possible

(Continued)

581

Immunization during Pregnancy (Continued)

IMMUNO-BIOLOGIC AGENT	RISK FROM DISEASE TO PREGNANT WOMAN	RISK FROM DISEASE TO FETUS OR NEONATE	TYPE OF IMMUNIZING AGENT	RISK FROM IMMUNIZING AGENT TO FETUS	INDICATIONS FOR IMMUNIZATION DURING PREGNANCY	DOSE SCHEDULE*	COMMENTS
			INACTIVATED VIRUS VACCINES				
Influenza	Possible increase in morbidity and mortality during epidemic of new antigenic strain	Possible increased abortion rate; no malformations confirmed	Inactivated virus vaccine	None confirmed	Women with serious underlying diseases; public health authorities to be consulted for current recommendation	One dose IM every year	
Rabies	Near 100% fatality; not altered by pregnancy	Determined by maternal disease	Killed virus vaccine	Unknown	Indications for prophylaxis not altered by pregnancy; each case considered individually	Public health authorities to be consulted for indications, dosage, and route of administration	

582

Vaccine	Effect of pregnancy on disease	Effect of disease on pregnancy	Type of vaccine	Risk to fetus	Indications	Dose	Comments
Hepatitis B	Possible increased severity during third trimester	Possible increase in abortion rate and prematurity; neonatal hepatitis can occur; high risk of newborn carrier state	Recombinant vaccine	None reported	Pre- and post-exposure for women at risk of infection	Three- or four-dose series IM	Used with hepatitis B immune globulin for some exposures; exposed newborn needs vaccination as soon as possible

INACTIVATED BACTERIAL VACCINES

Vaccine	Effect of pregnancy on disease	Effect of disease on pregnancy	Type of vaccine	Risk to fetus	Indications	Dose	Comments
Cholera	Significant morbidity and mortality; more severe during third trimester	Increased risk of fetal death during third-trimester maternal illness	Killed bacterial vaccine	None confirmed	Indications not altered by pregnancy; vaccination recommended only in unusual outbreak situations	Single dose SC or IM, depending on manufacturer's recommendations when indicated	
Plague	Significant morbidity and mortality; not altered by pregnancy	Determined by maternal disease	Killed bacterial vaccine	None reported	Selective vaccination of exposed persons	Public health authorities to be consulted for indications, dosage, and route of administration	

(Continued)

Immunization during Pregnancy *(Continued)*

IMMUNO-BIOLOGIC AGENT	RISK FROM DISEASE TO PREGNANT WOMAN	RISK FROM DISEASE TO FETUS OR NEONATE	TYPE OF IMMUNIZING AGENT	RISK FROM IMMUNIZING AGENT TO FETUS	INDICATIONS FOR IMMUNIZATION DURING PREGNANCY	DOSE SCHEDULE*	COMMENTS
Pneumococcus	No increased risk during pregnancy; no increase in severity of disease	Unknown	Polyvalent polysaccharide vaccine	No data available on use during pregnancy	Indications not altered by pregnancy; vaccine used only for high-risk individuals	In adults, 1 SC or IM dose only; consider repeat dose in 6 years for high-risk individuals	

| Typhoid | Significant morbidity and mortality; not altered by pregnancy | Unknown | Killed or live attenuated oral bacterial vaccine | None confirmed | Not recommended routinely except for close, continued exposure or travel to endemic areas | *Killed:* *Primary:* 2 injections SC at least 4 weeks apart. *Booster:* Single dose SC or ID (depending on type of product used) every 3 years. *Oral:* *Primary:* 4 doses on alternate days *Booster:* Schedule not yet determined |

(Continued)

Immunization during Pregnancy *(Continued)*

IMMUNO-BIOLOGIC AGENT	RISK FROM DISEASE TO PREGNANT WOMAN	RISK FROM DISEASE TO FETUS OR NEONATE	TYPE OF IMMUNIZING AGENT	RISK FROM IMMUNIZING AGENT TO FETUS	INDICATIONS FOR IMMUNIZATION DURING PREGNANCY	DOSE SCHEDULE*	COMMENTS
			TOXOIDS				
Tetanus-diphtheria	Severe morbidity; tetanus mortality 30%, diphtheria mortality 10%; unaltered by pregnancy	Neonatal tetanus mortality 60%	Combined tetanus-diphtheria toxoids preferred: adult tetanus-diphtheria formulation	None confirmed	Lack of primary series, or no booster within past 10 years	*Primary:* 2 doses IM at 1–2-month interval with a 3rd dose 6–12 months after the 2nd. *Booster:* Single dose IM every 10 years, after completion of primary series	Updating of immune status should be part of antepartum care

SPECIFIC IMMUNE GLOBULINS

Hepatitis B	Possible increased severity during third trimester	Possible increase in abortion rate and prematurity; neonatal hepatitis can occur; high risk of carriage in newborn	Hepatitis B immune globulin	None reported	Postexposure prophylaxis	Depends on exposure; consult Immunization Practices Advisory Committee recommendations (IM)	Usually given with HBV vaccine; exposed newborn needs immediate postexposure prophylaxis
Rabies	Near 100% fatality; not altered by pregnancy	Determined by maternal disease	Rabies immune globulin	None reported	Postexposure prophylaxis	Half dose at injury site, half dose in deltoid	Used in conjunction with rabies killed virus vaccine
Tetanus	Severe morbidity; mortality 21%	Neonatal tetanus mortality 60%	Tetanus immune globulin	None reported	Postexposure prophylaxis	One dose IM	Used in conjunction with tetanus toxoid

(Continued)

Immunization during Pregnancy (Continued)

IMMUNO-BIOLOGIC AGENT	RISK FROM DISEASE TO PREGNANT WOMAN	RISK FROM DISEASE TO FETUS OR NEONATE	TYPE OF IMMUNIZING AGENT	RISK FROM IMMUNIZING AGENT TO FETUS	INDICATIONS FOR IMMUNIZATION DURING PREGNANCY	DOSE SCHEDULE*	COMMENTS
Varicella	Possible increase in severe varicella pneumonia	Can cause congenital varicella with increased mortality in neonatal period; very rarely causes congenital defects	Varicella-zoster immune globulin (obtained from the American Red Cross)	None reported	Can be considered for healthy pregnant women exposed to varicella to protect against maternal, not congenital, infection	One dose IM within 96 hours of exposure	Indicated also for newborns of mothers who developed varicella within 4 days prior to delivery or 2 days following delivery; approx. 90–95% of adults are immune to varicella; not indicated for prevention of congenital varicella

STANDARD IMMUNE GLOBULINS

	Effect of pregnancy on disease	Effect on fetus/neonate	Immune globulin	Adverse effects	Indications	Dose	Comments
Hepatitis A	Possible increased severity during third trimester	Probable increase in abortion rate and prematurity; possible transmission to neonate at delivery if mother is incubating the virus or is acutely ill at that time	Standard immune globulin	None reported	Postexposure prophylaxis	0.02 ml/kg IM in one dose of immune globulin	Immune globulin should be given as soon as possible and within 2 weeks of exposure; infants born to mothers who are incubating the virus or are acutely ill at delivery should receive one dose of 0.5 ml as soon as possible after birth
Measles	Significant morbidity, low mortality; not altered by pregnancy	Significant increase in abortion rate; may cause malformations	Standard immune globulin	None reported	Postexposure prophylaxis	0.25 ml/kg IM in one dose of immune globulin, up to 15 ml	Unclear if it prevents abortion; must be given within 6 days of exposure

*Abbreviations: SC = subcutaneously; PO = orally; IM = intramuscularly; ID = intradermally.

†Two doses necessary for adequate vaccination of students entering institutions of higher education, newly hired medical personnel, and international travelers.

‡Inactivated polio vaccine recommended for nonimmunized adults at increased risk.

Source: American College of Obstetricians and Gynecologists. Immunization during Pregnancy. ACOG Technical Bulletin No. 160. Washington, DC. Copyright © 1991.

Appendix B

Ultrasound Values in Pregnancy

Table 1. Estimation of Gestational Age from Biparietal Diameter

BIPARIETAL DIAMETER (MM)	GESTATIONAL AGE (WK)*	BIPARIETAL DIAMETER (MM)	GESTATIONAL AGE (WK)*
20	12.0	60	23.9
21	12.0	61	24.2
22	12.6	62	24.6
23	12.8	63	24.9
24	13.2	64	25.3
25	13.5	65	25.6
26	13.7	66	26.0
27	14.0	67	26.4
28	14.3	68	26.7
29	14.5	69	27.1
30	14.8	70	27.5
31	15.1	71	27.9
32	15.3	72	28.3
33	15.6	73	28.7
34	15.9	74	29.1
35	16.2	75	29.5
36	16.4	76	30.0
37	16.7	77	30.3
38	17.0	78	30.8
39	17.3	79	31.2
40	17.6	80	31.6
41	17.9	81	32.1
42	18.2	82	32.6
43	18.5	83	33.0
44	18.8	84	33.5
45	19.1	85	34.0
46	19.4	86	34.5
47	19.6	87	35.0
48	20.0	88	35.5
49	20.3	89	36.1
50	20.6	90	36.6
51	20.9	91	37.2
52	21.2	92	37.8
53	21.5	93	38.3
54	21.9	94	39.0
55	22.2	95	39.7
56	22.5	96	40.3
57	22.8	97	41.0
58	23.2	98	41.8
59	23.5		

*GA: 12.0 to 17.9 wk, +/−1; 18.2 to 23.9 wk, +/−1.5; 24.2 to 29.5 wk, +/−2; 30.0 to 41.8 wk, +/−3.

Source: Adapted from Goldberg BB, Kurtz AB, Atlas of Ultrasound Measurements. Chicago, IL: Yearbook Medical Publishers; 1990.

Table 2. Length of Fetal Long Bones in Relationship to Gestational Age

WEEK NO.	HUMERUS PERCENTILE			ULNA PERCENTILE			RADIUS PERCENTILE			FEMUR PERCENTILE			TIBIA PERCENTILE			FIBULA PERCENTILE		
	5	50	95	5	50	95	5	50	95	5	50	95	5	50	95	5	50	95
11	—	6	—	—	5	—	—	5	—	—	6	—	—	4	—	—	2	—
12	3	9	10	—	8	—	—	7	—	—	9	—	—	7	—	—	5	—
13	5	13	20	3	11	18	—	10	12	6	12	19	4	10	17	—	8	—
14	5	16	20	4	13	17	8	13	19	5	15	19	2	13	19	6	11	10
15	11	18	26	10	16	22	12	15	21	11	19	26	5	16	27	10	14	18
16	12	21	25	8	19	24	9	18	21	13	22	24	7	19	25	6	17	22
17	19	24	29	11	21	32	11	20	29	20	25	29	15	22	29	7	19	31
18	18	27	30	13	24	30	14	22	26	19	28	31	14	24	29	10	22	28
19	22	29	36	20	26	32	20	24	29	23	31	38	19	27	35	18	24	30
20	23	32	36	21	29	32	21	27	28	22	33	39	19	29	35	18	27	30
21	28	34	40	25	31	36	25	29	32	27	36	45	24	32	39	24	29	34
22	28	36	40	24	33	37	24	31	34	29	39	44	25	34	39	21	31	37
23	32	38	45	27	35	43	26	32	39	35	41	48	30	36	43	23	33	44
24	31	41	46	29	37	41	27	34	38	34	44	49	28	39	45	26	35	41
25	35	43	51	34	39	44	31	36	40	38	46	54	31	41	50	33	37	42
26	36	45	49	34	41	44	30	37	41	39	49	53	33	43	49	32	39	43
27	42	46	51	37	43	48	33	39	45	45	51	57	39	45	51	35	41	47
28	41	48	52	37	44	48	33	40	45	45	53	57	38	47	52	36	43	47
29	44	50	56	40	46	51	36	42	47	49	56	62	40	49	57	40	45	50
30	44	52	56	38	47	54	34	43	49	49	58	62	41	51	56	38	47	52

593

Table 2. *(Continued)*

WEEK NO.	HUMERUS PERCENTILE			ULNA PERCENTILE			RADIUS PERCENTILE			FEMUR PERCENTILE			TIBIA PERCENTILE			FIBULA PERCENTILE		
	5	50	95	5	50	95	5	50	95	5	50	95	5	50	95	5	50	95
31	47	53	59	39	49	59	34	44	53	53	60	67	46	52	58	40	48	57
32	47	55	59	40	50	58	37	45	51	53	62	67	46	54	59	40	50	56
33	50	56	62	43	52	60	41	46	51	56	64	71	49	56	62	43	51	59
34	50	57	62	44	53	59	39	47	53	57	65	70	47	57	64	46	52	56
35	52	58	65	47	54	61	38	48	57	61	67	73	48	59	69	51	54	57
36	53	60	63	47	55	61	41	48	54	61	69	74	49	60	68	51	55	56
37	57	61	64	49	56	62	45	49	53	64	71	77	52	61	71	55	56	58
38	55	61	66	48	57	63	45	49	53	62	72	79	54	62	69	54	57	59
39	56	62	69	49	57	66	46	50	54	64	74	83	58	64	69	55	58	62
40	56	63	69	50	58	65	46	50	54	66	75	81	58	65	69	54	59	62

Source: Jeanty P. Fetal limb biometry. Radiology 1983; 147(2):602.

Table 3. Fetal Femur Length in Relationship to Gestational Age

FEMUR LENGTH (MM)	MENSTRUAL AGE (WK)	FEMUR LENGTH (MM)	MENSTRUAL AGE (WK)
10	12.8	45	24.5
11	13.1	46	24.9
12	13.4	47	25.3
13	13.6	48	25.7
14	13.9	49	26.1
15	14.2	50	26.5
16	14.5	51	27.0
17	14.8	52	27.4
18	15.1	53	27.8
19	15.4	54	28.2
20	15.7	55	28.7
21	16.0	56	29.1
22	16.3	57	29.6
23	16.6	58	30.0
24	16.9	59	30.5
25	17.2	60	30.9
26	17.6	61	31.4
27	17.9	62	31.9
28	18.2	63	32.3
29	18.6	64	32.8
30	18.9	65	33.3
31	19.2	66	33.8
32	19.6	67	34.2
33	19.9	68	34.7
34	20.3	69	35.2
35	20.7	70	35.7
36	21.0	71	36.2
37	21.4	72	36.7
38	21.8	73	37.2
39	22.1	74	37.7
40	22.5	75	38.3
41	22.9	76	38.8
42	23.3	77	39.3
43	23.7	78	39.8
44	24.1	79	40.4

Source: Hadlock FP, Harrist RB, Deter RL, et al. Fetal femur length as a predictor of menstrual age: Sonographically measured. AJR 1982; 138:877.

APPENDIX B

Table 4. Estimation of Fetal Weight*

BIPARIETAL DIAMETER	ABDOMINAL CIRCUMFERENCE											
	15.5	16.0	16.5	17.0	17.5	18.0	18.5	19.0	19.5	20.0	20.5	21.0
3.1	212	219	227	236	244	253	262	272	282	292	303	314
3.2	218	226	234	243	252	261	270	280	290	301	312	323
3.3	225	233	242	250	260	269	279	289	299	310	321	333
3.4	232	241	249	258	268	277	287	298	308	319	331	343
3.5	239	248	257	266	276	286	296	307	318	329	341	353
3.6	247	256	265	274	284	294	305	316	327	339	351	364
3.7	254	263	273	283	293	303	314	325	337	349	361	374
3.8	262	271	281	291	302	312	324	335	347	359	372	385
3.9	270	280	290	300	311	322	333	345	357	370	383	397
4.0	278	288	299	309	320	331	343	355	368	381	394	408
4.1	287	297	308	318	330	341	353	366	379	392	406	420
4.2	296	306	317	328	340	352	364	377	390	404	418	433
4.3	305	315	326	338	350	362	375	388	401	416	430	445
4.4	314	325	336	348	360	373	386	399	413	428	443	458
4.5	323	334	346	358	371	384	397	411	425	440	455	471
4.6	333	344	356	369	382	395	409	423	438	453	469	485
4.7	343	355	367	380	393	407	421	435	450	466	482	499
4.8	353	365	378	391	404	418	433	448	463	479	496	513
4.9	364	376	389	402	416	431	445	461	477	493	510	527
5.0	374	387	401	414	428	443	458	474	490	507	524	542
5.1	386	399	412	426	441	456	472	488	504	521	539	558
5.2	397	410	424	439	454	469	485	502	519	536	554	573
5.3	409	422	437	452	467	483	499	516	533	551	570	589
5.4	421	435	449	465	480	496	513	531	548	567	586	606
5.5	433	447	463	478	494	511	528	546	564	583	602	622
5.6	446	461	476	492	508	525	543	561	580	599	619	640
5.7	459	474	490	506	523	540	558	577	596	616	636	657
5.8	472	488	504	520	538	555	574	593	612	633	654	675
5.9	486	502	518	535	553	571	590	609	629	650	672	694
6.0	500	516	533	550	568	587	606	626	647	668	690	712
6.1	514	531	548	566	584	604	623	644	665	686	709	732
6.2	529	546	564	582	601	620	641	661	683	705	728	751
6.3	544	561	580	598	618	638	658	679	701	724	747	772
6.4	559	577	596	615	635	655	676	698	721	744	768	792
6.5	575	594	613	632	653	673	695	717	740	764	788	813
6.6	592	610	630	650	671	692	714	737	760	784	809	835
6.7	608	628	648	668	689	711	733	757	780	805	831	857
6.8	626	645	666	686	708	730	753	777	801	827	853	879
6.9	643	663	684	705	727	750	774	798	823	848	875	902
7.0	661	682	703	725	747	771	795	819	845	871	898	926
7.1	680	701	722	745	768	791	816	841	867	894	921	950
7.2	699	720	742	765	789	813	838	863	890	917	945	974
7.3	718	740	763	786	810	835	860	886	913	941	970	999
7.4	738	760	783	807	832	857	883	910	937	966	995	1,025
7.5	758	781	805	829	854	880	906	934	962	991	1,020	1,051
7.6	779	803	827	851	877	903	930	958	987	1,016	1,047	1,078
7.7	801	825	849	874	900	927	955	983	1,012	1,042	1,073	1,105
7.8	823	847	872	898	924	952	980	1,008	1,038	1,069	1,100	1,133
7.9	845	870	895	922	949	977	1,005	1,035	1,065	1,096	1,128	1,161

ABDOMINAL CIRCUMFERENCE												
21.5	22.0	22.5	23.0	23.5	24.0	24.5	25.0	25.5	26.0	26.5	27.0	27.5
325	337	349	362	375	388	402	417	432	448	464	481	498
335	347	359	372	386	400	414	429	445	461	478	495	513
345	357	370	384	397	412	427	442	458	475	492	509	528
355	368	381	395	409	424	439	455	471	488	506	524	543
366	379	393	407	421	436	452	468	485	503	521	539	559
377	390	404	419	434	449	465	482	499	517	536	555	575
388	402	416	431	446	462	479	496	514	532	551	571	591
399	413	428	443	459	476	493	510	528	547	567	587	608
411	426	441	456	473	489	507	525	543	563	583	603	625
423	438	453	470	486	503	521	540	559	579	599	620	642
435	451	467	483	500	518	536	555	575	595	616	638	660
448	464	480	497	514	533	551	571	591	612	633	656	679
461	477	494	511	529	548	567	587	607	629	651	674	697
474	491	508	526	544	563	583	603	624	646	669	692	716
488	505	522	541	559	579	599	620	642	664	687	711	736
502	519	537	556	575	595	616	637	659	682	706	731	756
516	534	552	572	591	612	633	655	678	701	725	750	776
531	549	568	588	608	629	650	673	696	720	745	771	797
546	564	584	604	625	646	668	691	715	740	765	791	819
561	580	600	621	642	664	687	710	734	760	786	812	840
577	596	617	638	660	682	705	729	754	780	807	834	862
593	613	634	655	678	701	724	749	774	801	828	856	885
609	630	651	673	696	720	744	769	795	822	850	879	908
626	647	669	692	715	739	764	790	816	844	872	901	932
643	665	687	710	734	759	784	811	838	866	895	925	956
661	683	706	730	754	779	805	832	860	888	918	949	981
679	702	725	749	774	800	826	854	882	912	942	973	1,006
698	721	745	769	795	821	848	876	905	935	966	998	1,031
717	740	764	790	816	843	870	899	929	959	991	1,023	1,057
736	760	785	811	837	865	893	922	953	984	1,016	1,049	1,084
756	780	806	832	859	887	916	946	977	1,009	1,042	1,076	1,111
776	801	827	854	882	910	940	970	1,002	1,034	1,068	1,103	1,138
797	822	849	876	905	934	964	995	1,027	1,060	1,095	1,130	1,166
818	844	871	899	928	958	989	1,020	1,053	1,087	1,122	1,158	1,195
839	866	894	922	952	982	1,014	1,046	1,079	1,114	1,150	1,186	1,224
861	889	917	946	976	1,007	1,039	1,072	1,106	1,142	1,178	1,215	1,254
884	912	941	970	1,001	1,033	1,065	1,099	1,134	1,170	1,207	1,245	1,284
907	936	965	995	1,027	1,059	1,092	1,126	1,162	1,198	1,236	1,275	1,315
931	960	990	1,021	1,052	1,085	1,119	1,154	1,190	1,227	1,266	1,305	1,346
955	984	1,015	1,046	1,079	1,112	1,147	1,183	1,219	1,257	1,296	1,337	1,378
979	1,009	1,041	1,073	1,106	1,140	1,175	1,212	1,249	1,287	1,327	1,368	1,410
1,004	1,035	1,067	1,100	1,133	1,168	1,204	1,241	1,279	1,318	1,359	1,400	1,443
1,030	1,061	1,094	1,127	1,161	1,197	1,233	1,271	1,310	1,350	1,391	1,433	1,477
1,056	1,088	1,121	1,155	1,190	1,226	1,263	1,302	1,341	1,382	1,424	1,467	1,511
1,083	1,115	1,149	1,184	1,219	1,256	1,294	1,333	1,373	1,414	1,457	1,501	1,546
1,110	1,143	1,177	1,213	1,249	1,286	1,325	1,364	1,405	1,447	1,491	1,535	1,581
1,138	1,172	1,207	1,242	1,279	1,317	1,356	1,397	1,438	1,481	1,525	1,570	1,617
1,166	1,201	1,236	1,273	1,310	1,349	1,389	1,430	1,472	1,515	1,560	1,606	1,653
1,195	1,230	1,266	1,303	1,342	1,381	1,421	1,463	1,506	1,550	1,595	1,642	1,690

Table 4. *(Continued)*

	ABDOMINAL CIRCUMFERENCE											
BIPARIETAL DIAMETER	15.5	16.0	16.5	17.0	17.5	18.0	18.5	19.0	19.5	20.0	20.5	21.0
8.0	868	893	919	946	974	1,002	1,031	1,061	1,092	1,124	1,157	1,190
8.1	892	918	944	971	999	1,028	1,058	1,088	1,120	1,152	1,186	1,220
8.2	916	942	969	997	1,026	1,055	1,085	1,116	1,148	1,181	1,215	1,250
8.3	941	967	995	1,023	1,052	1,082	1,113	1,145	1,177	1,211	1,245	1,281
8.4	966	993	1,021	1,050	1,080	1,110	1,142	1,174	1,207	1,241	1,276	1,312
8.5	992	1,020	1,048	1,078	1,108	1,139	1,171	1,203	1,237	1,272	1,307	1,344
8.6	1,018	1,047	1,076	1,106	1,136	1,168	1,200	1,234	1,268	1,303	1,339	1,377
8.7	1,046	1,074	1,104	1,134	1,166	1,198	1,231	1,265	1,300	1,335	1,372	1,410
8.8	1,073	1,103	1,133	1,164	1,196	1,228	1,262	1,296	1,332	1,368	1,405	1,444
8.9	1,102	1,132	1,162	1,194	1,226	1,259	1,294	1,329	1,365	1,402	1,439	1,478
9.0	1,131	1,161	1,193	1,225	1,257	1,291	1,326	1,361	1,398	1,436	1,474	1,514
9.1	1,161	1,192	1,223	1,256	1,289	1,324	1,359	1,395	1,432	1,470	1,509	1,550
9.2	1,191	1,223	1,255	1,288	1,322	1,357	1,393	1,429	1,467	1,506	1,545	1,586
9.3	1,222	1,254	1,287	1,321	1,355	1,391	1,427	1,464	1,503	1,542	1,582	1,624
9.4	1,254	1,287	1,320	1,354	1,389	1,425	1,462	1,500	1,539	1,579	1,620	1,661
9.5	1,287	1,320	1,354	1,388	1,424	1,461	1,498	1,536	1,576	1,616	1,658	1,700
9.6	1,320	1,354	1,388	1,423	1,460	1,497	1,535	1,574	1,614	1,655	1,697	1,740
9.7	1,354	1,388	1,423	1,459	1,496	1,533	1,572	1,611	1,652	1,694	1,736	1,780
9.8	1,389	1,424	1,459	1,496	1,533	1,571	1,610	1,650	1,691	1,733	1,776	1,821
9.9	1,425	1,460	1,496	1,533	1,571	1,609	1,649	1,690	1,731	1,774	1,817	1,862
10.0	1,461	1,497	1,534	1,571	1,609	1,648	1,689	1,730	1,772	1,851	1,859	1,905

	ABDOMINAL CIRCUMFERENCE											
BIPARIETAL DIAMETER	28.0	28.5	29.0	29.5	30.0	30.5	31.0	31.5	32.0	32.5	33.0	33.5
3.1	517	535	555	575	596	617	640	663	687	712	738	765
3.2	532	551	571	591	613	635	658	682	707	732	759	786
3.3	547	567	587	608	630	653	677	701	726	753	780	808
3.4	563	583	604	626	648	672	696	721	747	774	802	831
3.5	579	600	621	644	667	691	715	741	768	795	824	853
3.6	595	617	639	662	685	710	735	762	789	817	847	877
3.7	612	634	657	680	705	730	756	783	811	840	870	901
3.8	629	652	675	699	724	750	777	804	833	863	893	925
3.9	647	670	694	719	744	771	798	826	856	886	918	950
4.0	665	689	713	738	765	792	820	849	879	910	942	976
4.1	684	708	733	759	786	813	842	872	903	934	967	1,002
4.2	703	727	753	779	807	835	865	895	927	959	993	1,028
4.3	722	747	773	801	829	858	888	919	951	985	1,019	1,055
4.4	742	767	794	822	851	881	911	943	976	1,011	1,046	1,082
4.5	762	788	816	844	874	904	936	968	1,002	1,037	1,073	1,110
4.6	782	809	838	867	897	928	960	994	1,028	1,064	1,101	1,139
4.7	803	831	860	890	920	952	985	1,019	1,055	1,091	1,129	1,168
4.8	825	853	883	913	945	977	1,011	1,046	1,082	1,119	1,158	1,198
4.9	847	876	906	937	969	1,003	1,037	1,073	1,109	1,148	1,187	1,228
5.0	869	899	930	961	994	1,028	1,064	1,100	1,138	1,177	1,217	1,259
5.1	892	922	954	986	1,020	1,055	1,091	1,128	1,166	1,206	1,247	1,290
5.2	915	946	978	1,012	1,046	1,082	1,118	1,156	1,196	1,236	1,278	1,322

ABDOMINAL CIRCUMFERENCE

21.5	22.0	22.5	23.0	23.5	24.0	24.5	25.0	25.5	26.0	26.5	27.0	27.5
1,225	1,260	1,297	1,335	1,374	1,414	1,455	1,497	1,541	1,585	1,632	1,679	1,728
1,255	1,291	1,329	1,367	1,406	1,447	1,489	1,532	1,576	1,621	1,668	1,716	1,766
1,286	1,323	1,361	1,400	1,440	1,481	1,523	1,567	1,612	1,658	1,706	1,755	1,805
1,317	1,355	1,393	1,433	1,473	1,515	1,559	1,603	1,648	1,695	1,744	1,793	1,844
1,349	1,387	1,426	1,467	1,508	1,551	1,594	1,639	1,686	1.733	1,782	1,832	1,884
1,382	1,420	1,460	1,501	1,543	1,586	1,631	1,676	1,723	1,772	1,821	1,872	1,925
1,415	1,454	1,495	1,536	1,579	1,623	1,668	1,714	1,762	1,811	1,861	1,913	1,966
1,449	1,489	1,530	1,572	1,615	1,660	1,705	1,752	1,801	1,850	1,901	1,954	2,007
1,483	1,524	1,565	1,608	1,652	1,697	1,744	1,791	1,840	1,891	1,942	1,995	2,050
1,519	1,560	1,602	1,645	1,690	1,736	1,783	1,831	1,881	1,931	1,984	2,037	2,093
1,554	1,596	1,639	1,683	1,728	1,775	1,822	1,871	1,921	1,973	2,026	2,080	2,136
1,591	1,633	1,677	1,721	1,767	1,814	1,862	1,912	1,963	2,015	2,069	2,124	2,180
1,628	1,671	1,715	1,760	1,807	1,854	1,903	1,953	2,005	2,058	2,112	2,168	2,225
1,666	1,709	1,754	1,800	1,847	1,895	1,945	1,996	2,048	2,101	2,156	2,213	2,270
1,705	1,749	1,794	1,840	1,888	1,937	1,987	2,038	2,091	2,145	2,201	2,258	2,316
1,744	1,788	1,834	1,881	1,930	1,979	2,030	2,082	2,135	2,190	2,246	2,304	2,363
1,784	1,829	1,875	1,923	1,972	2,022	2,073	2,126	2,180	2,235	2,292	2,350	2,410
1,824	1,870	1,917	1,966	2,015	2,066	2,117	2,171	2,225	2,281	2,339	2,397	2,458
1,866	1,912	1,960	2,009	2,059	2,110	2,162	2,216	2,271	2,328	2,386	2,445	2,506
1,908	1,955	2,003	2,052	2,103	2,155	2,208	2,262	2,318	2,375	2,433	2,493	2,555
1,951	1,998	2,047	2,097	2,148	2,200	2,254	2,309	2,365	2,423	2,482	2,542	2,604

ABDOMINAL CIRCUMFERENCE

34.0	34.5	35.0	35.5	36.0	36.5	37.0	37.5	38.0	38.5	39.0	39.5	40.0
792	821	851	882	914	947	981	1,017	1,054	1,092	1,131	1,172	1,215
814	844	875	906	939	973	1,008	1,045	1,082	1,122	1,162	1,204	1,248
837	867	899	931	965	1,000	1,036	1,073	1,112	1,152	1,194	1,237	1,281
860	891	924	957	991	1,027	1,064	1,102	1,142	1,183	1,226	1,270	1,316
884	916	949	983	1,018	1,055	1,093	1,132	1,173	1,215	1,258	1,304	1,350
908	941	975	1,010	1,046	1,083	1,122	1,162	1,204	1,247	1,292	1,338	1,386
933	966	1,001	1,037	1,074	1,112	1,152	1,193	1,236	1,280	1,325	1,373	1,422
958	992	1,028	1,064	1,102	1,142	1,182	1,224	1,268	1,313	1,360	1,408	1,459
984	1,019	1,055	1,093	1,131	1,172	1,213	1,256	1,301	1,347	1,395	1,445	1,496
1,010	1,046	1,083	1,121	1,161	1,202	1,245	1,289	1,335	1,382	1,431	1,481	1,534
1,037	1,074	1,111	1,151	1,191	1,233	1,277	1,322	1,369	1,417	1,467	1,519	1,573
1,064	1,102	1,140	1,181	1,222	1,265	1,310	1,356	1,404	1,453	1,504	1,557	1,612
1,092	1,130	1,170	1,211	1,254	1,298	1,343	1,390	1,439	1,489	1,542	1,596	1,652
1,120	1,160	1,200	1,242	1,285	1,330	1,377	1,425	1,475	1,527	1,580	1,635	1,692
1,149	1,189	1,231	1,274	1,318	1,364	1,411	1,461	1,512	1,564	1,619	1,675	1,734
1,179	1,220	1,262	1,306	1,351	1,398	1,447	1,497	1,549	1,603	1,658	1,716	1,776
1,209	1,250	1,294	1,338	1,385	1,433	1,482	1,534	1,587	1,642	1,698	1,757	1,818
1,239	1,282	1,326	1,372	1,419	1,468	1,519	1,571	1,625	1,681	1,739	1,799	1,861
1,270	1,314	1,359	1,406	1,454	1,504	1,555	1,609	1,664	1,721	1,780	1,842	1,905
1,302	1,346	1,392	1,440	1,489	1,540	1,593	1,647	1,704	1,762	1,822	1,885	1,949
1,334	1,379	1,426	1,475	1,525	1,577	1,631	1,687	1,744	1,804	1,865	1,929	1,994
1,366	1,413	1,461	1,510	1,562	1,615	1,670	1,726	1,785	1,846	1,908	1,973	2,040

Table 4. *(Continued)*

BIPARIETAL DIAMETER	ABDOMINAL CIRCUMFERENCE											
	28.0	28.5	29.0	29.5	30.0	30.5	31.0	31.5	32.0	32.5	33.0	33.5
5.3	939	971	1,004	1,038	1,073	1,109	1,146	1,185	1,225	1,267	1,310	1,354
5.4	963	996	1,029	1,064	1,100	1,137	1,175	1,215	1,256	1,298	1,342	1,387
5.5	988	1,021	1,055	1,091	1,127	1,165	1,204	1,245	1,286	1,330	1,374	1,420
5.6	1,013	1,047	1,082	1,118	1,156	1,194	1,234	1,275	1,318	1,362	1,407	1,454
5.7	1,039	1,074	1,109	1,146	1,184	1,224	1,264	1,306	1,350	1,395	1,441	1,489
5.8	1,065	1,100	1,137	1,175	1,213	1,254	1,295	1,338	1,382	1,428	1,475	1,524
5.9	1,092	1,128	1,165	1,203	1,243	1,284	1,326	1,370	1,415	1,462	1,510	1,560
6.0	1,119	1,156	1,194	1,233	1,273	1,315	1,358	1,403	1,449	1,496	1,545	1,596
6.1	1,147	1,184	1,223	1,263	1,304	1,347	1,391	1,436	1,483	1,531	1,581	1,633
6.2	1,175	1,213	1,253	1,293	1,335	1,379	1,424	1,470	1,517	1,567	1,618	1,670
6.3	1,204	1,243	1,283	1,325	1,367	1,411	1,457	1,504	1,553	1,603	1,655	1,708
6.4	1,233	1,273	1,314	1,356	1,400	1,445	1,491	1,539	1,588	1,639	1,692	1,746
6.5	1,263	1,304	1,345	1,388	1,433	1,478	1,526	1,574	1,625	1,677	1,730	1,786
6.6	1,294	1,335	1,377	1,421	1,466	1,513	1,561	1,610	1,662	1,714	1,769	1,825
6.7	1,325	1,367	1,410	1,454	1,500	1,548	1,597	1,647	1,699	1,753	1,808	1,865
6.8	1,356	1,399	1,443	1,488	1,535	1,583	1,633	1,684	1,737	1,792	1,848	1,906
6.9	1,388	1,432	1,476	1,522	1,570	1,619	1,670	1,722	1,776	1,831	1,888	1,947
7.0	1,421	1,465	1,511	1,557	1,606	1,656	1,707	1,760	1,815	1,871	1,929	1,989
7.1	1,454	1,499	1,545	1,593	1,642	1,693	1,745	1,799	1,854	1,912	1,971	2,032
7.2	1,488	1,533	1,580	1,629	1,679	1,730	1,784	1,838	1,895	1,953	2,013	2,075
7.3	1,522	1,568	1,616	1,666	1,716	1,769	1,823	1,878	1,936	1,995	2,055	2,118
7.4	1,557	1,604	1,653	1,703	1,754	1,808	1,862	1,919	1,977	2,037	2,098	2,162
7.5	1,592	1,640	1,690	1,741	1,793	1,847	1,903	1,960	2,019	2,080	2,142	2,207
7.6	1,628	1,677	1,727	1,779	1,832	1,887	1,943	2,001	2,061	2,123	2,186	2,252
7.7	1,665	1,714	1,765	1,818	1,872	1,927	1,985	2,044	2,104	2,167	2,231	2,297
7.8	1,702	1,752	1,804	1,857	1,912	1,968	2,026	2,086	2,148	2,211	2,276	2,344
7.9	1,740	1,791	1,843	1,897	1,953	2,010	2,069	2,130	2,192	2,256	2,322	2,390
8.0	1,778	1,830	1,883	1,938	1,994	2,052	2,112	2,173	2,237	2,302	2,368	2,437
8.1	1,817	1,869	1,923	1,979	2,036	2,095	2,155	2,218	2,282	2,348	2,415	2,485
8.2	1,857	1,910	1,964	2,021	2,079	2,138	2,200	2,263	2,327	2,394	2,463	2,533
8.3	1,897	1,951	2,006	2,063	2,122	2,182	2,244	2,308	2,374	2,441	2,511	2,582
8.4	1,937	1,992	2,048	2,106	2,165	2,226	2,289	2,354	2,420	2,489	2,559	2,631
8.5	1,978	2,034	2,091	2,149	2,210	2,271	2,335	2,400	2,468	2,537	2,608	2,681
8.6	2,020	2,076	2,134	2,193	2,254	2,317	2,381	2,447	2,515	2,585	2,657	2.731
8.7	2,063	2,120	2,178	2,238	2,300	2,363	2,428	2,495	2,564	2,634	2,707	2,781
8.8	2,106	2,163	2,222	2,283	2,345	2,410	2,475	2,543	2,612	2,684	2,757	2,832
8.9	2,149	2,208	2,267	2,329	2,392	2,457	2,523	2,592	2,662	2,734	2,808	2,884
9.0	2,194	2,252	2,313	2,375	2,439	2,504	2,572	2,641	2,711	2,784	2,859	2,936
9.1	2,238	2,298	2,359	2,422	2,486	2,552	2,620	2,690	2,762	2,835	2,911	2,988
9.2	2,284	2,344	2,406	2,469	2,534	2,601	2,670	2,740	2,812	2,887	2,963	3,041
9.3	2,330	2,391	2,453	2,517	2,583	2,650	2,720	2,791	2,864	2,938	3,015	3,094
9.4	2,376	2,438	2,501	2,566	2,632	2,700	2,770	2,842	2,915	2,991	3,068	3,147
9.5	2,423	2,485	2,549	2,615	2,682	2,750	2,821	2,893	2,967	3,043	3,121	3,201
9.6	2,471	2,534	2,598	2,664	2,732	2,801	2,872	2,945	3,020	3,096	3,175	3,256
9.7	2,519	2,583	2,648	2,714	2,782	2,852	2,924	2,997	3,073	3,150	3,229	3,310
9.8	2,568	2,632	2,698	2,765	2,833	2,904	2,976	3,050	3,126	3,204	3,283	3,365
9.9	2,618	2,682	2,748	2,816	2,885	2,956	3,029	3,103	3,180	3,258	3,338	3,420
10.0	2,668	2,733	2,799	2,867	2,937	3,009	3,082	3,157	3,234	3,313	3,393	3,476

*Log(BW) = −1.599 + 0.144(BPD) + 0.032(AC) − 0.111(BPD$_2$ × AC)/1,000. S. D. = + OR − 106.0 Gm. per kilogram of body weight.

Source: Warsof SL, Gohari P, Berkowitz RL, et al. Fetus, placenta, and newborn. Am J Obstet Gynecol 1977; 128(8): 886–891.

ABDOMINAL CIRCUMFERENCE

34.0	34.5	35.0	35.5	36.0	36.5	37.0	37.5	38.0	38.5	39.0	39.5	40.0
1,400	1,447	1,496	1,547	1,599	1,653	1,709	1,767	1,826	1,888	1,952	2,018	2,086
1,433	1,482	1,532	1,583	1,637	1,692	1,749	1,808	1,868	1,931	1,996	2,064	2,133
1,468	1,517	1,568	1,621	1,675	1,731	1,789	1,849	1,911	1,975	2,041	2,110	2,181
1,503	1,553	1,605	1,658	1,714	1,771	1,830	1,891	1,954	2,020	2,087	2,157	2,229
1,538	1,589	1,642	1,697	1,753	1,812	1,872	1,934	1,998	2,065	2,133	2,204	2,277
1,574	1,626	1,680	1,736	1,793	1,853	1,914	1,977	2,043	2,110	2,180	2,252	2,327
1,611	1,664	1,719	1,775	1,834	1,894	1,957	2,021	2,088	2,156	2,227	2,301	2,377
1,648	1,702	1,758	1,816	1,875	1,937	2,000	2,066	2,133	2,203	2,275	2,350	2,427
1,686	1,741	1,798	1,856	1,917	1,979	2,044	2,111	2,179	2,251	2,324	2,400	2,478
1,724	1,780	1,838	1,898	1,959	2,023	2,088	2,156	2,226	2,298	2,373	2,450	2,530
1,763	1,820	1,879	1,939	2,002	2,067	2,133	2,202	2,273	2,347	2,423	2,501	2,582
1,803	1,860	1,920	1,982	2,046	2,111	2,179	2,249	2,321	2,396	2,473	2,552	2,634
1,843	1,901	1,962	2,025	2,090	2,156	2,225	2,296	2,370	2,445	2,524	2,604	2,687
1,883	1,943	2,005	2,068	2,134	2,202	2,272	2,344	2,419	2,495	2,575	2,657	2,741
1,924	1,985	2,048	2,113	2,179	2,248	2,319	2,393	2,468	2,546	2,627	2,710	2,795
1,966	2,028	2,091	2,157	2,225	2,295	2,367	2,441	2,518	2,597	2,679	2,763	2,850
2,008	2,071	2,136	2,202	2,271	2,342	2,415	2,491	2,569	2,649	2,732	2,817	2,905
2,051	2,115	2,180	2,248	2,318	2,390	2,464	2,541	2,620	2,701	2,785	2,871	2,960
2,094	2,159	2,226	2,294	2,365	2,438	2,513	2,591	2,671	2,754	2,839	2,926	3,017
2,138	2,204	2,271	2,341	2,413	2,487	2,563	2,642	2,723	2,807	2,893	2,981	3,073
2,183	2,249	2,318	2,388	2,461	2,536	2,614	2,693	2,776	2,860	2,947	3,037	3,130
2,228	2,295	2,365	2,436	2,510	2,586	2,665	2,745	2,828	2,914	3,002	3,093	3,187
2,273	2,342	2,412	2,485	2,559	2,636	2,716	2,798	2,882	2,969	3,058	3,150	3,245
2,319	2,388	2,460	2,533	2,609	2,687	2,768	2,850	2,936	3,023	3,114	3,207	3,303
2,366	2,436	2,508	2,583	2,659	2,738	2,820	2,904	2,990	3,079	3,170	3,264	3,361
2,413	2,484	2,557	2,633	2,710	2,790	2,872	2,957	3,044	3,134	3,227	3,322	3,420
2,460	2,532	2,606	2,683	2,761	2,842	2,926	3,011	3,099	3,190	3,284	3,380	3,479
2,508	2,581	2,656	2,734	2,813	2,895	2,979	3,066	3,155	3,247	3,341	3,438	3,538
2,557	2,631	2,707	2,785	2,865	2,948	3,033	3,121	3,211	3,303	3,399	3,497	3,598
2,606	2,681	2,757	2,836	2,918	3,001	3,087	3,176	3,267	3,360	3,457	3,556	3,658
2,655	2,731	2,809	2,888	2,971	3,055	3,142	3,231	3,323	3,418	3,515	3,615	3,718
2,705	2,782	2,860	2,941	3,024	3,109	3,197	3,287	3,380	3,475	3,573	3,674	3,778
2,756	2,833	2,912	2,994	3,078	3,164	3,252	3,343	3,437	3,533	3,632	3,734	3,838
2,807	2,885	2,965	3,047	3,132	3,219	3,308	3,400	3,494	3,591	3,691	3,794	3,899
2,858	2,937	3,018	3,101	3,186	3,274	3,364	3,457	3,552	3,650	3,750	3,854	3,960
2,910	2,989	3,071	3,155	3,241	3,330	3,420	3,514	3,610	3,708	3,810	3,914	4,021
2,962	3,042	3,125	3,209	3,296	3,385	3,477	3,571	3,668	3,767	3,869	3,974	4,082
3,015	3,096	3,179	3,264	3,352	3,442	3,534	3,629	3,726	3,826	3,929	4,035	4,143
3,068	3,149	3,233	3,319	3,407	3,498	3,591	3,687	3,785	3,886	3,989	4,095	4,204
3,121	3,203	3,288	3,374	3,463	3,555	3,649	3,745	3,844	3,945	4,049	4,156	4,265
3,175	3,258	3,343	3,430	3,520	3,612	3,706	3,803	3,902	4,004	4,109	4,216	4,326
3,229	3,313	3,398	3,486	3,576	3,669	3,764	3,861	3,961	4,064	4,169	4,277	4,388
3,283	3,368	3,454	3,542	3,633	3,726	3,822	3,920	4,020	4,123	4,229	4,338	4,449
3,338	3,423	3,510	3,599	3,690	3,784	3,880	3,979	4,080	4,183	4,289	4,398	4,510
3,393	3,479	3,566	3,656	3,748	3,842	3,938	4,037	4,139	4,243	4,349	4,459	4,571
3,449	3,535	3,623	3,713	3,805	3,900	3,997	4,096	4,198	4,302	4,410	4,519	4,632
3,505	3,591	3,679	3,770	3,863	3,958	4,055	4,155	4,257	4,362	4,470	4,580	4,692
3,561	3,647	3,736	3,827	3,920	4,016	4,114	4,214	4,317	4,422	4,529	4,640	4,753

Table 5. Birth Weight Percentiles Based on Gestational Age

GESTATION		ESTIMATED CENTILE BIRTH WEIGHTS (G)					
		FEMALES			MALES		
(WEEKS)	(DAYS)	10TH	50TH	90TH	10TH	50TH	90TH
27	189	708	840	997	726	852	999
28	196	869	1031	1223	896	1051	1232
29	203	1030	1222	1450	1065	1250	1466
30	210	1191	1413	1676	1235	1448	1699
31	217	1352	1604	1903	1404	1647	1932
32	224	1513	1795	2129	1574	1846	2166
33	231	1674	1986	2356	1744	2045	2399
34	238	1835	2177	2582	1913	2244	2632
35	245	1996	2367	2809	2083	2443	2865
36	252	2156	2558	3035	2252	2642	3099
37	259	2317	2749	3262	2422	2841	3332
38	266	2478	2940	3488	2591	3040	3565
39	273	2639	3131	3715	2761	3238	3798
40	280	2800	3322	3941	2931	3437	4032
41	287	2961	3513	4168	3100	3636	4265
42	294	3122	3704	4394	3270	3835	4498
43	301	3283	3895	4621	3439	4034	4732

Source: Secher NJ, Hansen PK, Lenstrup C, et al. Birthweight-for-gestational age charts based on early ultrasound estimation of gestational age. Br J Obstet Gynaecol 1986; 93:131.

Index

Abdominal circumference (AC), 246–248
ABO-incompatible pregnancies, 254
Abortion
congenital anomalies and, 197–199
isoimmunization and, 255
psychological sequelae of, 546–547
spontaneous, 304, 434, 499
Abruptio placentae, 331, 335–339
Accelerated fetal growth (AFG), 249–251
Acquired immunodeficiency syndrome (AIDS), 274–278
breast-feeding and, 87
Active phase of labor, 46, 130, 132–133
Activity
cardiovascular disease and, 357–358
during puerperium, 78
Acute fatty liver of pregnancy, 426–427
Acute tubular necrosis, 388–389
Addison's disease, 449–450
Admitting orders, 15–17
Adrenal disease, 449–453
Adrenocortical insufficiency, 449–450
AIDS-related complex, 276
Alcohol abuse, postpartum, 551
Alder's sign in appendicitis, 413
Alleles, 175–178
Ambulatory patient, care of, 14–15
Ambulatory uterine contraction monitoring, 285–286
Amniocentesis, 189
anxiety about, 547–548
isoimmunization and, 257, 259–260
premature labor and, 286–287
premature rupture of membranes and, 298
Amnioinfusion in prolonged pregnancy, 320–321
Amnionitis. See Chorioamnionitis

Amniotic band syndrome, 207
Amniotic fluid analysis, 309, 327
Amniotic fluid embolism (AFE), 570–572
Amniotic fluid factors, endometritis and, 323
Analgesia
epidural, pelvic, 139
during labor, 102–107
caudal epidural block and, 107
lumbar/caudal epidural block and, 104–107
paracervical block and, 103–104
in preeclampsia, 374
psychological, 102
systemic medications for, 102–103
psychological, 102
transplacental passage of drugs and, 98–99
Anemia, 457–471, 500
folate deficiency and, 461–463
glucose–6-phosphate dehydrogenase deficiency and, 468–470
hereditary spherocytosis and, 465–468
iron deficiency, 458, 461
pyruvate kinase deficiency and, 470–471
sickle cell. See Sickle cell anemia
vitamin B_{12} deficiency and, 463–465
Anencephaly, 206–207
Anesthesia, 95–110
allergic reactions to, 101
for delivery, 107–110
effect on labor and delivery, 98–99
local anesthetic intoxication and, 99, 101
physiologic changes during pregnancy and, 95, 97–98
in preeclampsia, 374

Anesthesia (*Cont.*)
  regional, 99, 101
  transplacental passage of drugs and,
    98–99
Aneurysms, "berry," 514–515
Angiogranuloma, 559–560
Angiotensin-converting enzyme (ACE)
  inhibitors, 381
Antacids, 109–110, 408, 409
Antibiotics
  in acute pyelonephritis, 387
  in appendicitis, 414
  in asthma, 398
  in asymptomatic bacteriuria, 385
  in chorioamnionitis, 327
  in endometritis, 324, 326
  in pancreatitis, 412–413
  in pneumonia, 400
  premature rupture of membranes
    and, 299–300
  prophylactic, 119, 359, 361
  in syphilis, 272
Anticoagulants, 155, 358, 364–366,
    495–496
Anticonvulsants, 155, 512
Antihistamines, 529, 531
Antihypertensives, 155–156, 379–381,
    520
Antithrombin III (AT III) deficiency,
    495–496
Antithyroid drugs, 444–445
Anxiety, 546–548
  about amniocentesis, 547–548
  during labor and delivery, 556
Anxiety attacks, 550–551
Aortic stenosis, 361
Apgar score, 64–65, 143
Appendicitis, 412–414
Arrhythmias, 288
Asherman's syndrome, 342
Asphyxia
  intrauterine, 248–249
  neonatal, 68, 75
Asthma, 396–398
Asynclitism, 45–46, 135
Atrial septal defects (ASDs), 359–360
Autonomic hyperreflexia, 519–520
Autosomal dominant inheritance, 176
Autosomal recessive inheritance, 176–
    178
Azathioprine (Imuran), 418, 501, 504

Bacteriuria, asymptomatic, 384–386
Bag and mask ventilation of newborn,
    69–70

Balanced translocation, 182
Banana sign, 204, 205
Barrier contraceptive methods, 80
Bell's palsy, 521
Beta-adrenergic blockers, 358, 380,
    398
Beta sympathomimetics, 287–289
Bilateral renal agenesis (BRA), 212–
    213
Biliary colic, 428
Biochemical testing, antenatal, 220–
    221
Biophysical profile, 230–233
Biophysical testing, 221–234
  biophysical profile and, 230–233
  contraction stress test and, 225–
    230
  fetal acoustic stimulation and, 233–
    234
  fetal movement and, 221–223
  nonstress test and, 223–225
Birthing rooms/centers, 56–62
  in-hospital, 56–57, 59
  patient's perspective on, 58–59
  provider's perspective on, 59
  quality of care and, 62
  types of, 56–57
Bleeding. *See* Hemorrhage
Blood pressure
  postpartum hemorrhage and, 342–
    343
  during pregnancy, 28, 357
  (*See also* Hypertension; Hypoten-
    sion)
Blood transfusion
  intrauterine, isoimmunization and,
    261–262
  placenta previa and, 334
  in postpartum bleeding, 345
Blood volume, changes during preg-
    nancy, 356
Bonding, 549–550, 552
Bradley method, 36
Breast cancer, 537–539
Breast examination, 6
Breast-feeding
  diet for, 83
  initiating, 83–84
  let-down reflex and, 84
  maintenance of milk supply for, 84
  nipple care and, 83
  positioning for, 84
  problems with, 85–88
  psychological issues related to, 89–
    90

weaning/suppression and, 90–91
working mothers and, 88–89
Breech presentation, 117, 141–148
Bromocriptine, 90–91
Brow presentation, 144, 146, 148–149

Calcium channel blockers, 309, 381
Calcium metabolism, 446
Cancer. *See specific cancers*
Cardiac anomalies, 215–217
Cardiac arrest, 574–577
Cardiac surgery, pregnancy subsequent to, 363
Cardiomyopathy, 361–362
Cardiopulmonary resuscitation (CPR), 576
Cardiopulmonary system during puerperium, 76
Cardiovascular disease, 355–363
general management guidelines for, 357–359
endocarditis prophylactic, 359
patient classification and, 355–356
(See also specific disorders)
Cardiovascular system
changes during labor and delivery, 356–357
changes during pregnancy, 95, 97, 356–357
Carpal tunnel syndrome, 522
Cell division, 171–172
Cephalometry, 245–248
Cephalopelvic disproportion (CPD), 130
Cerclage, 120–121
Cerebellum, absent, 204, 205
Cerebral embolism, 515–516
Cerebral venous thrombosis, 516
Cerebrovascular accidents, 514–516
Cervical carcinoma, 535–537
Cervical dysplasia, 536
Cervical infections, premature labor and, 283
Cervical priming, 319–320
Cervical ripening
premature labor and, 284
in prolonged pregnancy, 317
Cervix
cerclage and, 120–121
examination of, 11
during puerperium, 76

Cesarean section, 116–120
abnormal presentations and, 147–148
classification of, 116–117
complications of, 119–120
contraindications for, 118
eclampsia and, 377
endometritis and, 323
indications for, 117–118
in inflammatory bowel disease, 418
placenta previa and, 334
procedure for, 118–119
Childbirth education, 35–36
Chlamydial infection, endometritis and, 324
Cholelithiasis, 427–428
Cholera, immunization against, 583
Cholestasis of pregnancy, 425–426
Chorea gravidarum, 523
Chorioamnionitis
amniocentesis and, 286–287
intraamniotic, 326–327
premature labor and, 283
premature rupture of membranes and, 294, 300
Chorionic villus sampling (CVS), 190–192
Christmas disease, 492–493
Chromosome abnormalities, 182–186
Chromosomes, 173–175
Circumcision, 67
Coagulation studies
in abruptio placentae, 337
placenta previa and, 333
in preeclampsia, 372
Coarctation of aorta, 360–361
Colitis, ulcerative. *See* Inflammatory bowel disease
Colorectal cancer, 541–542
Colposcopy, cervical carcinoma and, 536
Compound presentation, 142, 144, 146, 149
Compression neuropathies, 522
Congenital adrenal hyperplasia, 451–453
Congenital anomalies, 195–217
abortion before 24 weeks' gestation and, 197
abortion or nonaggressive management of pregnancy after fetal viability and, 197–199
breech presentation and, 144
diabetes mellitus and, 434
multifetal pregnancy and, 306

Congenital anomalies (*Cont.*)
  placenta previa and, 331
  premature rupture of membranes
    and, 294
  route of delivery and, 199–200
  in utero therapy and, 199
  (*See also specific anomalies*)
Congenital heart block, 499
Conization in cervical carcinoma,
  536–537
Contraception
  diabetes mellitus and, 439
  postpartum, 80–81
  in systemic lupus erythematosus,
    502
Contraction stress test (CST), 225–230
Conversion disorder, 553
Cord accidents, breech presentation
  and, 144
Cord blood, collection of, 66
Cord management, 53–54
Cord problems, multifetal pregnancy
  and, 306
Cord prolapse, 569–570
Corticosteroids
  in asthma, 398
  in immune thrombocytopenic pur-
    pura, 486
  in papular eruptions, 529
  in rheumatoid arthritis, 504
  in sarcoidosis, 403
Crossing-over, 172
Cushing's syndrome, 450–451
Cytogenetic analysis, 173–174
Cytomegalovirus (CMV) infection,
  268–270

Dark-field microscopy, in syphilis,
  272
Death, sudden, maternal, 552
Decalcification, dental, 561
Deep vein thrombosis (DVT)
  in pregnancy, 364–365
  during puerperium, 80
Delivery
  abruptio placentae and, 338–339
  algorithm for, in prolonged preg-
    nancy, 317–319
  anesthesia/analgesia during. *See* An-
    algesia; Anesthesia
  cardiovascular system changes dur-
    ing, 357
  cesarean. *See* Cesarean section
  chorioamnionitis and, 327

in chronic hypertension, 381
  cord management and, 53–54
  in diabetes mellitus, 438
  eclampsia and, 377
  fetal distress and, 242
  forceps, 121–126
  location of, premature rupture of
    membranes and, 299
  of placenta, management of bleed-
    ing following, 344–348
  placenta previa and, 334
  preeclampsia and, 373
  pregnancy-aggravated hypertension,
    382
  preterm, 291
    multifetal pregnancy and, 304
    premature rupture of membranes
      and, 293
    psychological effects of, 549
    systemic lupus erythematosus
      and, 499
    (*See also* Labor premature)
  route of, congenital anomalies and,
    199–200
  spontaneous, 52–55
  vacuum extractor in, 127–128
Dental disease, 558–562
Depression, 547, 550, 552
  fetal death and, 549
  management of, 555–557
Dermatologic disease. *See specific disorders*
Dermatomyositis, 506–507
Descent disorders, 131, 133
Diabetes insipidus (DI), 454
Diabetes mellitus, 430–439
  cause of, 430–431
  complications of
    fetal, 434–435
    maternal, 432–434
  contraception and, 439
  diagnosis of, 431–432
  gestational, 438–439
  incidence of, 430
  interpregnancy care and, 439
  morbidity and mortality and, 430
  pathogenesis and pathophysiology
    of, 431
  pregnancy management and, 435–
    439
  screen, prenatal, 29–30
Dialysis, 392, 501
Diaphragmatic hernia, 211–212
Diet
  for breast-feeding, 83

cardiovascular disease and, 357
in diabetes mellitus, 436
during puerperium, 78
Diphtheria, immunization against, 586
DNA, 168–169, 171–172, 179–180
DNA analysis, 179–181
Doppler velocity studies, in diagnosis
of intrauterine growth retardation, 248
Down syndrome (trisomy 21), 183
Drug(s)
breast-feeding and, 86
preoperative, 19–20
suppression and, 90–91
teratogenic, 154–161
therapeutic, preoperative, 20
thrombocytopenia and, 484
(See also Anesthesia; Analgesia;
Drug therapy)
Drug abuse, postpartum, 551
Drug therapy
in acute pyelonephritis, 387
in adrenocortical insufficiency,
450
in appendicitis, 414
in asthma, 397–398
in asymptomatic bacteriuria, 385
in cardiovascular disease, during
pregnancy, 358
in cholestasis, 425–426
for dental disease, during pregnancy, 562
in eclampsia, 377
in gastroesophageal reflux, 408
in group B beta-hemolytic streptococcal infection, 273
in hemorrhage, following cesarean
section, 119
in immune thrombocytopenic purpura, 486
in inflammatory bowel disease,
417–418
in nausea and vomiting, 406
newborn and, 73–74
in pancreatitis, 412–413
in peptic ulcer, 409
in polymyositis and dermatomyositis, 507
in postpartum bleeding, 345, 347–348
in preeclampsia, 373–375
in premature labor, 287–291
in psychiatric disorders, 554–557
in rheumatoid arthritis, 504
in schizophrenia, 554

in scleroderma, 506
in seizure disorders, 512–514
in syphilis, 272
in systemic lupus erythematosus,
500–502
in toxoplasmosis, 266
in tuberculosis, 401–402
in upper respiratory tract infection,
396
Dystocia, 130–139
definitions and, 130
as indication for cesarean section,
117–118
normal, 130
passageway abnormalities and,
137–139
passenger abnormalities and, 135–137
power abnormalities and, 131–135
shoulder, 563–569

Eclampsia, 369, 375–377
Edema
during pregnancy, 27, 28, 34, 527
pulmonary, 288–290
Eisenmenger's syndrome, 360
Electronic fetal monitoring (EFM), continuous, 238–240
Encephalocele, 207–208
Endocarditis, prophylactic antibiotics
for, 359
Endocrine system, changes during
pregnancy, 97–98
Endometritis, 322–326
Endotracheal intubation of newborn,
70–72
Engorgement, breast-feeding and, 85
Episiotomy, 52–53, 79, 565
Erythema, palmar, 526
Erythroblastosis fetalis, 252
Estimated date of confinement (EDC),
determination of, 315–316
Estimated fetal weight (EFW), 28, 248,
596–601
Estriol, antenatal measurement of,
220–221
Eye care, newborn, 66

Face presentation, 142, 144, 146,
148
Failed forceps, 125
False labor, premature labor versus,
285

Fatigue
  during first trimester, 545
  postpartum, 550
Femoral nerve neuropathy, 522
Ferning test, premature rupture of
    membranes and, 295, 296
Fetal acoustic stimulation, 233–234
Fetal assessment
  abruptio placentae and, 338
  antenatal, 220–234
    biochemical testing in, 220–221
    biophysical testing in. See Bio-
      physical testing
    indications for, 220
    prolonged pregnancy and, 316–
      317
  in asthma, 398
  in chronic hypertension, 381
  in diabetes mellitus, 437
  intrapartum, 236–242
    fetal heart rate monitoring and,
      237–240
    fetal scalp pH assessment and,
      240–241
    meconium staining and, 241
    pathophysiology and, 237
    relationship of intrapartum events
      to subsequent neurological defi-
      cit and, 236
    umbilical cord blood acid/base
      assessment and, 241–242
  during labor, 49, 51, 52
  in preeclampsia, 372
  premature rupture of membranes
    and, 299
Fetal death
  as contraindication for cesarean sec-
    tion, 118
  diabetes mellitus and, 435
  grief reaction and, 548–549
  stillbirth, systemic lupus erythemato-
    sus and, 499
Fetal distress, 117, 124, 242, 282,
    294
  intrapartum fetal assessment and.
    See Fetal assessment, in-
    trapartum
Fetal growth, 244–251
  altered, accelerated fetal growth
    and, 249–251
  intrauterine growth retardation and,
    244–249, 304–305, 331
  prolonged pregnancy and, 314–315
Fetal heart rate monitoring, 237–240
Fetal lie, 28

Fetal lung maturity, amniocentesis
    and, 286
Fetal scalp pH assessment, 240–241
Fetal skin sampling, 192–193
Fetal weight, estimated, 28, 248,
    596–601
Fetopelvic relationships, 43–45
Fetus
  accommodation to maternal pelvis,
    141–142
  activity of
    assessment of, 221–223
    in multifetal pregnancy, 307
  adaptations to pelvis, 45–46
  attitude of, 44
  isoimmunization and. See
    Isoimmunization
  large-for-gestational-age, 249–251
  lie of, 43
  metastatic disease to, 542
  position of, 44–45
  presentation of, 43–44
  skull of, diameters of, 40
  small-for-gestational-age
    (See also Intrauterine growth
      retardation)
  teratogens and. See Teratogens
Fluid management
  in abruptio placentae, 338
  in nausea and vomiting, 406–407
Fluid status in preeclampsia, 371
Folate deficiency, 461–463
Foley catheter, cervical priming and,
    319–320
Food preferences during first trimester,
    546
Forceps delivery, 121–126
Frank breech presentation, 142
Fundal height, 28, 315–316

Gamma globulin, 486
Gastroesophageal reflux, 407–408
Gastrointestinal diseases during preg-
    nancy, 405–418
Gastrointestinal system, changes dur-
    ing pregnancy, 97, 405
Gastroplasty, 415
Gastroschisis, 210–211
Genetics, 168–186
  cell division and, 171–172
  chromosome abnormalities and. See
    Chromosome abnormalities
  DNA and, translation and, 171
  DNA structure and, 168–169

heritability and. *See* Heritability
RNA and, 169, 171
screening, 187–188
transcription and, 169, 171
translation and, 171
Genotype, 175
German measles, 266–268, 581
Gestational age
    birth weight percentiles based on,
        602
    estimation from biparietal diameter,
        592
    fetal femur length in relation to,
        595
    length of long fetal bones in relation
        to, 593–594
Gingivitis, 558–559
Glucose monitoring in diabetes melli-
    tus, 436
Glucose–6-phosphate dehydrogenase
    (G6PD) deficiency, 468–470
Glucose tolerance test, diabetes melli-
    tus and, 432
Glucosuria, diabetes mellitus and, 433
Granuloma, pyogenic, 527, 559–560
Granuloma gravidarum, 559–560
Graves' disease, 443–445
Grief reaction, fetal death and, 548–
    549
Group B beta-hemolytic streptococcal
    infection, 273, 300
Growth, fetal, 244–251
    accelerated fetal growth and, 249–
        251
    intrauterine growth retardation and,
        244–249, 304–305, 331
    prolonged pregnancy and, 314–315
Guillain-Barré syndrome, 520–521

Hair, changes during pregnancy, 525–
    526
Hand-foot syndrome in sickle cell
    anemia, 472
Headache
    prenatal, 35
    "spinal," 107
Heartburn, prenatal, 35
Heart rate
    changes during pregnancy, 356
HELLP syndrome, 490
Hematocrit
    in multifetal pregnancy, 308
    prenatal, 29
Hematology, placenta previa and, 333

Hemoglobin
    fetal, placenta previa and, 333
    prenatal, 29
Hemoglobin A1C, diabetes mellitus
    and, 434
Hemoglobinopathies, 471–477
Hemoglobin SC disease, 475–476
Hemolytic disease
    antibodies causing, 252–254
    (*See also* Isoimmunization)
Hemolytic uremic syndrome (HUS),
    488–490
Hemophilia, 490–493
Hemoptysis, pulmonary emboli and,
    365
Hemorrhage
    abruptio placentae and, 335–339
    as complication of cerclage, 121
    as complication of cesarean section,
        119–120
    fetomaternal, 331, 337
    general approach to, 329–330
    as indication for cesarean section,
        118
    placenta previa and, 330–335
    postpartum, 340–350
        cause of, 340–341
        diagnosis of, 342–343
        early, 340, 341
        incidence of, 340
        late, 340–341
        management of, 343–350
        morbidity and mortality and,
            342
        pathogenesis of, 341
Hemorrhoids, prenatal, 35
Hepatitis, 421–425
    breast-feeding and, 87–88
    cause of, 422
    diagnosis of, 424
    differential diagnosis of, 424
    immunization against, 583, 587,
        589
    incidence of, 421
    morbidity and mortality and, 421–
        422
    pathogenesis and pathophysiology
        of, 422–423
    prenatal screening for, 25–26
    prevention of, 424–425
    treatment of, 424
    viral pathophysiology of, 423–424
Hepatobiliary disease, 421–428
    (*See also specific disorders*)
Hereditary spherocytosis, 465–468

Heritability, 175–182
  autosomal dominant, 176
  autosomal recessive, 176–178
  DNA analysis and, 179–181
  mitochondrial, 179
  polygenic/multifactorial, 181–182
  X-linked, 178–179
Hernia, diaphragmatic, 211–212
Herpes gestationis (HG), 529–531
Herpes simplex virus (HSV) infection
  breast-feeding and, 88
  during pregnancy, 270–271
Hiatal hernia, 407
Hirsutism, 525, 526
Home birth, 57
Hormone antagonists, teratogenic,
    158–159
Hospitalized patient, 15–22
  postpartum and postoperative con-
    siderations and, 20–22
  preoperative considerations and,
    17–20
  routine admitting orders and, 15–17
Human chorionic gonadotropin (HCG)
  in multifetal pregnancy, 308
Human immunodeficiency virus (HIV),
    87, 274–278
Human placental lactogen (HPL)
  antenatal measurement of, 221
  in multifetal pregnancy, 308
Hydatiform mole, multifetal pregnancy
    versus, 307
Hydramnios, 306, 307, 433
Hydrocephalus, 200–202
Hydrops fetalis
  isoimmunization and, 261
  nonimmune, 214–215
11B-Hydroxylase deficiency, 452–453
21-Hydroxylase deficiency, 451–452
Hyperemesis gravidarum, 546
Hyperlipidemia, physiological, of
    pregnancy, 410
Hypermagnesemia, magnesium sulfate
    and, 290
Hyperparathyroidism, 447–448
Hyperpigmentation, 524–525
Hyperreflexia
  autonomic, 519–520
  in preeclampsia, 371
Hypersomnia, postpartum, 550
Hypertensive disorders, 368–383
  chronic, 369, 377–381
  classification of, 368
  definitions and, 368–369
  diabetes mellitus and, 433

gestational/transient, 369, 383
  pregnancy-aggravated, 369, 381–
    383
  pregnancy-induced, 368–369
  (See also Preeclampsia; Eclampsia)
Hyperthyroidism, 442–445
Hypnosis during labor, 102
Hypnotics, preoperative, 19
Hypogastric artery ligation in postpar-
    tum bleeding, 348–350
Hypoglycemia
  diabetes mellitus and, 432
  intrauterine growth retardation and,
    249
  neonatal, diabetes mellitus and, 435
  in newborn, 74
Hypokalemia, beta sympathomimetics
    and, 289
Hypoparathyroidism, 448–449
Hypopituitarism, 453–454
Hypotension, 106–107
Hypothalamic-pituitary-ovarian axis
    during puerperium, 76
Hypothyroidism, 445–446
Hypoxia, neonatal, sequelae of, 74
Hysterectomy in postpartum bleeding,
    350

Idiopathic hypertrophic subaortic sten-
    osis (IHSS), 362–363
Imaging, preoperative, 17–18
Immune thrombocytopenic purpura
    (ITP), 485–487
Immunizations
  against cytomegalovirus infection,
    270
  during pregnancy, 579–590
  during puerperium, 77–78
  against rubella virus, 268
Immunocompromised patients, en-
    dometritis in, 323
Immunosuppressive therapy
  in immune thrombocytopenic pur-
    pura, 486
  in rheumatoid arthritis, 504
  in systemic lupus erythematosus,
    501
Indirect Coombs' test, isoimmuniza-
    tion and, 256
Infanticide, 551
Infantile polycystic kidney disease
    (IPKD), 214
Infection
  breast-feeding and, 87–88

complicating AIDS, 276–277
as complication of cerclage, 121
as complication of cesarean section, 119
of episiotomy, 79
maternal, premature rupture of membranes and, 294
perinatal, 264–278
peripartum, 322–327
premature labor and, 283
(See also specific infections)
Inflammatory bowel disease, 415–418
Influenza, immunization against, 582
Informed consent, 18, 60
Inhalation anesthetics, transplacental passage of, 98
Insulin shifts, diabetes mellitus and, 432–433
Insulin therapy in diabetes mellitus, 437
Intervertebral disk herniation, 521–522
Intraamniotic infection (IAI), 326–327
Intrapartum infection. *See* Chorioamnionitis
Intrauterine device (IUD), postpartum, 80
Intrauterine growth retardation (IUGR), 244–249, 304–305, 331
Intrauterine transfusion, isoimmunization and, 261–262
In utero therapy, congenital anomalies and, 199
Iron deficiency anemia, 458, 461
Isoimmune thrombocytopenia, 487–488
Isoimmunization, 252–263
abruptio placentae and, 337
cause of, 255–256
definition of, 252
diagnosis of, 256
differential diagnosis of, 256
incidence of, 252, 254
management of, 256–262
during first sensitized pregnancy, 257, 259–260
in patient with previous immunized pregnancy, 260–261
prediction of severity of fetal disease and, 256–257
severely affected fetus and, 261–262
morbidity and mortality and, 254–255
placenta previa and, 331

prevention of, 262
prognosis of, 262–263

Jaundice, cholelithiasis and, 428
Jejunoileal bypass, 415

Ketoacidosis in diabetes mellitus, 438
Klinefelter syndrome (47,XXY phenotype), 186
Kyphoscoliosis during pregnancy, 402–403

Labor
abnormal. *See* Dystocia
anesthesia/analgesia during. *See* Analgesia; Anesthesia
cardiovascular system changes during, 357
early, management of, 38
false labor, 285
first stage of, 46, 49, 51, 99, 130
fourth stage of, 47, 54–55
impending, signs of, 38
length of, endometritis and, 322
management of, 38, 49–55, 359
mechanics of, 39–46
mechanisms of, 47–49, 141
membrane rupture and. *See* Membrane rupture
normal, definition of, 130
premature, 281–291
cause of, 282–284
chorioamnionitis and, 326
as complication of cerclage, 121
definition of, 281
in diabetes mellitus, 438
diagnosis of, 284–285
differential diagnosis of, 285
incidence of, 281
management of, 285–286, 309
morbidity and mortality and, 282
in multifetal pregnancy, 309
threatened, 285
treatment of, 286–291
second stage of, 46–47, 51–52, 99, 130
third stage of, 47, 54
Labor/delivery room, 56–57
Lactation, 82–91
(See also Breast-feeding)
Lamaze method, 35, 102

Laminaria tents, cervical priming and, 319
Laparoscopy in appendicitis, 414
Large-for-gestational-age (LGA) fetuses, 249–251
Latent phase of labor, 46
  prolonged, 130–132
Lemon sign, 204
Leopold's maneuvers, 145
Lethargy during first trimester, 545
Leukemia, 542
Liability, inheritance and, 181–182
Lie, 141
  (See also specific lies)
Lithium, 555
Liver damage, neonatal, sequelae of, 75
Liver function tests (LFTs) in pre-eclampsia, 371–372
Local anesthetics, transplacental passage of, 98–99
Lochia, 77
Low forceps delivery, 123
Lumbosacral cord neuropathy, 522
Lymphoma, 542
Lyon hypothesis, 178

McDonald procedure, 120
McRobert's maneuver, 565
Macrocytosis, in pyruvate kinase deficiency, 471
Macrosomia
  diabetes mellitus and, 434–435
  passenger abnormalities and, 135–136
  prolonged pregnancy and, 314
Magnesium sulfate, 289–290, 309, 373–375, 377, 573
Malmstrom extractor, 127–128
Manic-depressive psychosis, 550, 555
Marfan's syndrome , 362
Mastitis, 79, 85–86
Maternal assessment
  during labor, 49, 51
  premature rupture of membranes and, 298–299
Maternal serum alpha fetoprotein (MSAFP), 188, 308
Maternal support during labor, 51
Meckel's syndrome, 207
Meconium aspiration, prevention of, 321
Meconium staining, 241
Megaloblastic anemia, 461–465

Meiosis, 172
Melanocytic nevi, 532–533
Melanoma, 539
  malignant, 532–533
Melasma, 524–525
Membrane rupture
  as complication of cerclage, 121
  endometritis and, 323
  premature, 293–301
    cause of, 294–295
    chorioamnionitis and, 326
    diagnosis of, 295–296
    differential diagnosis of, 295
    incidence of, 293
    management of, 296–300
    morbidity and mortality and, 293–294
    term, 300–301
Mercury, teratogenic effect of, 161
Messenger RNA, 171
Metabolic acidosis in newborn, 73
Metabolic disorders, neonatal, sequelae of, 75
Metastatic disease to fetus and placenta, 542
Methylergonovine (Methergine), 54, 345, 347–348
Midforceps delivery, 123
Mitochondrial inheritance, 179
Mitosis, 171–172
Mitral commissurotomy, pregnancy subsequent to, 363
Mitral stenosis, 361
Mitral valve prolapse, 362
Mityvac extractor, 127, 128
Molluscum gravidarum, 527
Mood lability, postpartum, 550
Mortality, premature labor and, 282
Mosaicism, 182
Multifactorial inheritance, 181–182
Multifetal pregnancy, 303–311
  cause of, 307
  diagnosis of, 307–308
  differential diagnosis of, 307
  incidence of, 303
  management of, 308–311
  morbidity and mortality and, 303–306
  predisposing factors for, 303
Multiple sclerosis, 517–518
Mumps, immunization against, 580
Mutant allele, 175–178
Mutation, 175
Myasthenia gravis, 517

Myocardial dysfunction, neonatal, sequelae of, 75
Myocardial infarction, 363
Myocardial ischemia, beta sympathomimetics and, 288

Narcotics, neonatal depression and, 73
Natural childbirth, 102
Nausea, 34, 405–407, 546
  cholelithiasis and, 428
  epidural opioids and, 114
  in multifetal pregnancy, 307
Neonate
  accelerated fetal growth and, 250
  cytomegalovirus infection in, 269
  hypoglycemia in, diabetes mellitus and, 435
  isoimmunization and, 262
  magnesium sulfate and, 290
Neural tube defects (NTDs), 202–209
  diagnosis of, 203–206
  prognosis of, 206–209
Neurological deficit, relationship of intrapartum events to, 236
Neurologic diseases, 509–523
  diagnosis of, 509
  physiologic changes related to pregnancy and, 509
  (See also specific disorders)
Neurosyphilis, 273
Nevi, melanocytic, 532–533
Newborn
  Apgar score and, 64–65
  bathing and circumcision of, 67
  collection of cord blood and, 66
  depressed, 67–75
  eye care and, 66
  identification procedures for, 66
  minimization of heat loss and, 65–66
  normal, care of, 63–67
  normal physiology and pathophysiology of, 67–68
  resuscitation of, 68–75
  vitamin K and, 66
New York diagnostic criteria, for rheumatoid arthritis, 503
Nipples, breast-feeding and, 83, 85
Nitrazine test, premature rupture of membranes and, 295, 296
Nondisjunction, 182
Nonimmune hydrops fetalis (NIHF), 214–215

Nonstress test (NST), 223–225, 316–317
Norplant, postpartum, 80–81
Northern blotting, 181

Obesity, 323, 414–415
Obstetric emergencies, 563–577
  (See also specific emergencies)
Obstetric factors, premature labor and, 283–284
Obturator neuropathy, 522
Oligohydramnios, 213–214, 248, 315
Omphalocele, 209–210
Oophorectomy in breast cancer, 538
Ophthalmologic examination in diabetes mellitus, 437
Oral contraceptive pills (OCPs), postpartum, 80
Orders
  admitting, 15–17
  postoperative, 20–22
Osmotic fragility in hereditary spherocytosis, 466
Osteomyelitis in sickle cell anemia, 472–473
O'Sullivan technique in acute uterine inversion, 574
Outlet forceps delivery, 123
Ovarian artery ligation, in postpartum bleeding, 348–350
Ovarian cancer, 540–541
Ovulation, resumption of, 80
Oxytocin, 54, 320, 345, 347–348

Pain management, postoperative, 110–115
Palmar erythema, 526
Pancreatitis, 409–412
Panic attacks, 550–551
Pap smear, 11–12
Papular eruptions during pregnancy, 528–529
Paracervical block during labor, 103–104
Parathyroid disease, 446–449
Parenteral hyperalimentation in pancreatitis, 413
Patent ductus arteriosus (PDA), 360
Paternal antigen status, isoimmunization and, 257
Patient-controlled analgesia (PCA), postoperative, 110–112

Patient education
childbirth, 35–36
prenatal, 31–34
Pelvic artery embolization, in postpartum bleeding, 350
Pelvic contracture, dystocia and, 137–138
Pelvic examination, 8–11, 25, 145, 315, 324
Pelvic fractures, dystocia and, 138
Pelvic tumors, dystocia and, 138
Pelvimetry, 11
Pelvis
fetal adaptations to, 45–46, 141–142
planes and diameters of, 40–42
shapes of, 42–43
Peptic ulcer, 408–409
Percutaneous umbilical blood sampling (PUBS), 192, 260
Perfusion (Q) scan, pulmonary emboli and, 366
Perineal care during puerperium, 77
Periodontitis, 558–559
Peroneal neuropathy, 522
Phenobarbital, 426
Phenotype, 175
Physical agents, teratogenic, 161–162
Physical examination, 5
abruptio placentae and, 337
chronic hypertension and, 378
eclampsia and, 376
face presentation and, 146
in multifetal pregnancy, 307–308
placenta previa and, 332
preeclampsia and, 370–371
premature rupture of membranes and, 295
prenatal, 25
pulmonary emboli and, 365
Physiological hyperlipidemia of pregnancy, 410
Pitocin, 54, 134
Pituitary disease, 453–455
Pituitary tumors, 454–455, 520
Placenta
delivery of, management of bleeding following, 344–348
low-lying, 330
metastatic disease to, 542
removal of, in postpartum hemorrhage, 343–344
Placenta accreta, 330–331
Placental abruption. See Abruptio placentae

Placental dysfunction syndrome, prolonged pregnancy and, 314–315
Placental migration, 333
Placental problems, multifetal pregnancy and, 306
Placenta previa, 330–335
Plague, immunization against, 583
Plasmapheresis
in cholestasis, 426
in immune thrombocytopenic purpura, 486
in pancreatitis, 413
in rheumatoid arthritis, 504
in systemic lupus erythematosus, 501
in thrombotic thrombocytopenic purpura and hemolytic uremic syndrome, 489
Pneumococcus, immunization against, 584
Pneumonia, 398–400
Poliomyelitis, immunization against, 581
Polycystic kidney disease, infantile, 214
Polygenic inheritance, 181–182
Polyhydramnios. See Hydramnios
Polymerase chain reaction (PCR), 181
Polymyositis, 506–507
Polyploidy, 182
Polyps, endocervical, placenta previa and, 331
Position, fetal, 141
Postdate pregnancy, definition of, 313
Posterior urethral valve (PUV) anomaly, 213–214
Postmaturity, definition of, 313
Postoperative care, 20–22
Postpartum blues, 551, 552, 556
Postpartum psychosis, management of, 556–557
Postterm pregnancy, definition of, 313
Prednisone (Deltasone; Meticorten)
in adrenocortical insufficiency, 450
in Bell's palsy, 521
in immune thrombocytopenic purpura, 486
in inflammatory bowel disease, 417, 418
in polymyositis and dermatomyositis, 507
in rheumatoid arthritis, 504
in sarcoidosis, 403

in systemic lupus erythematosus, 500–501
Preeclampsia, 305–306, 369–375, 499, 547
(See also Hypertensive disorders)
Prenatal care, 23–30
    initial visit for, 23–27
    subsequent routine visits for, 27–30
Prenatal diagnosis, 186–193
    of accelerated fetal growth, 250
    amniocentesis in, 189
    chorionic villus sampling in, 190–192
    fetal skin sampling in, 192–193
    genetic screening and, 187–188
    indications for, 186–187
    of intrauterine growth retardation, 245–248
    of isoimmunization, 257, 259–260
    percutaneous umbilical blood sampling in, 192
    of α thalassemia, 479–480
Preoperative evaluation, 17–18
Preoperative preparation, 19–20, 118
Presentation, 141
    abnormal, 141–149
        cause of, 145
        diagnosis of, 145–146
        fetal accommodations to maternal pelvis and, 141–142
        incidence of, 142–143
        as indication for cesarean section, 117
        management of, 146–149
        morbidity and mortality and, 143–144
    (See also specific presentations)
    dystocia and, 135
Preterm birth prevention programs, 285
Prolonged pregnancy, 313–321
    cause of, 313–314
    definitions of, 313
    incidence of, 313
    management of, 317–321
    morbidity and mortality and, 314–315
    patient assessment and, 315–317
Prostaglandin synthetase inhibitors, 290–291, 309
Prosthetic valves, pregnancy subsequent to, 363
Protein C deficiency, 496–497
Protein S deficiency, 496–497
Proteinuria, 501

Prurigo gestationis, 528–529
Pruritic urticarial papules and plaques of pregnancy (PUPPP), 530–532
Pruritus gravidarum, 527–528
Pseudoseizures, 553
Pseudotumor cerebri (PC), 518–519
Psychiatric disease
    complicated by pregnancy, 550–557
        cause of, 552
        diagnosis of, 553–554
        differential diagnosis of, 553
        incidence of, 551
        infant distress and, 552
        management of, 554–556
        morbidity and mortality and, 551–552
        prognosis of, 557
    pregnancy-associated, 545–550
        during first trimester, 545–547
        postpartum, 549–550
        during second trimester, 547–548
        during third trimester, 548–549
Psychosis, postpartum, 550, 552
Psychosocial history, 24–25
Psychotropic drugs
    in anxiety, 556
    in depression, 556
    in postpartum psychosis, 557
    in schizophrenia, 554
    during second trimester, 547
    side effects of, 554
    teratogenic, 159–160
    toxic reactions to, 554
Pudendal block during delivery, 107–110
Puerperium, 76–81
    clinical care during, 77–78
    complications during, 78–80
    definition of, 76
    physiology of, 76
    postpartum contraception and, 80–81
Pulmonary disease, 394–403
    respiratory physiology and, 394
    (See also specific disorders)
Pulmonary edema, 288–290
Pulmonary emboli (PE), 365–366
Pulmonary hypoplasia, premature rupture of membranes and, 294
Pulmonary maturity, steroids for induction of, 299
Pulmonary system, changes during pregnancy, 97

Pulmonary vasoconstriction, neonatal, sequelae of, 74
Pyelonephritis, acute, 386–387
Pyogenic granuloma, 527, 559–560
Pyruvate kinase deficiency, 470–471

Quickening, 27, 316

Rabies, immunization against, 582, 587
Radiation, teratogenic effect of, 161–162
Radiation therapy, in rheumatoid arthritis, 504
Regional anesthesia, 99, 101
Regional enteritis, 415–418
Renal agenesis, bilateral, 212–213
Renal cortical necrosis, 389
Renal disease
  during pregnancy, 384–393
  (See also specific disorders)
Renal failure
  acute, 387–391
  chronic, 391–392
  neonatal, sequelae of, 74
Renal function in preeclampsia, 371
Renal stone disease, 392–393
Renal system
  changes during pregnancy, 98
  during puerperium, 76
Renal transplantation, 393
Reproductive genetics. See Genetics
Respiratory support of newborn, 69–72
Restriction endonuclease, 179
Restriction fragment length polymorphism (RFLP), 179–181
Resuscitation
  maternal, drugs and equipment for, 96
  of newborn, 74–75
Reticulocytes, in pyruvate kinase deficiency, 471
Retina
  chronic hypertension and, 378
  in preeclampsia, 371
Retinopathy, diabetes mellitus and, 433–434
Reverse transcriptase, 274
Rheumatoid arthritis, 502–504
Rh immunoglobulin (RhIG), isoimmunization and, 262
Rh sensitization. See Isoimmunization

Rickets, dystocia and, 138
Ritodrine (Yutopar), 287–289, 309
Robertsonian translocation, 182
Rubella virus infection, 266–268
  immunization against, 581

Sarcoidosis during pregnancy, 403
Schizophrenia, 550, 552, 554
Scleroderma, 505–506
Scoliosis, dystocia and, 138
Seizure disorders, 510–514
Serologic testing
  in cytomegalovirus infection, 270
  hepatitis and, 424
  rubella virus infection and, 267–268
  in syphilis, 272
  toxoplasmosis and, 265–266
Sex chromosome abnormalities, 184–186
Sexual history, 5
Sheehan's syndrome, 342
Shirodkar operation, 120
Shock, hypovolemic, postpartum hemorrhage and, 342
Shoulder dystocia, 563–569
Sickle cell anemia, 471–475
Sickle cell β thalassemia, 476–477
Skin
  changes during pregnancy, 524–525
  disorders of. See specific disorders
  in preeclampsia, 371
  systemic lupus erythematosus and, 499
Small-for-gestational-age (SGA) fetuses. See Intrauterine growth retardation
Smoking, 402
Socioeconomic factors
  endometritis and, 323
  premature labor and, 283
Southern blotting, 179–181
Spangler's papular dermatitis of pregnancy (PDP), 528–529
Speculum examination, 9–11
Spermicides, postpartum, 80
Spherocytosis, hereditary, 465–468
Spina bifida, 204, 208–209
Spinal cord injuries, 519–520
Spinal cord tumors, 520
Splenectomy, 467–468, 471, 486
Status epilepticus, 513–514
Sterilization, postpartum, 81
Steroids
  endometritis and, 324

in herpes gestationis, 531
intraarticular, in rheumatoid arthritis, 504
in premature labor, in multifetal pregnancy, 309
premature rupture of membranes and, 299
in pruritic urticarial papules and plaques of pregnancy, 532
Striae, 526
Stroke volume, changes during pregnancy, 356
Subarachnoid block during delivery, 108–109
Suicide, 551, 555–556
Surgery
in appendicitis, 414
in "berry" aneurysms, 515
in breast cancer, 538
cardiac, pregnancy subsequent to, 363
in cervical carcinoma, 536–537
cesarean section and. See Cesarean section
in colorectal cancer, 542
in hemorrhage, following cesarean section, 119–120
in hereditary spherocytosis, 467–468
in immune thrombocytopenic purpura, 486
in inflammatory bowel disease, 417–418
in mitral stenosis, 361
in ovarian cancer, 540–541
postoperative pain management and. See Analgesia, postoperative
in postpartum bleeding, 348–350
preoperative antacids and, 109–110
pulmonary emboli and, 366
in pyruvate kinase deficiency, 471
in rheumatoid arthritis, 504
in vascular malformations, 515
Sympathetic blockade, lumbar/caudal epidural block and, 106
Sympathomimetic agents, in asthma, 397
Synclitism, 45–46
Syncope, prenatal, 35
Syphilis, 271–273, 283, 324
Systemic lupus erythematosus (SLE), 498–502
Systemic sclerosis, 505–506

Tachypnea, pulmonary emboli and, 365
Telogen effluvium, 525–526
Teratogens, 153–162, 266
Terbutaline (Brethine), 287–289, 397, 573
Tetanus, immunization against, 586, 587
Tetralogy of Fallot, 360
Thalassemias, 477–484
Theophylline, 397–398
Threshold, inheritance and, 182
Thrombocytopenia, 484–490, 501
Thromboembolic disease, 363–366
Thrombolytic therapy, pulmonary emboli and, 366
Thrombophlebitis, superficial, 363–364
Thrombotic thrombocytopenic purpura (TTP), 488–490, 501
Thyroid disease, 441–446
Thyroiditis, acute, 443, 445
Tocolytic therapy, 287–291, 299, 309, 334, 414
Tooth decay, 560–561
Toxic delirium, 553
Toxoplasmosis, perinatal, 264–266
Transcription, 169, 171
Transfusion reactions, 342
Translation, 171
Translocation, 182
Transverse lie, 117, 142, 144, 146, 148
Trauma
breech presentation and, 144
placenta previa and, 332
Travel, prenatal, 35
Trial forceps, 125
Triplets, 311
Trisomy, 182–184
Tuberculosis, 400–402
Tumors
cerebral, 520
cutaneous, 527
pelvic, dystocia and, 138
pituitary, 454–455, 520
pregnancy, 559–560
spinal cord, 520
Turner's syndrome, 185
Twins
dizygotic, 303, 307
intrauterine death of, 306
locking of, 311
monozygotic, 303, 307
presentation of, 310–311

Twins (*Cont.*)
  twin-to-twin transfusion, 306
  undiagnosed, 306
  (*See also* Multifetal pregnancy)
Typhoid, immunization against, 585

Ulcerative colitis, 415–418
Ultrasonography, 26–27
  abruptio placentae and, 337–338
  in appendicitis, 414
  breech presentation and, 145–146
  in chronic hypertension, 381
  determination of estimated date of
    confinement and, 316
  in diabetes mellitus, 437–438
  fetal, in prolonged pregnancy, 316
  in multifetal pregnancy, 308–309
  in pancreatitis, 411
  placenta previa and, 332–333
  values for, 591–602
Umbilical cord blood acid/base assess-
    ment, 241–242
Upper respiratory tract infection (URI),
    394–396
Uremia, 390
Urinary tract
  anomalies of, 212–214
  during puerperium, 77
Urinary tract infection
  diabetes mellitus and, 433
  during pregnancy, 384–387
  premature labor and, 283
Urinary tract obstruction, in acute
    pyelonephritis, 387
Urine studies
  chronic hypertension and, 378–379
  in diabetes mellitus, 437
  in preeclampsia, 371
  premature rupture of membranes
    and, 298
  prenatal, 28–29
  in systemic lupus erythematosus,
    500
Uterine abnormalities, premature labor
    and, 283–284
Uterine activity
  ambulatory uterine contraction
    monitoring and, 285–286
  premature labor and, 284–285
Uterine artery ligation in postpartum
    bleeding, 348–350
Uterine atony, 341
Uterine bleeding, delayed, during
    puerperium, 78–79

Uterine compression, bimanual, in
    postpartum bleeding, 345
Uterine contractions
  abruptio placentae and, 337
  prenatal, 27
Uterine massage, 77
Uterus
  examination of, 11
  exploration of, in postpartum bleed-
    ing, 347
  integrity of, postpartum hemorrhage
    and, 341
  inversion of, acute, 573–574
  involution of, 77
  overdistention of, premature labor
    and, 284
  during puerperium, 76
  tenderness of, abruptio placentae
    and, 337

Vacuum extractor, 127–128
Vaginal discharge, 27
Vaginal examination, 146, 323, 346–
    347
Vaginal infections, premature labor
    and, 283
Vaginal sample for Pap smear, 11
Vaginitis, prenatal, 35
Varicella, immunization against, 588
Varicella zoster virus infection, breast-
    feeding and, 88
Varicose veins
  prenatal, 35
  vulvar, placenta previa and, 332
Vasa previa, 332
Vascular changes, dermatologic, dur-
    ing pregnancy, 526–527
Vascular malformations , 515
Vascular proliferation, 526
Vascular resistance, systemic, changes
    during pregnancy, 357
Vascular spiders, 526
Ventral wall defects, 209
Ventricular septal defects (VSDs) , 360
Version as prophylaxis for abnormal
    presentations, 147
Vertex presentation, 47–49, 127, 310,
    311
Vitamin B_{12} deficiency , 463–465
Vitamin K, newborn and, 66
Vomiting, 34, 405–407, 546
  cholelithiasis and, 428
  epidural opioids and, 114
  in multifetal pregnancy, 307
Von Willebrand's disease, 493–495

Weaning, 90–91
Western blotting, 181
Woods Screw procedure, 566
Worm procedure, 120

X inactivation, 178
X-linked inheritance, 178–179
45,X phenotype (Turner syndrome), 185
47,XXX phenotype, 186

47,XXY phenotype (Klinefelter syndrome), 186
47,XYY phenotype, 186

Yellow fever, immunization against, 581

Zavanelli maneuver, 566
Zygosity, multifetal pregnancy and, 306